THE HEALTHY HOUSEHOLD

A complete guide for creating
a healthy indoor environment

Lynn Marie Bower

The Healthy House Institute

Published by:
The Healthy House Institute
430 North Sewell Road
Bloomington, IN 47408

Copyright © 1995 by Lynn Marie Bower

Book and cover design by Lynn Marie Bower

Printed on recycled paper with soy-based ink.

10 9 8 7 6 5 4 3 2 1

DISCLAIMER: The information contained in this book should not be considered medical advice. Sensitive individuals should always contact a physician first before making any changes in their home environment.

Publisher's Cataloging-in-Publication Data.
Bower, Lynn Marie
The Healthy Household: A complete guide for creating a healthy indoor environment.
Includes bibliographical references, list of sources.
1. Consumer product safety—Popular works. 2. Housing and Health. 3. Indoor air pollution—Health aspects.
 I. Bower, Lynn Marie. II. Title.
TX335.B69 1995
645.042

Library of Congress Catalog Card Number: 94-096634
ISBN 0-9637156-3-1 $17.95 Softcover.

This book is dedicated to my husband John for his love and encouragement.

ACKNOWLEDGMENTS

I would like to thank my husband John for being the dedicated, caring person he is. Over the many years I've had MCS (Multiple Chemical Sensitivity), he's provided support in every way possible. While I was writing this book, he gave me objective criticism and suggestions—and taught me how to use a computer. A great deal of the information written in the Home Workshop section of Chapter 12 was gleaned from his prior research and writing.

I also would like to express my appreciation to the research librarians at various Indiana University departmental libraries and the Monroe County Public Library who were always ready to find all types of facts and figures. Others who supplied needed answers along the way were county extension agents and scores of technical advisors and representatives from various manufacturers, dealers, and trade associations. Finally, I'd like to thank those special friends who offered ideas, information, inspiration, and other help, and Bob Baird for an excellent job of copy editing.

CONTENTS AT A GLANCE

TABLE OF CONTENTS

CHAPTER 3: CLOTHING   67

CHAPTER 5: INTERIOR DECORATING   109

Table of Contents

CHAPTER 8: HOUSEKEEPING   235

CHAPTER 9: INDOOR AIR   293

INTRODUCTION

An April 1989 Massachusetts Special Legislative Commission report concluded that "Indoor air pollution is a growing problem in the United States and accounts for 50% of all illness." At first, this may sound simply unbelievable. How could our indoor environments be making so many people sick? Actually, the answer lies in two major housing trends. First, there is an ever-greater reliance on synthetic and petrochemical ingredients in building materials, furnishings, cleaning products, and personal items we commonly use indoors. Second, most homes are being made tighter to increase energy efficiency, yet many of them don't have mechanical ventilation systems specifically designed to bring in fresh air.

As a result of these two trends, a majority of Americans live in stale indoor environments filled with harmful emissions from carpeting, cabinets, cosmetics, laundry products, and clothing. Consequently, many of us breathe dangerous levels of formaldehyde and hundreds of other potentially harmful chemicals daily. Of course, dust, pollen, combustion by-products, mold spores, radon, and animal dander are also commonly a part of this toxic mix. Some people are able to live in this polluted air with no apparent ill effects. Growing numbers of us cannot.

Unfortunately, most Americans are still not aware of the potential dangers within their own home environments. While they may have health complaints such as sinus irritation, sore throat, tiredness, mild depression, and insomnia, these symptoms are usually attributed to viruses, old age, hormones, or stress. Sometimes these factors really do figure into these maladies. However, it's now believed that many symptoms are actually the consequence of breathing polluted indoor air. Even very serious conditions such as Multiple Chemical Sensitivity (MCS), chronic asthma, some birth defects, and even certain cancers have been linked to living in unhealthy houses.

The good news, however, is that you have the ability to choose to be less at risk. You can decide to live a healthier lifestyle that goes beyond just eating better food and exercising—you can choose a healthy, less-toxic household. That's what this book is all about. It is your complete guide to learning likely sources of dangerous indoor contamination and opting for healthier alternatives. In fact, *The Healthy Household* offers hundreds of suggestions and sources for less-toxic services and products. You'll find information on unscented and natural personal-care items, healthful housekeeping procedures, natural fiber clothing, safer pest-control measures, non-toxic interior decorating, as well as material on electromagnetic fields, air and water filtration, and much, much more. *The Healthy Household* explores so many subjects because they all impact your home and your health. The truth is: Everything you bring into your house, every activity you perform in it, and all that is on your body affects your home's indoor air quality.

Admittedly, this sounds rather intimidating. Some of you may feel that changing your present unhealthy household to an alternative, healthy one is just too big a job. However, this book will help you learn where to order, and how to sample, test, and experiment with new products and living patterns. Actually, all this isn't difficult to do; it just requires a certain degree of desire and commitment. Obviously, you probably already have these traits—else you wouldn't be reading right now. Some of you may also fear changing from a familiar (but unhealthy) lifestyle to something new out of fear of being labeled eccentric. Using alternative products definitely places you among the minority. Most of your neighbors and family will probably question you about your new changes, while they continue to use and do what "everyone else does." However, instead of feeling different or even odd, view your healthy modifications as signs of maturity, individuality, and good common sense. You may even inspire others to follow your example.

However, at the same time, you should have realistic expectations concerning the transition towards your new, healthier lifestyle. You need to know from the beginning that you'll probably occasionally get frustrated along the way. Also, you should anticipate that you may need to discard some of your early choices and may have to make some imperfect compromises. Yet, for the most part, you'll likely experience very satisfying results. Best of all, your efforts will ultimately provide you with better control over your own future and that of your family. By choosing a less-toxic lifestyle, you'll very likely enjoy many years of better health ahead.

It should be pointed out that very few, if any, readers will follow all the suggestions and advice available in the following chapters and appendices. As human beings we all tend to be selective. Also, you should know that you don't have to make all the desired changes at once. For many people, transforming how they live is a gradual process. They start by switching to healthier personal care-items or laundry products. Then, as time and finances allow, they expand into other areas. You can do this too—and if you continue to make changes over time—you'll eventually have the healthy household you wanted sooner than you ever imagined. In the end, each person must decide what changes to make and in what order to make them.

It is hoped *The Healthy Household* will enable you to transform your toxic interior environment into one that brings both pleasure and good health.

Introduction

Typical modern lifestyles are making too many people sick. I know—I am just one of thousands of individuals who has been made seriously ill by their homes. I became ill fifteen years ago during a major home restoration and remodeling project. My husband and I used common construction materials. We finished the inside with typical carpets, fabrics, furniture, and paints. We also wore typical clothing and cleaned, using widely advertised products. Like many renovated houses, ours was newly insulated and caulked—and it had no planned ventilation system. As a result of this very average life and home, I acquired MCS, which resulted in respiratory problems, joint and muscle pain, gastrointestinal problems, ringing in the ears, and a host of other symptoms—some more debilitating than others. My hair became brittle, I got acne, and I became hypersensitive to synthetic fragrances, printing ink, and common cleaning products. Eventually, building a healthy house and creating a healthy household within it helped me significantly—although optimum health has never completely returned. I'm telling you this because I am far from an isolated case. I am aware that thousands of others have similar stories to tell.

Sadly, you too could be made ill by your present lifestyle—if it's like the typical one most people are currently living. However, you have the power to change your own home environment. You can make your home less toxic as an important preventive measure. And for those who are already sick, you can create a healthier lifestyle and regain some measure of well-being and sense of control over your life again. Remember, each less-toxic choice you make is one step toward better health.

Lynn Marie Bower

HOW TO USE THIS BOOK

The Healthy Household is presented as a reference book, in an easy-to-use manual format. Therefore, background facts, developmental history, production-method explanations, operational descriptions, and product listings are given under many topic headings. This approach was used to help you understand why certain products have been suggested—and why some are not perfect solutions. All this information is included so you can make more informed decisions as you create your new healthier household. However, if you want to know specific product suggestions immediately, the introductory background material can be skipped. Of course, it can always be returned to at a later time, if you wish.

As you read this book, you may find some of the information is repeated in different chapters. This is because each heading is designed to be fairly complete in itself. Therefore, persons not reading the book straight through should find their questions satisfactorily answered simply within the particular sections they choose to look up. For the same reason, there are no sidebar stories or case examples which sometimes can be missed. However, where it seemed appropriate under certain headings, I have included suggestions for additional information that can be found elsewhere in the book. These references are written in *italics* within parentheses.

Furthermore, you should be aware that within each of the twelve chapters, only a limited number of products and dealer suggestions are given under each heading. This was done to provide a manageable sampling of options—not to overwhelm readers by listing all the choices that are currently available. In addition, the products and suppliers shown in **bold type** have their addresses and telephone numbers printed in at least one appendix. By the way, the appendices list many other sources for both alternative products and dealers whom you may also wish to contact.

As a very brief summary of the book, *Chapter 1: Getting Started* covers basic information on choosing and buying healthy products. *Chapter 2: Personal Care* provides material on such things as cosmetics and toiletries, and *Chapter 3: Clothing* discusses natural fibers, leather, stuffing, and specific clothing suggestions. Bedding and towels are covered in *Chapter 4: Linens*, a wide variety of home furnishing and decorating ideas are considered in *Chapter 5: Interior Decorating*, and stationery, hobbies, telephones, and exercise equipment are treated in *Chapter 6: Lifestyle*. *Chapter 7: Cleaning* gives information on products and techniques for various cleaning jobs, while *Chapter 8: Housekeeping* is filled with tips on storage ideas, appliances, and pest control. *Chapter 9: Indoor Air* discusses common indoor air pollutants and how to remove them, and *Chapter 10: Home Water* covers typical water quality problems, testing, and how to improve your water. *Chapter 11: Electromagnetic Fields* explores what electromagnetic fields are, common sources of high levels in homes, and how to reduce them. Finally, *Chapter 12: Home Workshop and Garage* addresses finishes, glues, lubricants, and woods—as well as suggestions for garages and cars.

There are four appendices. *Appendix 1: The Safe Haven* is a thorough, step-by-step discussion on how to create a livable oasis for those who are severely affected by allergies or Multiple Chemical Sensitivity. *Appendix 2: Utility and Government Help* supplies contact information for various utilities and governmental agencies in order to acquire free or low-cost services and products. *Appendix 3: Resources for a Healthy Household* includes listings for printed material, organizations, and product sources. The final appendix, *Appendix 4: Resources for Infants and Children*, has been included to address youngsters' special needs inasmuch as most of the book focuses on adults. However, it should be remembered that all healthy household changes will benefit children as well.

Even if you don't plan to read this book from cover to cover, it's highly recommended that most everyone first read *Chapter 1: Getting Started*. The basic information provided in the first chapter should help you in making decisions regarding suggested products and materials listed under all the headings of later chapters. In the end, my hope is that *The Healthy Household* will empower you—so you will feel more confident in the options you choose for your home and lifestyle. Best of luck to each of you as you begin to create your own healthy household.

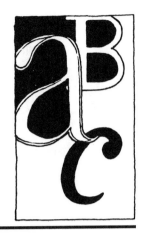

CHAPTER 1
GETTING STARTED

Now that you are seriously considering creating a healthy household, this chapter supplies the basic information you'll need to get started.

TOXIC CONSEQUENCES

Is our modern American lifestyle so bad that we really need to change it? Yes, at least some of it. Admittedly, this is in some ways unfortunate. Most consumer products are designed to be convenient to use, to make our housekeeping jobs easier, to provide comfort and pleasure. However, another side of the equation is rarely considered—even by people who are committed to recycling, saving whales, and preserving rain forests. That is the impact our modern way of living has on our health. Sadly, "better" and "more convenient" products made of synthetic materials and petroleum-based chemicals can create very harmful indoor surroundings. In fact, our home environments are commonly five to ten times more polluted than any outdoor environment—and this includes major cities. As a result, most houses and apartments have the potential to cause negative health consequences to their occupants.

In the *Introduction*, I mentioned several health problems that have been associated with poor indoor air. These included sore throats, insomnia, headaches, and mild depression, among others. Here are some specific examples of typically used products and their suspected medical outcomes. For instance, new synthetic carpeting can give off *xylene, ethylbenzene,* and *methacrylic acid.* Chemicals from carpeting have been shown to cause neurological impairment and even death in laboratory mice. *Formaldehyde,* given off by everything from particleboard closet shelving, permanent-press clothing, some types of paper, and certain personal-care items, can irritate the mucous membranes and eyes. Formaldehyde can also cause menstrual irregularities, provoke asthma, and depress the central-nervous system. Some synthetic scents used in particular personal-care items, paper goods, laundry products, and cleaning supplies are *neurotoxic* (capable of damaging the nervous system including the brain and spinal cord). In addition, *combustion gases* (including *carbon monoxide*) given off by wood stoves have been shown to cause a dramatic increase in the incidence of breathing problems in children. And our poor air quality isn't the only problem within our homes. There is also evidence that *chlorinated* drinking water increases the likelihood of bladder cancer. Sadly, the list of products, materials, devices, and practices commonly used in houses and apartments and their accompanying adverse health effects could go on and on.

Because most homes don't have adequate ventilation, most of us breathe indoor contaminants continually. Therefore, every minute of every day, year after year, we expose ourselves to these potentially harmful influences. Unfortunately, as stated in a December 1988 Congressional Research Service report to Congress, entitled *Indoor Air Pollution: Cause for Concern?*, "...[N]o one is immune to the effects of indoor air pollution." Incidentally, it should be mentioned that even in houses where there is an adequate air exchange, if the outdoor air is contaminated, the indoor air will be, too—unless it's properly filtered. Like a growing number of experts and concerned consumers, I firmly believe we should end the complacency of how most of us presently live. It's time to make our home environments healthier.

With so many stresses and problems already present everywhere, I know many people simply don't want to hear that their own homes could be making them sick. I realize that many people would like to think that at least in their homes, they are safe from the worries of the world. Well, it would be nice if the dangers of pollution were all "out there"—at some abandoned oil refinery, mismanaged landfill, or polluted inner city. However the sad truth is, there are likely many dangers inside your house right now that you should become aware of. Seemingly innocuous grease-cutting cleaners, foam-filled lounge chairs, stain-resistant cut-pile floor coverings, and wrinkle-free clothes could be endangering your health and that of your family at this very moment. This is neither fiction nor exaggeration—just reality.

MCS, A NEW MEDICAL CONDITION

Since World War II, increasing numbers of people have become ill with a host of baffling symptoms. For example, joint pain, mental confusion, digestive complaints, and skin rashes may be reported by a single individual, while others report their own set of seemingly unrelated problems. To make diagnoses even more difficult, common tests frequently used to determine the nature of many medical conditions are often unable to provide any sure indication of what these people have or why they have it. Because of this, most of the medical community has dismissed those unfortunate enough to have such mysterious conditions as hypochondriacs, neurotics, menopausal, overly stressed, or just plain flaky. *However, that does not mean it is not a real medical condition.* It simply means that it has *not yet* been validated by the mainstream medical establishment. After all, common conditions such as premenstrual syndrome (PMS), impotence, epilepsy, and depression have not always been known to have a physical cause.

At the same time, it should be noted that patients complaining of several simultaneous symptoms were first described decades ago in a 1962 ground-breaking book, *Human Ecology and Susceptibility to the Chemical Environment,* by Theron G. Randolph, M.D. This physician did not arbitrarily dismiss his patients' complaints as delusional. Instead, he believed that the varied effects were due to one general cause—the effects of exposure to low levels of chemicals in the home, workplace, and food. Randolph termed the condition *Ecological Illness.* A minority of other health professionals have agreed with Randolph's assessment.

Since the publication of Randolph's first book, Ecological Illness has been called by a number of other names—Twentieth Century Disease, Total Allergy Syndrome, Chemical Allergies, Chemical Sensitivity, and Chemical Hypersensitivity. Currently, the most widely accepted term is *Multiple Chemical Sensitivity,* or *MCS.* By the way, it's suspected that some cases of Chronic Fatigue Syndrome (severe and persistent tiredness) and Sick Building Syndrome (MCS-like symptoms temporarily exhibited by certain persons when inside a particular building) may be forms of MCS.

THE NATURE OF MCS

What exactly is MCS? Despite the myriad reported symptoms, MCS is now considered by some experts to be a single condition: one that results from chemical injury. A number of theories have been proposed which attempt to explain how toxic chemicals could affect certain individuals in so many different ways. These are generally written in complex physiological/biochemical language which can be difficult for most of us. However, very simply put, our bodies frankly haven't had enough time to evolve into forms able to successfully coexist with the thousands of chemicals with which we now surround ourselves—compounds which never existed before in human history. We know that trees in Germany's Black Forest have turned brown and sickly from acid rain, that great numbers of fish in the Great Lakes have tumors, and that certain bird species now lay thin-shelled eggs that often break before chicks ever hatch. All these are fellow lifeforms unable to thrive within polluted environments. Why do we humans think we are exempt?

Many of you may be wondering, "Why do some people get MCS or some other serious illness, while others seem to be doing okay?" The answer is, *we are never all equally susceptible.* A particular individual's susceptibility is actually due to a number of factors including age (the very young and the very old have less-functional immune systems), other previous or presently existing medical conditions (those with allergies or other illnesses have already-compromised immune systems), work exposure (those employed in petrochemical industries, those involved with pesticides, or those who work in sick buildings), genetic make-up (some individuals just have stronger constitutions than others), your home's proximity to toxic-waste sites—and just plain luck. One person can acquire MCS as the result of a one-time toxic event while others may acquire it as the result of an accumulation of small exposures over several years.

Often, persons report initially becoming ill after they moved into a new house, mobile home, or apartment. If they were in older buildings, a feeling of sickness might have set in following the installation of new kitchen cabinets or living room carpeting. MCS has also been associated with painting a master bedroom, newly-applied termite treatments—or with any other major or minor chemical exposure in the home (or elsewhere).

Some who have MCS have noted that, at first, it seemed they simply had the flu. However, unlike the flu, the achiness, tiredness, and general malaise did not go away within the expected week or two—and their former sense of well-being never returned. Instead, the sense of being "under the weather" lingered, then progressed into a variety of new symptoms.

Whatever the originating cause (whether singular, a combination of factors, or simply unknown), an affected individual may soon find he or she now feels sick around perfume, typical cleaning products, cigarettes, gas heat, vinyl, new clothing, etc. In many cases of MCS, the number of intolerable substances tends to increase, while at the same time, the levels of exposure capable of producing symptoms decrease. This effect is known as *increased sensitivity* or *hypersensitivity*. Some individuals also find they've acquired food allergies and/or an intolerance to electromagnetic fields (EMFs) (See *Chapter 11: Electromagnetic Fields*). In severe cases of MCS, a great many synthetic and even natural items will provoke a multitude of symptoms if inhaled or ingested.

You should be aware that each individual with MCS has his or her own set of unique symptoms—each with its own degree of severity and duration. These particular symptoms can manifest themselves physically, psychologically, or both. This shouldn't be seen as odd or remarkable—many petrochemicals are actually neurotoxic and affect the brain. Interestingly, some MCS complaints mimic already-established medical conditions such as arthritis. Actually, MCS symptoms have been associated with virtually every organ, body system, or mind function. The following is a limited list of some of the reported symptoms:

> Nausea, headache, hives, insomnia, depression, anxiety, gastrointestinal problems, urinary tract inflammation, menstrual irregularities, sinus inflammation, respiratory distress, heartbeat irregularities, mental confusion, chemical hypersensitivity, coma, loss of coordination, memory impairment, joint pain, tremors, muscle aches, blurred vision, sensitivity to light, ringing in the ears, changes in normal perspiration, and anaphylactic shock.

MCS TREATMENT

The recognition and treatment of Multiple Chemical Sensitivity varies enormously from doctor to doctor. The following will acquaint you with common medical responses.

MAINSTREAM RESPONSE TO MCS

Today, perhaps as many as two million people in the United States have symptoms both severe and persistent enough to be called Multiple Chemical Sensitivity (MCS). This illness is increasingly being recognized by state and federal authorities as a legitimate medical condition. For example, MCS has been included in the U.S. Social Security Administration's Social Security Income Benefit guidelines (see *Acquiring SSI Benefits* in *Appendix 2: Utility and Government Help*). Despite the growing numbers of those affected, some government recognition, and Dr. Theron Randolph's pioneering writing and work, some physicians remain unfamiliar with the condition—and many continue to dismiss it as not a "real" medical condition. Actually, the assessment and lack of positive help MCS patients commonly receive from their doctors is understandable. After all, MCS is a condition most physicians never studied in medical school, treated during medical training, read much about in medical journals, heard about at conferences, or discussed with colleagues. Few, if any, pharmaceutical salesman ever offered them samples of drugs or devices to treat MCS.

On such matters much of the medical community tends to be relatively traditional or conservative. This may be surprising to many, but it is reality in most of the medical community. Why this is so isn't out of fear of the prospect of malpractice lawsuits. Accepted medical knowledge, as with most other fields, usually changes though slow evolution—not rapid revolution. It's not uncommon for decades to pass between the time new information, procedures, drugs, and practices are first proposed and the time they're routinely implemented by local family physicians. Doctors with busy schedules can read, absorb, and change only so much. New drugs or surgical techniques that promise dramatic results with easy-to-understand illnesses are far more likely to generate interest than MCS with all its uncertainties. At the same time, it also appears that some physicians and major medical associations (and is especially true of traditional allergists and their associations) are simply adamantly opposed to the concept that everyday chemical exposures can cause negative reactions—in spite of increasing evidence to the contrary. These doctors believe there isn't enough proof (double-blind studies, convincing medical tests, etc.) to show that MCS is anything but a dramatic expression of an innate fear of chemicals in any form.

PHYSICIANS WHO RECOGNIZE AND TREAT MCS

Fortunately for individuals with Multiple Chemical Sensitivity (MCS) who seek medical help for their condition, there are physicians who are not only familiar with MCS but also offer treatment programs. For example, some occupational medicine practitioners are beginning to diagnose chemical-injury illnesses resulting from exposures in the workplace. However, these doctors may not use the term Multiple Chemical Sensitivity. Physicians who are members of the **American Academy of Otolaryngologic Allergists** recognize and treat MCS. These doctors are ear, nose, and throat allergy specialists. In addition, there are specialized physicians who have dedicated their practices to treating MCS. These are *clinical ecologists* or *environmental medicine specialists* and most belong to the **American Academy of Environmental Medicine.** Interestingly, many of this group's members became interested in MCS only when they themselves, a family member, or a friend came down with the condition.

What does MCS therapy entail? Actually, the therapy prescribed varies with each doctor and each patient. However, it often includes strategies to strengthen the immune system, desensitizing drops or shots to counteract (or *neutralize*) specific exposures and symptoms, antioxidant supplements (vitamin C, etc.), and detoxification regimes to reduce the levels of accumulated toxins in the body. Most individuals find that avoiding synthetic chemicals and other illness-provoking substances is also necessary. In fact, for many people with MCS, living a less-toxic lifestyle often makes a real and dramatic difference in the quality of their lives.

FINDING MORE INFORMATION ON MCS

A number of fine sources are available for information on MCS. A good introductory article is "Multiple Chemical Sensitivity" by Betty Hileman which appeared in *Chemical and Engineering News* (July 22, 1991, 69 (29), pp. 26–42). Reprints are available for $10.00 a copy by writing to: Distribution, Room 210, American Chemical Society, 1155 16th St. NW, Washington, DC 20036.

Two highly recommended books on MCS that have been in print for some time are *An Alternative Approach to Allergies* by Theron G. Randolph, M.D. and Ralph W. Moss, Ph.D. and *Coping with your Allergies* by Natalie Golos and Frances Golos Golbitz. A newer book written by both a physician and Ph.D. researcher is *Chemical Exposures: Low Levels and High Stakes* by Nicholas A. Ashford and Claudia S. Miller. It contains charts, graphs, and a great deal of detailed technical information

Furthermore, a number of mail-order companies handle books dealing with MCS. A few include **E.L. Foust Co., Inc., N.E.E.D.S., Body Elements/ TerrEssentials**, and **The Living Source**. Also, over fifty reprinted articles dealing with environmental medicine and MCS are available at low cost through the **American Environmental Health Foundation, Inc.** In addition, support groups such as **HEAL (Human Ecology Action League), AGES (Advocacy Group for the Environmentally Sensitive)**, the **National Center for Environmental Health Strategies (NCEHS)**, and **Share, Care and Prayer** offer newsletters and other written information.

THE LESSONS OF MCS

Today, the number of individuals who have Multiple Chemical Sensitivity (MCS) is still relatively small—that is, when compared to many other conventional medical conditions. However, the ranks are growing. And it's important to know that many patients are convinced that their home's poor indoor air quality was a major factor in contracting MCS.

Because MCS symptoms are often debilitating and long-term, it's wise to take measures to prevent you and your family from acquiring this condition. Unfortunately, you cannot remove all the possible risk factors. For example, we all have a less developed immune system when young, most of us will have a declining immune system as we age, and we can't change our basic genetic make-up. At the same time, some of us may not realize our homes are situated near buried toxic-waste sites. We have little control over these and other factors. However, it's generally within our own homes where we encounter the worst air—the very place many with MCS suspect originally made them sick. Fortunately, we all can do something to make our interior environments healthier.

As I mentioned in the *Introduction*, some experts now believe that one-half of all illness is caused by indoor air pollution. Feeling tired or having a headache, muscle ache, anxiety, and/or insomnia are so commonplace these days we often say "That's life." However—if researchers are right—many of these symptoms are the direct result of polluted indoor air. Therefore, if you decide to create a healthy household, you'll not only reduce the chances of acquiring a serious condition such as MCS, but you'll also very likely increase the odds of feeling better in general.

WHAT IS SAFE OR HEALTHY?

Of course, to create a healthier indoor environment, you'll need to choose healthier items to put in it. However, there are different ways to define the word *healthy*—and manufacturers and advertisers often project a healthy image by whatever convoluted means possible. Right now, *healthy* sells.

Some products may very well have real, positive health aspects—but in regards to "hot-button" issues such as landfills, the ozone layer, endangered species, fur-bearing animals, or old-growth forests. While these products may be healthy for the earth in some respect, they may or may not be the healthiest choices for the interior of your house or apartment. In this book, I will stress buying and using products that are, above all, designed to be healthy for you personally.

HEALTHY DEFINITIONS

Following are some terms that are often applied to *healthy* household products. You may want to consider them carefully because some of the meanings are probably not as clear as you may have thought.

ALL-COTTON

All-cotton refers to stuffing or fabric consisting of 100%-cotton fibers. However, this term doesn't always mean such items are all-natural or nontoxic products. Because of conventional American farming practices, cotton production uses tremendous quantities of pesticides, herbicides, and other toxic agricultural chemicals. Inevitably, some residues from these chemicals get on cotton fibers.

In addition to cultivation-acquired chemical contamination, permanent-press chemicals (which can be *formaldehyde-based resins*), synthetic dyes, stain-resistant treatments, and other compounds are often added to cotton fibers during the milling process (see *Formaldehyde* in *Chapter 9: Indoor Air*). As a result, all-cotton fabric can be, in many cases, very chemically laden (see also *Cotton* in *Chapter 3: Clothing*).

ALL-NATURAL

All-natural means "derived solely from materials or substances in their native state." These products are neither synthetically nor artificially created. Many natural products are quite benign, but some are not. Lead, radon, and asbestos are natural products and they're potentially quite dangerous. Turpentine, made from pine trees, and mint oil are both natural as well. However, they can be very bothersome to sensitive or allergic persons.

BIODEGRADABLE

Biodegradable is defined as "the ability of natural biological decay processes to break down complex compounds into simple molecules." This is truly an asset for any product to have—especially if it's to be composted. However at the present time, most potentially biodegradable trash is buried in landfills, and because of the manner in which landfills are constructed, virtually nothing in them can ever biodegrade. The tight compaction of alternating layers of trash and clay in typical landfills generally won't permit the breakdown of materials, even when they have the innate capacity under normal circumstances to do so.

Interestingly, in a surprising reversal of popular trends, some products are now actually said to be healthy for the environment because they will not biodegrade. Non-biodegradability is promoted as a positive feature because it helps prevent leachate (seepage) from leaving landfill sites and contaminating water supplies.

MADE FROM RECYCLED MATERIALS

Made from recycled materials is a phrase often used when all or part of an item is made from a previously manufactured material or product. Corrugated cardboard boxes, some papers, and many glass bottles often have labels stating they're made from recycled material. This is highly commendable. However, the percentage of recycled material used in certain products is often quite low.

Sadly, at this time, only a limited number of items are created of 100% post-consumer material. Many products labeled "made from recycled materials" have actually been made from scrap material left over from factory production. Using material swept up from the factory floor rather than throwing it away makes good environmental sense, but calling it recycled is misleading.

NONTOXIC

Nontoxic is defined as not being harmful at concentrations normally used. However, most people believe that it means a substance is harmless—and this just isn't so. Actually, according to the U.S. Federal Hazardous Substances Act, a substance can legitimately be called "nontoxic" if it does not cause acute (sudden-onset) health effects. By this narrow, legal definition, some products that could cause long-term problems such as cancer or birth defects, or are slow-acting or accumulating poisons, can be called nontoxic.

NO PRESERVATIVES OR BIOCIDES

No preservatives refers to the fact that nothing has been added to a product in order to prevent or slow the decay process. *No biocides* means nothing has been added to kill microorganisms. Many preservatives and biocides commonly used are bothersome to sensitive people, so they routinely avoid all of them, as do many other individuals wanting to live an eco-conscious, chemical-free life.

However some preservatives, such as vitamin C, are generally considered both safe and naturally derived. Small amounts of such relatively harmless preservatives are often appropriate in products that otherwise would have very short shelf-lives. This is especially true for foods in order to prevent possible food poisonings. Also keep in mind that, if you use biocide-free wallpaper paste or bathtub caulking, you risk unwanted fungal or bacterial growth. Therefore, less-toxic biocides in some products is actually a very good idea.

NO VOLATILE ORGANIC COMPOUNDS (VOCS)

No *volatile organic compounds (VOCs)* means that a product does not contain a class of chemicals made up of certain hydrocarbons which are able to rapidly evaporate (see *Volatile Organic Compounds* in *Chapter 9: Indoor Air*). VOCs often found in solvents, paints, caulking materials, household cleaning products, etc., can be harmful and some are extremely dangerous. However, natural VOCs are released by onions, oranges, and baking bread that are reasonably safe.

RECYCLABLE

Recyclable means an item is able to be reused in its present state or form, or is able to be broken down and reformulated into another manufactured product. This is seen almost universally as a positive attribute. Yet, many companies are not fully utilizing the recyclable items that municipal sanitation departments are amassing through recycling projects, and far too many communities don't even have recycling programs. Therefore, many potentially recyclable materials continue to be buried in landfills, shipped to and dumped in Third World countries, or incinerated. Although being recyclable is obviously an ideal, much of the material that is called recyclable is currently not being recycled because of cost factors, technological limitations, and/or lack of interest.

UNSCENTED

Unscented would seem to indicate that a product contains no natural or synthetically derived scent. However, some manufacturers use this term or *scent-free* when the scent has been altered so it can't be smelled. In some cases—especially with detergents—certain major companies use an additional *masking fragrance* to cover up or counter the odor of the original fragrance. Obviously, this type of labeling can be somewhat confusing, if not misleading. Unfortunately, for some very sensitive persons, the presence of the original odor and the masking fragrances will have an adverse effect on them because the chemical composition of the scents are what's bothersome—not just the odors themselves.

PROBLEMS OF PERSONAL TOLERANCE

Obviously, the *healthy* definition list above isn't complete. However, it's long enough to show you that word meanings and manufacturers' advertising can be misleading. As a result, unless you are very cautious, you can easily buy products you really wouldn't want—if you really knew all the facts. Therefore, it's important to read catalog descriptions, product literature, and labels carefully—and skeptically—in order to make informed purchasing decisions. Remember, the main criteria for anyone buying any product should be how it will affect your personal well-being and that of your family.

For healthy individuals, choosing items based on a thorough reading of product literature may be all that is necessary to create their healthy household. However, it should be noted that if you are already allergic or hypersensitive, reading labels will probably not be enough. Because we are each unique biological beings, we will each have our own set of personal tolerance levels. For those with Multiple Chemical Sensitivity (MCS) or allergies, the degree of tolerability is often very low to a wide range of synthetic—and sometimes even natural—products. Therefore, all readers must keep in mind that what one person may find healthy may actually be entirely inappropriate for someone else.

If you already know you have tolerability problems, you'll need to follow some special precautions when choosing healthier household products. First, you'll want to consult with your physician or other health-care professional in order to create a list of what he (or she) suggests you must avoid in order to prevent a bad reaction—and also what you can buy and safely use. For example, you should find out if there are certain natural herbs that you should stay away from or whether there are particular animal proteins that could be dangerous to you. On the other hand, you should determine whether you'll be able to tolerate some products containing man-made chemicals if they have minimal odor, and so on. With this information, you can narrow the selection of available choices to ones that will likely be suitable for you. I realize that some people will simply select the most-inert, least-toxic products available, yet for many hypersensitive individuals, it will still be essential to test all products for personal tolerability.

TESTING

For those of you who are allergic or hypersensitive, it's extremely important to test all products you have never used before. Of course, if you have a history of encountering severe negative reactions to substances, make sure to consult your physician first prior to testing any untried product at home. By the way, I believe testing is probably a good practice for anyone trying new items. After all, no one can absolutely rely on the recommendations of others that a particular product will be safe for them. Only by testing will you know for certain whether or not you'll experience a negative reaction. And because testing is relatively easy to do, it won't take up much of your time or be too complicated to master.

Actually, simple at-home tolerance testing can be done in a number of ways, depending on the product (see also *Testing Finishes, Testing Adhesives, Testing Lubricants,* and *Testing Woods* in *Chapter 12: Home Workshop and Garage*). The process usually involves a brief initial exposure to a new product to determine if there are any undesirable symptoms. For example, a bottle of a previously untried dish soap can be opened and lightly sniffed to determine if the odor is troublesome or not. If there is concern about possible skin reactions, a small amount of the dish soap can be placed on the inside of your lower arm to see if contact dermatitis erupts. For latent effects, your hands can be washed with the dish soap and the product not used again for four to seven days. As it turns out, most delayed reactions—if they are going to occur—will have become evident within that time period. To further test a product's tolerability, you can place a sample on your bedside table overnight. A good night's sleep generally indicates good tolerance. A restless night often means intolerance.

Of course, testing can provide information besides tolerability. It can be used to compare the effectiveness and cost of similar (and tolerable) products. By the way, you can save money while testing several brands by purchasing sample-size packages or the smallest sizes available. When testing, you'll want to make a written chart. On it should be the testing date, place of purchase, brand name, size, cost, and your observations and comments. Of course, both tolerability testing and effectiveness testing can be done at the same time. In the end, the best alternative products will be those that produce no negative reactions—and that perform their job well. Price is also an important consideration, but it should always be considered secondary to personal tolerability.

BUYING IN QUANTITY

Once you have found an item that seems to suit your needs, you should consider buying it in quantity if you plan to use it regularly. As you probably know, some products come in a variety of package sizes. This is especially true for certain cleaning products whose manufacturers (and their dealers) offer them in sizes ranging from a few ounces to a gallon or more. Naturally, the price per ounce when buying a gallon is almost always much cheaper than when buying in smaller amounts. By the way, also keep in mind that shipping costs will tend to be lower with one large order than with the accumulated total from several small ones. Minimum shipping fees can quickly add up.

Another important reason to buy in large amounts is that manufacturers sometimes change product formulations, create new packaging, or "improve" items in ways you may find additionally objectionable. Companies also occasionally drop certain products from their lines. You should be aware, too, that many firms making less-toxic or all-natural products are relatively small and, as with many small enterprises, it's not uncommon for them to go out of business. If any of these events should happen, a once-relied-upon, acceptable product may no longer be available when you need to reorder. Therefore, purchase in bulk when an item is currently in an acceptable form and you have a place to properly store it.

STORAGE CONCERNS

If you buy in bulk, it is important that the products be stored correctly. Do you have the necessary space? Will the temperature, light, and humidity be acceptable? Will you forget what you stored?

As a general rule, do not buy more of an item than you'll actually use within a year. If there is an expiration date, do not purchase more than you'll be able to use before that date. Otherwise, all your good intentions may sour, rot, come out of solution, or in a myriad other ways become useless and expensive garbage. To determine the best conditions and length of storage time for any particular product, you'll want to check the label, contact the dealer, or consult the manufacturer directly. To remember what you have purchased, you might want to keep a storage list with the brand names and date of purchase, then not buy any replacement items until you first check the list. Finally, remember to rotate your stock. When you purchase a new quantity of an item, put it on the back of the shelf so that the oldest products will end up being the easiest to retrieve and, therefore, first used.

FINDING HEALTHIER PRODUCTS

Where do you go to find sources of safer, less-toxic, more-natural, alternative-living products? For local suppliers, you can check the classified section of your phone directory for health-food stores and co-op groceries. Also, you can ask people you know who are already living a healthier lifestyle. Often, they're more than willing to share their personal experiences. In addition, your physician or health-care professional may offer some suggestions. By the way, even discount stores can yield some healthy products—if you know what you are looking for. Actually, finding local sources of healthier products is getting easier all the time. Fortunately, there is a business trend today to target the expanding, environmentally aware market. However, be careful that the particular definition of healthy used by others to describe a product will be one that is both applicable and acceptable to you.

Furthermore, there are now a number of books and magazines available on healthier lifestyles that contain mail-order and/or homemade sources for alternative products. Of course, this book, *The Healthy Household*, is just one example, but there are others. For example, *Clean & Green,* by Annie Berthold-Bond, contains 485 suggestions (recipes and product suppliers) for cleaning your home and yourself. *Non-toxic, Natural & Earthwise*, by Debra Lynn Dadd, lists a wide variety of less-harmful clothing, furnishings, make-up, and cleaning products and gives addresses where to purchase them. Anita Guyton's *The Natural Beauty Book: Cruelty Free Cosmetics to Make at Home* contains over 180 pages of homemade formulas for nontoxic face creams, shampoos, and other cosmetics. Also, the *Safe Home Digest Healthy Building Resource Guide* has an extensive resource listing. *The Healthy House* and *Healthy House Building,* both by John Bower, offer extensive information on healthier construction practices, materials, and suppliers. Bookstores and local libraries will likely have these and other helpful books (see also *Printed Material* in *Appendix 3: Resources for a Healthy Household*).

Organizations such as **HEAL** (a national support group for the chemically sensitive) and the **Washington Toxics Coalition** (a Seattle-based foundation for friendlier environmental living) offer fact sheets on a variety of subjects, some including listings of product sources. Consultants, such as **The Healthy House Institute** (which primarily deals with home construction), also can supply you with alternative ideas along with manufacturer and dealer addresses and phone numbers (see also *Organizations and Consulting Services* in *Appendix 3: Resources for a Healthy Household*).

You should also be aware of a growing number of mail-order companies that primarily focus on serving chemically sensitive and allergic people. They include **N.E.E.D.S.**, **The Allergy Store**, **The Living Source**, **The Cotton Place**, and **Janice Corp.**, among many others. Then, too, certain mail-order firms, such as **The Body Shop by Mail** and **Deva Lifewear**, target the eco-conscious consumer market. Alternative-product catalogs often focus on a single type of merchandise (such as clothing or cosmetics), while others carry a wide range of merchandise.

Quite a few catalogs geared to a more diversified customer-base also offer a number of healthy product choices. In this category, the classic outdoorsy catalogs (for example, **L.L. Bean, Inc.** and **Lands' End, Inc.**) often have good selections of untreated natural-fiber clothing (see also *Product Sources* in *Appendix 3: Resources for a Healthy Household*).

COST

It's not unusual for natural or less-toxic products to cost more than most of their less-healthy, but commonly available, counterparts. This is because the ingredients used in alternative items are often of a higher grade or quality and may be more difficult to obtain and/or process. In addition, small manufacturers have a much lower volume of production than large corporations which produce popular, name-brand items. However, it should also be noted that some companies actually charge more for healthier products out of a sense that people will be willing to pay extra for them.

On the other hand, some healthy products actually cost less than typical store-bought brands. This is especially true for simple, homemade alternatives. For example, inexpensive baking soda can be used as a scouring powder instead of a nationally advertised cleanser. Also, a solution of hydrogen peroxide and water can be substituted for conventional bottled mouthwash (Many of these low-cost alternatives will be covered in the chapters that follow). However, as a rule, you should expect healthy products to cost more. Of course, if their use results in better health and fewer visits to your doctor or other health-care professional, then the extra expenditure will have been well worth it.

MAKING CHOICES

The remainder of this book deals with specific information on how you can create a healthy household. It should be noted that improving indoor air quality will be of primary concern. This is because, as previously noted, some synthetically derived fragrances are neurotoxic, and odors given off by many new carpets, cleaners, man-made wood products, and paints have the potential to be carcinogenic or mutagenic. Even scents derived from natural and nontoxic sources can be intrusive and bothersome to certain people. Therefore, you'll find that suggested products and practices are often unscented, odor-free, or have only a minimal odor.

However, while improving indoor air is the major focus, other heath issues such as water quality, electromagnetic fields, "naturalness," and issues related to planetary health are also discussed and taken into account. It is hoped that, after you read through the information offered in the following chapters and appendices, you'll feel better equipped to choose what is appropriate for you and your family or household. Remember, what is offered are only suggestions—the ultimate decisions are yours. With that in mind, let's begin.

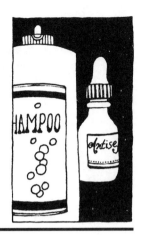

CHAPTER 2
PERSONAL CARE

Personal-care products you use on your body have the potential to create either healthy or unhealthy effects for you—and your home. Not only do they come in direct contact with your body, they also continually give off their own particular odors—odors that you inhale and become absorbed into your clothing, bedding, furnishings, and walls. These unique smells may be barely noticeable to one person, pleasant to someone else, slightly bothersome to a third individual, or life-threatening to someone who is hypersensitive. Actually, the particular resulting health effects are determined by the specific product ingredients, the duration of exposure, and the individual's personal tolerability.

It is important, therefore, to choose your personal-care items very carefully. To help you, this chapter begins with a section on scents—both natural and synthetic. Following are sections that will provide you with information on a variety of common cosmetics, toiletries, and other personal-care items—including product suggestions.

SCENTS AND SCENTED PRODUCTS

The aromas given off by many modern personal-care preparations are bothersome to a quite a few people. These odors can arise from several types of sources within each product. For example, some products have a particular smell because of the basic ingredients used in them: Citrusy is the odor of some natural lemon-juice shampoos and oily is the predominate smell of petroleum-derived mineral oil-based moisturizers. However, in addition, most hair and body products also contain very concentrated natural and/or synthetic scents. These fragrances usually have absolutely nothing to do with product effectiveness. Rather, their purpose is to create an intentionally conspicuous atmosphere surrounding their use.

WHAT ARE SCENTS?

Scents are often defined as aromatic compounds obtained from plants and other substances. Generally, their unifying characteristic is their capacity to be readily noticed, to linger, and to spread. Scents in concentrated forms (such as *essential oils*), as well as perfumes, magnify these traits.

Originally, many experts believe scents were aromatic substances connected with sacred ritual ceremonies. However, in time they became popular for secular and personal uses. Surprisingly, far from being an ancient phenomenon, what we now know as perfume (essential oils and other ingredients diluted in alcohol) did not make its appearance until fourteenth century Hungary. Soon afterward, perfume quickly became popular among the nobility and well-to-do. This may have been partially due to the lifestyle common in that era—one in which bathing was generally infrequent. Perfume may have provided a more appealing atmosphere than unwashed human bodies.

Eventually, the use of perfume and perfumed products expanded to the middle classes. By the end of the nineteenth century, fragrances were a part of many women's feminine wardrobe along with fine clothing and jewelry. Fragrance use has since expanded dramatically—especially since the creation of cheap, artificial scents. Scents (natural and/or synthetic) are now added to nearly all manufactured cosmetics and toiletries.

NATURAL ESSENTIAL OILS AND PERFUMES

Until relatively recently, virtually all perfumes and scented products used naturally derived *essential oils*. The adjective *essential* refers to the medieval alchemist's belief that these extracts were the very essence of certain plants. Since that time, chemists have scientifically analyzed essential oils. They're actually complex organic compounds—mostly mixtures of particular hydrocarbons known as *terpenes*.

To extract essential oils, steam distillation is commonly used. In this procedure, volatile compounds evaporate from plant materials (leaves, flowers, bark, seeds, roots, or wood) in the presence of hot vapor and then condense in water. Further processing removes this water, leaving a highly concentrated essential oil. Today, there are approximately two hundred commercially produced essential oils. Three very popular ones are orange blossom, jasmine, and rose.

The perfumes of the past and the natural ones of today not only contain essential oils but also other ingredients derived from nature. These may include some resins (plant solids or semisolids that don't readily evaporate) and animal substances such as civet (cat scent), musk (deer scent), castor (beaver scent), and ambergris (sperm whale intestinal secretions). Other possible ingredients are balsams, which are fragrant fluids from certain tree species. Perfumes also usually have fixatives which help bind all these components together and equalize their evaporation rates. By the way, some fixatives are the same previously mentioned fragrant plant resins and animal ingredients; it isn't unusual for a substance to serve dual purposes within a perfume formula.

Once a satisfactory blend of essential oils, resins, and animal substances, is achieved, it's then diluted with alcohol, chilled, filtered, and aged. Perfume has the highest concentration of non-alcohol ingredients, while cologne has a lower concentration. The lowest concentration of non-alcohol ingredients is in toilet water.

SYNTHETIC SCENTS AND PERFUMES

Today, natural scents are generally being replaced by synthetic ones. These man-made counterfeits are used in everything from pine-tree car deodorizers and kitchen garbage bags, to the most exquisite designer perfumes. No longer associated with special ritual, religion, wealth, or even sexual seduction, cheap synthetic scents and products using them are now virtually omnipresent. They're stock ingredients in the vast majority of manufactured personal-care products.

For the most part, synthetic scents have existed for only about a hundred years. However, since the first ones were created, a synthetic fragrance (and flavor) industry has developed and expanded rapidly. The reason is simple. The cost savings of producing synthetics, compared to finding, growing, gathering, and processing naturally aromatic ingredients into essential oils is enormous. A pound of natural ingredients (tuber rose for example) can cost as much as four thousand times more than a pound of a synthetic version.

Today, with gas chromatography and mass spectroscopy, scientists can map out the chemical structures of almost any natural ingredient. With this information, they're then able to create close copies by manipulating simple organic-molecule building blocks. These *builder molecules* are often originally derived from petroleum. Once a prototype synthetic essence has been achieved, it can be duplicated on a commercial basis.

While some natural aromas (such as coffee) cannot yet be synthesized, other natural fragrances continue to be analyzed and simulated. Two popular laboratory creations are synthetic wild cherry (benzaldehyde) and synthetic rose (B-phenylethyl alcohol). These two fragrances have relatively simple formulations, but many synthetic scents contain hundreds of individual components. Interestingly, some of the newer scents no longer attempt to mimic natural ones. Instead, they convey such intangibles as *fresh* and *clean*.

No matter what their price tags, most perfumes today are probably made with at least some synthetic scents. Some perfumes may also contain synthetic fixatives and other man-made additives such as methyl ethyl ketone, formaldehyde, etc. (see *Formaldehyde* in *Chapter 9: Indoor Air*). These synthetic components are often considered by the fragrance industry to be safe, but a number of them have already been shown to have negative health effects. Unfortunately, the truth is that many modern scent and perfume ingredients have had only minimal toxicity testing—or none at all.

PROBLEMS WITH SCENTS

Anymore, the majority of Americans accept fragrances, scents, incense, potpourri, etc. as a part of daily life. In fact, many people feel that scents are not only pleasurable, but also beneficial. Popular therapies now focus on applying certain aromatic oils to the body or heating particular fragrant oils so they'll evaporate into the room air to be inhaled. However, there is another side to fragrances and scents that needs to be seriously considered. That is, while most people are not aware of any ill effects, any natural or synthetic odor has the capacity to be unpleasant or irritating—at least to some people. Certain fragrances, aromas, and perfumes can also provoke allergic or asthmatic responses. In fact, the U.S. Food and Drug Administration (FDA) has reported that perfume-provoked respiratory symptoms are experienced by 72% of all asthmatics. And a great many people with MCS (Multiple Chemical Sensitivity) (see *MCS, A New Medical Condition* in *Chapter 1: Getting Started*) also report that they, too, experience negative reactions when they breathe in scents and perfumes. But that's still not the full extent of the possible ill effects from being exposed to fragrances.

In "Patient Education: Scents Make No Sense" in the Fall 1991 issue of *The Environmental Physician*, author Irene Ruth Wilkenfeld wrote that in 1989 The National Institute of Occupational Safety and Health (NIOSH) recognized 884 of 2,983 substances (both naturally and synthetically derived) used in the fragrance industry as toxic. Some of these ingredients actually act as *neurotoxins*—that is, they're capable of harming the central nervous system. For example, linalool (a clear fragrant terpene alcohol compound obtained from several types of essential oils) has been reported to cause ataxic gait (an abnormal stride due to loss of muscle coordination in the extremities) and depression. Methyl ethyl ketone (a colorless, flammable solvent that's commonly synthesized) has the capacity to induce stupor and unconsciousness. Cyclohexanol (a clear flammable synthesized solvent with a peppermint-like odor) can inhibit motor activity and instigate spasms, and generally depresses the central nervous system. On and on. While the majority of people have not been obviously or severely impacted from being exposed to these ingredients, it is also probably true that increasing numbers of people are being affected by them—at least to some lesser degree. In any case, many of the compounds used in scents and perfumes don't appear to be innately safe or healthy for humans.

As fragrances and scented products have become popular (it has been estimated that the average consumer uses about twenty scented personal-care items each day), the interiors of our homes have been absorbing more of these potentially bothersome (and/or illness provoking) odors. Unfortunately, fragrances which are designed to quickly spread are often extremely difficult to remove from skin, hair, walls, floors, and furnishings. It's no wonder then that the term *ineluctable* has been applied to the use of scents. This big word conveys the simple idea that fragrances are now virtually impossible to evade—at least totally. By the way, many people don't realize that some of the various scent ingredients can actually chemically interact with each other—creating new, totally unplanned synthetic compounds. No one can even guess what health effects these compounds could ultimately induce.

Interestingly, negative sensory and aesthetic consequences are usually seldom, if ever, discussed as problems associated with perfumes and scents—but from all indications they should be. Because fragrances can be found nearly everywhere all the time, many people are unable to perceive that a background of perfume and scent odors is even present. Surrounded and saturated by no-longer-discernible odors, some individuals (usually women, but increasingly men) further feel they must apply large amounts of bottled perfume to their bodies in order to know they even have it on. The resulting wafting odor is often unpleasantly strong to those people who have been trying to avoid scents, or at least minimize their exposure to them. By the way, the intensity of the perfume would probably be unpleasantly strong to those same perfume wearers if they, too, were trying to avoid using or being around scented products for a few weeks and reacquired their normal sense of smell.

Also, from an aesthetic standpoint, being constantly in the presence (consciously or unconsciously) of scents could tend to diminish some of life's special moments. For example, being in the presence of a magnificent blooming lavender bush or at the edge of a pounding ocean could be sensed just as "nice" smells amid the ever-present daily barrage of other "nice" smells—from hand lotion, eye shadow, bath beads, and toilet tissue. As a result, real-world events can be lost or at least watered down by the banal and contrived olfactory experiences of everyday life.

Perhaps not surprisingly, there are individuals who have decided they'd like to avoid the many scents to which others have grown accustomed. This decision is often reached when they find their own personal health has been (and usually continues to be) seriously affected by fragrances. Unfortunately, it requires real determination to limit scent and perfume exposure—especially in situations outside your own home. The truth is, you probably will have very little control over what products are used in public buildings, public transportation, other dwellings, or on other people. Even within your own residence, if you decide to create a scent-free environment, it'll take a great deal of resolve and personal commitment. However, it can be done—and using unscented personal-care products is key to doing this. (Using unscented cleaning products is another significant source over which you have some control. See *Chapter 7: Cleaning*.) Therefore, before buying, making, or using any personal-care preparation, seriously consider the probable odor consequences.

COSMETICS AND TOILETRIES

Cosmetics and toiletries as preparations that soothe, alter, or enhance the face, skin, and hair, generally fall into several commonly recognized classifications. These include powders (minute granular materials which adhere to skin and absorb moisture), emulsions (oil particles dispersed in water such as creams and lotions), lipsticks (semisoft compounds consisting of oils, waxes, and pigments), eye make-up (generally similar to lipsticks or powders), and miscellaneous products (depilatories, deodorants, hair preparations, nail care products, etc.).

Cosmetics have a long history, traceable to prehistoric rituals. Later, like scents, they became commonly used simply for personal pleasure. By the 1700s (sometimes known as the Age of Artifice), upper-class European men and women routinely whitened their faces, drew blue vein lines on their skin, and wore other forms of make-up. The Victorian Era ushered in a period of austerity in cosmetic and toiletry use. However, by the end of the nineteenth century the use of personal-care items, particularly cosmetics worn by women, greatly increased. This was due to several factors, including the beginnings of large-scale manufacturing and advertising, combined with a growing middle-class. Today, cosmetic and toiletry production and use continues to rise, especially since the creation of inexpensive synthetic ingredients. Men are also using more personal-care preparations and cosmetics, though not nearly to the same degree as women. Another trend is the use of make-up and toiletry items by girls at ever-earlier ages.

EARLY NATURAL AND CHEMICAL INGREDIENTS

During most of human history, the ingredients in personal-care products and cosmetics were derived from minerals, plants, and animals. Although they originated naturally, not all these products were safe. For example, lead dust was used for thousands of years as white face powder. Later, early chemists brought other dangerous ingredients into the public's hands—red mercuric sulfide (lip colorant), sulfuric acid (hair bleach) and sublimate of mercury (wart and freckle lightener) to name just three. Surprisingly, these toxic products were often extremely popular, despite the risk of poisoning and disfiguring. Fortunately, most of the early hazardous preparations are now outlawed. However, surprisingly, a few highly noxious ingredients are still allowed limited use in certain applications (see *Government Regulations* below).

TYPICAL MODERN INGREDIENTS

Some of the ingredients used in today's personal-care preparations remain natural. Most of these are considered quite safe, but some do cause health problems. For example, talc—the natural mineral hydrous magnesium silicate—can cause lung problems if breathed over time (talcosis). Other natural ingredients, such as certain plant oils, can produce skin and mucous-membrane irritation or pose other health risks.

While a few manufacturers use natural substances exclusively, the majority of today's cosmetics and toiletries contain synthetically derived ingredients. In many cases, these ultimately originate from petroleum or coal tar. A few of the more common synthetic-ingredient categories are dyes, flavoring agents, base components, preservatives, and scents. Many of the actual synthetic compounds used have unpronounceable polysyllabic names combined with hyphenated numbers. However, while an intimidating name sometimes coincides with the potential for causing negative side effects, this is not always the case. As was discussed earlier, *healthy* isn't a word with a simple, clearcut definition nor is it an effect or condition that's universally agreed upon and understood (see *"Healthy" Definitions* in *Chapter 1: Getting Started*).

Of course, many natural ingredients have desirable properties—and they definitely have an aura of goodness about them. After all, some individuals choose to use only naturally derived products for very valid ecological, philosophical, medical, or spiritual reasons. But not every synthetic ingredient is bad; in fact, each varies considerably from one to another. Like natural ingredients, each synthetic ingredient has its own appearance, consistency, odor, effect on the environment, and toxicity. The known possible negative effects of synthetic personal-care substances ranges from none at all, to mild skin irritation, to chromosomal damage—and yes—even cancer.

Of course, the precise heath effects of any ingredient (natural or synthetic) on a particular individual will depend on many factors. Some of these include the chemical make-up of the substance, the quantity used, the duration of use, and the innate susceptibility of the person using it. For example, the synthetic colorant FD&C Blue No. 1 can cause allergic reactions in some people while others seem to be unaffected. However, this same dye has been shown to be carcinogenic in animals when they're intentionally exposed to relatively large amounts over time. How will this same product affect you? No one can predict for sure.

At the same time, it should be kept in mind that many recently created synthetic ingredients have been used by the consuming public for only a few short years. As a result, there hasn't been enough time to establish a true history of what negative outcomes conceivably could occur. Thus, while it *appears* certain synthetic substances have not caused any health problems so far, the long-term effects are often relatively unknown. Because cosmetic and toiletry regulations are minimal, nonexistent, or poorly enforced, each of us must educate him- or herself to determine what to use and what to avoid. One source of in-depth information about specific personal-care ingredients is *The Consumer's Dictionary of Cosmetic Ingredients* by Ruth Winter. This book should be available in your local library and bookstores.

As final note, many sensitive individuals are able to tolerate low-odor, mild, undyed, synthetic personal-care products better than all-natural formulations that contain aromatic essential oils. Remember that no expert can really say what is best for you, especially if you are allergic or sensitive. That is only gauged by your own personal research, testing, and experience.

ALTERNATIVE COSMETICS AND TOILETRIES

A growing number of individuals find scents and typically available personal-care products intolerable. To meet their needs, alternative preparations are being marketed, ranging from name-brand items formulated without the usual fragrances added, to completely all-natural product lines. Certain books can also help you create your own homemade preparations.

SCENT-FREE AND HYPOALLERGENIC PRODUCTS

Today, people who find scents and perfumes bothersome or intolerable often try name-brand toiletries labeled *scent-free* or *fragrance-free*. These generally have formulas similar to the standard varieties, but they contain no scent additives. For many individuals, these are very acceptable alternatives.

In addition, complete product lines of specially created *hypoallergenic* cosmetic and personal-care items are available. In most cases, however, only the most commonly allergenic substances are left out of these formulations—ingredients such as fragrances and/or lanolin. Unfortunately, sometimes other ingredients many people would consider undesirable remain. For example, until very recently, at least one hypoallergenic shampoo was still made with formaldehyde. By the way, both scent-free versions of conventional products, as well as those labeled hypoallergenic, often contain many synthetic compounds.

ALL-NATURAL PRODUCTS

A few companies now produce skin and hair-care preparations that are *all-natural*. Unfortunately, it seems that this term is rather loosely defined. Therefore, some products labeled as having all-natural ingredients may actually contain components considered synthetic by some experts. Two such ambiguously classified ingredients are sodium lauryl (an emulsifier) and methyl paraben (a preservative).

Another potential concern with many all-natural products is that they often contain essential oils or other highly aromatic ingredients. This may be a problem for certain allergic or sensitive individuals or for those who have simply decided to avoid fragrances.

HOMEMADE PREPARATIONS

Instead of purchasing ready-made body-care preparations, you can create them yourself at home from scratch. Because you select the ingredients yourself, you will have complete knowledge and control over what will be applied to your skin or hair. If you want, you can use only organic ingredients.

Remember, of course, that making homemade products will require you to first obtain the necessary vegetables, fruits, grains, clays, etc. It'll also be necessary for you to take the time to cut, mash, mix, or do whatever else is necessary for proper preparation. Also, you should keep in mind that your homemade products could have very short shelf-lives; in many cases they could become quickly contaminated by mold and bacteria. Therefore, without preservatives, certain homemade preparations may need to be stored in a refrigerator, then heated on a warm stove each time you use them.

If you decide to make your own skin and hair-care preparations, it's undoubtedly easiest to use already established formulas and methods. One book you may find helpful is *The Natural Beauty Book: Cruelty Free Cosmetics to Make at Home* by Anita Guyton. In print for many years, this British guide provides a wide variety of natural cosmetic recipes.

GOVERNMENT REGULATIONS

Many Americans believe the cosmetics and toiletries industry has volumes of strict regulations it must follow. It's also commonly believed that products and production lines are continually being monitored by government agencies. Unfortunately, these are wrong assumptions. In reality, the laws protecting citizens from potentially dangerous personal-care products remain absent, minimal, or rarely enforced.

For many centuries, there were no laws concerning cosmetics and toiletries whatsoever. Finally, government regulation began with the passage of the 1938 U.S. Federal Food, Drug, and Cosmetic Act. Its purpose was to stop mislabeling and product adulteration (the addition of dangerous or impure substances). A number of regulations have since followed. Now, clear, accurate labeling of all cosmetic ingredients (*except* flavorings, fragrances, and colors) is required. Also, laws forbid the use of known cancer-causing ingredients and the inclusion of particular dangerous substances in certain products. For example, compounds containing mercury can no longer be used in skin preparations.

Despite these federal regulations, ingredients some researchers and consumers consider potentially harmful still remain in some cosmetics. This is due to several factors, a major one being that cosmetic manufacturers are not required to register their company, products, ingredients, or adverse reactions with the Food and Drug Administration. Instead, experts on an industry-created Cosmetics Ingredient Review Board determine product safety. Even if the Board decides to take some action, company compliance is only voluntary. Even in situations where regulations require the Food and Drug Administration itself to get involved, cosmetic-industry surveillance is still very limited because of budgetary and personnel limitations. Therefore, in many respects, government supervision and enforcement is only superficial at best.

Actually, many personal-care items, as well as certain ingredients in otherwise regulated products, are under little or no government requirements or restrictions at this time. As it turns out, many toiletries, such as soap, are not legally classified as cosmetics, and, therefore, are unregulated. Also, as previously noted, fragrance, dye, and flavoring ingredients, even if in a legally classified cosmetic preparation, are exempt from product-labeling regulations. Unfortunately, this is particularly distressing because the word fragrance on a product label can mean that hundreds of individual chemical components have been added—but exactly what they are, no consumer will ever know. Finally, some product ingredients can remain unknown to the public because they're legally defined as *proprietary trade secrets*.

PERSONAL-CARE PRODUCT SUGGESTIONS

Ideally, personal-care products should be readily available (either easy to find in local stores or through mail-order suppliers, or easy to make at home), convenient to use, effective, affordable, odor-free, nontoxic, biodegradable, organic, and simple in formulation. It would also be nice if they contained no endangered plant or animal by-products, were not tested on animals, contained no preservatives, had an inherently long shelf-life, and were packaged in recycled natural materials that could, in turn, be recyclable. That is a long wish list. While there are a few such products, in most cases, compromises have to be made.

However, with the increasing variety of alternative products now being manufactured and with the knowledge of how to make homemade ones, it's possible for even sensitive individuals to satisfactorily meet most of their personal-care needs. By the way, you'll want to check local pharmacies and health-food stores from time to time to see what acceptable choices they have in stock. After all, new products that may be suitable for you are coming out every day. Also, your local bookstores and library should have available several books with natural, do-it-yourself personal-care product recipes.

It's important to give yourself the freedom to experiment with preparations that are new to you. However, be sure to test any new product first, whether manufactured or homemade. This step is absolutely critical for sensitive or allergic individuals. (Remember, many personal-care formulas, especially homemade ones, contain food substances.) For those who have experienced severe reactions in the past, such testing should only be done under the supervision of a physician or health-care professional (see *Testing* in *Chapter 1: Getting Started*).

The following listings of the most essential personal-care items include specific suggestions for using them. These suggestions are ones that are likely to be tolerable for even very sensitive and allergic persons and tend to have minimal odor. However, a number of all-natural preparations that happen to contain essential oils or aromatic base-ingredients are also included as alternative choices. However, as has been pointed out, this book stresses indoor air quality. Therefore, while other characteristics were taken into account, unscented or low-odor products were given priority.

It is hoped the suggestions that follow will work well for you. Don't forget the many additional catalogs and suppliers handling a wide variety of alternative personal-care products that are listed in *Appendix 3: Resources for a Healthy Household.*

ASTRINGENTS

Astringents sold in stores are usually alcohol-based. These should be avoided, not only because their of the odor (which many sensitive persons would find bothersome), but also because of their drying effect on skin. A good alcohol-free astringent can be made simply with equal amounts of hot water and apple-cider vinegar. Other homemade options include cold chamomile tea, fresh lemon juice in cool water, strained cucumber juice, and strained tomato pulp. If you plan to use tomato pulp, you'll want to leave it on your skin a few minutes. Then, you can rinse it off with tepid water. Generally, refrigerating any of your natural preparations will allow them to keep for a few days.

BATH SOAKS

By dissolving $1/2$ cup of baking soda in a tub of tepid water, you can create a soothing bath able to neutralize perspiration odors. You might also want to try pouring $1/2$ gallon of milk in a tub of tepid bath water, followed by a shower to rinse, to help nourish your skin.

BLACKHEAD THERAPY

If you have acne or severe blackheads, it would be best for you to consult a physician. However, for milder conditions you may want to try a number of simple solutions. For example, a mixture made of equal parts of baking soda and water can be gently rubbed on the face to loosen blackheads. Also, fresh lemon juice can help remove blackheads, and at the same time, lighten the presence of any that remain. Another option is to boil 2 teaspoons of rosemary in a pint of distilled water. You can then carefully place your face in the resulting steam to open the pores.

COMBS, BRUSHES, AND SCRUBBERS

Combs made of metal, bone, or wood are excellent all-natural choices, often both attractive and long-lasting. The same goes for boar-bristle brushes with hardwood handles. To purchase natural combs and brushes, check the **Eco Design Co.**, **Simmons Handcrafts**, and **Natural Lifestyle Supplies**. Also, **The Vermont Country Store** sells boar-bristle brushes. Natural animal-hair make-up brushes are made by **Ida Grae's** under the Nature's Colors brand (available from **N.E.E.D.S.** and other catalogs).

After you've purchased natural brushes, you'll occasionally need to wash them—gently so they aren't damaged. You'll find that using a mild shampoo works well to clean away dirt and body oil without harming the brush fibers. Afterwards, you should rinse the brushes with clear warm water, shake out the excess water, shape any soft fibers with your fingers, then allow to air-dry.

For scrubbing, natural *loofa* scrubbers work well. They're actually made of the interiors of certain dried fibrous tropical gourds. Other good natural scrubbers, commonly available, are made from woven grasses. To find natural scrubbers, you'll want to see what your local health-food store handles. If you prefer mail-order, **Simmons Handcrafts** offers loofa scrubbers, facial buffs, wood-handled/natural-bristle bath brushes, and nail brushes, as well as sea sponges, undyed cellulose sponges, and a good selection of *ayates* (Mexican natural-fiber washcloths). Loofas with wooden handles, loofa mitts, wooden-handled sisal bath brushes, and other natural scrubbers are available through **The Body Shop by Mail**.

(See *Dental Care* below for toothbrushes and *Shaving Creams* for shaving brushes.)

DENTAL CARE

Baking soda (sodium bicarbonate) has been used successfully for many years as a toothpowder. So has table salt. Both of these are low-cost, effective, and safe dentifrices you may want to try—as long as you're not on a low-sodium diet. In addition, baking soda can be mixed with 3% dilution hydrogen peroxide (the concentration usually sold in pharmacies) to be used as a good tooth whitener.

You might already be aware that a number of alternative dental products are now being marketed. Peelu (**Peelu-Floss Lifelong Products**) is one. It's a tooth powder derived from *salvadora perisia* shrub fiber. In the Mideast and Asia, where the plant grows, it's been used to clean teeth for centuries. Peelu is actually a beige, slightly gritty powder that is normally marketed with natural mint oil as a flavoring agent. If you don't care for tooth powders, Peelu also comes in toothpaste form. To purchase it, you'll want to check with your local health-food stores.

Of course, there are several other all-natural toothpastes you might want to try. A popular one is Tom's of Maine Natural Toothpaste (**Tom's of Maine**) which is available with or without fluoride in several natural flavors. This particular product is commonly sold in heath-food stores. You should be aware that the **Natural Lifestyle Supplies** catalog handles Tom's of Maine, as well as a number of other alternative toothpastes. This mail-order company also offers natural-bristle toothbrushes with pear-wood handles.

Most dental floss today is made of nylon. Fortunately, this is a material which is generally well-tolerated by many allergic and sensitive persons. This is especially true for unwaxed and unflavored types. One national brand, Tuff-Spun dental floss (**John O. Butler Co.**), is available unwaxed and unflavored in disposable plastic packages. In addition, the company offers a small, plastic, barrel-shaped dispenser designed to be refillable. Interestingly, the refills still come on wooden spools. The refills may have to be specially ordered for you by your pharmacist.

As a rule, most typical mouthwashes are mostly artificially dyed and flavored alcohol solutions. However, an all-natural, inexpensive mouthwash is simply a solution of water with a pinch of dissolved table salt. One teaspoon of baking soda added to a half glass of water will also help neutralize mouth odors. If you're on a low-sodium diet, you might prefer to gargle using equal parts of 3% dilution hydrogen peroxide and water. Another choice you may want to try is Tom's of Maine Natural Mouthwash (**Tom's of Maine**), which contains aloe and vitamin C—and it's alcohol-free. You'll also want to check your local health-food stores to see if it's available.

DEODORANTS

Many of the deodorants and antiperspirants on the market are scented and/or contain potentially bothersome ingredients—and they usually are expensive, too. Fortunately, there are better alternatives. For example, baking soda makes a good, low-cost, natural deodorant powder. However, it has a tendency to leave a white ring on dark clothing. Cornstarch can be substituted—but it can be messy, too.

Instead, you may want to try one of the unscented, hypoallergenic deodorants or antiperspirants. These are sold in pump, cream, or roll-on forms under nationally distributed brand names in many drugstores. However, you should be aware that hypoallergenic deodorants and antiperspirants usually contain a variety of synthetic ingredients, and in most cases, aluminum as well. As you probably already know, aluminum deposits found in the brain have been associated with Alzheimer's disease. Until more is understood about the connection of aluminum to this disorder, it might be wise to avoid personal-care products containing this ingredient.

If you're seeking an alternative deodorant that is effective, non-marking, natural, unscented, and aluminum-free a good choice is Le Crystal Naturel (**French Transit Ltd.**). It's actually just a fist-sized chunk of alum mineral salts. Since it was originally marketed, other similar products have become available. Some of these are packaged in smaller sizes or in stick dispensers. These all-alum mineral products act as deodorants, but not antiperspirants. They work by inhibiting bacterial growth on the skin rather than stopping wetness. Interestingly, it's the by-products of bacterial metabolism which are the source of body odor—not the perspiration itself. **The Living Source** and **N.E.E.D.S.** are two catalog sources for crystal deodorants. They're also commonly available at health-food stores.

Another all-natural aluminum-free choice is Le Stick (**Nature de France, Ltd.**). It's a compressed product containing baking soda, clay, chlorophyll and a few other ingredients. You'll want to check your local health-food stores to see if they handle it. There are also quite a few natural, liquid deodorants on the market made with herbs. One popular brand is Tom's of Maine Natural Deodorant Unscented (**Tom's of Maine**). It's a combination of aloe, lichen, and coriander and is commonly sold at health-food stores. It's also offered for sale in the **Natural Lifestyle Supplies** catalog.

DUSTING POWDER

Breathing dust of any kind can be damaging to the respiratory system, so dusting powder is often not recommended. However, if you really want to use a dusting powder, try using a light sprinkling of baking soda. Corn and rice starches are other possibilities you might want to use.

EYE CARE

For puffiness around the eyes, you might want to try the following procedure. Lie down and place cold cucumber slices on your closed eye lids for approximately 15 minutes. By the way, cooled, steeped tea bags will also help.

To temporarily tighten the skin around your eyes and to minimize lines and wrinkles, you can simply apply a small amount of egg white. In addition, a tiny amount of olive oil lightly dabbed to the area will provide gentle moisturizing. Be sure to take special care to keep all preparations out of the eyes themselves.

FACIAL SCRUBS

Baking soda sprinkled on a washcloth works well as an inexpensive, all-natural facial scrub. Another option is to mix a little oat flour and water in the palm of your hand and apply the mixture to your face with a gentle scrubbing action. After applying a facial scrub, you'll want to rinse it off with tepid water.

FEMININE HYGIENE

Some women simply can't tolerate most of the nationally distributed brands of menstrual pads and tampons. One major reason for this is that commonly available feminine napkins and tampons have likely been treated with chemicals to increase absorbency and to mask menstrual odors. Even if a woman purchases unscented pads, these can still be odorous and, thus, bothersome because they often absorb fragrances from the boxes of scented pads that sat adjacent to them on store shelves.

Fortunately, truly unscented mini, maxi, and panty-shield pads can be ordered from mail-order companies such as **The Seventh Generation**. Besides being unscented, they're also dioxin-free. (Dioxin is a toxic chemical commonly found in minute quantities in paper goods that have been bleached with chlorine.) Another often-tolerable option is New Day's Choice feminine napkins (**Confab**). These are carried by some alternative groceries and health-food stores, but if you can't find them locally, call the company for the nearest dealer. New Day's Choice napkins are constructed of a thin upper layer of 100% cotton and are available in regular and thin maxi sizes.

However, if even these alternative paper-based pads prove to be too irritating or otherwise unacceptable, washable 100%-cotton cloth feminine napkins are available that you can launder and reuse. Through mail order, you can obtain 100%-organic washable cotton pads from **The Richman Cotton Company**. In addition, **The Seventh Generation** sells both non-organic and organic 100%-cotton washable types. Incidentally, 100%-cotton pointelle-knit menstrual panties in two styles are available from **The Vermont Country Store**. These have a protective plastic liner sandwiched between the cotton fabric in the crotch.

For women who choose to douche, it's wise, of course, to use only a naturally mild solution. One you might try is a weak dilution of apple cider vinegar and tepid water. You might even use warm water by itself, too. (Before using any douching solutions, be sure to check with your physician for his (or her) recommendations concerning safe products and ingredients for you.)

FIRST AID

An excellent antiseptic for minor cuts and scrapes is simply a 3% solution of hydrogen peroxide (the type commonly available at drugstores). Besides having germicidal properties, it is low-cost, colorless, and virtually odorous. In addition, Zephiran (**Winthrop Pharmaceuticals**) is often tolerated by sensitive individuals as an antiseptic; however, it does have a mild medicinal odor. Zephiran is a brand name for a benzalkonium chloride solution which can be specially ordered for you by your local pharmacist or you can mail-order it directly from **The American Environmental Health Foundation, Inc.**

Another often-tolerable first-aid preparation is aloe vera. This is actually the juice from the leaves of the water-aloe plant, a succulent member of the lily family. It's often available in bottles at health-food stores. Aloe vera has the ability to soothe many minor burns and skin irritations. Another simple first-aid solution is a paste made from three parts baking soda and one part water. It can be applied to poison ivy outbreaks and insect bites to help relieve itching. You'll want to allow the paste to dry, then later gently wash it off with warm water. (Note, if redness, irritation, and/or swelling persists or increases after a few days using any remedy, you should always consult your personal physician.)

Unfortunately, plastic bandage strips are often bothersome to sensitive individuals. However, many find that cloth bandage strips or sterilized cotton gauze held into place with first-aid tape are better tolerated. These items are available in most drugstores. By the way, if available, you may want to simply use sterile cotton cloth that has been torn into strips. These can be tied around small wounds on fingers or limbs in place of tape.

FOOT CARE

A number of foot preparations are available or that can be made that are generally well-tolerated by sensitive individuals. For example, your feet can be soaked for 10–20 minutes in a solution consisting of nothing more than 4 tablespoons of baking soda in a quart of warm water. This acts as a skin soother and at the same time neutralizes foot odors and softens calluses. Another unscented foot bath consists of 1 teaspoon of San-O-Zon in a quart of warm water. You'll want to soak your feet in this solution for 10–20 minutes for a relaxing effect that also neutralizes foot odors. San-O-Zon is a patented form of sodium-borax powder. One mail-order source is **Cottontails OrganicWear**.

After soaking your feet, you may also want to safely remove calluses or toughened skin by gently rubbing your feet with a pumice stone. (Pumice is actually a frothy-appearing, hard, volcanic glass.) These stones can be ordered from **Simmons Handcrafts**. Afterwards, you can rub in a few drops of olive oil or other well-tolerated vegetable oil.

To help absorb foot perspiration and odor, you can lightly dust your soles with baking soda. Another option to help control foot odor is to apply an alum mineral product such as Le Crystal Naturel (**French Transit Ltd.**) or another similar product. To use a crystal deodorant, just wet the crystal and rub it across the soles of your feet. **The Living Source** and **N.E.E.D.S.** are two catalog sources for crystal deodorants. They're also commonly available at health-food stores.

HAIR COLORANTS

Powdered leaves of the henna shrub have been used for centuries as a semi-permanent reddish hair colorant. The common auburn shade is sold both prepackaged and in bulk at some health-food stores. Light Mountain (**Lotus Brands**) markets henna in shades from black to blond. These are sold in some heath-food stores and pharmacies. They can be mail-ordered through the manufacturer's catalog.

Another option is to try Vita Wave hair color (**Vita Wave Products**) that uses vegetable dyes and no harsh chemicals. The colors available range from Bright Red to Medium Brown to Golden Blond. Vita Wave hair colors are sold through **Natural Lifestyle Supplies** and **N.E.E.D.S.**

HAIR CONDITIONERS

Many conventional hair conditioners contain scents and/or other ingredients that can be bothersome to allergic or sensitive persons. Fortunately, you can make your own excellent hair conditioners at home. One simple conditioner is a small amount of a tolerable brand of mayonnaise that you rub into your hair. After 20 minutes or so, you then rinse it off using warm water.

In addition, an egg yolk beaten with a few drops of tolerated oil works well as a hair conditioner. Again, you'll want to rub the preparation into your hair and leave it on for about 20 minutes before rinsing with warm water.

HAIR SPRAYS

Often, one very intolerable product for those with sensitivities or allergies is hair spray. This is of little wonder when you consider that many conventional products contain lacquer and a host of synthetic ingredients including synthetic scents. If you are unable to tolerate typically available hair sprays, you may be able to tolerate some of the hypoallergenic brands available in certain drugstores. If not, you might want to purchase hair spray made and sold by **The Living Source**. It contains "no lacquer, toxic chemicals, or fragrance."

Incidentally, homemade hair spray can be made using $1/4$ teaspoon powdered gelatin dissolved in $1/3$ cup of very hot water. Pour a small amount of the solution into a spray bottle and make sure to use it before the gelatin cools. If any is remaining, refrigerate it. You should be aware that this cooled hair spray solution must be reheated before it can be reused. Those with food allergies should know that, although gelatin can be derived from certain plants (such as agar from some seaweeds), it's most commonly an animal by-product, usually from cattle.

For those who can tolerate the fragrance of natural lemon, you can put one roughly chopped, unpeeled lemon in a saucepan, add 2 cups water, or enough to cover the lemon, and boil the mixture down to 1 cup. Then, cool the solution and strain it through cheesecloth. Finally, pour the mixture into a spray bottle. (You may need to thin it down with additional water before using.) This homemade hair spray will keep for several days—that is, if you store it in the refrigerator.

HAIR-SETTING SOLUTIONS

Many of the hair-setting products available—like most cosmetics and toiletries—contain scents. To avoid these, you may want to purchase hair spray made and sold by **The Living Source** which can also be used to set your hair. A simple homemade recipe you can make at home is 2 tablespoons of flaxseed dissolved in 1 cup warm water (You'll need to strain the solution before using). Another homemade formula is to use a solution consisting of 2 tablespoons of superfine white sugar dissolved in $1/2$ cup warm water, which you apply to your hair while the solution is still warm.

MAKE-UP

Several make-up lines sold nationally in department and drugstores are marketed as being hypoallergenic. Such products are generally free of the harshest irritants and allergy-provoking ingredients—perfume and lanolin, for example. However, they usually contain a number of synthetic ingredients and/or substances that could still provoke a negative reaction—but in a smaller percentage of the population. For some sensitive and allergic people, hypoallergenic cosmetic brands work quite acceptably, but for others, they discover they must use, not only unscented products, but also ones containing all-natural ingredients.

Fortunately, a few companies do make totally natural, unscented products. For instance, Indian Earth Original (**Indian Earth Cosmetics**) is completely natural and unadulterated. It's made of only one ingredient—a natural, deep reddish/orange unrefined powdered clay. It comes packaged in small earthenware pots with cork lids. Indian Earth Original can be used as an eye shadow, cheek blush, and lip color. It's relatively expensive, but a tiny amount goes a very long way. This product can be ordered through **The Cotton Place** or directly from the company. As a note of caution, some firms making simple natural make-up products such as clay blushers often also make other products which are scented or contain synthetic ingredients. This includes Indian Earth Cosmetics. Therefore, you'll want to make sure you read the ingredient list of every cosmetic you intend to buy—no matter who manufactures it.

One cosmetic line with which you'll probably want become familiar is **Ida Grae's** Nature's Colors. This company produces many unscented all-natural products including Earth Rouge (iron oxide and silicate), colored powder eye shadows, and a translucent face powder. Nature's Colors are sold in a number of catalogs including **N.E.E.D.S.** Another natural cosmetic line is Colorings, available from **The Body Shop by Mail**. Some of the items offered under this label are eye shadows, rouges, lipsticks, mascaras, foundations, and powders. However, most of these items contain natural scents in the form of essential oils (concentrated scents). Yet another all-natural cosmetic line is Paul Penders which is handled by **N.E.E.D.S.** and other catalogs. You might also be able to purchase it at some local health-food stores, department stores, and pharmacies.

An excellent lip gloss you might want to try is Nanak's Lip Smoothee, Unscented (**Golden Temple Natural Products**). Its ingredients are just natural oils and beeswax. This product works well alone, or as a gloss over an application of natural powdered clay such as Indian Earth Original. Actually, this particular combination makes a very good substitute for conventional lipsticks. By the way, Nanak's Lip Smoothee is also a good moisturizer—able to prevent or treat chapped lips. You can often purchase this product at local heath-food stores. Other often-tolerable clear glosses are available from **Indian Earth Cosmetics** and **Nature's Colors Cosmetics**. In addition, just using a small amount of petroleum jelly on your lips often works well as a gloss. Despite obviously being a petroleum-based product, petroleum jelly tends to be tolerable for a number of sensitive individuals.

Of course, many women will want to use other brands, types, and colors of make-up. Several catalogs, including **Natural Lifestyle Supplies** and **Janice Corp.**, sell a good variety of alternative cosmetics you may want to try. In addition, *Appendix 3: Resources for a Healthy Household* lists many other mail-order companies handling make-up. For new products available locally, you'll want to remember to check the cosmetic counters of nearby health-food stores, department stores, and pharmacies from time to time.

MOISTURIZERS

A moisturizing product which seems to have no detectable odor is Moisture Guard (**Granny's Old Fashioned Products**). Like most products offered by this manufacturer, it's inexpensive, has a simple formula, and is available packaged in a variety of sizes. Granny's line is often sold in health-food stores and also handled by several catalogs including **The Living Source** and **N.E.E.D.S.**

There are now dozens of national brands of popular conventional-formula moisturizers that also come in unscented, hypoallergenic forms. These lotions may moisturize effectively but generally contain many synthetic chemicals, some of which could be bothersome to certain individuals. However, one such product you may want to consider is Oil of Olay Beauty Fluid for Sensitive Skin, which is sold at most drug-, discount, and department stores. Oil of Olay not only effectively moisturizes, it is also absorbed quickly into the skin and is *non-commodious* (won't clog your pores). Another product you might try is a moisturizer produced by a small hypoallergenic-cosmetic company. Chap Cream (**Ar-Ex, Ltd.**) has a thick formulation and comes packaged in a tube. It's sold in some pharmacies and may be ordered directly from the company.

Of course, some natural oils such as lanolin, apricot, or jojoba can be used as moisturizing fluids. Probably the best time to use these oils (or any type of moisturizer for that matter) is immediately after showering or bathing. This is because a small amount of oil applied at that time helps retain the water that was just absorbed by your skin. Unfortunately, a drawback to natural oils is that they tend to be greasy. As a result, they could contribute to clogging your skin pores and staining your clothes, so use them sparingly. **Common Sense Products** offers lanolin as well as a selection of other natural oils derived from plants through its catalog. Natural oils are also usually available at local health-food stores.

PERMANENTS

Most at-home and salon permanents contain potentially harmful chemicals. These ingredients are designed to alter the molecular structure of your hair shafts. Fortunately, a far less toxic product is available: Vita Wave permanent (**Vita Wave Products Co.**), which is still able to give bounce and curl to your hair. However, it should be noted that it does contain fragrance. Catalog sources for Vita Wave include **Natural Lifestyle Supplies** and **N.E.E.D.S.**

To avoid the use of permanents all together, you might consider a hairstyle that is able to work attractively with your hair's own innate texture and curling ability. To find an appropriate style, look in hairstyle booklets, guides, magazines, and books—or consult with a professional hairstylist.

SHAMPOOS AND RINSES

Many sensitive persons have trouble finding a tolerable shampoo. This can be a serious concern because hair will retain the odor of whatever you put on it for some time. Fortunately, some individuals have found that all-natural, unscented Castile soaps can often work well as shampoos. Dr. Erlander's Jubilee Castile Soap (**Dr. Erlander's Natural Products**) is one of several liquid shampoos you may wish to try. It can be purchased directly from the company. Sirena Fresh Coconut (**Tropical Soap Co.**) is a Castile bar soap which also works well on hair. It's often handled by local health-food stores and can be ordered by mail through **Janice Corp.**

By the way, liquid or bar Castile soaps work especially well for fine or thinning hair. With coarse or thick hair, Castile soap oils can sometimes build up. A cleansing rinse of apple-cider vinegar or lemon juice mixed with water should help solve this, but these rinses will leave their characteristic smells on your hair. If you are bothered by these odors or have allergies to apples or lemons, it may be best to avoid them.

Of course, there are usually a number of all-natural shampoos available at most local health-food stores, drugstores, and cosmetic departments. While some contain sea kelp, vitamins, and/or proteins which have minimal odor, the majority of these shampoos are made with herbs, spices, and natural scents. You might have to experiment with these types of shampoos to see if one or more will be appropriate for you.

There are also a few unscented alternative shampoos available that contain few ingredients other than a mild synthetic *surfactant* (natural or synthetic) and water (see *Soaps versus Detergents* in *Chapter 7: Cleaning* for more on surfactants). Certain brands of these have proven to be quite tolerable for some sensitive people. One that lathers well, despite its inexpensive price, is Rich & Radiant (**Granny's Old Fashioned Products**). This product comes in a range of package sizes. Granny's also makes a simple conditioning rinse, Soft 'N Silky, that you may want to try. Both products are commonly available in health-food stores. Two mail-order sources for them are **The Living Source** and **N.E.E.D.S.**

Still another shampoo you might consider is a concentrated simple-formula product available from **N.E.E.D.S.** under its label. This particular shampoo is unscented and coconut-oil free. SafeChoice Satin Touch (**American Formulating and Manufacturing**) is yet another unscented synthetic-surfactant shampoo option. It's handled by **The Living Source** and other catalogs.

One product that you may find quite acceptable as a shampoo is Green (**Neo-Life Products of America, Inc.**). This item is actually promoted as a mild personal cleaner, but it can work on hair as well. Green is made with sea kelp and has often been recommended for sensitive individuals. It can be mail-ordered from **The American Environmental Health Foundation, Inc.**

Other unscented shampoos can be found among hypoallergenic cosmetic lines in drug and department stores. Although perfumes may not have been added to these products, they can contain other ingredients that sensitive persons may find bothersome. Only by testing will you know whether certain hypoallergenic shampoos will be acceptable for you (see *Testing* in *Chapter 1: Getting Started*). For a good selection of often-well-tolerated shampoos, rinses, and conditioners, check out **The Living Source, N.E.E.D.S.** and **Natural Lifestyle Supplies** catalogs.

You can also create your own shampoo at home. One old-fashioned hair cleaning method is to simply rub a beaten egg vigorously into your hair and scalp. (The egg can also be first beaten with one to two cups of cool water before applying.) A final rinse with a dilute lemon juice/water solution is suggested. For dry shampooing, you can vigorously rub $1/2$ cup cornmeal or oat flour into your hair and scalp—then, brush it out. You'll probably find that doing this outdoors makes clean-up afterwards much easier.

SHAVING CREAMS

To avoid shaving-cream intolerance, you might consider using only an electric shaver. However, if you just don't like using an electric shaver, other options available may be acceptable.

One national brand of unscented shaving cream is Colgate Fragrance Free (**Colgate-Palmolive Co.**) It's sold through most grocery stores and pharmacies. However, because this product contains a number of synthetic ingredients, it may be intolerable for certain sensitive individuals. For those of you who want all-natural ingredients, Tom's of Maine Natural Shaving Cream (**Tom's of Maine**) may be a better choice. However, this product does not come in an unscented formula; it's marketed only with added mint or honeysuckle. Generally, Tom's Shaving Cream is handled by local health-food stores. You can also order it from **Natural Lifestyle Supplies**, which handles other shaving products you may be interested in. The Body Shop Shaving Cream (**The Body Shop by Mail**) is another all-natural, but scented, product. It's actually made with a coconut-oil base with added sandalwood fragrance, and is sold through its catalog, in both tubes and jars.

Shaving cream substitutes that are less effective but unscented and 100%-natural can be made at home. For example, you can create a thick lather using a tolerable, natural unscented soap, or you can dissolve 4 tablespoons of baking soda in 1 pint hot water and apply.

For those who like using a shaving brush, natural badger-hair shaving brushes are still available. Two mail-order sources are **The Vermont Country Store** and **The Body Shop by Mail**. After each use, however, you'll need to rinse it thoroughly. Then, if possible, allow the shaving brush to hang-dry by placing the handle in a shaving brush stand. This will greatly prolong the life of your brush's bristles.

SOAPS

A number of soaps are marketed today that sensitive people generally find tolerable. One of the most common is Castile soap. Castile soap was originally made from olive oil in Castile, Spain. Today, Castile soaps are made everywhere and the definition has been expanded to include natural soaps made with a combination of vegetable oils. You'll find that Castile soaps are sold in two basic forms: liquid and bar.

Liquid Castile soaps are usually sold in health-food stores and through alternative health catalogs. Some of these liquid formulas have almond, mint, or other natural scents added. Dr. Erlander's Jubilee Castile Soap (**Dr. Erlander's**

Natural Products) is one popular unscented liquid Castile soap you can order directly. Another low-odor liquid Castile soap is Baby-Liquid Castile Soap (**Dr. Bronner**), commonly found in health-food stores. However, if you are unable to locate it, you can order it directly from the company.

Unlike liquid Castile soaps, Castile bar soaps are often made with palm or coconut oils, whose solid fats permit hardening. Other vegetable oils may be included as well. One 100% coconut-oil bar soap that is particularly good is Sirena Fresh Coconut (**Tropical Soap Co.**). It contains no perfume, deodorant, coloring, animal fat, or synthetic additives of any kind. It's also reasonably priced. You can usually purchase Sirena Fresh Coconut at some of your local pharmacies and health-food stores. In addition, **Janice Corp.** is a mail-order source.

Also, you might consider using natural soaps containing oatmeal or vitamins. Simmons Pure Unscented Oatmeal Soap (**Simmons Pure Soaps**), available from **Simmons Handcrafts**, is one worth trying. Sirena Miracle E (**Tropical Soap Co.**) is an unscented, coconut bar soap enriched with vitamin E. You may find it's especially helpful for moisturizing dry skin. Sirena Miracle E is sold in some local pharmacies and health-food stores, and can be ordered from **Janice Corp**.

Other soaps you may want to try are those made primarily of unscented glycerin. Glycerin (also known as glycerol) is a sweet, syrupy substance specially derived from certain fats and oils. While glycerin soap is available in liquid form, more commonly it's sold as translucent orange-brown bars. Although mild, glycerin bar soaps have a major drawback: They tend to dissolve quickly. Thus, after using a bar, be sure to set it in a soap dish to permit it to air-dry. Otherwise, the bar will turn into gooey glop. Unfortunately, some of the liquid and bar varieties of Castile soap tend to be relatively expensive. If you'd like to try glycerin soap, you'll find that most local drugstores generally sell one or more brands. One very popular unscented Castile soap is Neutrogena (**Neutrogena Corporation**).

Anymore, you'll find that most local health-food stores carry a large selection of alternative soaps—far more than can be mentioned here. Catalogs such as **The Living Source** and **Natural Lifestyle Suppliers** also have quite a variety from which to choose. If you want to experiment with several types, you might consider ordering the Soap Sampler from **Janice Corp.**, containing several different brands of alternative bar soaps.

By the way, because alternative soaps are often costly, you might want to try this conservation tip when using flat bars of the same brand. When an old bar is nearly used up, you simply wet both it and the new replacement bar with water. Then rub them together back to back to create a small amount of lather, press the two bars firmly together, and set them aside until they're dry. This will bond both the bars together, creating a single slightly-larger one— so you won't have any wasted slivers.

Besides soap, other options are available to wash your skin. One alternative is Green (**Neo-Life Products of America, Inc.**), a mild cleaner often recommended for sensitive individuals. The **American Environmental Health Foundation, Inc.** is one mail-order source. For those of you with extremely dry skin who can't use any soaps or cleaners, try applying olive oil or some other well-tolerated oil to your skin. Then, gently remove the oil with cotton balls or gauze. You may want to follow this procedure with a facial scrub. Finally, you'll need to rinse your skin with clear water and pat it dry.

For especially ground-in grime, sprinkle baking soda on a wash cloth and gently rub soiled skin. Scrubbing with Bon Ami Cleaning Bar (**Faultless Starch/ Bon Ami Company**)—containing unscented soap and ground feldspar—also works well. It's handled by some health-food stores and grocery stores. One mail-order source is **The Living Source**.

(For more on soaps, see also *Soaps* in *Chapter 7: Cleaning*.)

SUNSCREENS AND SUNBLOCKS

Sunscreens have the ability to protect your skin from cancer-causing sun rays. However, you may not know that skin that has been repeatedly treated with sunscreen solutions apparently produces lower quantities of vitamin D—an essential vitamin needed by the human body. There is also the concern that people using sunscreens may overestimate the protective capacities of these products and, therefore, unknowingly overexpose themselves to sunlight. For these and other reasons, one of the best defenses against ultraviolet (UV) radiation is to simply limit the amount of time you spend in the sun. Above all, the most important times to avoid direct sunlight are between 11 AM and 2 PM. When you are outdoors, a good way to avoid sun rays is to wear a large brimmed hat and other protective clothing.

If you feel you must use a sunscreen, choose one that does the job effectively. Sunscreens (and sunblocks) are rated according to their sun protection factor (SPF). The higher the SPF number, the greater the protection. Ratings of 2 to 15 are typical for sunscreens. (Sunblocks have much higher ratings.) Therefore, try to use a product with a 10 SPF or above—especially if you have fairer skin. By the way, many, if not most, sunscreens and sunblocks are made with para-aminobenzoic acid (PABA) as their active ingredient, although other substances will also block UV rays.

One low-odor, sun-protecting product you might consider is SkinSaving Sunblock (Lily of the Desert). It comes in a 3-fluid ounce tube and contains no PABA. It is also nongreasy and waterproof. This brand has a very high SPF of 40. It's available in some drug- and health-food stores. You may also want to try the unscented, hypoallergenic brands of sunscreens and sunblocks found in some pharmacies, or organic products sold in some alternative grocery and health-food stores.

Interestingly, an application of sesame-seed oil to your skin can act as a simple sun protector, reputedly screening out some 30% of the sun's UV rays.

TONING MASKS

All-natural homemade facial masks are easy to make. A simple one is made with a raw egg white, or the egg white can be mixed with a drop or two of olive oil. (The egg white can be whipped if desired.) After applying it to your skin, leave the mask on for around 30 minutes, then rinse it off with warm water.

Another toning mask you might try is uncooked rolled oats combined with enough honey to make the mixture sticky. After you've mixed it, pat the concoction on your face and leave it on for 20–30 minutes. (Lying down is best during this time.) Then, you'll want to rinse it off with warm water. This mask is admittedly a bit messy, but it can be very beneficial to your skin.

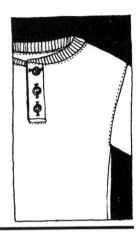

CHAPTER 3
CLOTHING

Because clothing is continually in direct contact with your skin, you'll want to consciously choose garments that contribute to your health and well-being—not items that compromise it. This chapter gives you the information you need to do that.

NATURAL FIBERS

Many people have learned that untreated natural-fiber clothing offers a number of benefits they simply can't get from synthetic alternatives. For example, natural-fiber garments actually "breathe," thus allowing the wearer's perspiration to readily evaporate. Natural fibers are also biodegradable and made from renewable resources. In addition, the appearance and feel of natural-fiber clothing is often more visually and tactually pleasing than with synthetic items.

Very importantly, untreated natural-fiber clothing can't outgas low-level, potentially bothersome odors often associated with synthetic clothing. Finally, some sensitive people have noticed that odors from tobacco smoke and perfume can often be more easily removed from natural-fiber items than from those made of most synthetic fibers—either by laundering or airing.

NATURAL-PLANT FIBERS

Natural plant fibers include cotton, ramie, linen, jute, and hemp. These particular fibers are used to create the majority of the natural-fiber garments currently available. To help you become more knowledgeable about these materials, the sections below provide background information on cultivation, milling, fiber traits, etc. The most complete descriptions are for cotton—perhaps the most popular fabric with people concerned about minimizing harmful effects.

COTTON

Although cotton is by far the most popular natural fiber today, few of us realize how many steps (and possible chemical treatments) are involved between planting cotton seeds and purchasing a finished cotton garment. Unfortunately, many of these steps can make some cotton garments intolerable for sensitive persons.

Cotton Cultivation

Because cotton is so widely used, it has been called the "universal fiber." Cotton is popular for several reasons: It is widely cultivated, processing and milling are relatively easy, and the cotton fibers themselves are soft, fairly strong, and can be manipulated in a variety of ways. Unlike most other natural fibers—which have rather limited uses—cotton fibers can be woven, knit, made into lace, tufted (chenille is an example of tufting), and formed into nonwoven fabrics with chemical resins. Cotton also takes dyes, soil resistance, fire retardance, and other chemical treatments well. Finally, most cotton items are easy to clean.

Cotton is actually a subtropical plant of the mallow family. It has been cultivated for thousands of years in Egypt, Asia, and South America. Today, it's grown in warm climates around the world, wherever its soil and moisture needs can be met. While wild cotton is a perennial, as a cultivated crop it's planted annually. As cotton plants mature, they eventually grow three to six feet tall. The cotton fibers appear as soft, fluffy "hair" (lint) surrounding cotton seeds within the pods (bolls). Each fiber is a long, cylindrical single cell.

There are three main commercial cotton species, each with a number of varieties. Of all the cotton types grown, the finest (such as Pima) produce the longest, strongest, and silkiest fibers. By the way, all cotton varieties, besides having longish cotton fibers, have very short, stout fibers known as *linters*. Linters are considered the very lowest quality of cotton. However, they're commonly used as stuffing in upholstery and mattresses, as well as raw material in cotton-content papers.

Between the planting of cotton seeds and finished fabric, many steps abound. First, the seeds are planted in the spring. During the growing season, large amounts of fertilizer and pesticide are usually applied to the fields. The pesticides are targeted against boll weevils and pink boll worms. Unfortunately, because weevils are so persistent, newer and deadlier chemicals continue to be used against them. Incidentally, some once-popular pesticides are no longer used because of health concerns associated with them or because weevils have become resistant to them. Actually, the now-problematic pink boll worm only became a serious pest when potent anti-weevil pesticides killed the insects that naturally kept pink boll worm numbers in check. Because of the potential for serious negative health effects with most chemical pesticides, synthetic pheromones that mimic female insect sex-attractant chemicals are beginning to be used in some areas as an alternative pest-control method. However, chemical attack remains the most popular approach.

When the cotton plants are mature, their bolls burst open. After the cotton fibers air-dry, they then become ready for harvesting. In the U.S.—and in other countries harvesting cotton mechanically—it's common practice to spray chemical defoliants on the plants before the picking equipment goes into the fields. Defoliants cause the leaves to wither and fall off, leaving only the bolls on the stems. Herbicide applications or flame jets may then also be used to kill surrounding weeds. Once the cotton fibers are finally harvested, they're further dried. Then they're cleaned of debris and seeds by gins. The last pre-milling step is to compress the cotton into bales.

Typical Cotton-Mill Processing

At the mills, cotton bales are transformed into rolls of flat batting (laps). Carding machines then align the fibers within these laps. As a result, the cotton takes on the appearance of rope-like strands, known as *slivers*. To produce *combed cotton*, the slivers go on to mechanical combers to further straighten and align the fibers. Finally, the slivers are sent to spinner machines to be transformed into yarn or thread.

In cotton cloth manufacturing, yarns or threads are woven by mechanical looms. The fabric produced is termed *raw, gray cloth*, or *greige* at this stage. The cloth then may undergo quite a few treatments before it's considered done. For example, it may be *kier boiled*—to further clean it and remove any natural plant waxes. The cloth may also be bleached (usually with chlorine) to whiten it. In addition, it may be *mercerized* (a process using a caustic soda solution) to add luster, strength, and dyeability.

After these treatments, the fabric is then generally *tentered* (stretched into proper proportions) and sheared to remove any surface nubs. At this point, most cotton cloth is dyed by a process called *piece dyeing*—the simplest and cheapest method to of dyeing. (By the way, *yarn dyed* means that the cotton threads or yarn had been dyed just prior to weaving. Had the dyeing occurred still earlier—when the cotton was still in raw fibers—it would have been termed *stock dyed*.) Today, the majority of dyes are made of synthetically derived ingredients.

However, dyes are not the only synthetic chemicals usually applied to cotton cloth. In fact, most of the fabric now produced undergoes a series of additional treatments. These are designed to add wrinkle-resistance, soil-resistance, flame-resistance, mildew-resistance, rot-resistance, and/or water-repellence. The chemicals used for these often include formaldehyde (see *Formaldehyde* in *Chapter 9: Indoor Air*) and some other potentially bothersome compounds.

Alternative Cotton and Cotton Processing

Not surprisingly perhaps, some consumers are demanding cotton clothing made with fewer chemicals—or no chemicals at all. To cater to this market, some specialty growers are now raising *certified organic cotton*. Certification is usually made by state agencies enforcing strict regulations in order for crops to be legally classified as organic. Interestingly, a few growers are even producing organically grown cotton with naturally occurring pastel shades of color. One popular brand name of such cotton is Foxfibre.

A relatively new trend in the cotton industry is the manufacture of *green cotton*. In this case, *green* doesn't refer to the color of the cotton or mean the cotton has been organically raised. Instead, green cotton is commonly defined as cotton fabric that has gone through processing and manufacturing without chemical treatments. Therefore, green cotton items are unbleached, undyed, and have no added formaldehyde. However, they were made with cotton that was chemically treated during cultivation.

You should also be aware that some cotton fabric is described as *unbleached*. This is cotton in its natural beige color. Cotton labeled unbleached may or may not have undergone other chemical treatments. On the other hand, *non-permanent press cotton* simply indicates that no wrinkle-resisting treatments were applied. (A formaldehyde-resin application can be used as a wrinkle-resistance treatment.)

Cotton Garments

Of all the natural fibers, cotton is undoubtedly the most affordable and easiest to find in clothing. A real plus is that most 100%-cotton garments can be machine or hand-washed as well as machine- or line-dried. However, not all clothing made of 100% cotton can be laundered safely at home. Some specialty cotton items may come with a label recommending "dry-clean only." This is likely to be especially true for lined items, tailored pieces, or garments with embellishments.

If you plan to wash your cotton clothing at home, remember to be careful. Cotton has the capacity to shrink, sometimes a great deal. To minimize shrinkage, follow the care-instructions on labels explicitly (see *How Much Shrinkage Should be Expected?* below).

By the way, for those people who want washable, untreated-cotton garments but just don't like ironing, consider buying textured cottons. Deva cloth is one such fabric. It has a permanent pebble-like surface. Deva cloth is sold by **Deva Lifewear**—both as yardage and in finished clothing. Other minimal-care cotton options include gauze, voile, and seersucker fabrics. In addition, most cotton corduroys, knits (jersey and interlock, for example), and flannels can be easily smoothed by hand while they're still warm just out of the dryer.

LINEN

Linen cloth has a coarse, somewhat lustrous, nubby texture that is visually very appealing. Linen is a sturdier, cooler fabric than cotton and is relatively resistant to damage from sunlight. It also tends to soil less easily than cotton. However, untreated linen cloth tends to wrinkle easily.

Linen fabric actually has been used since ancient times. In fact, in medieval Europe linen was the most commonly used plant-derived fiber. However, newer methods of increasing production were few and far between as compared to cotton. When the cotton gin was invented, the manufacture of linen products plummeted.

The actual linen fibers come from the stems of fiber-flax plants. (There are also oil-flax plants that produce linseed oil.) Flax was originally cultivated around the Mediterranean Sea and in southern Asia. Today, it's grown around the world in temperate climates. Linen from Belgium is now considered to be among the finest linen cloth available.

In the fields, flax plants grow from one to four feet tall. The mature plants are eventually harvested after their stems have yellowed. Traditionally, the cut stalks are allowed to *ret*: a planned decomposing process in which the stems are immersed in a watery solution that causes woody tissues and plant gums to rot. Afterwards, the flax fibers are able to be pulled apart from most of the decayed by-products. Then comes *scutching*, a scraping procedure which removes any remaining woody plant portions. Next, the flax fibers are combed, cleaned, and readied for spinning. The final steps are dyeing and weaving.

As was mentioned, linen was once used extensively for clothing, as well as upholstery, draperies, tablecloths, and bedding (hence, the still-popular terms—*table linens* and *bed linens*). However, actual linen fabric is no longer commonly used in the manufacture of any of these. In fact, linen is now generally considered a luxury fiber. Therefore, most of the 100%-linen garments today are very expensive suits, dresses, and imported handkerchiefs. However, linen is being used more frequently in fabric blends, such as linen/cotton. Although some linen articles may be safely laundered at home, manufacturers often recommend dry cleaning (see *Is Dry Cleaning a Problem?* below). To ensure that you clean your linen items correctly, make sure to follow cleaning instructions on labels carefully.

RAMIE

Ramie is a soft, lustrous, light to mediumweight fiber that somewhat resembles linen. Ramie fibers are relatively strong, but lack elasticity. Therefore, ramie cloth can wear or abrade fairly easily.

Ramie fibers actually come from the inner stems of certain perennial Asian plants in the nettle family. These plants are bushy and fairly tall—up to six feet high. They are cultivated mostly in semitropical areas of the Far East, although some is now grown in the southern U.S. When they're mature, ramie stalks are either cut and stripped of their fibers by hand, or machine-harvested and stripped. No matter how they're separated from the surrounding bark, the fibers are next cleaned and readied for spinning. At this point, ramie fibers are sometimes called *China grass*. Dyeing usually follows—and ramie takes dyes very well. Finally, the fibers are ready for weaving.

One hundred percent ramie fabric (also known as *grass cloth*) isn't commonly made anymore. (Today, ramie is usually blended with cotton or other fibers.) When you do find it, its price range is generally between that of cotton and linen. Many items made of or with ramie can be hand-washed, though certainly not all. Often, ramie articles need to be dried flat. This is especially true for knit items. To be sure, you'll need to read the manufacturer's tags carefully. Interestingly, ramie shrinks very little.

JUTE

Jute is one of the lowest-cost natural fibers. Surprisingly, after cotton, it's the most-used plant fiber in the world. Unfortunately, it's also one of the weakest and tends to fall apart if exposed to prolonged moisture. Jute is actually a name that is applied to two tall annual plants of the Asiatic linden family. Almost all jute is grown in hot and humid areas of India and Bangladesh. Because its cultivation has not yet been mechanized, intense hand labor is usually required.

Jute plants grow to a height of 2–12 feet. After the mature plants have been cut, they're soaked in running water for several days to rot the outer-bark and loosen the inner jute fibers—a type of *retting* process (see *Linen* above). Afterwards, the stems are dried. Then comes *scutching:* hand-kneading and crushing that frees the fibers. Interestingly, a tremendous number of long fibers can be removed from just a single stalk. Next, the fibers are ready for spinning—and possibly bleaching and dyeing. However, most jute does not take bleach or dye particularly well. (When jute is dyed, the colors may be somewhat harsh-looking.) Finally comes weaving.

The finer grades of jute are similar to linen in appearance. They're sometimes used in wearing apparel, including fine suits. Lesser grades are sometimes used in shoes, handbags, tote bags, and carpet backing. Recently, area rugs made of jute have been marketed. Burlap is a type of cheap, coarsely woven jute fabric. To clean any jute item successfully, follow the manufacturer's directions closely.

HEMP

Recently, a few hemp clothing articles have become available in the U.S. Some international-aid groups have been encouraging hemp cultivation in poor countries to replace coca plant production. Actually, hemp is a generic term that is often applied to a group of unrelated plants. The only common trait these various plants have is that fibers are derived from their stalks. However, there is a *true* hemp plant: *Cannabis sativa* or cannabis.

In cultivation, mature hemp plants are cut and left on the ground to *ret.* (This is a rotting process of the unwanted plant materials.) Once the fibers are loosened and freed from the woody debris, they and then combed. This further cleans and aligns the individual fibers. At this point, the hemp fibers are ready to be spun into thread or yarn. The final steps involve dyeing and weaving.

Because there are several possible plants from which hemp fibers can be derived, it's impossible to describe the qualities of any particular hemp-made garment without knowing the original source. However, it can be said that true hemp (cannabis) sweaters are similar in appearance and feel to those of cotton. Because garment-grade hemp production is still low, prices are relatively high. For proper cleaning instructions, you'll need to read the information provided on manufacturers' tags.

NATURAL ANIMAL FIBERS

Besides natural plant fibers, of course important fiber sources are derived from animals. These include silk and several varieties of wool.

SILK

Silk is perhaps one of the world's most luxurious fabrics. It has always been prized for its naturally opulent look and feel, as well as its ability to take dyes. (No natural fiber dyes as well as silk.) However, despite its lightweight and fragile appearance, silk is extremely strong—as strong as synthetic nylon. Woven silk also breathes. In fact, it's the coolest fabric to wear in hot climates. Yet, woven silk has tremendous insulating properties; it's sometimes used in thermal underwear and thermal liners for gloves, etc. In addition, silk can absorb up to 30% of its weight in moisture and still not feel damp to the touch. If all that were not enough, silk is naturally heat-resistant—it'll burn only when a flame comes directly in contact with it.

The following sections will explain how this remarkable fiber is derived and ultimately woven into garments.

Sericulture and Silk Processing

Silk comes from the unraveling of cocoons spun by domesticated silk moth caterpillars, also known as silk worms (*Bombyx mori*). Silk-moth cultivation (*sericulture*) actually began thousands of years ago in China. At that time, the source of silk, and how it was produced, were state secrets; revealing information on this was punishable by death. Eventually, however, Byzantine emissaries learned the truth and smuggled silkworm eggs out of China. As a result, sericulture eventually spread to other countries.

In sericulture, silk moths are confined in order to lay harvestable eggs. The eggs then hatch into hungry caterpillars. After eating mulberry leaves (their only food) for about five weeks, the caterpillars crawl into specially built frames to spin their cocoons. Interestingly, each caterpillar produces not one but two slender filaments at once. These almost immediately become a single filament—bonded together by a sticky secretion known as *sericin*. The sericin also is responsible for gluing the cocoon together as it's being created by the silk worm.

Once the cocoons are completely spun, they're subjected to high heat that kills the insects inside without damaging the cocoons. The cocoons are then removed from the frames and bathed in hot water. This dissolves the sericin so that the cocoons can be unreeled.

Each cocoon actually produces a single filament from eight hundred to twelve hundred yards long. However, because it's so delicate and fine, several cocoons are unreeled at the same time and combined to create a single, stronger thread. The small amount of sericin remaining on the individual filaments holds this larger, united thread permanently together. At this point, the reeled silk thread is known as *raw silk*.

Other procedures may follow, such as *throwing* (in which several of the larger threads are twisted together), a *weight treatment* (in which oil or some other substance is added to the threads, although this is now less commonly done), dyeing, and/or steaming (to add luster). Finally, the processed silk is ready for weaving or knitting.

Silk Garments

Because of its sheen, softness, strength, and other properties, silk was, until fairly recently, popularly used despite its relatively high cost. However after World War II, less-expensive rayon, nylon, polyester, and other synthetic substitutes just about replaced silk in all its previous uses. However, in the last few years, silk production has increased enormously—and prices have come down substantially. As a result, today silk items are not only more commonly seen, they tend to be much more affordable.

Many people shy away from purchasing silk items because they're unfamiliar with, and somewhat afraid of, cleaning them. Actually, some silk articles can be safely cared for at home. For example, certain unlined sand-washed, raw, or noile silks are hand-washable. A few such pieces may sometimes even be laundered in the washing machine on a short, gentle cycle. After laundering, most washable silk items should be laid flat. However, to be safe, unless manufacturers' tags say otherwise, all silk items should probably be dry cleaned only. Otherwise, they could shrink or lose their shape.

WOOL

By far, wool is the most widely used animal fiber—and always has been. As you, no doubt, already know, wool has many excellent properties. For example, it can be easily spun into yarn or formed into matted felt. Of great importance is wool's tremendous ability to insulate. In fact, even when it's wet (and wool can absorb a lot of moisture), it still provides warmth to the person wearing it. Wool also is naturally attractive looking and also takes dyes well. In addition, wool is naturally fire-resistant and *resilient* (keeps its bounce or loft).

To help you learn more about this natural fiber, this section will provide information on different aspects of wool and wool production.

Typical Wool Production

Wool is often defined as the curly fleece of sheep and lambs. Interestingly, it has been estimated there are around 450 different domesticated wool-bearing sheep breeds. Each of these produces wool with its own particular characteristics. By the way, the term wool also refers to the fleece of alpacas, llamas, Kashmir goats (*cashmere*), angora goats (*mohair*), camels, etc.

It took herders centuries of selective breeding to produce the types of coats seen on domesticated sheep today: those with wool and very little hair. Wool is made of the same substance as hair—*keratin*—but wool fibers are constructed much differently. Hair is composed of aligned, adjacent cells. On the other hand, the cells that make up wool filaments are crimped and overlapped. Because wool's cells are shingle-like, they're actually able to enmesh with one another or mat (*felting*). In addition, because the filaments are crimped, they're naturally elastic. It should also be noted that raw sheep's wool is waterproof. This is due to the lanolin or *sheep grease* which is secreted by certain sweat glands in the sheep's skin and absorbed by the wool fibers themselves.

Unfortunately, domesticated sheep are often subjected to certain chemical treatments to minimize insect infestations. These treatments, known as *sheep dips*, generally involve leading the animals through tanks or pits filled with special solutions. Then, in early spring, just before the winter coats naturally shed, the fleeces are removed. While most wool is still removed by shearing, some ranchers are now using a hormone injection which allows the entire coat to be peeled off. After the fleece has been removed, the raw wool is graded. The best wool has the slenderest and longest filaments, the whitest color, and the thickest density. *Merino wool* is considered one of the finer grades. The lowest grade is *carpet wool* which often contains a fair quantity of hair fibers.

Typical Wool-Mill Processing

At mills, the raw wool is cleaned and possibly combed (to align the wool fibers). It's then commonly spun into thread or yarn, or made into felt. However, processing may also include bleaching, dyeing, and/or treatments to provide insect resistance, among others.

Actually, there are two major types of wool thread and yarn. *Worsted wool* thread consists of only combed, long fibers that have been spun together. Worsted wool thread is generally of very fine quality—able to be woven into smooth fabrics such as suits or even hosiery. On the other hand, *woolen processed* yarn uses no special combing. It consists of spun long and short fibers or simply just short fibers. The resulting yarn is coarser than worsted wool thread. It's often used to make blankets or bulkier, tweedy fabrics. By the way, if the wool is to be felted, it's soaked in a soapy water solution, rolled, and then pressed. Wool felt is commonly used to make hats.

Alternative Wools and Wool Processing

While most sheep fleeces are white, some wool-bearing animals are purposely bred for their gray, brown, tan, black, or mottled coats. Such wool is naturally colored and undergoes no bleaching or dyeing treatments. Icelandic sheep's wool items, as well as some Central- and South-American llama-wool articles, are often created using naturally colored wool.

There are also a few specialty sheep raisers who don't subject their animals or their sheared wool to synthetic chemicals. Wool of this type is often termed *organic wool*. When wool is said to be *untreated*, it generally means it has not been bleached, dyed, or undergone mothproofing treatments. In addition, some untreated wool may also never have had sheep-dipping treatments. However, because at this time there are no clearly accepted definition standards (including legal) for either organic or untreated wool, what these terms exactly mean on labels can be unclear.

Wool Clothing

Today, 100%-wool clothing is generally fairly expensive and relatively rare, compared to before World War II. Far more common now, wool is blended with less costly natural and/or synthetic fibers. Because wool can cause skin irritation, garments such as wool or wool-blend skirts and pants are usually lined with another less irritating fabric.

Incidentally, *virgin wool* means that the wool in your garment (or other wool items) has never been used in a previous manufacturing process. On the other hand, the term *shoddy* applies to reused wool—wool that was previously spun, knitted, or felted. Shoddy wool is sometimes added by manufacturers to increase fabric strength, especially in knits.

As you probably know, most wool items require special care—to both clean and store. This is because of wool's tremendous capacity to shrink, as well as its innate attractiveness to destructive clothing moths (see *How Much Shrinkage should be Expected?* below, and *Clothing Moths* in *Chapter 8: Housekeeping*). While some wool clothing items can be hand-washed and dried flat at home, most have manufacturers' tags recommending that they be dry-cleaned. Unfortunately, this not only means that dry-cleaning solvent odors will be in your newly cleaned wool items, but perhaps added moth-preventing chemicals as well. In fact, if you don't want moth-prevention treatments done to your woolens, you'll want to clearly specify this to your dry cleaner when you take them to be cleaned (see *Is Dry Cleaning a Problem?* below).

You should be aware though, that there are some garments made of *boiled wool* that can be washed at home, even in a washing machine, without ever shrinking them. This is possible because of the unique manner in which such articles are made. You see, to create boiled wool clothing, items are purposely produced oversized. Then they're boiled in water to shrink them to their final correct proportions. The resulting clothing is sturdy, dense, and virtually incapable of further shrinkage. However, boiled wool, like other types of wool, still needs to be protected from clothing moths.

LEATHER AND FUR

Leather and fur are more two natural animal materials used in clothing—but they're not fibers. Despite increasing concerns for animal rights, they still remain popular today, especially leather.

LEATHER

Leather is a natural material which typically undergoes many chemical treatments to process it and later maintain it. Not surprisingly, leather, especially new leather, can be bothersome to sensitive people.

LEATHER TYPES

By definition, leather is the tanned skin of any animal. Some popular leather choices include cow, calf, pig, sheep, lamb, goat (kidskin), snake, lizard, alligator, deer, and eel. When you purchase leather, there are several terms with which you'll want to become familiar to better help you know exactly what you are buying. Perhaps first, you should know that some thin leathers are used intact; these are said to be *unsplit*. However, many times thick hides, such as those from cattle, have several layers cut or *split* from them. *Full-grain* refers to leather that has the natural skin texture (*grain*), whether from an unsplit or split hide. *Top-grain* is the uppermost layer of a split hide. Top-grain is considered the best grade of split leather because it's the only one that is full-grain. *Genuine leather* simply means that it's not a synthetic product or a composite-leather material. Many times it suggests that the leather is from a split hide, but it's not top-grain.

On the other hand, *bonded-leather* is a composite leather material; it's actually made of finely shredded leather scraps held together with glue. Bonded-leather can often be stiff and is generally less durable than genuine leathers. Products made of bonded-leather are usually inexpensive, but they can be very odorous because of the adhesives used to make them. Therefore as a rule, bonded-leather should be avoided by sensitive people.

LEATHER PROCESSING

Leather can be *tanned* in a number of ways. Tanning is actually any treatment that transforms animal skins or hides into pliable, long-lasting forms. Occasionally, deerskin and other game hides are tanned using animal brains or other natural animal substances. A few leathers are also tanned using natural oils. Once a common natural tanning method, oak bark solutions (containing active *plant tannins*) are still sometimes used. However, most of today's commercial tanning processes use synthetic chemical solutions.

As you well know, the surfaces of many leathers are textured into a variety of distinctive forms. One favorite process to do this is with *embossing*, a relatively inexpensive stamping procedure. Embossing is often done on lower-costing leathers to mimic higher-priced or endangered animal leathers. To create *suede*, the inner sides of hides (sides that don't have grain) are mechanically rubbed or brushed to produce a velvety feel.

Also, colors (often synthetic) are routinely added to leather. This can be accomplished through *surface-dyeing* (when only the topside of a piece of leather receives dye), hand painting, or *vat-dyeing*. In vat-dyeing, whole hides are soaked in dye-filled tanks. Because the color completely saturates the leather, nicks, scratches, and wear are less noticeable on items dyed in this way.

LEATHER GARMENTS, FOOTWEAR, AND ACCESSORIES

As was mentioned earlier, new leather articles are often intolerable for sensitive individuals. This is likely due to a combination of factors: the natural odor of the leather itself and the processing chemicals used in tanning, texturing, and/or coloring. Of course, new genuine-leather items will lose most of their odor over time. However, it wouldn't be unusual for it to take up to two years of airing before some new leather items are tolerable for certain very sensitive individuals. Many times, finding a suitable site for this extended aging process to take place can be difficult. Therefore, it's wise to choose leather items carefully and well in advance of when they'll actually be needed.

In caring for your leather goods, more problems with intolerance can arise. One major reason is that leather clothing must usually be professionally cleaned using special leather-cleaning treatments performed by your dry cleaner. Unfortunately, the odors from the cleaning solutions (commonly solvents and other synthetic compounds) are absorbed by the leather. In any case, airing your newly cleaned items outdoors will help dissipate these bothersome odors. By the way, it should be said that professional leather cleaning can be costly.

Of course, you can usually care for your leather footwear at home. However, most shoe polishes and waterproofing products are made with strong-smelling—often very objectionable—petroleum-based ingredients. You may be interested that **Eco Design** and **Sinan Co.** both offer alternative Tapir German shoe polishes and waterproofing compounds. These natural-ingredient polishes are made with aromatic tree waxes and citrus solvents. However, certain sensitive individuals will likely find the relatively strong odors of these products still too bothersome, even though they are natural. Therefore, it might be a good idea to have a less sensitive person polish or waterproof your shoes or boots for you outdoors. Once your footwear has been treated, let them air outside until the odors are no longer noticeable.

Despite initial intolerability, leather can still be a good choice for many people, especially if the leather items are designed to require little maintenance. (For example, certain medium to medium-dark suede leather requires no polishing, shows little dirt or dust, and can often be simply brushed to clean.) After all, leather articles, including shoes, belts, wallets, handbags, and clothing, are naturally derived, long-lasting, and attractive to look at and touch.

FUR

Fur is soft, attractive, warm, and luxurious. However, there are a variety of negatives associated with it that usually make it less than ideal, especially for sensitive and allergic persons.

FUR TYPES AND PROCESSING

The garment industry defines fur as any hairy animal pelt resistant to shedding. Of course, fur is an ancient material; in fact, it was probably humankind's first clothing. Interestingly, it wasn't until the Middle Ages that fur was considered prestigious or special. About that time, laws were invoked to restrict commoners from wearing fur, and so it became reserved for the nobility and well-to-do. Today, fur still has those connotations linked to it.

These days, most furs are obtained from captive animals raised on farms, although a number of fur-bearing species are still trapped or hunted in the wild. Probably the most popular fur types are mink, rabbit, fox, squirrel, coyote, raccoon, beaver, lynx, seal, and sable. For temperate and polar-region species, their thick winter coats are known as *prime fur*. Pelts taken at other times of the year from such animals are considered *unprime*.

After a fur-bearing animal is killed, it's skinned. This *raw fur* is sent to *dressing processors*. There the pelts are *dressed* (cleaned and tanned) using a variety of chemical solutions. Afterwards, some furs are left in their natural hue while others are bleached and/or dyed. In some cases, natural dyes are used, but often the dyes are synthetically derived. The actual dyeing process may involve complete immersion (for total coloring), stenciling (to create a pattern), or *tipping*. (*Tipped-fur* has only the very ends of the fur hairs dyed.) After dyeing, furs are ready for shipment to *furriers* (fur clothing-makers) to be made into garments.

FUR GARMENTS AND ACCESSORIES

Although fur apparel is both soft and warm, it's usually expensive to purchase, store, and clean. In addition, fur can be quite odorous when new. This can be due to several factors: the innate smell of the fur itself, the dressing chemicals, the dyes, and/or the added insect-resisting treatments. Such odors can actually remain in fur hairs for long periods of time, despite lengthy airings outdoors. Unfortunately, when furs are worn, they can easily absorb other odors such as perfume and tobacco. In addition, professionally cleaned and/or stored furs will likely absorb more bothersome odors. All these accumulated odors, too, may be difficult to remove. Furthermore, some fur items may begin to shed after only a few years of use. Because of odor and shedding problems, fur items are not suggested for sensitive or allergic persons.

It should also be mentioned, that growing numbers of people today object to anyone involved with the production, sale, or wearing of fur. Such individuals believe, for personal and/or philosophical reasons, that killing any animal simply for its fur is distasteful, cruel, or even immoral. In fact, in certain places in this country, wearing fur can subject the wearer to verbal abuse or worse by outspoken, anti-fur advocates.

NATURAL STUFFINGS

Although many individuals consider natural fibers important in their clothing (as well as their furnishings), they often forget about batting, padding, and loose-fill material. Unlike most synthetic counterparts, natural stuffing allows moisture to evaporate, and because it's made from renewable resources, it's biodegradable.

COTTON STUFFING

Cotton is a fine stuffing material, is relatively inexpensive and washable, and has fairly good loft. However, it has largely been replaced by polyester, which is even cheaper and stays fluffier over time. Unfortunately, most of the cotton loose-fill stuffing and batting that is still available in fabric and craft stores has been bleached and chemically treated. However, organic, unbleached cotton batting is available from **Dona Designs, The Living Source**, and **Nontoxic Environments**.

WOOL STUFFING

Wool stuffing is also an excellent insulating material. Unlike cotton, wool retains heat even when it's wet. It's also naturally resilient and, therefore, keeps it's loft. However, because of wool's higher cost, it's being used less and less as stuffing, though it is being used in some futons and comforters. If you'd like to purchase wool stuffing, loose organic wool is available from **The Noon Family Sheep Farm** and untreated wool batting is handled by **Nontoxic Environments**.

FEATHERS AND DOWN

Although they both have many uses, feathers are less valuable than down. This is because down lacks the *barbicels* (minute hooks) that lock other feather types into stiff, definable shapes. As a result, down is extremely soft and fluffy. It actually has a free-form, three-dimensional configuration that can trap large volumes of air. This trapped air gives down its remarkable capacity to insulate.

Feathers and down are still used as stuffing in some coats, as well as some comforters, pillows, and furniture. White Peking ducks and white domestic geese are the two main feather and down sources. However, these products can be derived from other poultry as well. In the U.S., most feathers and down are actually by-products of poultry packing plants. In such plants, slaughtered birds undergo a series of processing steps leading to a dip in hot resinous wax. This wax is allowed to cool and harden so that it, along with the wax-embedded feathers, can to be pulled off together. The removed feathers are then washed to clean and sterilize them and to remove any natural oils. Drying under high heat further sterilizes the feathers by killing any remaining microbes. The feathers and down are then separated, sorted, and bagged. By the way, some clothing (or bedding or furniture) manufacturers may later add mildew-resisting and/or insect-resisting chemical treatments to the feathers or down.

Certain feather and down items can be safely laundered in the washing machine, if set on a gentle cycle. That is, unless the manufacturers' tags recommend dry cleaning, and the items are small enough to fit in your machine. Because the oils that naturally make feathers and down waterproof have been removed during processing, they will absorb a considerable amount of water when they become wet. Therefore, it's extremely important to dry all feather and down items thoroughly. You should be aware it's possible for outer fabric coverings to feel dry, while the feather or down stuffing inside is still slightly damp. Unfortunately, any remaining moisture could lead to fungal or microbial growth. (This is especially true if the feathers or down are untreated.)

Therefore, an extra cycle through your clothes dryer may be necessary for a truly complete drying. Incidentally, a clean, washable tennis shoe placed in the clothes dryer with a down-stuffed item will really help to fluff the down.

KAPOK

Kapok is the white, silky material surrounding the seeds of the large deciduous kapok tree (silk-cotton tree). At harvest time, each tree produces nearly 100 pounds of fiber. Original to Asia, kapok is now cultivated throughout the tropics. Once it was commonly used as a stuffing material, but it has now generally been replaced by synthetic.

Kapok fibers actually resemble those of cotton, but unlike cotton, kapok fibers can't be spun. However, they are naturally fluffy, buoyant, and waterproof. As a result, kapok is still used in some flotation equipment such as life preservers. Pillows and other items stuffed with kapok are now rare but still occasionally available.

ACCEPTABLE SYNTHETIC FIBERS

In the not-too-distant past, all clothing was made from natural fibers and stuffing, leather, and/or fur. Today, many garments are manufactured with synthetic fibers and stuffing ultimately derived from petroleum, natural gas, or coal. These man-made materials are easy to care for and usually less expensive than their natural counterparts. However, they have a number of drawbacks that many consumers commonly fail to consider. While they may realize that the majority of synthetic fibers are made of non-biodegradable, nonrenewable resources, there are other concerns of which they may not be fully aware.

One such problem is that synthetic clothing generally doesn't breathe (moisture doesn't readily evaporate), so wearers can become unnecessarily hot and sticky. Also, some synthetic fabrics and stuffing emit low levels of potentially bothersome odors. In addition, some sensitive persons have found that certain synthetic clothing seems to retain perfume, tobacco, and other odors, despite repeated cleaning and airing.

NYLON

While many synthetic fibers are bothersome to sensitive individuals, nylon is often an exception. Nylon was actually the first truly synthetic fiber ever produced. In 1935, during an experiment at E.I. DuPont De Nemours and Co., a long, glossy fiber was accidentally created. The material was a *polymer* (a compound created from many small molecules). When the specific molecular composition of the fiber was determined, it was trademarked as Nylon—an arbitrary name that included the *-on* suffix so as to be reminiscent of the man-made fiber rayon. One of the earliest uses for Nylon was as a silk substitute. Eventually, Nylon became the generic term *nylon* after several different nylon types were developed.

Nylon fibers are extremely tough and resilient. Probably because of this, they give off very little synthetic chemical odor. Some sensitive persons have also reported that nylon seems to retain fewer fragrance and tobacco odors after cleaning than most other synthetic fibers. Nylon fabric is also easy to care for—washing either by hand or in a machine. Some nylon garments can even be dried in the dryer, though most must be line-dried. However, nylon does have its drawbacks. It doesn't breathe and it's not biodegradable.

Today, 100% nylon is often used to make hosiery, lingerie, coats, sportswear, and linings. It's also the fabric of some ties, dresses, blouses, and skirts. In addition, nylon is used as the covering material on many boots and athletic shoes. Unfortunately though, most outerwear and shoe manufacturers have begun to routinely add water-repelling chemicals to their nylon products. For example, in the case of nylon winter boots, the boots may have a vinyl, urethane, or other type of synthetic resin coating. Such chemical treatments may make otherwise tolerable nylon clothing intolerable for many sensitive people. Therefore, you'll want to read manufacturers' tags carefully before purchasing any nylon item to see if it's water-repellent or not. By the way, many fabric blends contain a portion of nylon. Nylon is included to add either sheen or strength, or both.

RAYON

Another man-made fiber that is often well-tolerated by sensitive people is rayon. Rayon has a relatively long history. Back at the 1889 Paris Exposition, inventor Count Hilaire de Chardonnet first revealed his *Chardonnet silk* to the public, later known as rayon. By the way, rayon is a coined word with no particular meaning other than an intended allusion to the sun for some reason. At any rate, rayon was originally created as an silk substitute.

Strictly speaking, rayon isn't a synthetic fiber. It's actually reworked *cellulose*, the natural material that makes up the cell walls of plants. To make rayon, very short cellulose fibers are transformed through special processes into long silky strands. Unlike a true synthetic material, the cellulose isn't altered at the molecular level into a new substance; it merely changes its physical shape.

During the actual manufacturing process, wood pulp or other plant material is bleached. Then it's mixed with certain chemical solutions that break down the tough cellulose making up the plant cell walls. (The particular chemicals used depends on the type of rayon being produced.) The cellulose/chemical solution is next filtered, aged, and eventually mixed with a coagulating liquid to cause it to solidify. Finally, rayon threads are extruded by *spinnerets* (devices with tiny holes through which the congealing solution is forced). The hardened threads are then ready for dyeing and weaving.

Rayon is often well-tolerated by many sensitive individuals. Like other natural fibers, it's able to breathe and it's biodegradable. Some items made of rayon can be machine- or hand-washed—especially those in rayon challis. Washable rayon clothing is usually laid flat or hung up to dry. Many rayon garments, however, must be dry-cleaned, so you should check manufacturers' labels carefully.

Rayon has traditionally been used for blouses, dresses, and lingerie because of it's lightweight, lustrous feel, and its excellent dyeing capacity. For many years though, rayon products were often considered to be of poor quality. However, today's better technology has created modern rayons that better retain their shape, have improved appearance, and clean more satisfactorily. As a result, rayon is becoming more widely used again.

SPECIFIC CLOTHING CONCERNS

Natural fiber clothing has many pluses. However, there are several special considerations that should be kept in mind. The following sections will discuss some of these.

HOW NATURAL ARE SOME NATURAL-FIBER CLOTHING?

It's important to point out that just because a fiber or stuffing is naturally derived *does not* mean it hasn't been subjected to chemical treatments; sometimes a lot of them have been used. This fact is sometimes overlooked. Many natural-fiber crops, such as cotton, are commonly grown using huge amounts of fertilizers, herbicides, and pesticides. During the manufacturing process, bleaches, synthetic dyes, as well as wrinkle-resisting, soil-resisting, insect-resisting, mildew-resisting, water-repelling, and/or flame-retarding treatments, among others, using formaldehyde or other petrochemicals may have been applied (see *Formaldehyde* in Chapter 9: *Indoor Air*).

Therefore, be aware of what you are buying, especially if you are a sensitive person. Some of these chemical treatments are difficult, or even impossible, to remove. As a result, those people who are extremely sensitive are strongly advised to only buy natural-fiber garments that have undergone as few chemical treatments as possible; ideally, they should have had none.

HOW MUCH SHRINKAGE SHOULD BE EXPECTED?

A common concern with natural-fiber clothing is shrinkage when it's washed. While ramie is one of the exceptions, most natural fibers will shrink during laundering. Of these, cotton and wool are probably the two fibers of most concern, especially because they make up the majority of most natural-clothing wardrobes and are often cared for at home.

COTTON SHRINKAGE

Most washable cotton clothing can be successfully laundered at home, if proper care is taken. For example, certain garments should be hand-washed rather than put in the machine. As a rule, these would include cotton knit sweaters, delicately woven items, and embellished pieces. After washing, these generally should be dried flat. (See *Hand Laundering* in Chapter 7: *Cleaning.*) Of course, most manufacturers' tags and labels should provide this information.

If cotton items are machine washable, make sure to choose an appropriate water temperature at which to wash them. As a rule, the cooler the temperature, the less shrinkage and the better the color retention. However, cleaning can be less effective in cool or cold water. After machine washing, some cotton clothing should be line-dried or dried flat. Sturdier garments are usually able to hold up well when dried in a warm or hot dryer.

Commonly, with machine washing and drying, cotton clothing may shrink 3–15%, unless it was preshrunk during the manufacturing process. However, how much a particular cotton garment actually shrinks depends on whether it's knit or woven, the looseness of the knit or weave, the type and size of the thread or yarn used, and the temperatures used in both washing and drying. Therefore, for cotton items that are untreated and not preshrunk, it's often a good idea to buy one size larger to account for any shrinkage. For items such as thermal knits and muslin slips, buying two sizes larger is suggested.

WOOL SHRINKAGE

Wool clothing has a well-earned reputation for tremendous shrinkage. This is because the crimped structure of the fibers have the ability to tightly contract. If wool items are not made of boiled-wool (see *Wool* above) and you want to clean them at home, you must usually gently hand-wash them in cool water, then dry them flat (see *Hand Laundering* in *Chapter 7: Cleaning*).

IS DRY CLEANING A PROBLEM?

It takes time and effort to properly clean your natural-fiber clothing at home. In spite of this, very sensitive individuals should probably purchase only those items they can care for themselves, rather than items that will require dry cleaning. This is because dry-cleaning chemicals are often intolerable to sensitive people. Actually, the term *dry-cleaning* is a bit of a misnomer. The process is called *dry* only because water isn't used. Instead, a liquid petroleum-based solvent is the primary cleaning solution. (Sometimes special soaps and detergents are used along with the solvent.)

Professional dry cleaning has been around for about a century and a half. It began in France when kerosene and turpentine were used to cut grease stains and clean clothes. Since that time, carbon tetrachloride, benzine, benzol, naphtha, and even gasoline have been used as dry-cleaning solvents. However, the dangers of fire and explosion from these fluids were so great that less-combustible *chlorinated hydrocarbon solvents* were eventually developed in the 1930s. One of those, *perchloroethylene* (*perc*) is the most common dry-cleaning solvent used today.

When a garment is dry cleaned, it's first sorted by color, fabric, and weight. Then it's placed in a solvent-filled rotating cleaning drum. After a specific period of time, the excess fluid is spun out. Hot air then evaporates the remaining liquid fluid in the clothes. Finally, the garment is ready for pressing and customer pickup. By the way, certain items, such as leather and fur, have their own special cleaning processes.

Unfortunately, when dry-cleaned clothing is brought home, solvent residues often remain on the fabric fibers. In many cases, these emit solvent odors which can be dangerous to breathe, even for the healthiest of individuals. Therefore, if you have a garment that has just been dry cleaned, be sure to remove it from it's protective plastic bag and hang it outdoors as soon you bring it home. You'll need to air it out at least several hours, or until the characteristic dry-cleaning odor has dissipated.

As a service to their customers, some professional dry cleaners routinely add mothproofing chemicals to all wool items. To avoid these potentially bothersome chemicals, you'll want to specify clearly that you don't want your wool items treated against moths.

WHY IS 100%-COTTON DENIM OFTEN INTOLERABLE?

Although most of the denim used in jeans, vests, jackets, coats, tote bags, etc. is untreated 100%-cotton (all-cotton fabric which has not undergone wrinkle-resisting, waterproofing, etc. treatments), it's often intolerable when new for many sensitive people. The main reason is often the dye. While blue denim can be colored with natural indigo or synthetic indigo-color dyes, it seems the real problem isn't the source of the dye but the fact that such large quantities of it are absorbed by the cotton fibers.

As it turns out, many traditional dark-blue denim items are dyed using a process known as *range-dyeing*. In range-dyeing, cotton yarns, which are used to weave the denim, first go through a soaking indigo dye bath. Then, they're air-dried. This particular dyeing method allows the deep-blue tint to gradually fade through repeated launderings. However, if you choose blue denim items labeled faded, stone-washed, acid-washed, or bleached, much of the indigo will have already been removed at the mill. Therefore, such denim pieces are often tolerable, even when they're first purchased.

IS ACCEPTABLE CLOTHING HARD TO FIND?

Many sensitive people believe it's extremely difficult to find tolerable clothing. Actually, it's becoming easier all the time. This is because natural-fiber clothing has become more popular with the general public in recent years. Therefore, more of it can be found in local stores to meet this demand. This is particularly true in the cases of 100%-cotton and 100%-silk items.

Acceptable clothing made from a variety of natural fibers may also be purchased through popular mail-order companies such as **L.L. Bean, Inc.**, **Eddie Bauer**, and **Lands' End, Inc.** However, the best selections are usually found in natural-fiber specialty-clothing catalogs such as **Deva Lifewear**, **The Cotton Place**, **Richman Cotton Company**, and **Winter Silks**. These types of mail-order companies often handle everything from bras to outer coats (see *Specific Clothing Suggestions* below).

In addition, you can often find natural-fiber garments at secondhand shops and garage sales. However, for sensitive individuals, buying at these places often has to be avoided. That's because most used clothing has accumulated over months or years a great deal of perfume, scents from laundry products, and/or tobacco odors (see *Problems with Scents* in Chapter 2: *Personal Care*). Very often these contaminating odors will cause tolerance problems. While repeated laundering and airing may help, they often don't help enough.

Unfortunately, many new, untreated natural-fiber clothes can also be intolerable, at least initially. This is likely due to all the chemicals typically added during milling. Surprisingly, even organic-fiber pieces can sometimes be unwearable at first. Commonly, when new, organic cotton has a rather strong grainy odor that can be bothersome. In addition, *any* new piece of clothing can be intolerable because of the perfume and/or tobacco odors the item picked up between the time it left the mill and when it was purchased. Fortunately, in many, if not most, cases, odors in new, untreated, washable natural-fiber garments can be removed through airing and special laundering procedures (see *Removing New Clothing Odors* in Chapter 7: *Cleaning*).

By the way, if you go to the effort and expense to find and buy natural-fiber clothing, make sure you care for it properly. This includes laundering all washable items using only tolerable cleaning products (Unscented brands are preferable for most sensitive individuals.) (see *Testing* in Chapter 1: *Getting Started* and *Alternative Laundry Products* in Chapter 7: *Cleaning*). Also, make sure your closets, drawers, and other storage areas are as free from dust, mildew, and potentially contaminating odors as possible (see *Closets* in *Chapter 8: Housekeeping*). Finally, store your natural-fiber clothes in such a way that there will be no damage from clothing moths (see *Clothing Moths* in *Chapter 8: Housekeeping*).

SPECIFIC CLOTHING SUGGESTIONS

Most of the clothing suggestions given in this section are ones that have proven satisfactory for a number of sensitive persons. While only a few mail-order companies are listed here, many others that also offer acceptable clothing can be found in *Appendix 3: Resources for a Healthy Household.*

WOMEN'S CLOTHING

Obtaining attractive *and* tolerable garments can be easier than you think, as long as you know where to look. Here's an alphabetical listing of basic clothing items with several sources of where to purchase them to help get you started in creating a healthy wardrobe. These suggestions are generally items that many sensitive individuals can tolerate.

ACCESSORIES

Ideally, you should probably choose metal, natural fabric, or leather belts (but not bonded leather). Casual, 100%-cotton canvas and leather belts are usually available by mail order from **L.L. Bean, Inc.**, and **Lands' End, Inc.** Also, **Deva Lifewear** offers a variety of attractive untreated natural-cotton sashes and cummerbunds. Of course, most department stores will have a greater selection of belts—including dressier styles.

Scarves of 100% silk, cotton, rayon, or nylon are good choices and are widely available in many local stores. If you want handkerchiefs, untreated all-cotton ones are handled by **The Cotton Place**. Elegant 100%-cotton and 100%-linen handkerchiefs are often sold in upscale women's clothing stores.

BRAS

Untreated natural-fiber bras "breathe" and aren't made of created materials that could innately give off bothersome odors. Interestingly, large brassiere companies usually manufacture a few 100%-cotton bras, even though most of their lines are synthetic-fabric bras. You'll need to check your local department stores for these cotton models, which are often labeled as sport bras. On the other hand, **Decent Exposures**, a very small company run by women, produces custom-made 100%-cotton bras. In fact, they'll make bras to fit any cup or figure type.

In addition, catalogs specializing in all-cotton clothing, such as **The Cotton Place** and **Janice Corp.**, always offer a good selection of all-cotton bras. A few 100%-cotton bras are also sold by **The Primary Layer**. Green-cotton bras in a number of styles can be purchased from **The Seventh Generation**. Remember: All 100%-cotton bras will likely shrink unless they're labeled otherwise, so you'll want to select your size accordingly.

Silk bras are perhaps the ultimate in softness, but their high cost is often a drawback. To find them locally, you'll need to check lingerie stores and women's foundations in fine department stores. Also, the **Winter Silks** catalog offers all-silk brassieres, many of which are affordably priced. Of course, nylon bras are commonly available everywhere. However, nylon doesn't permit the rapid evaporation of moisture. Therefore, in hot, humid conditions, they can be uncomfortable.

COATS

Acceptable coats that are attractive, tolerable, and easy to care for, especially winter ones, are not usually easy to find. Therefore, if you own one, it's extremely important to take good care of it so it won't need to be replaced until absolutely necessary.

However, a few good coat options are still worth considering. Locally, many department stores handle 100%-cotton denim jackets, dusters, and coats. Also, unlined, mediumweight, 100%-cotton jackets and coats are available from **Deva Lifewear**. All these cotton choices are usually not only generally tolerable, but machine washable and dryable as well.

Of course, wool coats are an old favorite, but most of them will require dry cleaning and proper storage to prevent moth damage. You should be aware that some new wool items are pretreated with mothproofing chemicals, so be sure to check the garment's tags. Generally, most fine apparel shops and department stores offer at least some 100%-wool coats. In addition, unusual ethnic-style, full-length coats are offered by **The Daily Planet/Russian Dressing**. These come in both 100% wool and 100% cotton.

Recently, silk casual jackets have become popular. Therefore, you may be able to find them in local stores. Nylon coats filled with down have often proven acceptable for many sensitive people. However, you'll want to check first to see if the coat is labeled as water-resistant. If so, it was probably treated with chemicals that could become bothersome. Generally, nylon coats are available in local sports, clothing, and department stores. Also, you'll want to check the **L.L. Bean, Inc.**, **Eddie Bauer**, and **Lands' End, Inc.** catalogs for their current availability.

Leather coats can be good choices if the odor of the new leather isn't overly objectionable. Often, airing a new leather coat will reduce this initial odor problem. However, completely removing the odor may take months or years if you are extremely sensitive. You should also be aware that some leather outerwear could have been treated with waterproofing chemicals, which can be bothersome to certain individuals. If a leather item is water-resistant, it often states this on the manufacturer's tag. Therefore, you'll need to read all labels and catalog descriptions carefully. To find a leather coat, check out local leather shops and department stores. By mail order, **The Deerskin Trading Post** offers a good selection of coats made from a variety of leather types.

DRESSES, BLOUSES, SKIRTS, SWEATERS, PANTS, ETC.

Fortunately, 100% natural-fiber clothing is now available in many local stores as well as catalogs. You'll find that mail-order companies, such as **L.L. Bean, Inc.**, **Lands' End, Inc.**, and **Eddie Bauer** have casual outdoorsy lines that are often both comfortable and affordable. In addition, two women's-wear catalogs with good selections are **James River Traders** and **Newport News**. Other sources for 100%-cotton clothing are **The Cotton Place** and **Janice Corp.**

Deva Lifewear offers a large inventory of untreated all-cotton clothing. Interestingly, they design and produce much of the line themselves from fabrics that are often preshrunk and require little or no ironing. **The Richman Cotton Company** also designs and sews most of what they sell from organic, unbleached 100%-cotton. This company's clothing is colored using less-toxic dyes. One mail-order company, **Reflections**, sells *only* women's-wear made of organically raised cotton fabric.

Catalogs devoted to third-world ethnic-style clothing, such as **Marketplace of India** and **The Daily Planet/Russian Dressing**, offer unusual natural-fiber garments, many of which are all-cotton. However, with this type of clothing you'll need to be cautious. Some items may not have been made using colorfast dyes. Therefore, it is essential to read all the garment labels carefully and wash such clothing correctly to avoid color bleeding or running.

All-cotton sweaters, or a blend of cotton/ramie, are sold in most department stores. Also, a number of catalogs carry them. You may want to check **L.L. Bean, Inc.**, **Eddie Bauer**, **Lands' End, Inc.**, **James River Traders**, and **Newport News** to see what's currently available.

All-wool items are usually found in local department stores and specialty clothing shops. However, they will require special measures to both properly clean and store them (see *Wool* above). In addition, silk clothing is often sold in fine-quality, upscale stores. Two excellent mail-order sources of silk items are **Winter Silks** and **The Silk Collection**. On the other hand, all-rayon or all-nylon garments are generally available in most local outlets. Leather skirts, dresses, and vests are sold through the **Deerskin Trading Post** catalog. Also check your area department stores and leather specialty shops.

LEOTARDS AND BATHING SUITS

Untreated 100%-cotton leotards are available from **Janice Corp.** You'll also want to also check the **Back to Basics** catalog. One hundred percent cotton leotards may also be available in your local sports shops and department stores. If you'd like a cotton and spandex (synthetic elastic fiber) bathing suit, these are sold by **Hanna Anderson** (listed in *Appendix 4: Resources for Infants and Children*). Green-cotton body suits are handled by **The Seventh Generation**.

NURSING-MOTHER CLOTHING

If you're interested in 100%-cotton clothing for nursing mothers, such as dresses, casual wear, slacks, sleepwear, and undergarments, these are sold by **Motherwear**. You might also want to check your local department and maternity stores.

PANTIES

Of course, panties of 100%-cotton can be found in most stores and catalogs Panties of this type will "breathe;" therefore, they may help prevent the emergence of vaginal yeast infections. Mail-order sources include **Back to Basics**, **Janice Corp.**, and **The Cotton Place**. Also, fine-quality, all-cotton panties are available from **The Primary Layer**. The **Richman Cotton Company** offers unbleached 100%-cotton panties in both brief and hipster styles. Green-cotton panties in several styles are handled by **The Seventh Generation**.

All-silk panties are available from **Winter Silks** and in some finer stores. Nylon panties, even those with cotton crotch linings, are not recommended. This is because they don't "breathe," so they can't allow natural evaporation to take place.

(For menstrual panties with absorbant linings, see *Feminine Hygiene* in *Chapter 2: Personal Care*.)

SHOES AND BOOTS

If you are a sensitive person, you should realize that most new shoes and boots, no matter what they're made of, will require an extended airing period. This will help dissipate often bothersome "new" odors. However, some footwear choices are better than others. These include shoes made of 100%-cotton canvas or a fairly tolerable leather. Also, untreated nylon shoes are usually low-odor items. However, nylon footwear doesn't "breathe," so there can be a buildup of perspiration.

While leather boots are readily available, they often require waterproofing treatments (see *Leather* above). These treatments usually contain highly odorous compounds and generally must be reapplied every so often. Untreated nylon is a good boot choice, but many nylon boots are now chemically waterproofed during the manufacturing process (see *Nylon* above). These treatments can be bothersome to some sensitive individuals.

Therefore, if you need boots, especially for damp or winter conditions, you might be more tolerant of all-rubber or all-vinyl boots that are inherently waterproof. However these, too, can pose tolerance problems because vinyl and rubber odors can be bothersome to some individuals. As you can see, finding tolerable boots can be a real problem. As a result, when not in use, boots are often best stored in an enclosed porch or "mud room." In this way they are separated from the actual living space when not being worn, but are still within easy reach.

Of course, many local outlets are available for shoes and boots. By mail order, **The J.C. Penny Company, Inc.**, **L.L. Bean, Inc.**, **Deerskin Trading Post**, and **Newport News** catalogs offer a good selection.

SLEEPWEAR

Natural-fiber sleepwear items can be found in many local stores. However, you'll want to check to see if they've been treated with fire-retardant chemicals, which can be bothersome to sensitive individuals. Cotton, rayon, and nylon sleepwear are also popular items in department, clothing, and even discount stores. By mail order, attractive 100%-cotton gowns are sold by **The Primary Layer**, and **The Seventh Generation** have pajamas made of 100% green cotton. **Deva Lifewear**, **The Cotton Place**, **Janice Corp.**, and **The Richman Cotton Company** all carry untreated all-cotton sleepwear. All-silk sleepwear is sold by **Winter Silks**.

In addition, 100%-cotton bathrobes are available from **The Cotton Place**, **Deva Lifewear**, and **The Vermont Country Store**, just to name a few. **The Vermont Country Store** also has a good selection of women's slippers in 100%-cotton terry and in boiled wool. Organic-cotton slippers are offered by **The Seventh Generation**.

SLIPS

Slips of 100% cotton are occasionally available in local stores. They can also be purchased by mail order from **Deva Lifewear** and **The Cotton Place**. Attractive slips made from silk are available from some fine local department stores or from **Winter Silks**. Nylon slips are sold almost everywhere.

SMOCKS AND APRONS

All-cotton duck aprons and smocks can be found in many kitchen specialty departments and shops. Also, you might want to look in kitchen/cooking catalogs such as **Colonial Garden Kitchens**. In addition, untreated 100%-cotton denim aprons are sold by **The Living Source**.

By the way, all-cotton, untreated white twill laboratory coats are sold by **The Cotton Place**. These make great kitchen cover-ups because your clothes are completely protected from neck to knee as well as down to your wrists. These particular items shrink tremendously if you wash them in hot water and dry them in a hot dryer. Therefore, you'll need to order two to three sizes larger than your normal size.

SOCKS AND HOSIERY

Natural-fiber socks "breathe" so they're usually very comfortable to wear. If you need socks for hiking or cold weather, you might consider wearing wool socks. Wool can actually absorb a large percentage of its weight in moisture and still provide insulating warmth. Of course, most department stores, sport shops, and women's clothing stores will carry a selection of at least some all-cotton socks. By mail order, all-cotton socks are handled by **The Cotton Place**, **Janice Corp.**, and **The Vermont Country Store**. Unbleached 100%-cotton socks and all-wool socks are sold by **The Richman Cotton Company**. Organic-cotton socks, in naturally grown colors of natural, brown, and green, are offered by **The Seventh Generation**.

By the way, breathable cotton panty hose are available from **The Vermont Country Store**. Also, **The Seventh Generation** sells tights in natural or black colors made from a blend of 70% organic-cotton and regular cotton, with a small amount of Lycra to add elasticity. In addition, **The Vermont Country Store** handles 100%-cotton and all-wool hosiery, some having elastic tops while others require a garter belt. Cotton garters are sold by **The Cotton Place** and **The Vermont Country Store**.

SWEATWEAR

Much of the sweatwear that is marketed is made, either partially or entirely, of synthetic materials. However, **The Richman Cotton Company** sells tops, vests, pants, and hooded sweatshirts of untreated 100%-cotton fleece. One hundred percent organic sweatshirts and pants are available from **Cottontails OrganicWear**.

THERMAL UNDERWEAR

Finding all-natural-fiber thermal wear can be difficult. Fortunately, all-cotton long johns and tops are sold by **The Richman Cotton Company** and **The Cotton Place**. All-silk versions are offered by **Winter Silks**.

WINTER GLOVES, HATS, AND SCARVES

Probably the vast majority of winterwear accessories are now made of acrylic. However, 100%-cotton scarves and gloves are being manufactured by a company called **Tom Tom**. If you'd like to purchase its products, you'll need to contact them for a mail-order or a nearby retail source. If you'd like all-wool caps, scarves, and gloves, these are sold by **The Vermont Country Store**. Wool items are a good choice because they can provide insulation despite getting wet. However, they'll need to be properly cleaned and stored.

MEN'S CLOTHING

Unfortunately, natural (and tolerable synthetic) clothing choices for men are more limited than the choices available for women. However, there are a few sources of acceptable items that should meet most of your needs. Many of the suggestions given below are satisfactory to many sensitive persons.

BELTS

Leather belts (except bonded leather) and especially those made of 100%-cotton canvas are generally healthy choices. Locally, most men's clothing stores and department stores should carry a good selection. In addition, 100%-cotton canvas belts in several colors are usually sold in army/navy surplus stores. Mail-order companies such as **L.L. Bean, Inc.**, and **Eddie Bauer** handle a variety of casual belts. Dressier belts are sold in the **J.C. Penny Company, Inc.** catalog, among others.

COATS

Finding tolerable outerwear (especially for cold weather) can often be extremely difficult for sensitive people. Therefore, if you have a coat or jacket that is acceptable, try to keep it in as good a shape as possible for as long as you can. However, there are a few sources where you may be able to buy an acceptable replacement coat. For example, casual all-cotton denim coats are sold in most men's-wear departments. Simple Amish-style, untreated, all-cotton work jackets (unlined or lined with 100%-cotton flannel) are offered by **Gohn Brothers**. In addition, **Deva Lifewear** offers a few unlined, washable, mediumweight, 100%-cotton jackets that are untreated.

If you want a 100%-wool coat, these can be few and far between, except for expensive overcoats which are often chemically mothproofed. However, used boiled-wool European military jackets are sometimes handled by local army-navy surplus stores. These are actually washable and may not have been mothproofed. (However, mothproofing information may not be available on used clothing.) Also, **The Daily Planet/Russian Dressing** offers uniquely styled full-length unisex coats in all-wool as well as in all-cotton. Remember, if you purchase a wool coat, it will have to be properly cared for in both cleaning and storage.

If it's not too bothersome, a new leather coat can be a good choice; that is, after it has aired over an extended period of time. (This could be months or years depending on the coat and how sensitive you are.) To find leather coats and jackets, you'll want to look in local department stores, men's clothing stores, and leather shops. By mail order, **The Deerskin Trading Post** sells a number of styles made from several types of leather.

Unlined, lightweight, nylon jackets—and those that are cotton-lined—are available in some local stores. These can make ideal jackets for sensitive persons unless the nylon has been treated with potentially bothersome water-repelling chemicals. (Be sure to read the tags and labels to see if the coat is water-resistant before you purchase it.) By the way, untreated nylon jackets filled with down are good choices for wintertime. You'll want to look in the **Land's End, Inc.**, **Eddie Bauer**, and **L.L. Bean, Inc.** catalogs to see what they currently offer.

HANDKERCHIEFS

Nonpermanent press, untreated, 100%-cotton handkerchiefs are sold through most local men's departments and clothing stores, and they can also be ordered from **The Cotton Place** and **Janice Corp.** Linen handkerchiefs and silk pocket handkerchiefs are sometimes available at finer men's clothing stores.

SHOES AND BOOTS

Usually new footwear (especially if it's made of leather) needs to be aired for an extended period of time before it can be worn; that is, if you are a sensitive person. Saying that though, one of the better shoe materials from an outgassing standpoint is untreated 100%-cotton canvas. Interestingly, untreated nylon is often relatively low at emitting potentially bothersome odors. But then, nylon can't breathe. Therefore, nylon shoes (particularly unvented nylon shoes) can lead to foot perspiration and odor problems.

Unfortunately, finding acceptable boots is even more challenging than finding acceptable shoes. While damp- or winter-condition leather boots are commonly available, they generally need repeated waterproofing treatments, which can make them intolerable (see *Leather* above). On the other hand, vinyl and rubber boots are inherently waterproof, but they have their own inherent odors which can be bothersome to certain people. Nylon boots, which were once made from untreated material and, therefore, were quite tolerable, are now generally coated with a synthetic substance to make them waterproof (see *Nylon* above). In the end, it seems the best solution is to just buy boots made of the materials that seem to pose the least problems to you, then keep them stored in an enclosed porch or mud room away from the living space.

Leather shoes are also sold by **Huntington Clothiers & Shirtmakers**. The **L.L. Bean, Inc.**, **J.C. Penny Company, Inc.**, and **The Deerskin Trading Post** catalogs offer good shoe and boot selections (for slippers, see *Sleepwear*).

SLACKS, SHIRTS, SWEATERS, ETC.

Untreated all-cotton shirts and slacks can be found in a number of department stores and men's wear shops, although lately, wrinkle-free versions have begun replacing them. By mail order, **Eddie Bauer**, **Lands' End, Inc.**, and **L.L. Bean, Inc.** all offer 100%-cotton men's clothing. You might also check **The Cotton Place** and **Deva Lifewear**. A good variety of fine 100%-cotton shirts can be purchased from **Paul Federick's Menstyle**, and **Huntington Clothiers & Shirtmakers** has an excellent selection of all-cotton shirts and slacks. By the way, a few organic-cotton items are sold by **The Richman Cotton Company** and **Huntington Clothiers & Shirtmakers**. In addition, 100%-cotton or cotton/ramie sweaters are offered by **Eddie Bauer, Lands' End, Inc.**, and **L.L. Bean, Inc.**

Generally, 100%-wool clothing can be found in fine men's stores. However, some of it may have been chemically mothproofed. Reading the garment tags and labels may give you this information. One catalog source for non-mothproofed dressy wool-flannel slacks is **The Cotton Place**.

On another note, silk shirts are now becoming popular—and affordable. Often, your local department stores, men's clothing shops, and even some discount stores handle them. A number of silk shirts are sold by **Winter Silks**. They also offer men's silk sweaters.

SLEEPWEAR

Of course, all-cotton sleepwear can be found in a variety of stores and catalogs. However, sensitive persons should check for the addition of fire-retarding or wrinkle-resisting chemicals before purchasing them. By mail order, **The Vermont Country Store** carriers a number of 100%-cotton styles as does **The Primary Layer**. Another source is **The Cotton Place**. One hundred percent green-cotton pajamas are sold by **The Seventh Generation**. Silk sleepwear is generally offered by a few better local department stores, and it can be ordered though **Winter Silks**.

You should be able to find all-cotton bathrobes locally. However, if you'd like to mail-order them, they're available from **Deva Lifewear**, **The Primary Layer**, **The Cotton Place**, and **The Vermont Country Store**. Green-cotton flannel robes are offered by **The Seventh Generation**. All-cotton slippers, wool and leather slipper socks, and boiled-wool slippers are offered through **The Vermont Country Store**.

SOCKS

All-cotton sport socks are sold in many stores. Men's departments and specialty stores also usually carry cotton dress socks. Two catalogs that offer a variety of 100%-cotton men's socks are **The Primary Layer** and **The Vermont Country Store**. Unbleached all-cotton socks, as well as wool socks, are available from **The Richman Cotton Company**. Silk socks are sometimes found in finer men's shops and departments.

SPORT JACKETS AND SUITS

Sport jackets and suits made of 100% wool, cotton/linen blends, or 100% cotton are sometimes sold at local men's departments. A good selection is also offered by **Huntington Clothiers & Shirtmakers**. This particular company has fine tailored suits and jackets as well as unconstructed casual styles. They also sell 100%-wool tuxedos. All-cotton or all-wool suits and sport jackets are also sometimes available through **L.L. Bean, Inc.**, **Eddie Bauer**, and **Lands' End, Inc.** catalogs. You should be aware that virtually all the garments in this category must be dry-cleaned. However, **Deva Lifewear** offers 100%-cotton, mediumweight, unstructured, washable sport jackets in a variety of colors.

Some fine men's stores also occasionally handle suits and jackets made of rayon/natural-fiber blends or perhaps all-silk versions. In addition, local leather shops often feature sport jackets made from various leathers. Through its catalog, **The Deerskin Trading Post** offers leather sport jackets and vests.

SWEATWEAR

All-synthetic or synthetic-cotton blend sweatwear is, by far, the most commonly encountered. However, untreated 100%-cotton fleece tops, pants, vests, and hooded jackets are sold by **The Richman Cotton Company**. Also, **Cottontails OrganicWear** offers organic all-cotton sweatshirts and pants.

TIES

Ties in 100% cotton, rayon, and silk are widely available. **L.L. Bean, Inc.** and **Eddie Bauer** are two mail-order sources offering these items. Also, **Deva Lifewear** generally handles a few unique and casual all-cotton ties. An excellent selection of 100%-silk ties is sold by **Huntington Clothiers & Shirtmakers**

UNDERWEAR

T-shirts and undershorts made of 100% cotton are still very popular, and so are found in most local department and clothing stores. Mail-order sources include **The Vermont Country Store** and the **J.C. Penny Company, Inc.** Fine-quality 100%-cotton underwear is sold by **The Primary Layer**. Unbleached all-cotton briefs and T-shirts are handled by **The Richman Cotton Company**. Green-cotton underwear can be purchased from **The Seventh Generation** and silk underwear from **Winter Silks**.

WINTER GLOVES, HATS, AND SCARVES

Most winter accessories these days seem to be made of acrylic. However, cotton scarves and gloves are manufactured by **Tom Tom**. To purchase them you'll need to contact them for a mail-order source or nearby retailer. Wool caps, scarves, and gloves are sold by **The Vermont Country Store**. Incidentally, woolen items still keep you warm even if they get wet. Of course, wool gloves, etc. require proper cleaning and storage.

CUSTOM-MADE CLOTHES

You don't always have to search catalogs or local stores to find natural-fiber or acceptable synthetic clothing. You can create much of what you need right in your home. Even if you can't tolerate sewing machine odors, consider buying the patterns, materials, and notions and having a friend, family member, or professional seamstress do the actual work. However, remember to choose a person who doesn't smoke or use perfume, and who won't be working in an area where others do. Otherwise, your custom-made clothing could absorb these odors and end up being too bothersome for you to wear.

FINDING FABRICS AND NOTIONS

Local fabric shops often have several untreated natural fabrics from which to choose. However, catalog sources are also available for both natural-fiber materials and notions. For example, **The Cotton Place** offers a variety of untreated 100%-cotton fabrics. (Small fabric swatches are available.) In addition, **Deva Lifewear**, which primarily sells finished clothing, offers untreated 100%-cotton fabrics in several weights, solid colors, and textures. The company also offers some untreated, all-cotton novelty fabrics. These include hand-woven styles imported from Central America and a few Far Eastern batiks. (A fabric sample packet is sold at a nominal fee.)

Besides ready-made clothing, **The Richman Cotton Company** offers 100% natural-fiber yardage. Included are unbleached organic-cotton cloth in twill, gauze, sheeting, knit, flannel, and Peking varieties. These products are also available in several colors, having been dyed using less-toxic dyes. The company also offers some rayon and silk fabric. Furthermore, **Dharma Trading Company** offers both undyed 100%-cotton and silk fabrics. By the way, you might consider joining **The Natural Fiber Fabric Club**, from which, for an annual fee, members receive a selection of beautiful fabric swatches from which to order.

If you require 100%-cotton notions, such as thread, trim, or elastic, you'll want to check **The Cotton Place** catalog. Although wooden and metal buttons are commonly found, **The Richman Cotton Company** sells tauga-nut buttons. These are in a simple two-hole, one-half inch wide style you may find interesting to use as an alternative. (Tauga nuts are a hard, natural vegetable material that looks similar to ivory.) In addition, **Home-Sew** handles some all-cotton lace, trim, and notions. The **Nancy's Notions** catalog offers a huge variety of notions, many of which can't be found in local stores or other catalogs. However, most of these aren't made of all-natural materials.

For dyes that work well on natural fabrics, you'll want to check **The Richman Cotton Company** and **Dharma Trading Company**. You may also want to experiment making your own natural dyes. If so, you can look for books on the subject at your local library.

SEWING

Once you obtain your natural-fiber or acceptable synthetic fabric, it's best to wash and air it to remove any bothersome "new" odors (see *Removing New Clothing Odors* in *Chapter 7: Cleaning*). This step is essential for sensitive individuals, but everyone should make sure his or her yardage is preshrunk before sewing with it anyway. If you'd like to use a pattern but are bothered by the paper or printing ink, try unfolding the uncut pattern sheets and hanging them outside to air on a clothesline. Be careful though; while a light breeze will help the airing-out, a strong wind could easily damage them. Simply laying the paper sheets on the ground in the sun until they become tolerable is another approach. Of course, you'll need to use weights to hold the sheets in place.

If you've decided to do the sewing yourself but are a sensitive individual, try to have plenty of ventilation around you when you sew with a machine. Many sewing machines have plastic housings that can release synthetic chemicals. Hot sewing-machine motors can also give off odors, as can newly applied sewing-machine oil. Therefore, open nearby windows if possible. In addition, use an electric fan to blow air from behind or beside you toward the sewing machine and then away. These measures should help dissipate most of the troubling odors. You might also wear an activated-charcoal mask (see *Personal Facial Air Filters* in *Chapter 9: Indoor Air*). Furthermore, some sensitive individuals may find they'll still need to take frequent breaks away from the machine.

KNITTING AND CROCHETING

Of course, not all clothing is made of fabric. Knitted and crocheted items are also an important part of most people's wardrobes, and many persons find these items enjoyable to create themselves. Fortunately, it's not difficult to find acceptable yarns. Virtually all stores and catalogs that handle knitting and crocheting supplies will carry some yarns made of 100% natural-fibers. By mail order, a few all-cotton yarns are available from **The Cotton Place**.

In addition, **The Noon Family Sheep Farm** is a source of undyed, organic, wool yarns. The colors available are in natural-white, light-brown, and dark-brown shades derived from specially bred sheep. **Pueblo to People** offers hand-spun alpaca yarns in several natural colors as well. Furthermore, you can sometimes find organic and/or vegetable-dyed yarns at local yarn specialty shops. Sometimes the people working in such stores may also sell hand-spun natural-fiber yarns or they may be able to provide the names of spinners who will be able to sell their yarns directly to you. Homespun yarns can be exciting to see, feel, and work with, so it's often worth the effort and extra expense to find them.

If there is no specialty-yarn store in your area, ask your local library's reference department for help. Libraries often keep lists of local clubs and organizations, including those that do spinning, dyeing, weaving, or knitting. Your reference librarian can also help you find magazines devoted to natural fibers and natural dyeing. (Most public libraries subscribe to at least one such periodical.) Fiber-craft magazines often list advertisements and classifieds offering homespun natural yarns for sale.

For very sensitive or allergic persons, fine fibers or odors released into the air when working with any type of yarn (even organically raised yarn) may be bothersome. In that case, try working outdoors—or wear a protective charcoal-filled mask indoors (see *Personal Facial Air Filters* in *Chapter 9: Indoor Air*). If these measures are impossible or simply don't help enough, have someone else knit or crochet items for you. However, be sure to choose someone who will be careful not to work on your project if perfume, tobacco, or other strong odors are present. These can be easily absorbed by the yarn fibers.

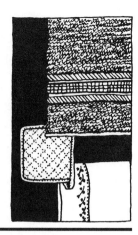

CHAPTER 4
LINENS

In creating an ideal healthy household, linens should be as toxic-free as possible. This should be especially true for sheets and bedding items, which are in direct contact with you from 6–10 hours daily. Fortunately, natural-fiber mattresses, sheets, pillow cases, blankets, quilts, comforters, and bedspreads are becoming more popular and available. Some of these are made of untreated or even organic materials.

In the following sections most of the product suggestions have been used successfully by sensitive individuals. However, other acceptable suppliers may also be found in *Product Sources* in *Appendix 3: Resources for A Healthy Household.*

BEDDING

Your bedding should promote both good sleep—and good health. It is hoped the following information will help you better accomplish this.

MATTRESSES

At one time, mattresses were little more than large cloth sacks filled with straw, wool, cotton, or rags. The forerunners of modern box springs were simply wood frames strung with grids of ropes. By comparison, today's mattresses and box springs are engineering marvels. Manufacturers now use secret specialized coils and patented support systems, combined with a variety of synthetic foams, battings, and covering materials. *Fire-retardant* (see *What is Fire?* in *Chapter 8: Housekeeping*) and stain-resistant chemicals are then generally added. Not surprising, many sensitive individuals can't tolerate typical conventional mattresses.

One of the more recent mattress innovations is the water bed. These large, vinyl bags, usually supported by particleboard or plywood frames, can outgas low-levels of bothersome odors that can be offensive to sensitive people. Built-in electric heaters can actually increase the outgassing rates.

Fortunately, a few very good all-natural bedding alternatives do exist, some of which are available without fire-retardant or stain-resistant chemicals. Among these are the all-cotton mattresses and box springs offered by **Janice Corp.** Also, both **Dona Designs** and **Nontoxic Environments** sell organic 100%-cotton mattresses and box springs in popular sizes. The fabric used to cover these is untreated, but to make them more tolerable, the fabric is washed in both vinegar and baking soda before being sewn. In fact, if you are extremely sensitive, **Dona Designs** will actually ship the covering materials directly to you. That way, you can wash and air them as much as necessary to make them personally tolerable for you. (Note that, mattresses are required to have fire-retardant treatments by law, but the suppliers listed above can omit them if your physician provides a prescription that states they can't be used for health reasons.)

You should be aware that most new cotton mattresses, especially organic cotton mattresses, have an innate odor that can be fairly strong. This is primarily the natural grainy smell of the cotton itself. Generally, it'll dissipate after a few months and become almost unnoticeable to even most sensitive individuals. However, for those who find the raw cotton odor bothersome, you might consider using *barrier cloth* mattress covers to help seal it in (barrier cloth is a special, extremely tight woven cotton) (see *Mattress Covers and Pads* below).

Heart of Vermont offers mattresses and box springs made with organic-wool cores surrounded by organic cotton. The ticking use is untreated cotton. Untreated (no mothproofing, flame-resisting, etc. chemicals) wool mattresses and box springs are also sold by **Nontoxic Environments**.

An unusual natural-bedding choice is the rye-straw mattress. Rye-straw mattresses are now being imported from Germany by **Sinan Co.**, but only in one size: a single (39" x 75") with no box spring. (It's recommended that the mattresses be placed on wooden-slat platforms.) These mattresses are actually constructed with an inner layer of heat-treated rye straw surrounded by untreated wool (the straw is heated to kill microbes). The covering fabric used is linen. Rye-straw mattresses will have a definite straw-like odor that could be bothersome to some individuals when new. However, it's likely that, as they age, the odor will lessen. If the odor is too objectionable, the mattresses can be encased in barrier-cloth mattress covers. Interestingly, no physician's prescription is usually necessary for purchasing either wool or wool/rye-straw mattresses because they're inherently flame-resistant.

As expected, all these alternative mattresses are relatively expensive. This is due to higher material costs, custom manufacturing, and factory-to-home freight charges. Therefore, if you purchase a special mattress, it's wise to protect your investment. If at all possible, use washable natural-fiber mattress covers and pads (see *Mattress Covers and Pads* below). By the way, you can lengthen your mattress's life considerably by flipping it over and rotating it occasionally. A good schedule is to flip it over on the first of January, May, and September and rotate it head to foot on the first of March, July, and November. By thumbtacking a small card with this schedule on it in your linen closet, you'll very likely be reminded to do this.

(For healthy headboards and frames, see *Solid Wood Furniture* and *Metal Furniture* in *Chapter 5: Interior Decorating*.)

MATTRESS COVERS AND PADS

Mattress covers and pads will help protect your mattresses from soiling. Now a days, most covers and pads are made of synthetic fibers such as polyester, but washable, 100%-cotton, untreated mattress covers and mattress pads are still made. In fact, heavyweight, zippered, unbleached, all-cotton, muslin covers for both mattresses and box springs are sold by **Mother Hart**. These are well-made and very affordable.

All-cotton *barrier cloth* covers are sold by **The Cotton Place**. Barrier cloth is an extremely tightly woven, untreated, 100%-cotton fabric. It was originally developed for medical use. However, the tight weave has also been found to be a good odor barrier by many sensitive people. By completely encasing your mattress and box springs in barrier cloth, most unwanted bedding odors are prevented from escaping into the room. This can often make some beds tolerable, even if they're made of synthetic battings, foams, and ticking, or have a strong natural odor from new, organically raised cotton. The main drawback to barrier-cloth mattress covers is their relatively high cost, but if they can make an otherwise intolerable bed acceptable, they are well worth the expense.

You may or may not be able to find all-cotton mattress pads locally. However, they're handled by **The Vermont Country Store**. Organic, untreated 100%-cotton pads are sold by **Dona Designs**. (A doctor's prescription is required to omit flame-retardant chemicals.) By the way, two or three untreated all-cotton flannel blankets can substitute for a mattress pad, and no physician's prescription is necessary. All-cotton chenille pads, made of green cotton, can be found in **The Seventh Generation** catalog.

In addition, 100%-wool shearling-fleece mattress pads are available. They too can be healthy choices, especially if they haven't been treated with moth-proofing chemicals. (You'll need to check the manufacturers' tags carefully for this information—and for proper cleaning procedures.) One mail-order source for wool mattress pads is **The Vermont Country Store**. Also, the **Aussie Connection** has wool-fleece mattress pads in two thicknesses for all bed sizes. Washable wool pads in twin through king sizes are handled by **The Seventh Generation**. Untreated, pure-lamb's-wool mattress pads with tufted cotton exteriors can be purchased from **Nontoxic Environments**.

FUTONS

Futons (also known as *shikibutons*) are thin, cotton-covered mattresses stuffed with cotton batting. They're the traditional bedding in Japan where relatively thin futons are unrolled directly onto the floor for sleeping. In the West, where futons are now becoming popular, they're generally placed on wooden frames. Some of these frames are specially designed to convert into sofas (see *Solid Wood Furniture* in *Chapter 5: Interior Decorating*).

Futon shops are found in some localities where futons can be purchased in several fabrics and materials. (Check your classified telephone directory.) By mail order, all-cotton futons are offered by **Futon Designs, Inc**. Also, organic 100%-cotton-filled futons are sold by **Heart of Vermont**, **Bright Future Futons**, and **Dona Designs**. In addition, 3" and 6" thick organic-wool futons are handled by **Nontoxic Environments**. This particular company recommends that its 3" wool futons be used on top of its 4" organic-cotton futons. (Six-inch organic-cotton futons are also available.) Futons with untreated-wool cores and organic-cotton outer layers are available from **Jantz Designs**. Futons with organic-wool cores surrounded by organic-cotton batting are sold by **Heart of Vermont**. Note, that all 100%-cotton futons not treated with fire-retardant chemicals will require a doctor's prescription before purchase. You should be aware that some wool futons may not have been treated because they're naturally flame-resistant.

If you want to make your own futon, **Nontoxic Environments** offers instructional pamphlets. They also handle tufting needles, organic-cotton batting and untreated-wool batting. In addition, the company sells 80" and 90" wide unbleached-cotton muslin fabric for covering. (For more on sewing, see *Custom-Made Clothes* in *Chapter 3: Clothing*.)

It should be pointed out that futons can be somewhat cumbersome. The thin, traditional Japanese-futons are lightweight and easily rolled up, but the 4" to 8" thick Western models are fairly weighty. Most are simply too bulky to wash at home. Therefore, it's important for you to air your futons frequently outdoors in uncontaminated air. It's also highly suggested that you use removable 100%-cotton futon covers, which can be taken off and laundered regularly.

FUTON COVERS

Protective covers for your futons are a great idea. Generally, companies that sell futons also handle covers that fit them (see *Futons* above). As a rule, futon covers are made of 100% cotton and some come in a variety of colors. One mail-order source for untreated, undyed 100%-cotton muslin futon covers is **Dona Designs**. Also, **Bright Future Futons** offers covers in both all-cotton and 100%-Irish linen varieties. For do-it-yourselfers, instructions and untreated cotton-muslin fabric for making futon covers are available from **Nontoxic Environments** (For more on sewing, see *Custom-Made Clothes* in *Chapter 3: Clothing*).

SHEETS

Undyed, 100%-cotton percale or muslin sheets, without permanent-press treatments, are excellent healthy bedding choices. Actually, cotton sheets come in several grades. *Combed-percale* refers to the best cotton sheeting fabric available. The finest-quality combed-percale sheets have a thread count of at least 200 threads per square inch and the threads used are the best available—thin and strong. This kind of thread, and the very tight weaving results in lightweight sheets with the smoothest, softest texture.

With at least 180 threads per square inch, *combed percale* is slightly coarser, so it's less expensive and not quite as luxurious. Even less costlier are *muslin* sheets. Muslin is woven of still thicker, coarser cotton yarns, with at least 128 threads per square inch. Although not as soft and smooth as percale, muslin is extremely durable and much more affordable.

All-cotton sheets are sold as bleached (white), unbleached (natural tan), or as green cotton (no chemical treatments added during the manufacturing process). Unfortunately, it's often difficult to find 100%-cotton sheets that have not been treated with permanent-press chemicals in local stores. However, **Mother Hart** often carries untreated white and unbleached percales in a variety of sizes. Sometimes this particular company also offers manufacturer's seconds—sheets with minor flaws. The good news about such sheets is that they're priced substantially lower than their first-quality counterparts. Green-cotton percale sheets in all sizes are handled by **The Seventh Generation.** Also, you can for look for untreated sheets in **The Vermont Country Store, The Cotton Place** and **Janice Corp.** catalogs.

Another healthy cotton-sheet option to consider is flannel. Although untreated 100%-cotton flannel sheets are somewhat less durable than percale or muslin, they're warm, cozy, easy to care for, and relatively inexpensive. Flannel sheets are commonly available during the fall and winter seasons in department stores and catalogs such as **L.L, Bean, Inc.** (*Home and Camp* catalog). A few companies, such as **Mother Hart** and **Janice Corp.**, offer them year-round. Organically raised, 100%-cotton flannel sheets are handled by **Heart of Vermont.**

Linen sheets are sometimes sold locally in a few very fine stores. However, the cost of linen sheets can often be extremely high. One mail-order source for 100%-Belgium linen, twin-size, flat sheets is **The Cotton Place.**

To get the most wear for your money, you might consider purchasing only flat sheets, rather than sets with both flat and fitted sheets. Flat sheets can be used in either the top or bottom bed-making position. This means your flat sheets are less likely to acquire the typical wear patterns that often occur in the centers of fitted sheets, which are always used in the bottom position. Also, the corners of flat sheets are less likely to rip than those of fitted-corner sheets whose seams must be continually stretched.

PILLOWS

Because your head is in direct contact with your pillow for 6-10 hours, it's really wise to choose a pillow that is naturally low in toxicity to help you get healthful, restful sleep. Feather or down-filled pillows can make good healthy pillow choices. However, sometimes these materials are chemically treated to prevent mold or insect damage (see *Feathers and Down* in *Chapter 3: Clothing*). These treatments could be intolerable for some sensitive persons, so you'll want to check the manufacturer's labels carefully before purchase. Your local department store should have feather and down pillows. However, if you want to order them by mail, **The Vermont Country Store** and **The Living Source** both handle feather and down pillows. And, one of the healthiest pillow ticking for covering your pillow is untreated 100%-cotton.

Although not commonly seen, 100%-cotton pillows with all-cotton covers are very acceptable bedding options. Sources include **KB Cotton Pillows** and **Mother Hart.** Also, **Janice Corp.** handles 100%-cotton pillows with either untreated all-cotton or barrier-cloth ticking. Pillows stuffed with organic 100%-cotton are available from **Dona Designs, The Seventh Generation,** and **The American Environmental Health Foundation.**

Note: Organic-cotton pillows generally have a strong, grainy smell when first purchased. This smell is actually the natural cotton odor, but it can be bothersome to some sensitive people. However, by hanging your new cotton pillows outside to air in dry, uncontaminated surroundings (no car exhaust, wood smoke, high pollen counts, etc.) for several days will help. Another approach is to place the pillows (no more than two at a time) in your clothes dryer on high heat for about thirty minutes. You can keep repeating the drying cycle until the pillows become tolerable. Yet another option is to use *barrier cloth* (special tightly woven cotton) pillow protectors over your pillows to help seal in odors.

Even more uncommon these days than cotton-filled pillows are pillows stuffed with wool, but they, too, can be a healthy choice. **Heart of Vermont** offers organic-wool pillows with untreated 100%-cotton covers. **Janice Corp.** sells untreated pillows with a wool core surrounded by cotton. These are also encased in untreated 100%-cotton ticking.

Odd-shaped (by American standards) traditional Japanese pillows stuffed with buckwheat hulls and covered in 100% cotton are sold by **Nontoxic Environments**. Cotton cases to fit are also available. Also, **The Seventh Generation** has 6" x 13" cylindrical Japanese pillows encased in organic cotton with removable green-cotton covers. **Nontoxic Environments** handles square kapok-filled pillows (see *Kapok* in *Chapter 3: Clothing*) with removable 100%-cotton cases. Sizes are 18", 24", and 28" square.

Tip: To freshen your natural-material filled pillows, hang them outdoors in uncontaminated air or place them in your clothes dryer for at least 15 minutes. To keep the ticking on your pillows cleaner, use removable, washable pillow protectors.

PILLOW CASES AND PROTECTORS

It's not easy anymore to find untreated 100%-cotton bleached and unbleached percale pillow cases. However, mail-order sources include **Mother Hart**, **The Cotton Place**, and **The Janice Corp.** Green-cotton pillow cases are sold by **The Seventh Generation**. All-silk and 100%-Belgium linen pillow cases are handled by **The Cotton Place.**

In addition to pillow cases, it's also a good idea to purchase pillow protectors. While the pillow ticking itself is usually permanently sewn shut, pillow protectors are commonly zippered. (In actual use, they're placed around the pillow with the pillow case going over them.) Pillow protectors should be removed and washed regularly, but that doesn't have to be done nearly as often as for the pillow cases. Two sources of untreated 100%-cotton muslin protectors are **Mother Hart** and **Janice Corp.** Barrier-cloth (special tightly woven cotton) protectors help keep ticking clean, as well as any bothersome pillow odors sealed in. Suppliers of these include **Janice Corp.**, and **The Cotton Place**.

BLANKETS

Ideally, your blankets should be comfortable, but also tolerable and easy to care for. Because many blankets can be expensive, choose them carefully and store them properly when not in use. However, refrain from placing them in cedar chests, especially if you are a sensitive person. Cedar chests can transfer potentially bothersome cedar odors into your blankets (Surprisingly, this odor apparently has little or no effect deterring clothing moths.) (see *Clothing Moths* in *Chapter 8: Housekeeping*).

ACRYLIC AND ELECTRIC-BLANKET CONCERNS

Acrylic blankets are soft, machine-washable, and machine-dryable. They're also inexpensive and clothing moths won't damage them. It's not surprising then that they've almost replaced natural-fiber blankets. However, blankets made of acrylic do have serious drawbacks—they can often lose their attractive initial appearance after only a few launderings, and worse, they have the potential to emit synthetic chemical odors from the acrylic fibers themselves. Of course, these blankets are also not made from renewable resources, nor are they biodegradable.

Electric blankets, which tend to be acrylic, are popular in very cold climates. However, they have an additional problem than do simple acrylic blankets alone: their embedded wiring. In older electric blankets, this wiring can produce unacceptably strong electromagnetic fields (EMFs) that can cause negative health effects (see *Chapter 11: Electromagnetic Fields*). Fortunately, newer electric blankets are wired in special patterns designed to counter most, but not all, of these electromagnetic fields.

However, even with reduced EMFs, warming up an acrylic blanket has the potential to increase the outgassing rate of odors originating from the acrylic fibers. Also, many electric blankets require special handling to clean them, so regular cleanings may be put off. Because of the negative health issues associated with acrylic and electric blankets, you are strongly urged to use untreated natural-fiber alternatives.

WOOL BLANKETS

All-wool blankets have always been popular. This isn't surprising; wool blankets are warm, comfortable, attractive, and long-lasting. Today, wool blankets are still relatively easy to find, but they've become quite expensive. Popular styles now available include trader stripes (blankets like these were originally exchanged for furs at frontier trading posts), plaids, and solid colors. However, there are two major drawbacks to wool blankets: They need to be protected from moth damage and they often require dry-cleaning.

Some manufacturers attempt to prevent moth damage by chemically treating their blankets with moth-repelling chemicals. Unfortunately, this "helpful" treatment may prove intolerable to sensitive individuals, so you'll want to check manufacturers' tags and literature before purchasing any new wool blanket to determine if mothproofing treatments have been applied. The real key to safely and effectively preventing moth damage is proper storage.

If your wool blankets require professional dry cleaning, ask your dry cleaner not to add mothproofing chemicals when you drop them off. (Some dry cleaners routinely mothproof wool items as a service to their customers.) After you bring your newly dry-cleaned blankets home, air them outdoors in uncontaminated surroundings to eliminate as much of the residual solvent odor as possible (see *Is Dry-Cleaning a Problem?* in *Chapter 3: Clothing*).

It's generally not too difficult to find wool blankets locally; most major department stores offer them. However, if you'd prefer mail-ordering them, wool trader-stripe blankets are sold by **L.L. Bean, Inc.** (*Home and Camp* catalog). **The Vermont Country Store** handles blankets in an eighty percent wool/twenty percent cotton blend. Hand-washable, undyed, untreated, wool blankets are offered by **The Seventh Generation**. They also offer other wool blankets, including lambs-wool thermals.

COTTON BLANKETS

Several types of 100%-cotton blankets are available today, with *thermals* being among the most common. Thermal all-cotton blankets are woven in specially designed open-weave patterns that are able to trap air. Trapped air in these blankets functions as an effective insulation. Most thermal cotton blankets are machine-washable, and many are machine-dryable, though some must be line-dried. One unfortunate characteristic of thermal blankets is their tendency to stretch out of shape.

All-cotton thermal blankets are often sold in local department stores and in many discount stores. Several catalog sources include **Mother Hart, L.L. Bean, Inc.** (*Home and Camp* catalog), and **Janice Corp.** Unbleached 100%-cotton thermals are available from **The Richman Cotton Company**. Green-cotton thermal blankets are sold through **The Seventh Generation**.

Thick 100%-cotton flannel blankets are also bedding options you might consider. Hospitals often use such blankets for their patients because they're relatively inexpensive, lightweight, comfortable, and they're machine washable and dryable. Unfortunately, flame-retardant chemicals may have been applied to some flannel blankets to meet certain hospital requirements. These treatments could be bothersome to sensitive people. Therefore, when buying flannel blankets, make sure to check the manufacturer's tags and literature carefully. (Unfortunately, chemical-treatment information may not always be listed, but it generally can be obtained by contacting the manufacturer directly.) Mail-order companies handling untreated, unbleached flannel blankets include **The Richman Cotton Company** and **Janice Corp.**

COMFORTERS

Comforters made of natural fibers and natural stuffing are good, healthy alternatives to blankets. Comforters are lightweight, attractive, and warm. Although most stores handle synthetic-fabric polyester-filled versions, natural-fiber comforters are again becoming more popular. Some of these are made with untreated 100%-cotton fabric with loose fillings of cotton, wool, feathers, down, or a combination of feathers and down. Of all the available choices, comforters filled with pure down are generally considered the warmest. They're also usually the most expensive. However, feathers and down may have been treated with chemicals to discourage insect or microbial infestations (see *Feathers and Down* in *Chapter 3: Clothing*). This can become a problem for some sensitive individuals.

Untreated, 100%-cotton-filled comforters encased in untreated, all-cotton muslin or barrier cloth are sold by **Janice Corp.** Organic, 100%-cotton comforters with untreated all-cotton covers are offered by **Dona Designs** and **Heart of Vermont**. Untreated-wool comforters with untreated all-cotton muslin or barrier-cloth covers can be purchased from **Janice Corp.** On the other hand, **Heart of Vermont** uses organic wool stuffing with untreated, 100%-cotton fabric.

An unusual, all-natural comforter option is to buy an Ogallala down comforter from **N.E.E.D.S.** These particular comforters are covered with 100%-

cotton fabric and stuffed with a combination of white goose down and milk-weed floss. Twin, queen, and king sizes are offered in two weights (normal and Arctic). In addition, **The Seventh Generation** offers silk-stuffed comforters with green-cotton covers at surprisingly reasonable prices in twin, full/queen, and king sizes.

To properly clean your natural fiber and stuffing comforters, be sure to follow the care-instruction tags that came with them. You may find that some manufacturers recommend dry cleaning (see is *Dry-Cleaning A Problem?* in *Chapter 3: Clothing*). Others may suggest you machine-wash the comforter. If possible when buying them, always choose comforters that are washable so you won't have to be exposed to solvent odors. (Hanging your recently dry-cleaned comforters outside in clean air will help dissipate these odors.) To help minimize the frequency for cleaning, consider using washable untreated-cotton comforter covers. To freshen your comforters between cleanings, hang them outdoors in uncontaminated air.

COMFORTER COVERS

All-natural comforters can be expensive; in fact, they usually are. To help protect your investment, encase them in washable, untreated 100%-cotton comforter covers. These are designed to be easily removed for regular launderings, so you don't need to clean the comforters themselves as often. High-quality, untreated, all-cotton covers with a 300-thread count are available from **Janice Corp.** Organic, 100%-cotton comforter covers are offered by **Heart of Vermont**. They also handle untreated 100%-cotton comforter storage bags.

QUILTS

The quilts produced in recent decades have usually been made with polyester/cotton fabric coverings, although a few are still made with all-cotton coverings. Many of these new quilt coverings have been chemically treated for wrinkle-resistance and/or stain-resistance. Almost all the quilts on the market, no matter what the coverings are made of, are filled with polyester rather than cotton batting. This is because polyester batting is apparently better at resisting balling, bunching, and flattening, and it's usually less expensive than cotton batting.

Therefore, unless you commission someone to make a quilt for you, or you make it yourself, it can be difficult finding new quilts made of untreated 100%-cotton—both inside and out (For more on sewing, see *Custom-Made Clothes* in *Chapter 3: Clothing*). However, one source of organic 100%-cotton, lightweight summer quilts is **Dona Designs**.

Another approach to acquiring an all-cotton quilt is to buy an older (pre-1960) quilt. Unfortunately, older quilts may be contaminated with perfume, tobacco, mildew, or scents from air fresheners and detergents. They also may retain odors from previous owners' soaps and shampoos. If you are a sensitive person, any or all of these odors can be very bothersome. However, if a quilt isn't heavily saturated, airing it outdoors in the shade can often help. Of course, be sure the air is fresh and clean. Note that, it's important not to expose valuable antique quilts to the sun. Exposure to ultraviolet light could damage dyes or fibers.

BEDSPREADS

Bedspreads these days seem to becoming more and more elaborate. As with most modern bedding, they are often made almost exclusively of chemically treated synthetic materials. Some are washable, but others require dry cleaning. Unfortunately, dry cleaning is often intolerable to sensitive individuals (see *Is Dry Cleaning a Problem?* in *Chapter 3: Clothing*). Although they are relatively few and far between, 100% natural-fiber bedspreads are still possible to find.

From a health standpoint, washable, untreated, all-cotton construction is an ideal choice for bedspreads. Corduroy, cording, woven plaid, print, and tufted chenille are a just a few of the 100%-cotton bedspread styles currently available. Of these, corduroy and cording spreads are particularly tough and durable. Prints and woven spreads, which come in so many colors and styles, can be pleasing to a wide range of personal preferences. Depending on the pattern, tufted-chenille spreads can appeal to traditional, colonial, or contemporary tastes.

To find washable 100%-cotton bedspreads, especially in tufted chenille, you should check your local department stores. If you'd like woven, hand-printed, or batik styles at a reasonable cost, these can often be found in import shops. Through its catalog, **The Vermont Country Store** sells a number of washable 100%-cotton bedspreads. Those from **Janice Corp.** are untreated all-cotton spreads. Also, very attractive green-cotton bedspreads are sold by **The Seventh Generation**.

Tip: Between washings you can occasionally tumble your bedspreads in a warm or hot dryer for about fifteen minutes. This will help to remove any light surface dust.

TOWELING

Natural-fiber towels are soft, absorbent, biodegradable, and, thank goodness, still readily available in stores and catalogs.

BATH TOWELS

All-cotton bath towels remain popular, despite the introduction of less-expensive synthetic-blend towels. While all-cotton towels are relatively easy to find in local department and discount stores, you should know that not all of them are created equal. Generally, the most expensive towels are made from high-grade cottons such as *Pima*. (High-grade cottons have very soft, long fibers.) Less-expensive towels commonly use lower-grade cottons. This results in toweling with a stiffer, scratchier feel.

Another consideration when buying towels is their texture. Bath towels now come in *terry* (complete loops) or *velour-style* (cropped loops). Many people find looped-terry towels are more absorbent, but they're relatively easy to snag. On the other hand, velour towels tends to be less absorbent, but they retain their appearance longer. No matter which type you choose, the more loops per square inch (the thicker the loop density), the better the quality of the toweling. By the way, you'll also want to check a towel's *underweave* (the yarns woven between the loop rows). A firm, tightly woven underweave usually indicates durability.

Of course, color is also important when you buy towels. Sensitive people who find dyes bothersome, however, should only purchase natural, ecru, or white towels; these have very little or no added dye in them. Another plus for light-colored towels is they cause minimal color-bleeding problems when washed. Unfortunately, white or off-white towels can look gray as they age, especially if they're washed in hard water. Darker towels have the advantage that stains are far less noticeable on them. Overall, darker towels just look better over time than most light-colored towels.

One hundred percent cotton bath towels should be readily available in your local department stores, discount stores, and bath shops. In addition, catalogs such as **J.C. Penny Company, Inc.**, always offer a good variety. Other mail-order sources of untreated 100%-cotton towels include **The Cotton Place** and **Mother Hart**, and green-cotton towels are sold by **The Seventh Generation**. If you prefer to make your own towels, **The Cotton Place** offers untreated, 100%-cotton toweling fabric (For more on sewing, see *Custom-Made Clothes* in *Chapter 3: Clothing*).

KITCHEN TOWELS AND POT HOLDERS

In the kitchen, 100%-cotton dish towels are highly suggested over towels made of synthetic blends. Towels made of cotton are both natural and extremely absorbent, and from an environmental standpoint, are often preferred over paper towels. Fortunately, all-cotton dish towels are still commonly available at most local department and discount stores. Also, **Williams-Sonoma** has a good selection of fine-quality kitchen towels made of 100%-cotton duck or flour-sack material. Other mail-order sources include **Janice Corp.**, **Lillian Vernon**, and **The Cotton Place**. **The Seventh Generation** sells green-cotton dish towels.

Locating all-cotton potholders was once easy to do. Now, it's becoming far more difficult. Synthetic fabrics and stuffings, nonstick coatings, and fire-retardant treatments are very common today. Fortunately, **The Cotton Place** has plain all-cotton potholders. Untreated 100%-cotton hot pads and oven mitts are also available from **Mother Hart**.

TABLECLOTHS, PLACEMATS, AND NAPKINS

Washable, natural-fiber table linens can add warmth to any home without synthetic-fiber odors. Even better, from a health point of view, are natural-fiber table linens without any stain or wrinkle-resistant chemical treatments. Sometimes your local department stores and kitchen shops will handle a few types. They're also occasionally available in kitchen catalogs such as **Williams-Sonama** and **Colonial Garden Kitchens**. However, **The Vermont Country Store** regularly offers tablecloths, placemats, and napkins made of 100% cotton fabric.

In addition, **Janice Corp.** handles all-cotton placemats and napkins without stain-resistant chemicals. In addition, green-cotton placemats and napkins are sold by **The Seventh Generation**. Of course, you can always make your own table linens (For sewing information, see *Custom-Made Clothes* in *Chapter 3: Clothing*).

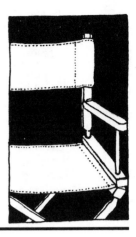

CHAPTER 5
INTERIOR DECORATING

Ever since men and women lived in caves, they've felt compelled to adorn their homes with paint and other materials, as well as objects, to add comfort and a sense of their own personalities to their interior surroundings. Most of the wall and window treatments, paints and stains, furniture, and floor coverings used today, while often attractive, can actually be sources of discomfort and illness. This is because many of the materials now used in decorating and furnishing are man-made creations that can outgas potentially harmful chemical odors.

As you begin to create your own healthy household, remember that while color and style are important, your primary decorating consideration should always be the potential health effects of what you put in your home. No matter what the current fashion dictates, your well-being and that of your family should always come first. Therefore, choosing less-toxic, low-odor finishes and materials is extremely important.

WALLS AND CEILINGS

In your house, you are surrounded by, and continually exposed to, hundreds of square feet of walls and ceilings. Because this represents a considerable surface area, it should be covered and decorated with materials that are as inert as possible.

WALL PAINT

Paints have been used since prehistoric times. For thousands of years, paint ingredients were natural substances. Most were fairly benign, but others, such as lead, were poisonous. As chemistry developed, and later as the use of petrochemical solvents and other compounds began to be used, paints continued to become potential sources of illness. Today, most typical paints can contain scores of ingredients including volatile organic compounds (VOCs) and synthetic biocides (see *Paints* in *Chapter 10: Home Workshop and Garage* and *Volatile Organic Compounds* in *Chapter 9: Indoor Air*).

Therefore, of all the interior decorating decisions you'll have to make, few will be as important as the wall paint you choose. You must keep in mind that once the paint is on the walls, it can't be easily removed, and putting another layer on top of it could cause even more problems as far as bothersome odors are concerned. You should be aware that all paint, even natural and low-toxicity brands, has a fairly strong odor when it's first applied. Then, too, you should keep in mind that the painting process itself can be expensive, disruptive, and labor-intensive. Therefore, before you decide to go ahead and paint, ask yourself if it is really necessary. You may decide that merely a thorough cleaning is all that's really needed.

If you decide to clean your walls rather than repaint them, consider using *trisodium-phosphate (TSP)*. This heavy-duty cleaner usually does a very good job of removing dirt and grime from painted surfaces. If you're unfamiliar with TSP, it's a white or clear crystalline powder that can be used as a powerful, unscented cleaning product. Usually, it's well-tolerated by most sensitive persons (For directions on cleaning walls with TSP, see *Cleaning Walls* in *Chapter 7: Cleaning*).

TESTING FOR LEAD

Surprising to many people, the existing paint on your walls could contain lead, and you don't have to live in a tenement house to have valid lead-paint concerns. The truth is, lead was still used as a paint ingredient up to the late 1970s. Fortunately though, if the paint is intact and not deteriorating, it may not be hazardous. However, if it's peeling, or if you plan to scrape or sand it, you must first make sure your wall paint is indeed lead-free.

LeadCheck Swabs (**HybriVet Systems, Inc.**) and Lead Alert (**Frandon Enterprises**) are two products that can be used to test paint for lead's presence. Both can be purchased directly from the manufacturers. If the lead test is positive, you should contact your local board of health for suggestions and regulations how to proceed. *Never* sand or scrape lead-containing paint yourself, especially without taking proper precautions. Lead particles that are ingested or inhaled can cause mental retardation in children and serious illness in adults (see *Lead* in *Chapter 9: Indoor Air*).

For additional information on lead, call the EPA's **National Lead Information Center** hot line at (800) 532-3394. The agency offers printed material about lead poisoning and preventive measures you can take. Also included is a list of state and local agencies that can provide further help.

CHOOSING THE RIGHT PAINT

Many people, especially sensitive individuals, ask, "What paint should I buy that will be safe for me and my family?" As it turns out, there are a growing number of alternative healthier brands you can choose from. (See *Paints* in *Chapter 12: Home Workshop and Garage*.) Because of personal tolerances, personal preferences (for example, all-natural ingredients or synthetic bright colors or neutral ones, and basic paint type such as latex or acrylic), as well as the particular requirements of the room (scrubbable walls for kitchens and moisture-resistant ones for bathrooms) there is no one single correct paint for all people for all jobs.

For very sensitive people, it's really best to purchase small samples of several different brands and test each one for personal tolerance (see *Testing Finishes* in *Chapter 12: Home Workshop and Garage*). In fact, sensitive people should probably *never* do any painting without first testing the product. Besides determining tolerability, testing helps you judge a paint's appearance (color and sheen), coverage, and scrubbability. Because test samples should air out for a period of time, testing should be started well in advance of any painting project. Sensitive people in particular should not expect to test a paint today and use it tomorrow. Testing takes time, sometimes several weeks, and if it's done early and thoroughly, the entire painting process should go much more smoothly.

While it's impossible to actually recommend a specific paint, in general most sensitive people seem to tolerate one or more of the alternative low-odor water-based paints currently on the market. These paints usually cover well, and they don't require turpentine, alcohol, or paint thinner for cleanup. As a rule, alternative water-based paints contain fewer additives than their typical paint-store counterparts. However, each manufacturer has his own idea of what ingredients to eliminate from conventional paint formulas. For example, Series 2000 interior latex paint (**Glidden Co.**) contains no volatile organic compounds (VOCs) (see *Volatile Organic Compounds* in *Chapter 9: Indoor Air*). Other paint manufacturers avoid biocides. Still others eliminate all synthetic ingredients.

Of course, whenever you choose a paint, color is an important consideration. If you pick a neutral color, such as white, almond, ecru, or pearl gray, you're more likely to be able to live with it for a long time. Unusual or intense colors, though exciting at first, can quickly grow tiresome. This may lead you to repaint after only two or three years. Another plus for neutral colors is that they provide the most decorating options, and they're always in style. In addition, neutral tones can be used as ceiling paints. This eliminates the need to buy separate wall and ceiling paints, while at the same time hastening the actual painting process. Using all neutral colors will also create a room that appears more spacious. By the way, some alternative water-based paints *only* come in neutral colors.

Still another paint consideration is its sheen. Products are often sold in *gloss*, *semigloss*, and/or *flat* formulas. Flat paint minimizes the appearance of any flaws or imperfections on walls. However, flat paints are usually not as durable or washable as gloss paints. Gloss paint works well on doors and trim. However on walls, its reflective qualities are often considered somewhat unattractive. As a compromise, many people find that semigloss paint works fine on both walls and woodwork. A flat paint often works out well on a ceiling. Note that, for kitchens and bathrooms, semigloss or gloss are good choices because they are better able to resist moisture and are easier to clean than flat paint.

You should be aware that most alternative paints must be ordered through the mail. One exception is the Series 2000 (**Glidden Co.**), which is often available through local Glidden dealers. (Contact the company for an outlet near you.) Whenever you're ready to begin a painting project, be sure to initially purchase enough paint so you won't run out while actually painting a room. Reordering can mean a delay while you wait for additional paint to arrive. This can be costly in terms of both labor and time, especially if the paint must be mail-ordered. There is also the possibility your new cans of paint could come from a different batch, resulting in slightly different colors. If that happens, it's possible your new paint may not perfectly match what's already been used so far.

Because all paint has an odor when first applied, you may have to make special arrangements during and after painting. Unfortunately, it isn't unusual for sensitive people to find fresh paint odors unacceptable for up to several weeks or even several months. Ideally, to help quicken the time for your newly painted walls to become tolerable, paint only during those months when you can have the windows open for long periods of time. In addition, you'll find that using window fans is often helpful. If you are extremely sensitive, you may actually need to find temporary accommodations elsewhere until the paint loses it's "newness."

THE PAINTING PROCESS

Before they're painted, any home's walls should be in good condition. This will guarantee a more attractive, long-lasting finish. If the walls are dirty, you can clean them with a solution of TSP (trisodium phosphate) in water, then rinse them. TSP is a white or clear crystalline powder that works as a powerful, unscented cleaner that even many sensitive persons can tolerate. (For more information how to clean walls with TSP, see *Cleaning Walls* in *Chapter 7: Cleaning*.)

After the walls have been cleaned, fill all the nail holes and imperfections with a low-odor product such as Murco Hi-po Drywall Compound (**Murco Wall Products, Inc.**). Murco is packaged as a dry powder in 25-pound bags. Even though you may only need a small amount for patching, it's relatively inexpensive and can be stored indefinitely, if it's kept dry. To purchase Murco drywall compound, simply order it directly from the manufacturer. (For other wall patching product choices, see *Drywall Compounds* in *Chapter 12: Home Workshop and Garage*.)

When you are ready to begin painting, remove as much of your furniture from the room as possible. Then protect what you can't take out, as well as the floors, with drop cloths. Washable, 100%-cotton canvas drop cloths are probably the best type. While old bed sheets are often used, they generally aren't thick enough to prevent paint from penetrating through them. Of course, plastic drop cloths are readily available in stores. They're inexpensive and can be thrown away after painting, but they can outgas bothersome odors when new. However in reality, they probably won't be as bothersome as the fresh paint itself.

It's important to make sure there's plenty of ventilation whenever the painting is in progress and until after all the odors have dissipated. It's also a good idea for the person actually doing the painting to wear a cartridge-type respirator mask. These masks can usually be found in local hardware stores. Other protective measures would include wearing a long-sleeved shirt and a hat (to prevent paint from dripping onto the body). If you plan to paint overhead, protective eyewear is highly recommended (see *Protective Gear* in *Chapter*

12: Home Workshop and Garage). As a rule, sensitive individuals should never actually apply the paint themselves, but have someone else do the work for them.

OTHER WALL TREATMENTS

Of course, there are other wall decorating options besides painting. The following sections will offer some examples and help to explain why some are healthier choices than others.

WALLPAPER

In Europe during the late 1400s, strips of decorative paper were first glued on the walls of a few homes. By the mid-1700s, the use of wallpaper became more commonplace. At that time, many types of wallpaper were available; nearly all were made by hand with block-printed designs. By 1850, most wallpapers consisted of continuous paper rolls rather than separate strips and the patterns were then printed by printing presses. Today, most wallpapers are still manufactured in basically the same way. Because of the wide array of designs, surface textures, etc., wallpaper is a more popular wall treatment than ever. Despite the fact that it's relatively inexpensive and a quick method to give any room a new look wallpaper is not often suggested for use in healthy households. Here's why:

Wallpaper Types

Truly healthy wallpapers are extremely difficult to find. This is because most of the wallpapers manufactured today are either all-vinyl or vinyl-coated. Unfortunately, vinyl wallpapers have the potential to outgas synthetic chemical odors which can bother sensitive people. Even if they're first unrolled in an uncontaminated garage to air a few weeks, often the remaining vinyl odors can still be a problem.

On the other hand, old-fashioned paper wallpapers don't give off vinyl odors, but they're often attacked by microorganisms and they can't easily be washed. Natural-fiber coverings, such as jute or grass, are sometimes available. However, they can be treated with potentially harmful chemical biocides to prevent insect or mold damage. Like paper wallpaper, these coverings are difficult to clean. Natural-fiber fabrics can be glued directly to walls, but they're also virtually impossible to care for.

Of all the varieties of wall coverings available, foil papers seem to be one of the better choices. Their aluminum foil surfaces are inert and they can often seal in odors originating from the paper backing, the paste, and even the walls themselves. Foil papers are also generally washable. However, wallpaper pastes may not dry quickly underneath foil papers, which could lead to hidden mold or mildew problems. You may have difficulty finding outlets that handle aluminum-foil-faced/paper-backed wallpapers.

You should be aware that the adhesives used to attach wallpapers or wall coverings can pose additional problems. For example, starch-based pastes can provide appealing food for mold, mildew, and other microorganisms. Also, some adhesives contain chemical biocides which can be intolerable for some sensitive individuals. Others that are used to glue heavy coverings are sometimes made of strong-smelling synthetic compounds.

An option to covering an entire wall with wallpaper or any other wall covering is to use decorative border strips. These minimize all the problems associated with wallpapering simply because they cover much less area. Border strips are now being manufactured in a wide variety of patterns and colors. Although they're just a few inches wide, they can add new visual interest to any room by providing an attractive band of color. Border strips are generally used on walls just below the ceiling, but you might consider other possibilities. For example, they can be used around all window and door frames, or to surround a room at chair-rail height.

The Wallpapering Process

If you decide to go ahead and use wallpaper, make certain the old, painted wall surfaces are properly prepared. First, a thorough cleaning is usually necessary to remove surface grease that could prevent good adhesion. One excellent cleaning method is to use a solution of TSP (trisodium phosphate) and water. TSP is a white or clear crystalline powder that can be used as a powerful, unscented cleaner. It's often well-tolerated even by very sensitive persons. (For directions on washing walls with TSP, see *Cleaning Walls* in *Chapter 7: Cleaning.*)

Next, fill any nail holes or other wall imperfections with a low-odor spackling compound. Many sensitive people find that Murco Hi-po Drywall Compound (**Murco Wall Products, Inc.**) works well for this job. Murco is sold in powdered form and is mixed with water just before being used. Murco can be ordered directly from the manufacturer. (For other products, see *Drywall Compounds* in *Chapter 12: Home Workshop and Garage.*) Some wallpaper manufacturers next recommend an application of *sizing* to the walls. Sizing is generally a starchy glue product that creates better adhesion. However, some of these materials may contain biocides that could be bothersome to sensitive individuals.

When you need to choose a wallpaper paste, consider Golden Harvest Wheat Paste (**Golden Harvest, Inc.**), sold by many local wallpaper stores. Surprisingly, Golden Harvest Wheat Paste is made almost entirely of natural vegetable starches and contains no fungicides. However, in those situations where mold and mildew growth could be a concern, you might want to add 1 tablespoon of boric acid powder to each quart of the paste. Boric acid is an effective mineral biocide that is generally less of a problem for sensitive individuals than are synthetic biocides. (See also *Wallpaper Pastes* in *Chapter 12: The Home Workshop and Garage.*) Note that, wallpapers with prepasted backings may contain bothersome ingredients, including synthetic chemical fungicides and glues.

Stripping Wallpaper

At some point, wallpapers usually need to be removed. As anyone who has done this can say, it can be a horrible, time-consuming, and messy job. Scraping the paper can create irritating and harmful dust, and it can damage the walls. Steam equipment is popular, but the heat and moisture can activate dormant mold spores and/or cause the release of biocides into the air. Very old wallpapers sometimes contained arsenic compounds to inhibit mold growth. Because of all these potential health concerns, wearing a cartridge-type respirator mask, rubber gloves, and protective eyewear, and having plenty of ventilation when tackling this chore is essential. (See *Protective Gear* in *Chapter 12: Home Workshop and Garage.*) This is definitely *not* a job for sensitive persons.

STENCILING AND MARBLEIZING

An interesting and usually much healthier alternative to wallpaper is *stenciling*. Actually, stenciling has been used to decorate walls for thousands of years. In the last few years, it's gained renewed popularity because it's such a simple and fun way to make large plain surfaces more exciting. In stenciling, paint is lightly dabbed over a cutout pattern (now usually made of clear plastic) to form a uniform surface design. Bands of stenciled patterns can be used around windows and doors, just below the ceiling line, or surrounding a room at chair-rail height. In some cases, a repeating pattern used all over the surface of a wall can create a visual statement similar to that of wallpaper. Actually, with stenciling you are only limited by your imagination. Other similar creative wall treatments include *marbleizing* (using paint in such a way as to imitate the color and veining of natural marble) and *texturizing* (using paint to give the illusion of wood or to create free-form designs). All these are often surprisingly easy to do.

Stenciling equipment such as plastic patterns, brushes, sponges, special texturizing tools, and instruction books can usually be purchased at your local wallpaper outlets and craft stores. Of course, sensitive people should only use paints that have been tested first for personal tolerance. (See *Testing Finishes* and also *Paints* in *Chapter 12: Home Workshop and Garage.*) Whenever you use paints, it's a good idea to wear proper protective gear including eye protection and a cartridge-type respirator mask and to have plenty of ventilation. If you are very sensitive, you'll probably need to have someone else do the work. In fact, you may need to be out of the house entirely while it's being done.

WOOD PANELING

Wood paneling can give a room an entirely new look, while at the same time covering damaged walls. However, for anyone wanting a healthy house, it's wise to avoid man-made wood paneling. Although it is relatively cheap and easy to install, virtually all types of man-made paneling are constructed with *urea-formaldehyde (UF)* glue. Unfortunately, UF glue emits high levels of harmful formaldehyde—much more than from the *phenol-formaldehyde (PF)*, which is commonly used in construction-grade products. (See *Formaldehyde* in *Chapter 9: Indoor Air* as well as *Man-Made Wood Products* in *Chapter 12: Home Workshop and Garage.*) In addition, man-made paneling is generally created, all or in part, from softwoods. Softwoods can give off strong natural *terpene* odors that can be bothersome to some sensitive people (see *Solid Wood* in *Chapter 12: Home Workshop and Garage*).

A healthier alternative to man-made paneling is traditional, solid-hardwood, tongue-and-groove boards. (Again, softwoods such as pine are sometimes not tolerable for sensitive people because of terpene odors.) Solid hardwood paneling has always been associated with the dining halls, dens, libraries, and other rooms of the well-to-do. As a result, most people today don't even consider using hardwood paneling because they just assume it's going to cost too much. However, it can be affordable, if you choose the right wood.

For example, tulip poplar is actually a relatively inexpensive hardwood species. It's also attractive and easy to work with (see *Solid Wood* in *Chapter 12: Home Workshop and Garage* for other wood choices). To further reduce your costs, you can the install the solid-wood paneling on just one wall, rather than on all four. Odds are, this will still provide the atmosphere you had in mind. Another less-costly wall paneling option is to use *wainscoting*. Typically, wainscoting is paneling that's applied to only the lower third of walls. It can be an excellent decorating choice for dens, family rooms, and dining areas. Simply applying chair-rail molding is even less expensive, and yet it can still dress up a room. Chair-rail molding is typically a 2–3" wide strip of decoratively cut and shaped solid wood. It's usually mounted horizontally, one-third of the way up the walls.

To find solid hardwood paneling and molding, check nearby lumberyards to see what they stock or can order for you. Also, there may be mills in your part of the country that can supply material made from locally grown wood. (Check your classified telephone directory.) You might also check with the Industrial Arts teacher at the local high school. When you are ready for installation, try to avoid using construction adhesives whenever possible. Instead, use only nails or screws. Construction adhesives can contain potentially harmful ingredients and they're nearly always very odorous. However, there are a few less-toxic water-based products that are now starting to appear on the market that you may want to try—if an adhesive must be used.

Wood stains can be bothersome to some sensitive people. To avoid the problem, simply leave the wood its natural color. To protect paneling or molding, it should be coated with a tolerable clear finish. Whoever does this work should wear proper protective gear and have plenty of ventilation. As with painting, this type of work should generally not be done by sensitive individuals themselves.

Tip: To minimize construction odors indoors, cut, stain, and finish your solid-wood trim or paneling outdoors or in a garage. If the prefinished wood is allowed to air out for an extended period of time afterwards, it may be inert enough to be installed inside without requiring a sensitive person to leave the premises.

FLOORING

Your choice of floor covering is extremely important, namely because it covers a large surface area, costs you a great deal of money, and has the potential to greatly affect your well-being. Health considerations regarding flooring are especially important, not only for certain sensitive adults, but also for all children. After all, children generally play for hours directly on the floor, so they are often closer to it than adults.

CARPETING

Most people are still not aware that carpeting can pose health dangers. This is too bad because it often can. Sadly, many individuals with Multiple Chemical Sensitivity (MCS) (see *MCS, A New Medical Condition* in *Chapter 1: Getting Started*) have attributed the onset of their illness to newly laid carpets. The truth is, you needn't put down carpeting just because everyone else does; there *are* other flooring options.

The following sections will discuss typical carpet and it's problems, and offer a few healthier carpeting choices—if you still feel that's what you want.

CARPET DEVELOPMENTS

Carpeting is defined as any heavy fabric that is permanently attached to a floor. Its use goes back thousands of years to the Orient. In the West, it periodically goes in and out of favor. Today, carpeting is fashionable. In fact, since World War II, wall-to-wall carpeting has become the norm in virtually all U.S. homes.

At one time, only natural dyes were used to color the yarns that made up carpeting. However, as early as the 1880s, synthetic *aniline dyes* started replacing the natural coloring agents (aniline is a toxic oily liquid derived from *nitrobenzene*).

Up until the 1950s, the carpet yarns themselves were still made almost exclusively of natural-fibers, such as cotton or wool. Then in the late 1950s, a revolution occurred in carpet manufacturing: New equipment became available that could *tuft* yarn into a backing material (a tuft is a loop of yarn fastened at its base). At about the same time, a new process was invented that allowed thin nylon yarns to take on a bulky quality called *loft*. These developments meant that new synthetic carpets could be produced much more quickly and sell for much less money than their traditionally made counterparts of the past.

Today, 97% of all machine-made carpets consist of synthetic fibers, and about 90% of these are tufted. Generally, the tufts are held into place with a latex compound. In addition, stain and wear-resistant treatments are commonly applied to the yarn fibers. Backing materials in modern carpets are either natural jute or man-made materials. Sometimes, the entire backing receives an additional vinyl coating or a layer of foam-cushioning. Carpets without a layer of foam attached to the back must generally have some other form of padding underneath in order to minimize carpet wear and provide comfort underfoot. Often, a synthetic foam material is used, although other types of padding are available.

TYPICAL CARPET AND PADDING CONCERNS

With all the synthetic components in new carpeting, it's not surprising that it often outgasses a hundred (or more) different chemical compounds including xylene, ethylbenzene, and methacrylic acid. Unfortunately, a number of these chemicals are known to be toxic. Interestingly, experiments performed at an independent laboratory (Anderson Laboratories Inc.) in Dedham, Massachusetts, have found that laboratory mice that breath air first blown across certain carpet samples suffered severe neurological symptoms as a result of their exposures. So severely were some of these mice affected, a few of them died. Some of the carpet samples that became *rodenticides* (mouse killers) were from brand-new synthetic carpeting—but others were taken from carpets as much as eight years old. On the October 29, 1992, broadcasts of the "CBS Evening News with Dan Rather" and "Street Stories," these findings were reported. However, despite this publicity, little has been done to resolve the problem of toxic carpets, and the popular media seems to have lost interest in the issue altogether.

Some people believe that if their carpeting is made of all-natural yarns, it's inherently safer and won't cause them any health problems. Unfortunately, even carpets made with 100% wool or 100% cotton can sometimes be intolerable for sensitive people. This is because of the chemicals used during the yarn and carpet milling processes (wool is often treated with mothproofing chemicals), and because of the odors that can be given off by carpet backing and padding, many of which are made of synthetic materials. In addition, all carpeting, whether all-natural or not, acts as a highly effective allergen reservoir. In fact, vast quantities of dirt particles and pollen grains, as well as tens of millions of microorganisms (mold spores, dust mites, and other microbes) are actually present in *each* square foot of carpet.

Another problem with carpeting is that it eventually wears out as the integrity of the surface yarns breaks down. When that occurs, the fibers making up these yarns become house dust. If they happen to be synthetic fibers and they come into contact with a hot surface (such as a furnace or baseboard heater), tiny amounts of *phosgene* (also known as chloroformyl chloride, a deadly nerve gas), or *hydrogen cyanide* (used in gas chambers) can be produced. Even though only very minute quantities would be formed, *no* amount of these gases is good to breathe.

Quite frankly, wall-to-wall carpeting is simply *not* a healthy flooring. Other options, such as solid wood or ceramic-tile floors, are long-lasting and usually pose minimal health risks. Although they can cost more to buy and to install than carpeting, the added expenses can be justified. Wood and tile usually last a very long time; they're often considered permanent. However, carpeting needs to be replaced about every eight years or so. Therefore, over a floor's lifetime, carpeting has a higher per-year-of-use cost than wood or tile floors. You should also keep in mind that if a new carpet causes you or a family member to have chronic ill health, you should factor in the costs of medical bills. Admittedly, this sounds a bit dramatic, but is new wall-to-wall carpeting really worth the risk? For even more information on carpet-related health issues, contact the **Toxic Carpet Information Exchange.**

HEALTHIER CARPET AND PADDING

Despite learning all the negatives associated with carpeting, some people still want it on their floors anyway. For those individuals, a few carpet choices tend to be healthier than others. Be aware though that despite outgassing fewer chemical compounds, these carpets still have the potential to become reservoirs for dirt, pollen, and literally millions of microorganisms.

Healthier Carpet Suggestions

One of the healthier options is to buy carpet made from 100%-wool yarn. Very fine local carpet stores may have some. However, a good mail-order source of wool carpet is **Hendericksen Natürlich Flooring and Interiors.** The company also sells carpeting made with sisal or jute yarns. An undyed, natural jute carpet called GoldSpun—available in 12' x 50' rolls—can be purchased from **World Fiber**. To order, call the company directly.

Another less-toxic choice is carpet made from 100%-cotton yarn. Again, a few local stores may possibly handle it. A mail-order source is **Nontoxic Environments**, which offers all-cotton carpet in an undyed, natural tone or custom-dyed in a variety of colors. **Carousel Carpet Mills** sells both Casual Trends and Cotton Trends natural-fiber carpeting, made without latex backings. However, this carpeting is quite expensive; expect to pay as much as $200 per yard.

Also, **Flowright International Products** offers nylon carpeting in a range of colors. Unlike most of the nylon carpeting sold in stores, the fibers of this carpet have not been subjected to chemical soil-resisting treatments. In addition, **Harbinger Carpet** is now actively involved in developing a conventional synthetic carpeting with reduced rates of chemical outgassing. If you're interested in these particular carpets, you can contact the companies for additional information.

You should be aware that unrolling any new carpeting where it can air for several weeks will help diminish, but probably not eliminate, many of its bothersome odors. Ideally, it's best to choose a place that's dry, uncontaminated by unwanted odors, and has good ventilation. After the carpet installation job, some people have applied a special coating designed to help seal in any remaining odors. One product of this type is SafeChoice Carpet Guard (**American Formulating and Manufacturing (AFM)**), which has been described as a "water soluble siliconate." It's sold by AFM dealers such as **N.E.E.D.S.**, **The Living Source**, and **Nontoxic Environments**. Unfortunately, the reported results from using odor-stopping carpet coatings are mixed.

Healthier Padding Suggestions

Ideally, the padding under your carpet should be as nontoxic and odor-free as the carpet itself. Some sensitive people assume that natural jute padding would be a healthy choice. Unfortunately, some jute padding can contain potentially bothersome binding agents made from synthetic resins, or biocides. However, in its favor, all-jute products are naturally fire-resistant. One jute padding you might find acceptable is Jute Carpet Felt (**World Fibre**) (test a sample first if you are a sensitive person, see *Testing* in *Chapter 1: Getting Started*). It's made of non-dyed waste jute thread and comes in 4.5' x 197.5' rolls. You'll need to call the company for purchasing information, but be aware that delivery could take as long as three months.

Another padding option is 100%-nylon padding, which is often tolerable for sensitive people. It's available in some local carpet stores. It can also be mail-ordered from **Hendericksen Natürlich Flooring and Interiors** as well as **Flowright International Products**.

HARDWOOD FLOORING

Hardwood flooring is an attractive, healthful option that has been available for years. So ancient is the use of wood flooring that it was probably one of the first permanent flooring materials to replace earthen floors. Today, hardwood floors are still being installed in homes, yet wood flooring is now far less popular that carpet or vinyl.

HARDWOOD FLOORING TYPES

Originally, hardwood floors were made with relatively thick solid-wood planks. Unfortunately, laminated-wood flooring products are more commonly used in new construction and remodeling. Laminated flooring is constructed of a thin, attractive, hardwood top layer glued to a less-costly plywood or other man-made wood-product base-layer. Laminated wood flooring nearly always comes both prestained and prefinished. There are several drawbacks to using these laminated wood products for flooring. First, unlike solid wood flooring, the thin top lamination layer can't be sanded or refinished in the future. Another minus is the fact that laminated floors often require an offensive adhesive product to hold them in place. (However, some laminated wood flooring can be adhered with a less-toxic white glue or a yellow carpenter's glue.) As a result, these floors have the potential to outgas bothersome chemicals emanating from the laminating glues, the synthetic finishes, and the flooring adhesives.

A healthier choice would be to use the more-costly solid-wood flooring. While initially more expensive to purchase, it's extremely long-lasting. In fact, if the surface of the solid-wood planks should ever become badly marred or damaged, they can simply be sanded and refinished. Another plus is that solid-wood floors usually don't require potentially bothersome adhesives; they can often be nailed down.

Today, solid hardwood flooring comes either unfinished or prefinished. If you purchase unfinished, you can use the tolerable finishes of *your* choice. The wood itself is available as long tongue-and-groove strips and planks, or as *parquet squares* (short strips or blocks of wood glued into decorative patterns). While parquet is attractive, the glues used to hold it together can be bothersome to sensitive persons, and some parquet flooring must be glued down (rather than nailed). Furthermore, parquet patterns often become tiring to look at over time.

You should be aware that solid-wood flooring (strips or planks) comes in several grades. *Clear grades* have no imperfections and a uniform color. On the other hand, *#2 or #3 grades* have more color variation and occasional knots, and they are much more affordable. In addition, the wider and longer the strips, the more expensive they'll be.

Ideally, if you are very sensitive, you'll want to choose a low-odor hardwood species for your floor, such as maple, birch, or beech. These have far less odor than the more commonly used red or white oak (see *Solid Wood* and also *Testing Woods in Chapter 12: Home Workshop and Garage*). Softwoods, such as yellow pine, can be less expensive. The naturally occurring pine-terpene odors can be unacceptable to some sensitive persons. However, softwood flooring is often an acceptable and less-costly flooring material for people who aren't chemically sensitive. Sometimes, solid hardwood (or softwood) flooring is available through local lumberyards, building centers, and flooring specialty stores. Also, in a few parts of the country local woodworking mills can supply flooring made from regionally grown timber. (To find such a mill, check your classified telephone directory under Woodworking, Lumber, or Flooring Manufacturers.)

FINISHING HARDWOOD FLOORS

Unfortunately, the stains and clear finishes used on hardwood floors can pose problems. While some prefinished wood flooring can be okay for sensitive individuals, it's generally better to apply finishes that have proven to be tolerable after the flooring has been installed. You may want to seriously consider omitting stain and letting the natural beauty of the wood show through. If you decide not to stain, you've certainly eliminated one potentially bothersome product. At any rate, some woods, such as maple, don't stain particularly well anyway. (If you choose to stain, see *Stains* in *Chapter 12: Home Workshop and Garage.*)

Because the clear protective finish applied to your hardwood floors is exposed directly to the living space, it must be chosen with care. As a general rule, water-based polyurethane floor finishes usually work very well for many sensitive individuals. These finishes tend to lose most of their odor within a week, and yet they're very durable. Aqua Zar (**United Glisonite Laboratories**) is one water-based polyurethane product that is widely available, but there are several similar brands on the market. (Clear finishes including waxes and other types of water-based products are discussed in *Chapter 12: Home Workshop and Garage.*)

Whenever any staining or finishing job is being done, the person doing the work should wear a cartridge-type respirator mask and eye protection and have good ventilation (see *Protective Gear* in *Chapter 12: Home Workshop and Garage*). Obviously, this isn't a project for a sensitive individual to do themselves. In fact, he or she may need to make arrangements to live elsewhere during the finishing process—and for several days or even weeks afterwards—until the outgassing chemical odors have dissipated.

LINOLEUM

At one time, *linoleum* was the most popular kitchen flooring and countertop material. Traditionally, it was made with oxidized linseed oil, ground cork or wood flour, and *rosin* (a type of resin formed from the distillation of oil of turpentine), or other plant resins. This mixture was then pressed onto a burlap or felt backing under high heat and pressure. Generally, it was available in rolls or square tiles.

Linoleum had many good qualities. Besides being all-natural, it was *resilient* (returns to its original shape after being compressed), dimensionally stable at varying temperatures and humidities, fairly easy to clean, resistant to burning, and less expensive than ceramic tile. However by the 1960s, linoleum began to be rapidly replaced by vinyl. This was primarily because vinyl flooring was available in brighter patterns and required less maintenance.

MODERN LINOLEUM

Surprising to many people, natural linoleum is still available today in rolls. It's gained renewed, but limited, popularity, primarily because it continues to have an all-natural ingredient list. Modern linoleum is still made of linseed oil, pine resins, powdered wood, and jute backing. Sometimes termed *battleship linoleum* (because of the drab, gray-colored material used for art projects and industrial applications over the years), linoleum flooring is now available in a variety of solid colors and marbleized patterns. These colors are not just surface treatments; they actually extend through the entire thickness of the material.

If you are considering linoleum for your floor, you should be aware that it's often not tolerated very well by sensitive persons, despite being an all-natural product. In addition, linoleum has a rather strong, innate odor that can be bothersome, and it is more susceptible to water damage than vinyl. If you'd like to purchase natural linoleum, it's handled by several companies, including **Forbo North America**, **Nontoxic Environments**, and **Hendricksen Natürlich Flooring and Interiors**.

LINOLEUM FLOORING INSTALLATION

In most installations, linoleum is glued directly to the surface of the subfloor. Many of the mastics and adhesives manufactured for this job are made of petrochemicals, which can be extremely odorous. Fortunately, **Nontoxic Environments** sells two alternative products, including an all-natural formula imported from Germany. However, even these products may prove too bothersome to some sensitive individuals (see *Testing Adhesives* in *Chapter 12: Home Workshop and Garage*).

Therefore, plenty of ventilation is advised if an adhesive is used. It is also a good idea for whoever is doing the actual installation work to wear a cartridge-type respiratory mask as a precaution. This type of work isn't recommended for sensitive persons to do themselves. Actually, it's often possible to install linoleum without any adhesives. To do this, first remove the room's baseboard molding. Then cut the linoleum to fit closely up to the walls. Finally, replace the molding; if it rests firmly on top of the linoleum, it will hold it in place. If you do this, you may need to install a threshold at doorways to hold the linoleum down.

Once laid, the linoleum's surface must be sealed to protect it against moisture and scuffing. These sealant coatings may also help reduce the natural odor of the linoleum, but they'll add their own characteristic odor which can be a problem in their own right. To purchase linoleum sealants, check with your linoleum supplier. Sensitive people should test both the linoleum and the sealer prior to installing an entire floor (see *Testing* in *Chapter 1: Getting Started* and *Testing Finishes* in *Chapter 12: Home Workshop and Garage*). It is often a good idea to test a piece of linoleum with the finish already applied. One sealing product you might try is One Step Seal and Shine (**American Formulating and Manufacturing (AFM)**). It's available from **Nontoxic Environments** and other AFM dealers.

VINYL FLOORING

Vinyl flooring has become commonplace in kitchens, bathrooms, utility rooms, and recreation rooms since the early 1960s. Vinyl has virtually replaced linoleum as a flooring material because it is fairly low in cost, attractive, simple to install, easy to care for, and available in many styles and patterns. (Most of the vinyl flooring now being made doesn't need sealants, protecting compounds, or special sheen products.)

VINYL FLOORING TYPES

Vinyl flooring is available in both sheet goods and individual tiles through local flooring stores and building-supply centers. Unlike linoleum, vinyl is made primarily of a synthetically derived resin, usually thermoplastic polyvinyl chloride (PVC). However, pure PVC is actually a very stiff material, so it's combined with noxious *plasticizing compounds* to make it soft and supple. Although the ingredients making up vinyl flooring can certainly outgas potentially bothersome chemical odors, these often cause fewer problems than those given off by carpeting. (Carpet can release one hundred or more different compounds for years.) With vinyl floors, you also get the advantage of having a relatively impenetrable, smooth surface: one that's water-resistant, unable to harbor millions of dust mites, pollen grains, and mold spores, and one that's easy to sweep or wash clean.

Several grades of vinyl flooring are available in stores. The more expensive types are fabricated with a thick clear top layer, a thick middle layer with an inlaid pattern, and a spongy foam backing on the bottom. The foam is added to provide better *resiliency* (the ability to return to its original form after being compressed), thus creating a cushioned surface that is more comfortable to walk on. Unfortunately, in order to manufacture cushioned floors, additional amounts of potentially bothersome plasticizers are added to the vinyl to prevent the floor from cracking. Incidentally, the foam backings themselves can outgas additional odors. However, the backing is usually sealed in by the upper vinyl layers, so the backing's odors don't usually reach the room air.

Of the various vinyl flooring options on the market, it's probably wise to choose harder vinyl products, at least from a health standpoint. This is because fewer plasticizing chemicals are used in their production. Self-sticking tiles should also be considered because they eliminate the need for more-odorous mastic compounds that are required to adhere other vinyl-flooring products in place.

VINYL FLOORING INSTALLATION

If you decide to use vinyl sheet flooring, your exposure to its outgassing chemicals can be reduced by first unrolling it in an unpolluted place. This can be outdoors, on a porch, in an empty garage, or anywhere that's dry and uncontaminated by objectionable odors. Generally, new vinyl flooring will need to air for at least several days. Some sensitive persons find it necessary to leave it unrolled for several weeks. Once the flooring has lost its odor, it can then be brought indoors and installed.

While most vinyl flooring is held in place by adhesives, it is possible to completely avoid them. In many cases the flooring can be held in place with just the baseboard molding that surrounds the perimeter of the room (see *Linoleum Flooring Installation* above). However, adhesives are sometimes necessary. They definitely are needed where two sheets of vinyl flooring abut each other. Actually, at these junctures the two edges are often *welded* together. This is accomplished using a special synthetic compound that dissolves the butting edges of both vinyl sheets. After the liquefied vinyl has cured, the seam becomes invisible. Seam-welding is actually accompanied by a several-inch-wide band of adhesive under each side of the seam.

In other installations, adhesives are used more extensively. But whenever they are necessary, they should always be water-based mastics and adhesives rather than solvent-based types. This is because the water-based versions are usually less toxic and less odorous. A number of water-based products are probably available through your local flooring supplier. One you may want to try 3-in-1 Adhesive (**American Formulating and Manufacturing (AFM)**) sold by **Nontoxic Environments** and other AFM dealers. Of course, the use of adhesives, mastics, or synthetic welding fluids *always* requires plenty of ventilation and use of a cartridge-type respirator mask. Sensitive individuals probably should not to do this type of installation themselves.

CERAMIC TILE

Ceramic tile is made of baked natural clays, sometimes with a glass-like glaze on the surface. It's actually one of the world's oldest flooring materials. Although it's been out of favor for awhile, it's now being used more and more. This is good news because ceramic tile can be one of the healthiest of flooring choices.

CHOOSING CERAMIC TILE

Ceramic tile has usually been thought of as a flooring for bathrooms and kitchens, but it can provide a natural, durable, easy-to-maintain floor for any room in the house. As a result, some healthy homes are now being built with ceramic-tile floors throughout. With tiles available in a wide variety of sizes, shapes, colors, and surface textures, ceramic-tile floors can be very attractive. While it's easier to lay ceramic tile directly on a concrete slab, it can be installed over other surfaces, so it's use is not limited by the type of subfloor your house has.

Many people assume that ceramic tile is out of their price range. However, there are generally less-expensive tile lines sold through building-supply centers. Often, *seconds* (tiles with minor surface imperfections) are available at a surprisingly low cost. In addition, if homeowners do the installation work themselves, labor costs are virtually eliminated. Actually, only a few tools are needed to cut and shape the tiles, and these are sold at tile stores. Tile cutters can also usually be rented at local rental shops. Be sure to wear protective eyewear whenever you cut tiles.

When you pick out your ceramic tile, you'll find that there are two basic types: unglazed and glazed. Unglazed tiles, and *Mexican pavers* (sun-baked tiles) are all-clay. As a result, the top surface must be coated with a protective sealer or finish after being installed or they'll absorb moisture and become easily soiled.

Glazed tiles have a glass-like top layer which requires no sealing. Glazed tile are naturally water-resistant, permanently retain their hard, colored surface, and need no additional sealers. Although they cost more than unglazed tiles, they're the better, healthier choice. To find glazed tiles, you'll want to check your local building centers, flooring centers, tile shops, and bathroom/kitchen outlets. Glazed-tile manufacturers include **American Olean Tile Co.**, **Summitville Tiles, Inc.**, and **Dal-Tile Co.**

Generally, glazed tiles are odorless. However, in rare cases, some tiles may have absorbed natural-gas odors from the gas-fired baking kilns or other odors from manufacturing and warehousing procedures. Therefore, it's important for sensitive people to test the tile for personal tolerance. To do this, first lightly sniff a sample tile. If it seems okay, place it on a table near your pillow. If you sleep well, you'll likely be able to tolerate it once it's on your floors. However, be aware that sometimes the sample tiles given to customers have been stored in offices where they could have become contaminated by tobacco smoke or perfume. If at all possible, always request a sample tile from an unopened box in the warehouse.

CERAMIC TILE INSTALLATION

Today, ceramic tiles are most commonly adhered to *subfloors* (the flooring surface below the tile) with products known as *thinset mortars* or *mastics*. Of the two materials, mastics are usually somewhat more odorous. Most thinset mortars consist primarily of Portland cement (which is relatively inert) and some synthetic additive compounds (which can be odorous). Actually, a few thinset mortars have a very strong odor when wet, and the odor can linger for extended periods of time, even after the tiles have been installed. However, there are also thinset products that are relatively odor-free and tolerable even for sensitive people.

A few low-odor thinsets are handled by **Nontoxic Environments**. However, it is generally possible to use a thinset from your local tile or building-supply store. Simply get a small sample, mix it with water, and see if it has a strong chemical odor; most don't. (For testing information, product brand names, and other sources, see *Chapter 12: Home Workshop and Garage*.)

The grout used to fill the spaces between the tiles is another cementitious product you'll need to test. (Do the same testing procedure as with thinset mortars above.) Actually, most locally available grouts consist simply of Portland cement, sand, and a few synthetic additives. As with thinset mortars, the additives are what can sometimes be odorous. While some locally purchased grouts can be acceptable, you may prefer to purchase an alternative product (at least one that is additive-free) from **Nontoxic Environments**.

In addition, you might like to know that you can actually make your own additive-free grout. The recipe is Portland cement, clean sand, and water. The proportions depend on the width of the grout joint—for joints under $1/_8$" wide mix 1 part cement with 1 part sand; for joints up to $1/_2$" wide use 1 part cement to 2 parts sand; for joints over $1/_2$" use 1 part cement to 3 parts sand. To create colored grout, you can add natural, mineral pigments. These powdered-rock colorants are often used by brick masons, so they're usually available wherever mortar is sold. They can also be ordered from **Nontoxic Environments**. Because there are no synthetic additives, the simple sand/Portland cement/water grout will require *damp-curing*. With damp-curing, a freshly grouted ceramic-tile floor is covered with plastic sheeting (plastic drop cloths) for three days to prevent rapid drying. (Rapid drying can cause the grout to become weak and crumbly.) After that, the plastic is removed and the tiles are scrubbed cleaned. Incidentally, the entire installation procedure for ceramic tile following this process is covered in text and photographs in *Healthy House Building* by John Bower. This book can be ordered directly from **The Healthy House Institute**.

To prevent stains, the cured grout joints can be sealed by carefully brushing them with a product called *water glass* (see *Water Glass* in Chapter 12: Home Workshop and Garage). Water glass is actually a clear, odorless sodium-silicate solution. Chemically, it's very similar to window glass, but in liquid form. When water glass is applied to grout, it chemically reacts with the calcium in the grout, forming a hard, transparent crystalline surface. One brand of water glass is Penetrating Water Stop (**American Formulating and Manufacturing (AFM)**). It's available from **The Living Source** and **Nontoxic Environments**, as well as other AFM dealers. Johnson's Super Seal is another brand manufactured by **Johnson's SuperSeal, Inc.**

RUGS

Rugs have been used for centuries to provide comfort and beauty to homes. In nomadic cultures, rugs were particularly popular because they could easily be rolled and moved, then unrolled in a new location to provide instant protection from the bare earth. Various cultures developed their own rug-making techniques and most of these are still used today, at least to some extent in some places.

However, most of the area rugs available in the U.S. today are manufactured *tufted* rugs. In tufting, small clusters of yarn are attached to a backing material and then held in place using a latex compound. An additional vinyl-cushioning layer is then often applied to the rug backs. Other rugs that can be purchased are made by needle-punching, hooking, or braiding. Woven rugs are also popular, usually made by machines in Europe and on hand looms in Asia.

Overwhelmingly, most of the rugs sold today are created with synthetic fibers, such as nylon or polypropylene (see *Carpeting* above), and nearly all rely on synthetic dyes for coloring. In addition, many rugs have chemical stain-resistant treatments. Despite their obvious similarities to wall-to-wall carpeting, rugs have one major advantage: They can be removed for thorough cleaning, not only to better remove dirt, but also to minimize a buildup of dust mites and other microorganisms.

Unfortunately, many sensitive people find new synthetic rugs intolerable. However, some of these individuals have found that if they repeatedly clean a bothersome rug with low-odor alternative cleaning products (see *Rugs and Carpets* in *Chapter 7: Cleaning*) and air it outside in dry, uncontaminated surroundings, their rug is far less a problem for them. Of course, the ideal solution is to purchase only untreated natural-fiber rugs that can be machine-laundered and machine-dried.

COTTON RUGS

Despite their often higher cost, untreated natural-fiber area and accent rugs can add a great deal of warmth and appeal to any room. They're especially attractive when laid over hardwood or ceramic tile floors. Many natural-fiber rugs are machine-made, but handmade imports are also readily available.

All-cotton rugs come in a variety of styles and sizes. Popular types include chenille, *dhurrie* (flat, woven non-pile rugs), and rag. Ideally, you'll want to choose machine-washable all-cotton rugs. That way, you won't require the services of either a professional rug cleaner or dry cleaner who might use odorous cleaning solutions. Remember though, if you plan to wash your rugs at home, carefully follow any manufacturer's recommendations listed on their tags or labels. Also, make sure to only use tolerable laundry products. You should be aware, too, that in many cases there will be some shrinkage of your rugs after their first laundering.

To find 100%-cotton rugs locally, check department stores, discount houses, and import shops. You can also order them from **Yankee Pride** and **Peerless Imported Rugs**, both of which carry a number of attractive rug varieties. **Home Decorators Collection** offers both all-cotton dhurrie and all-cotton braided-style rugs. Also, the **Pottery Barn** handles 100%-cotton woven and hooked rugs. **Heart of Vermont** and **Crate and Barrel** offer a few choices in all-cotton rugs as well.

Nontoxic Environments also offers commercial quality, all-cotton rugs in sizes from 17" x 24" to 27" x 48" and also a 36" round. These particular rugs come in natural tones, several solid colors, as well as in tweeds—and the rugs have no latex backings. The company also offers 100%-cotton, undyed, natural carpeting that can be custom-cut to any size and the edges bound with cotton binding.

WOOL RUGS

Wool is another good natural-fiber rug option. Wool rugs not only are beautiful and long-wearing, but some also are considered investments. Of course, rugs of this caliber are high in cost, yet they are generally very beautiful, extremely durable, and most likely one-of-a-kind handmade creations. Many of these are made with hand-spun yarns and natural vegetable dyes. This is especially true of fine Oriental and *rya* rugs (Scandinavian hand-loomed shaggy rugs).

However, other more-affordable wool rugs are also available. Although they may not be of interest to investors, they'll still provide an attractive, natural floor covering without breaking your budget. Included in this group are lesser-quality Oriental-style, native American, braided, hooked, and contemporary designer-look rugs. Usually these are machine-made, mass-produced designs using synthetic dyes.

Unfortunately, many wool rugs are treated with mothproofing chemicals that are often bothersome to sensitive persons. Sometimes the manufacturer's labels will provide this information. However, if a wholesaler or dealer has moth-treated a rug along the way, this information will probably not be listed with the rug. Airing bothersome rugs outdoors can help reduce some of these treatment odors, but in some cases it may not eliminate them all.

It's not difficult to find wool rugs for sale. Fine-quality wool rugs are usually sold in upscale department stores, decorator studios, and specialty rug shops. Because the cost of real Oriental rugs can be very high, you may want to read some books on the subject or talk with several reputable dealers before actually purchasing one. (Most libraries offer a number of such books.) One word of warning: Never buy an expensive Oriental rug from a transient dealer who rents store space for only a few weeks and then leaves the area. Often their rug prices are high, despite claims of unloading bankrupt dealers' inventories. Even if you get a good price, you may not be able to contact the seller if a problem arises at a later date.

If you are after a lower-cost wool rug, a number of styles are usually available at local import shops, as well as at moderately priced department stores and some carpet stores. One catalog source for wool rugs is **Home Decorators Collection**, which offers Oriental-style, braided, and hooked varieties. The **Yankee Pride** catalog also sells many affordable wool rugs, as does **Peerless Imported Rugs**. In addition, the **Pottery Barn** handles a few neutral-colored wool rugs.

Interesting wool-rug alternatives are *wool shearling rugs* (sheepskins). Besides being cozy and provocative, these rugs are often fairly inexpensive.

Sometimes they're even washable, but always read the manufacturers' tags first. One catalog source for wool shearling rugs is **The Aussie Connection**. They can also often be found in leather-craft shops.

Proper care is essential for your wool rugs. They should be vacuumed regularly or beaten on a line outdoors to remove particulate matter that can damage the wool yarns. To avoid solvent odors, you'll want to have your wool rugs professionally cleaned by carpet-cleaning firms or sent to the dry cleaners only when absolutely necessary. Although you may not be aware of this, some wool Oriental rugs can actually be hand-washed (see *Simple Rug Washing* in *Chapter 7: Cleaning*).

OTHER NATURAL-FIBER RUGS

Sometimes, natural-fiber rugs are made of sisal, jute, or hemp. These can be attractive, but in some cases difficult to clean. Therefore, you'll want to talk with your rug dealer and read the manufacturers' tags carefully before cleaning any with a water or solvent solution. You should also know that these rugs, especially jute, should not be placed where they'll receive direct sunlight. Sunlight can cause jute to deteriorate fairly quickly.

Check nearby import stores to see what natural-fiber rugs are available locally. By mail order, you can purchase attractive GoldSpun (**World Fibre**) jute rugs in a variety of sizes and patterns. Also, **The Sinan Co.** catalog offers several area rugs made of unusual natural-fibers, and **Pottery Barn** sells a fairly large selection of *coir* (coconut-husk fiber) rugs.

RUG GRIPS

Unfortunately, natural-fiber rugs without latex or vinyl backings may slip on slick, smooth flooring surfaces. To solve this common, but potentially dangerous, problem, manufacturers have created a variety of latex or vinyl rug-gripping products to securely hold rugs to the floor. Some of these rug grippers may be available in your local import stores, department stores, and rug shops. By mail order, **Home Etc.** sells washable latex rug-grip mats in several sizes from 2' x 4' to 9' x 12' and a 2' x 8' runner. **Heart of Vermont** handles what it terms *rug holds* made of washable natural rubber and jute. These can be cut to size. All-natural rubber rug grips are also sold by **The Seventh Generation**. These come in sizes including 3' x 5', 4' x 6', and 5' x 8', and a nice consideration is that they're washable. Still another option is Lok-Lift rug grip tape, which is sold by **Home Etc.** This product is available in 25' long rolls in two widths.

If latex and rubber odors are bothersome to you, other products on the market will hold rugs in place. One is a special Velcro "sticky-back" tape. To use it, simply apply the corresponding strips to both your floor and the rug's back. You'll want to read the manufacturer's label carefully before applying it so you'll know whether it can be used on washable rugs and whether the tape will be easy to remove from your floor at a later date. To find rug-holding Velcro tape, check your local carpet stores and rug shops.

CABINETS

Permanently installed cabinets are a relatively recent phenomenon. Prior to the turn of the century, in most cases kitchen supplies and utensils were stored in freestanding units (tables, bins, cabinets, etc.), or on wall shelves and hooks. Cabinets surrounding bathroom sinks didn't really become popular until the late 1950s and early 1960s. When the first permanently installed cabinets were put in, they were custom-built and made entirely of solid wood. Later, companies began manufacturing more-affordable wood or metal *stock units* (readily available separate cabinets that could be combined to create the look of a custom-cabinet job).

Today's cabinets come in a variety of styles with all types of special features, such as sliding trays, vegetable bins, etc. While a few are still made entirely of metal, the majority are made of a combination of wood products (manmade, veneer, and solid softwood or hardwood). Some cabinets are also made using woods and plastic laminate. Unfortunately, many people don't realize that most new cabinets now installed, except for all-metal cabinets and expensive solid-wood custom cabinets, can pose serious health dangers. This section explores some of these potential problems and offer several healthier cabinet alternatives.

TYPICAL MODERN CABINETS

As just noted, virtually all of the kitchen and bath cabinets installed in homes today are made with at least some man-made wood products. Even very expensive upscale cabinets with solid-wood doors and drawer fronts usually have drawer sides and bottoms, shelves, backs, and cabinet frameworks made of plywood or particleboard. While these man-made wood products are more stable (they shrink and expand less when the temperature and humidity fluctuates) and are cheaper than solid wood, they can pose real health risks. Here's why:

Cabinet-grade plywoods and particleboards are made primarily of thin layers or bits of softwoods, such as pine, held together with glue. The pine can give off fairly strong natural terpene odors (see *Man-made Wood Products* as well as *Solid Wood* in *Chapter 12: Home Workshop and Garage*). These are actually gaseous hydrocarbon compounds that can be irritating to your mucous membranes. Not surprisingly, many sensitive individuals find these airborne terpenes bothersome. People who are not highly sensitive are generally only bothered by terpene odors at high concentrations, such as might be released by turpentine.

A bigger concern with man-made wood products involves the glues used to construct them—especially urea-formaldehyde (UF) resins. UF glues can emit high levels of formaldehyde. To make matters worse, the clear finishes commonly applied to cabinets are made from urea-formaldehyde resins. As a result, kitchen and bath cabinets are often major sources of formaldehyde pollution in most homes. This is a serious situation that can lead to the development of a number of unhealthy symptoms. For example, formaldehyde can cause sinus and respiratory irritation, menstrual irregularities, and an acquired hypersensitivity to many other substances (see *Formaldehyde* in *Chapter 9: Indoor Air*).

It's been suggested that you can reduce terpene and formaldehyde gases from being released from your cabinets by simply coating all the exposed particleboard or plywood surfaces with a sealant product (see *Sealants* in *Chapter 12: Home Workshop and Garage*). However, even painting four coats will not be able to seal in all the bothersome gases completely. While they'll be greatly reduced, the remaining emission levels could still be intolerable, especially for sensitive individuals. Then too, sealants are often very odorous in their own right. In fact, they could take several months to lose their odor after being applied.

As an alternative to sealants, some people have tried stapling heavy-duty aluminum foil inside their cabinets. Generally, this won't form a perfect seal either. In most cases, terpene and formaldehyde odors will still be noticeable. Also, in time, the heavy-duty foil will likely tear. However, if you want to try this approach, *builder's foil* (aluminum on one or both sides of Kraft-paper) is a more durable choice. Two mail-order sources are **E.L Foust Co. Inc.** (DennyFoil brand) and **Nontoxic Environments** (two brands, each in a different thickness). Both companies also sell aluminum-foil tape that can be used to hold the foil sheets to the cabinets and to each another. (See *Tapes* and also *Foil Barriers* in *Chapter 12: Home Workshop and Garage.*)

As you can see, making problematic new cabinets tolerable is often difficult—maybe even impossible in many cases. Time may be a better cure, though it'll probably take several years before the emissions are significantly reduced. However, eventually the terpene and formaldehyde levels given off will decrease as the cabinets age. Obviously, the ideal approach would be to install healthier cabinets to begin with.

NEW ALTERNATIVE CABINETS

In any home-construction or remodeling project requiring new cabinetry, it's best to choose cabinets that won't compromise your own health or that of your family. In the following sections, some less-toxic cabinet suggestions are offered.

SOLID-WOOD CABINETS

Solid-wood cabinets can be a healthy choice—if the woods, glues, and finishes are carefully chosen. Such cabinets are attractive and long-lasting, but you should realize that they'll likely be quite expensive. This is not only because solid wood costs more than man-made wood products, but also because solid-wood cabinets will probably need to be custom-built. (Note: Some commercially made cabinets are advertised as being "made from solid wood," when, in fact, they contain plywood. If you ask about this discrepancy, the suppliers will usually claim that, by their definition, plywood *is* solid wood. However, no matter how they define *solid wood*, if plywood was used to construct the cabinets, they will contain formaldehyde glues— glues it's best to avoid if at all possible.)

To help locate a capable woodworker to make you *real* solid-wood cabinets, you can check in the classified sections of your phone book under Cabinet-makers, Wood Working, etc. Another good idea is to ask at local lumber-yards handling hardwoods, industrial/vocational education departments at local schools or colleges, and interior decorating shops for any suggestions or recommendations they may have. When you do find a prospective wood-worker, ask him (or her) for several of his clients you can contact and ask to see examples of his work. You'll also want to find out if the craftsperson is willing to use finishes that are tolerable to you, but which may be unfamiliar to him. Furthermore, you should request written estimates of the total project cost and how long the project will take for its completion. In addition, it's important to find out whether there could be smokers in the workshop whose tobacco smoke could permeate and contaminate your cabinets. This may be unlikely simply due to the danger of fire, but it's best to ask ahead of time anyway. After you have all this information, you can then make a well-informed decision whether you want to hire him or not.

The next step is to decide on the type of wood to be used in your cabinets. Some people may want to use softwood pine. It's certainly a low-cost choice and it's easy to find in local lumberyards. This is a viable option for most people; however, new pine gives off relatively strong natural terpene odors that can be too bothersome to some sensitive people. Ideally, a hardwood species that naturally has little odor should be chosen instead. Some low-odor hardwoods you might consider are maple, birch, and tulip poplar (see *Solid Wood* in *Chapter 12: Home Workshop and Garage*). Tulip poplar is often an especially good choice; it's fairly inexpensive and should fit in most budgets. Tulip poplar is also easy to work with and has an attractive, yet informal appearance.

"What can we use for drawer bottoms?" is a question often asked by people wanting all solid-wood cabinets. Actually, a simple solution is to use *galvanized sheet metal*. Galvanized sheet metal provides a washable, sturdy surface, eliminating the need for plywood or other man-made wood products that are normally used. You may not be familiar with it, but galvanized sheet metal is simply thin, zinc-coated steel (zinc coating is a finishing treatment to prevent rusting). Garbage cans are often made of galvanized sheet metal. Sheets of this material can be purchased and custom-cut at most sheet-metal shops. A 24-gauge thickness will generally provide cabinet drawers bottoms with adequate support, but for extra-wide drawers, it's better to use a slightly thicker material.

By the way, new galvanized metal may have a thin surface coating of oil on it. This is sometimes applied during the manufacturing process to aid the metal's passage though the rollers and other machinery. Fortunately, this oil coating can often be easily washed off by using a solution of trisodium phosphate (TSP) and water. TSP is a white or clear crystalline powder that can be used as a powerful, unscented cleaner that many sensitive persons tolerate well. You can purchase TSP at most local hardware stores and paint/wallpaper shops. One phosphate-free brand is Red Devil TSP/90 Heavy Duty Cleaner (**Red Devil, Inc.**). To use it, dissolve 2 level tablespoons of TSP in 1 gallon of warm water. Then, dip your sponge into the solution, wring it, and thoroughly wipe the metal. Finish up the process by rinsing with clear water. It should be mentioned that wearing rubber gloves to prevent skin inflammation is a good idea.

Another factor to consider with solid-wood cabinets is stain. Actually, stain is often unnecessary. Without any stain, a wood's natural beauty (color and grain) will clearly show through. At the same time, a possible source of intolerance is eliminated. Another point to decide on is what glue to use. Often, a low-order carpenter's glue makes a good choice. Finally you'll need to choose a tolerable and durable clear finish. (See also *Chapter 12: Home Workshop and Garage*.)

Remember, your new cabinets will likely have a "new" odor immediately after being made, no matter what materials, glues, and finishes you have chosen. This odor can actually persist for some time. Therefore, if possible, store your new cabinets in a dry, uncontaminated area for several weeks before their final installation. If you're a sensitive person, it's best not to put them in your kitchen or bathroom until they're completely odor-free.

ALTERNATIVE PARTICLEBOARD CABINETS

Medite and Medex II (**Medite Corp.**) are two particleboard products that can be used instead of solid wood when constructing new cabinets. Unlike typical particleboards, these are not made with formaldehyde-based glues. While Medite and Medex II cost more than other particleboards, they're much less expensive than using solid hardwood. Also, the skill required to work with them is much less than with solid wood. Therefore, labor costs should be lower. If you want to purchase **Medite Corp.** products, you can call the manufacturer for a dealer in your geographic area.

However, you should be aware that despite using healthier glues, these alternative particleboards are often still too bothersome to sensitive people. This is usually because they release natural hydrocarbon terpenes from the softwoods of which they're made. Softwoods also often contain a tiny amount of naturally occurring formaldehyde. Completely coating all the alternative particleboard's exposed surfaces with up to four coats of a sealant will help reduce these odors, but it will not completely eliminate them. Also, it's important to keep in mind that sealants are often very odorous in their own right. In any case, Medite and Medex II are currently only available as raw particleboard, they are not available with a veneer of oak, cherry, or other attractive wood.

To make alternative-particleboard cabinets more tolerable as well as attractive, all the surfaces can be covered with a hard-plastic laminate. Hard-plastic laminates will not only seal in most of the odors being released from the wood underneath, but will also give your cabinets a sleek, modern "European" look. If you choose to follow this approach, you should use a water-based contact cement as an adhesive. Elmer's Saf-T Contact Cement (**Elmer's Adhesives**) is one of the less-toxic brands. This particular product is often available at local hardware stores and building centers. Whenever laminating is being done, having plenty of ventilation and wearing a cartridge-type respirator mask as preventive safety measures are a good idea (see also *Protective Gear* in *Chapter 12: Home Workshop and Garage*).

Currently, **Enviro Safe Cabinets Co., Ltd.** is the only company manufacturing cabinets without formaldehyde-based glues whatsoever. For cases (ends, shelves, etc.), it uses a high quality particleboard made especially for them, and covers it with a plastic-laminate surface. The fronts of the cabinets, drawers, and doors are made of solid hardwood. These cabinets are very attractive and use European-style hardware. A Canadian company, Enviro-Safe also ships to the U.S. You can contact the company for further information.

ALTERNATIVE-PLYWOOD CABINETS

Cabinet-grade, furniture-grade, and hardwood plywoods are generally not suggested for the same reasons typical particleboards aren't. That is, they all release relatively high levels of formaldehyde from the urea-formaldehyde (UF) glues. However, if you really want to use plywood, you might consider choosing a construction-grade product.

Construction-grade plywood (either interior or exterior grade) is usually made of much-less-attractive fir or pine, but its layers are held together using a water-resistant phenol-formaldehyde (PF) glue. These products all have an American Plywood Association (APA) grade stamp. A PF glue emits much lower quantities of formaldehyde than the non-water-resistant urea-formaldehyde (UF) glue. To make construction-grade plywood even more tolerable, you might consider the various options discussed above for alternative-particleboard cabinets.

METAL CABINETS

Today, metal is an often overlooked but excellent choice for cabinets. Metal cabinetry can be attractive, low-odor, easy to clean, and very durable. However, many people continue to think of metal cabinets as the drab, white, cheap-looking products that were sold in the 1950s. But metal cabinets are now available that are much better looking with many more features than those earlier cabinets. This is especially true for metal cabinets manufactured by **St. Charles Manufacturing Co.** One kitchen and bath consultant/dealer who handles this line is **Kitchens and Baths by Don Johnson.** For the names of other St. Charles cabinet dealers, you'll want to contact the manufacturer.

St. Charles metal cabinets are offered with either smooth or textured baked-enamel finishes in a wide array of attractive colors. Even stainless steel is available. In addition, **Kitchens and Baths by Don Johnson** is one of the few dealers offering custom-made solid-hardwood doors and drawer fronts. These can be specially ordered made from any wood species. St. Charles cabinets have several hardware options, including chrome, brass, and wood in several styles. Surprisingly, **St. Charles Manufacturing Co.** has an all-metal cabinet version *especially* manufactured for chemically sensitive customers. These are called their Chemically Reduced Environment (CRE) cabinets. With the CRE option, the stiffeners inside the doors are metal instead of a composite material, and the door hinges and drawer rollers will be degreased upon request. It should be pointed out that St. Charles metal cabinets are fairly expensive, especially the CRE cabinets that need to undergo special procedures during their production. But they are quite sturdy and very well made. CRE cabinets are only available with a textured finish.

If you are interested in less-expensive metal cabinets, one line you might be interested in is manufactured and sold by **Davis Products Co.** This company's cabinets come in a number of baked, acrylic-enamel designer colors and all of the units have rigid insulation inside the doors to help deaden sounds. Whether this insulating material will be bothersome to sensitive people is difficult to predict. If you are a sensitive person, it would be best to actually test a finished cabinet (or just a door) yourself before ordering an entire kitchen's worth. By the way, **Dwyer Products Corp.** has metal cabinets of a similar quality.

Metal cabinetry is also offered by **Ampco.** These cabinets can be purchased with several options. For further information and to locate a nearby dealer, you'll need to contact the company. **Arctic Metal Products Corp.** makes simple metal cabinet styles that come in just a few colors. Some of their units are offered both with sound-deadening insulation and without. Sensitive individuals may want to choose uninsulated cabinets whenever possible. This eliminates the possibility that the insulating materials could prove bothersome. Unfortunately at this time, Arctic only sells its products at a few stores in the New York/East Coast area. You can call the manufacturer for a location near you.

ALTERNATIVE UPDATING OF OLD CABINETS

Maybe you've decided to keep your old wood cabinets, rather than installing new ones. Actually, giving sturdy old cabinets a new appearance, rather than replacing them, has real advantages. For one, the formaldehyde glue used in the manufactured man-made wood materials utilized in most cabinets has a *half-life* of 3 to 5 years. This means that after every 3 to 5 years, half the formaldehyde remaining in the cabinets will have dissipated. Because of this, older cabinets are much less potent formaldehyde emitters than typical new cabinets. Another reason for choosing to update your cabinets is that it's nearly always cheaper to redo existing cabinets than to purchase new ones.

PAINTING OLDER CABINETS

Painting your old cabinets with a tolerable, durable finish may be all that's needed to update them satisfactorily (see *Paints* in *Chapter 12: Home Workshop and Garage*). Of course, it's important to test several brands of paint first (see *Testing Finishes* in *Chapter 12: Home Workshop and Garage*). Besides the new paint itself, buying and installing attractive replacement hardware will easily, and affordably, add to the new look.

Before beginning to paint your old cabinets, you'll need to properly prepare them. This will ensure a more-attractive and longer-lasting finish. The first essential step is a thorough cleaning to remove any acquired grime, cooking grease, and perhaps layers of built-up wax. To remove these, one method is to go over all the cabinet surfaces with a strong concentration of TSP (trisodium phosphate) and water. TSP is a white or clear crystalline powder that's used as an unscented, heavy-duty cleaning powder. It's usually sold at paint, hardware, and wallpaper stores. One popular brand is Red Devil TSP/90 Heavy Duty Cleaner (**Red Devil, Inc.**), which is phosphate-free. To use TSP, dissolve 2 level tablespoons in 1 gallon of warm water. Dip a sponge into the solution and wring it, then wipe just a small section of your cabinets at a time. If the cabinets are particularly dirty, you'll need to rinse with clear water. By the way, you should wear rubber gloves to prevent any possible skin irritation.

Besides washing, you might take the additional step of lightly sanding the old cabinets. Fresh paint often adheres to sanded surfaces better. If you do sand, you'll want to wear a good-quality dust mask, such as a cartridge-type respirator (see *Protective Gear* in *Chapter 12: Home Workshop and Garage*). When you're finished sanding, thoroughly vacuum all surfaces of the cabinets with a soft dusting attachment. At this point, you're ready to paint using an appropriate brand you've pretested.

There's one additional matter you should be aware of: Some old cabinetry may have been polished with a silicone-containing product. If so, new paint may not stick to the cabinets properly. If you know silicone polish was, indeed, used, don't attempt to paint unless you first remove it from the cabinetry surfaces. Unfortunately, this can be difficult because silicone products are often waterproof. In many cases, they won't come off using typical wax removal techniques. If they don't, it may be necessary to sand the cabinets or even use a paint stripper. If you find that you'll have to strip the cabinets, a less-toxic water-based stripper such as Safest Stripper (**3-M Do-It -Yourself Division**) is a better choice than a traditional solvent-based product. Fortunately, water-based strippers are now generally available at most local hardware, building-supply, and paint stores. However, when using any type of stripper (water- or solvent-based), it's best to wear protective gear such as safety goggles, neoprene gloves, and a cartridge-type respirator mask, and to have plenty of ventilation.

You should keep in mind that painting your cabinets will be not only disruptive, but also odorous. Therefore, ideally, you should only do this type of work in those seasons when you can have the windows open. Using a window fan blowing outdoors from the room where the painting is taking place is also a good idea. Of course, if you're a sensitive person, this isn't a job for you to do personally.

OLDER CABINET FACELIFTS

While painting all the surfaces of your old cabinets is one option for updating them, there are others. One is to paint only the fronts of the cabinets' case frames and install new replacement solid-hardwood doors and drawer fronts. Naturally, these new door and drawer fronts will need to be coated with a durable, yet tolerable, clear finish. Remember, whenever you're doing any painting or coating, you need plenty of ventilation and to wear appropriate protective gear.

Another approach to modernizing your old outdated kitchen cabinets is to have new solid-wood doors and drawer fronts made, but instead of painting the existing cabinet case-frame fronts, you can have hard-plastic laminate applied to them. Of course, this project will require someone skilled with plastic laminates. To find such a person, you can ask for recommendations at your local kitchen cabinet shops and building-supply centers. You can also check in the classified section of your telephone book under Countertops or Kitchen Cabinets.

No matter who does the laminating work, a nontoxic water-based contact cement such as Elmer's Saf-T Contact Cement (**Elmer's Adhesives**) is best to use instead of noxious solvent-based brands. This particular product, as well as similar ones, are now often available at hardware stores and building centers. Having good ventilation during the laminating process and wearing appropriate protective gear, including a cartridge-type respirator mask, is still highly advised. By the way, the plastic laminate should only be applied to the cabinet surfaces after the cabinets have first been cleaned in order to ensure good adhesion.

COUNTERTOPS

Since the 1950s, almost all cabinet tops have been made of hard-plastic laminates. That is, until the last decade or so. Now there are a surprising number of countertop options. This section will cover several of the most common types now used.

HIGH-PRESSURE PLASTIC LAMINATES

Hard $1/16$" thick *high-pressure plastic laminate* is still probably the most popular countertop surface in the U.S. today. This isn't surprising; they're waterproof, inexpensive, attractive, and relatively easy to install. So common is their use that plastic laminates can be readily purchased at nearly all building centers and cabinet shops. One of the more familiar brands is Formica (**Formica Corp.**), but there are a number of others. Despite being plastic products, high-pressure plastic laminates are so hard and dense, they tend to release relatively few synthetic odors. Therefore, while they're still in sheet form at least, they're often tolerable for most sensitive people.

What exactly are plastic laminates? Plastic laminates are actually made of several layers of Kraft paper bonded together with plastic resins under heat and very high pressure. The topmost layer of resin-impregnated paper is colored or patterned; this gives the laminate sheet its particular appearance. Modern plastic laminates now come in a wide variety of designs, colors, textures, sheens, and grades. However, they're all subject to scorching and chipping to some degree.

Unfortunately, plastic laminate sheets are much too thin ($1/16$") and brittle to serve as countertops as they are; they must have a supporting surface beneath them. Therefore, plastic laminates are always permanently glued to thick, smooth, stable, solid, *substrates* (base materials). Generally, particleboard is used for this. Sadly, from a health standpoint, most particleboard gives off high levels of formaldehyde from urea-formaldehyde (UF) glues. Particleboard will also outgas potentially bothersome softwood terpene odors. However, alternative particleboards made without formaldehyde or construction-grade plywoods, which use a less problematic phenol-formaldehyde glue (PF), can be substituted. (Note, these still will emit terpenes.) Some people are tempted to use plastic laminates over solid wood, but this generally doesn't work very well because solid wood can warp and change dimensions too much as the humidity fluctuates with the seasons.

While it's usual practice to only apply plastic laminate to the top and front edge of the substrate, you might seriously consider covering *all* the sides—top, bottom, and each of the four edges. This encasement approach is especially important for sensitive individuals. If this is done, most of the polluting formaldehyde, as well as the natural pine terpene odors are sealed in.

If you choose not to apply plastic laminate to all sides, you may want to coat the exposed plywood or particleboard surfaces with a sealant (see *Sealants and Other Acrylic Water-Based Wood Finishes* in *Chapter 12: Home Workshop and Garage*). You should be aware though that sealants can't totally seal in formaldehyde emissions, even with four coats, and they're very odorous in their own right. Another option would be to glue or staple heavy-duty aluminum foil to the exposed plywood or particleboard base material. However, this isn't completely effective either, and the foil will likely tear. Builder's foil (Kraft-paper core with aluminum on one or both sides) is stronger and more durable. **Nontoxic Environments** offers two brands in two thicknesses. **E.L. Foust Co., Inc.** sells DennyFoil. They both also sell aluminum tape to hold the sheets together (see *Tapes* and also *Foil Barriers* in *Chapter 12: Home Workshop and Garage*).

For gluing plastic laminate to a substrate, it's best to use a low-toxicity contact cement. Elmer's Saf-T Contact Cement (**Elmer's Adhesives**) is one such product, and it's often available at local hardware stores and building centers. During the actual laminating process, there should be good ventilation and, of course, appropriate protective gear should always be worn.

BUTCHER-BLOCK COUNTERTOPS

Another countertop option is a wood *butcher block*, which is becoming more popular. Most butcher block countertops consist of narrow maple or oak strips held together with glue. Originally, butcher block surfaces were only made of *end grain* (wood cut across the width of the trunk) because it's much harder than wood cut parallel with the grain. Real butcher blocks had to withstand the abuse of cleavers and knives without easily chipping or splitting. However, today's butcher-block countertops usually don't receive this kind of daily assault. Therefore, many are not made with end-grain work surfaces. Incidentally, if you have the choice, it's best to choose maple over oak for your new butcher-block countertops, if you are a very sensitive person. This is because oak contains natural, strong-smelling *tannin compounds,* which can be irritating to the mucous membranes of susceptible people.

Unfortunately, the glues and surface-sealing treatments used in the manufacturing of certain butcher block countertops can also be intolerable to some sensitive people. Another point to consider is that although they're extremely attractive when new, many butcher-block counters eventually get stained by foods, especially if no sealant or clear finish was used on them, and scorched by hot pans. However, light stains and scorch marks can often be removed with light sanding.

Surprisingly, there are a number of butcher-block countertop manufacturers. Among these are **Balley Block Co., John Boos & Co.,** and **Taylor Wood-Craft, Inc.** You'll need to call each company to find dealers near you. There is also at least one company, **Block-Tops, Inc.,** which will custom-make countertops and ship them directly to your home without any intermediary dealer.

Sensitive individuals interested in having butcher-block countertops will want to ask for samples from at least two manufacturers. These samples should then be tested for personal tolerance (see *Testing* in *Chapter 1: Getting Started*). However, be aware that such tests will only give you general indications. This is because the samples you receive may be relatively old and, therefore, already aired out, or they may have been stored in offices or warehouses near smokers or persons wearing perfume. You should keep in mind that samples are generally quite small compared to the total square footage of installed countertops.

CORIAN COUNTERTOPS

After plastic laminate, the most popular countertops are probably mineral/acrylic countertops. Originally, these were available only in white, but now they come in a number of colors. At least one brand, Corian (**DuPont Co.**), has been successfully used by a number of sensitive individuals, but other similar brands are readily available.

Corian is actually a specific patented formulation made up of marble dust and synthetic resin. Despite the synthetic content, Corian seems to have only a slight odor, perhaps because it's so hard and dense. One very positive feature of Corian is that in many installations, it doesn't require a plywood or particleboard substrate (base material) for support. This eliminates formaldehyde glue and softwood terpene problems that are usually associated with these man-made wood products.

You should be aware that Corian is now available in two forms: a solid material or a laminated version with a thin Corian layer surrounding a man-made wood core. While the laminated type is less expensive, it could theoretically pose more of an intolerance problem. However, if the Corian *indeed* completely encases the inner man-made material, any formaldehyde and softwood terpene odors coming from this core material should be sealed in. On the plus side, Corian is relatively stain-resistant, and even if it does acquire some minor discolorations (or scratches), these can often be sanded out. Of course, this must be done very carefully. (Remember to follow any manufacturer's guidelines.) To purchase Corian countertops, you can check with your local kitchen/bath cabinet dealers. If necessary, you can call the company for a dealer near you.

CERAMIC-TILE COUNTERTOPS

One of the oldest countertop materials, ceramic tile, can still be an attractive countertop option for today's kitchens and bathrooms. Ceramic tile is beautiful, natural, durable, and generally well-tolerated by sensitive people. However, it's best to only choose glazed, kiln-fired ceramic tiles. This type of tile has a hard glass-like surface which doesn't require any sealing treatment (see *Choosing Ceramic Tile* under *Flooring* above). These days, ceramic tiles are available in a variety of sizes, patterns, colors, and shapes to give your countertops an attractive and personal touch. In addition, many manufacturers produce them. A few companies include **American Olean Tile Co.**, **Dal-Tile Co.**, and **Summitville Tiles, Inc.** To find suitable ceramic tile locally, check the classified section of your phone book under Ceramic Tile for dealers in your area.

However, it should be stated that there could be a few potential problems with ceramic-tile countertops. One is with the substrate (base material) used beneath the tiles themselves. Commonly, ceramic tile is adhered to a construction-grade plywood substrate using a thinset mortar. Unfortunately, some thinset mortar products can be bothersome to sensitive individuals. For such people, testing is essential.

Another concern is with the substrate material itself. Construction-grade plywood emits formaldehyde from phenol-formaldehyde (PF) glue and natural hydrocarbon terpenes from the softwoods that can be bothersome. A healthier substrate option is to use two layers of $1/2$" *cement board* (a cementitious product sold in sheets). Unfortunately, even this material is fairly odorous. However, some sensitive persons find they can tolerate cement board better than construction-grade plywood. Cement board is available through some building centers and lumberyards, and through ceramic-tile suppliers. There are several different brands on the market, including Wonder-Board (**Modulars, Inc.**) and Durock (**USG Industries, Inc.**). You can call these companies for their nearest dealers.

To help block any objectionable emissions from either a plywood or cement-board substrate, you could coat the exposed underside surfaces with a sealant. Four coats will often seal in most odors, but not all. Cement board can often be sealed by coating the exposed surfaces with a layer of thinset mortar. Another option would be to cover any exposed plywood or cement-board surfaces with an aluminum-foil product.

Yet another common worry with ceramic-tile countertops is the grout. Many prepackaged grouts contain chemical additives which can be bothersome to some sensitive people. However, a simple grout with no additives can be made by merely mixing clean sand, water, and Portland cement (see *Ceramic Tile Installation* under *Flooring*, above). To add color, you can use a small amount of natural mineral pigments. These can usually be bought locally wherever mortar is sold. They can also be mail-ordered from **Nontoxic Environments**. Because it's additive-free, this grout must be *damp-cured*. This means that the newly grouted tile countertop will have to be covered with plastic sheeting (plastic drop cloths) for three days. This is done to prevent rapid drying that would prevent the grout from becoming strong and durable. Afterwards, the plastic is taken off. Then, the tiles are scrubbed to remove any grout film. (For compete information on tile installation, see *Healthy House Building* by John Bower, which can be ordered from **The Healthy House Institute**.)

Many people are also afraid that stains and mold growth will get on the grout lines. Actually, you can greatly minimize these problems by laying the ceramic tiles very close together. In addition, after installation, the grout itself can be sealed by carefully brushing it with *water glass* (sodium silicate). Water glass is a colorless, odorless liquid that is chemically similar to window glass. When it's applied to grout, it chemically reacts with the calcium in it to form an impermeable crystalline structure in the surface of the grout (see *Water Glass* in *Chapter 12: Home Workshop and Garage*). One brand of water glass is Penetrating Water Stop (**American Formulating and Manufacturing (AFM)**), which is available from **Nontoxic Environments**, **The Living Source**, and other AFM dealers.

VITREOUS CHINA COUNTERTOPS

An excellent countertop alternative for bathrooms is *vitreous china*. (The term *vitreous* refers to a surface that has the hardness and gloss of glass.) This ceramic material is actually what toilets and freestanding sinks are made of. Vitreous china is naturally stain resistant, durable, and inert.

Universal Rundle Corp. is one manufacturer that makes one-piece vitreous china countertops with molded sinks. These are both attractive and easy to clean but they come in only a few colors and sizes. Sometimes these types of countertops are available through local lumberyards, building centers, and plumbing-supply shops. If you can't find them, you can contact the company for its nearest dealer.

STAINLESS-STEEL COUNTERTOPS

One of the healthiest countertop choices is *stainless steel*. It's been used in commercial kitchens for years but it's just now being used a little more commonly in residential applications. It is hoped it will become even more widely used as people realize that its sleek modern appearance is, indeed, appropriate in their own home kitchen.

What exactly is stainless steel? Stainless steel is defined as any steel alloy that has at least a 12% chromium content. Chromium gives steel tremendous rust and corrosion resistance. Nickel, molybdenum, or other elements may also be used in certain stainless-steel alloys. Currently, the most popular stainless steel is called 18-8. This grade contains 18% chromium, 8% nickel, and 0.15% carbon. This particular alloy of stainless steel is generally used in flatware, cooking utensils, plumbing fixtures, and it works very well for kitchen countertops.

One drawback to stainless-steel countertops is that they're relatively expensive. First, the stainless-steel sheets themselves can be quite pricey, and then you have to add in the cost of having them custom-made into countertops by skilled fabricators. Yet, stainless steel's advantages are considerable. Stainless steel is virtually indestructible and it won't support microbial growth. It's also stain-resistant, scorch-resistant, and not subject to cracking or peeling. In other words, stainless-steel countertops will last forever and probably never have to be replaced.

Because stainless-steel countertops are almost always custom-made, you can have finished countertops manufactured with many special features. For example, you can choose to have extra-tall backsplashes, or none at all, and perhaps a seamless integral countertop sink. Though they're more expensive, integrated sinks offer a clean, streamlined look. This is because all integral components of a stainless-steel countertop are welded together and the rough weld seams are ground and polished so they become invisible. Therefore, an integrated countertop sink eliminates the sink/counter seams created by typical drop-in sinks, which could eventually become traps for food particles or microbial growth.

It should be pointed out that when you're having your stainless steel countertops made, you can specify that they be fabricated using a particular *gauge* (thickness). It's best for sensitive people to choose a gauge that's relatively heavy because with thin stainless steel, a plywood or particleboard substrate (support base) is required. This man-made wood material can release formaldehyde from formaldehyde-based glues and softwood terpene odors. (For more on man-made wood substrates, see *High-Pressure Plastic Laminate* above.) To eliminate the substrate altogether, stainless steel with at least a 14-gauge thickness will have to be used. Stainless-steel countertops of that thickness will probably only need a few solid-wood braces underneath for sufficient support. If you are a very sensitive individual, consider using a hardwood such as tulip poplar for the braces rather than pine, to avoid any terpene odors.

To find a company in your area that can fabricate stainless-steel countertops, you can check your telephone classified section under Commercial Kitchen Suppliers. If none are listed there, ask at local restaurants and other commercial kitchens to find out where their countertops were made. When you find a fabricator, make certain that his work will be of sufficient quality to be in your kitchen. Also you'll want to get a total cost estimate which will include materials, labor, shipping, etc., as well as an expected date your countertop should be completed. You should be aware, however, that some fabricators do not actually install countertops. In that case, you'll have to make arrangements with someone else to install them. Remember to be extremely careful when giving countertop measurements to your stainless steel fabricator. Any mistakes can mean very expensive countertops that don't fit. Stainless-steel countertops can't be easily modified once fabricated, so accurate measurements are mandatory.

FURNITURE

Furniture originated as simple utilitarian necessity. However, with time, the decorative aspects became more and more prominent. As designs and construction techniques improved and evolved, professional furniture-making became an occupation—and sometimes an art. For centuries, skilled craftsmen and their assistants made individual pieces by hand.

However, during the 1800s, factories began mass-producing furniture. While the prices went down, the quality sometimes did, too. With the proliferation of cheap man-made materials after World War II, most furniture began being made with at least some synthetic components. Today, the use of man-made materials is greater than ever. For the most part, the furniture now sold isn't particularly well-made, aesthetically pleasing, or long-lasting. Actually, a great deal of the furniture made in the last four or five decades is throwaway furniture. Completely hand-crafted pieces using solid woods, natural fabrics, and stuffing are now quite rare, and often very expensive. Fortunately, there are a few furniture-making companies that do produce affordable furniture using *real* materials.

TYPICAL MODERN MANUFACTURED FURNITURE

Today, furniture is often constructed with some solid wood (often a softwood such as pine, or a very inexpensive hardwood), as well as some composite man-made materials (hardboard, particleboard, or plywood). In factories, furniture parts are machine-cut and sanded, then quickly assembled with mechanical nailers, screw guns, staplers, and quick-drying glues. Some pieces may also have hardwood *veneers* (very thin layers of solid wood) and/or plastic laminates, permanently attached to them with the use of synthetic adhesives. The use of sprayed-on synthetic stains and finishes is routine on most exposed wood parts.

Soft pieces (sofas, etc.) are usually upholstered with synthetic stuffing and fabrics. Frequently, upholstery materials are chemically treated to repel dirt and stains. Interestingly, furniture sold in California may now have to meet mandated flame-retardant standards—meaning the addition of synthetic fire-retardant chemicals.

Therefore, it's not surprising that most new furniture releases many potentially harmful chemical gases, including formaldehyde. Man-made wood products, finishes, stains, glues, stuffing, fabrics, and special treatments all emit a variety of compounds that can pollute a home's indoor air. As a result, typical new furniture is often intolerable for most sensitive individuals.

ACCEPTABLE NEW MANUFACTURED FURNITURE

Fortunately, healthier furniture selections do exist. The following sections offer some alternatives for you to consider.

SOLID-WOOD FURNITURE

Solid-wood furniture can be a healthy furnishing choice, and luckily there are still a few companies and individuals making it. The styles now available range from traditional, colonial, and Shaker, to modern contemporary. The most commonly used woods are probably pine and oak. Unfortunately, for some very sensitive individuals, both of these woods can be a problem because of the natural terpenes in softwoods and the tannins in oak. These natural compounds can be both odorous and irritating. However, there are furniture-makers who work with solid maple, beech, birch, or cherry, which are usually more tolerable wood choices.

You may be able to find some finished solid-wood furniture at your local furniture stores. However, there are a number of mail-order sources if you can't. For example, **Shaker Workshop** offers Shaker-style benches, bookcases, stools, platform beds, end tables, rockers, and dining room tables and chairs constructed of solid maple and other solid hardwoods. Also, **Shaker Shops West** sells similar furniture, while **Sturbridge Yankee Workshop** carries all-cherry beds. Reproduction tables, beds, chairs, and benches in pine, maple, and cherry can be purchased from **Cohasset Colonials**. In addition, **Bartley Collection** has reproduction beds, dressers, wardrobes, chairs and tables in solid cherry and mahogany, though veneered plywood (plywood with a thin top layer of hardwood) is sometimes used, too.

L.L. Bean, Inc. (in its *Home and Camp* catalog) sells solid-oak rockers and solid-ash Mission-style tables, maple beds, and cherry dining room tables. **The Crate & Barrel** handles solid-oak tables and beech stools. Solid-pine tables and wardrobes and and all-beech dining chairs and barstools are offered by **Pottery Barn**. Solid-oak Mission-style tables and solid-maple Adirondack furniture are sold by **Home Decorators Collection**. In addition, check garden and patio catalogs such as **Smith & Hawken**. This particular company has some solid teak and redwood furniture. (Redwood is a softwood, but it's usually better tolerated by sensitive people than pine or fir.)

Attractive, contemporary, solid-cherry and solid-maple beds, dressers, end tables, and convertible futon sofas and chairs are available from **Jantz Designs**. The **Sinan Co.** has all-hardwood school desks, bookcases, beds, and cribs finished with Auro natural-resin oils and plant waxes (see *Clear Finishes* in *Chapter 12: Home Workshop and Garage*). Also, **Dona Designs** sells solid-oak end tables, lawyer's bookcases, futon bed frames, and convertible futon bed/couches protected with beeswax finishes.

Of special note is **Pompanoosuc Mills**, which has a complete solid-hardwood furniture line in a number of species: oak, birch, maple, cherry, and walnut. The company also has dining room sets, benches, living room seating options, desks, coffee tables, and bedroom suites. The styles available are colonial, country, and contemporary. Of special note, this company welcomes sensitive clients. In fact its catalog specifically states that the company "offers special materials, stains, and finishes for chemically sensitive individuals." According to a company representative, it'll even create custom pieces for you, if the designs are similar to ones they usually make.

(For more solid-wood furniture options, see *Unfinished and Kit Furniture* as well as *Custom Furniture* below.)

METAL AND METAL WITH GLASS FURNITURE

Metal furniture can be an excellent healthy choice for your home's interior. Often, manufacturers combine metal with glass, both of which are generally inert. More popular then ever, brass, wrought iron, painted steel, stainless steel, and chrome pieces are easy to find at most local furniture stores, bedroom shops, and import stores. You can also buy metal desks, bookcases, and chairs at many office-supply stores. These particular pieces often work very well in your den or home office.

Also, a number of companies offer metal furniture through the mail. One is **The Crate & Barrel**, which sells attractive metal racks. Metal headboards and baker's racks are sold by **Sturbridge Yankee Workshop** as well as by **Home Decorators Collection**. **The Brass Bed Shoppe** handles brass headboards and daybeds in all sizes.

A catalog that sells very attractive metal furniture is **Ballard Designs**. This company offers designer wrought-iron tables, steel beds, benches, stools, dining chairs, and dining room tables. It also handles heavy glass tops in $1/2$" and $3/4$" thicknesses with two different edge treatments. The size and shape assortment is vast, including glass rounds, ovals, rectangles, squares, and octagons; even glass shelving is sold. For a beautiful selection of designer steel and wicker chairs and tables, check out the **Pottery Barn** catalog.

One classification of metal furnishings you may not have considered is patio furniture. Actually, this furniture can often be suitable for most rooms in your house. However, to make it more homey, as well as healthier, replace any vinyl and synthetic foam seat cushions with washable, removable, natural-fabric-covered cushions filled with natural-fiber batting (see *Natural Fibers*, *Natural Stuffing*, and *Custom Made Clothes* in *Chapter 3: Clothing*). You can purchase metal patio furniture locally in patio shops, as well as many furniture, department, and discount stores. Also, good-looking metal pieces are often available in garden catalogs. One example is **Smith & Hawken**, which sells both cast-iron and steel patio furniture.

Note: Metal furniture that has been painted or lacquered (brass items are often coated with a clear lacquer) will often require some time to air out in uncontaminated surroundings before being brought indoors. If possible, choose only products with a baked-on finish because they usually require less airing.

WICKER FURNITURE

Many people assume that wicker and reed furniture, which is made of natural grasses, would be good choices in a less-toxic home. These pieces do have certain pluses, such as being appropriate for most rooms and often being relatively inexpensive. However, there can be some problems with this kind of furniture. Particular parts, for example, shelves or seat bottoms, are likely to have been made of plywood or other man-made wood products. These materials can emit formaldehyde from formaldehyde-containing glues, as well as softwood terpene odors that can be bothersome to some sensitive people. Also, it's possible that mold or mildew may have contaminated some reed or wicker pieces. This is understandable if you realize that, in most cases, these materials are damp when they're woven. (To make sure a piece you're interested in has not been contaminated by fungus, you'll need to check the bottom and back for telltale dark fungal discolorations.) Finally, another concern is that some wicker and reed pieces are rather difficult to thoroughly clean.

If you're interested in this type of furniture, you'll want go to wicker shops, import stores, and furniture stores to see what's available locally. If you'd prefer to order through the mail, **Pottery Barn** handles very attractive wicker tables and camelback chairs. The company also has a good selection of designer rattan and steel end tables, dining tables, chairs, and barstools.

CERAMIC FURNITURE

Ceramic or plaster seats, pedestals, and end tables can be exciting home additions. This is because they're commonly made in unusual shapes such as elephants, columns, or even winged lions. However, there can be other advantages to owning ceramic and plaster items: They tend to be virtually odorless and they're also easy to clean.

Locally, import shops and furniture stores may handle a few plaster or ceramic furniture items. Garden and decorator catalogs often carry them, too. In fact, both the **Ballard Designs** and **Home Decorators Collection** offer a great many ceramic and plaster pieces. (For glass tops for ceramic and plaster bases, see *Metal and Metal with Glass Furniture* above.)

UNFINISHED AND KIT FURNITURE

Unfinished furniture is another furnishing option you might seriously consider. Today, it's getting easier to find these pieces because there are growing numbers of stores and catalogs offering them. Actually, this isn't surprising; unfinished furniture often costs much less than comparable finished pieces. By the way, you'll find that virtually all unfinished furniture constitutes "hard" pieces, such as benches, rockers, cabinets, etc. In most cases, the furniture is completely assembled and all you have to do is apply paint, or stain (if desired) and clear finish. This gives you complete control of the finishing products actually used on your furniture, a real plus for sensitive individuals.

Another do-it-yourself option is *kit furniture*. While most unfinished furniture comes assembled, kit furniture doesn't. Therefore, this furniture is often termed *knockdown* or *KD furniture*, meaning it comes to you in separate pieces. However, most kit furniture can be easily put together using a few screws, clamps, and a tolerable carpenter's glue. One popular brand is Elmer's Professional Carpenter's Glue (**Elmer's Adhesives**). It's sold at many hardware stores and building-supply centers. Once your kit furniture is assembled, it should be lightly sanded, vacuumed, and then stained and finished with tolerable products.

The quality, materials, style, and cost of both unfinished and kit furniture varies enormously. However, you'll want to avoid, especially if you are sensitive, very cheap pieces made with tempered hardboard, plywood, particleboard, or solid softwoods such as pine. While pieces constructed with these materials are readily available and cheap, they'll most likely give off bothersome formaldehyde from formaldehyde-containing glues and softwood terpene odors. Also, it's often wise for sensitive people to avoid solid-oak kit furniture—unless you've personally tested oak and found it tolerable for you.

This is because new oak tends to release natural tannin compounds, which some people can find irritating.

Fortunately, some companies offer fine-quality unfinished and kit furniture in more tolerable hardwoods; some even handle museum-quality reproductions. By mail order, **Heart of Vermont** offers contemporary unfinished cherry or ash convertible futon/couch frames, ottomans, end tables, futon frames, and mattress beds. They also have kits for casual maple horizontal-slat chairs, tables, and benches. Also, the **Sinan Co.**'s hardwood furniture is sold unfinished. In addition, **Cohasset Colonials** and **Bartley Collection** offer reproduction kits. Kits are also available from **Sturbridge Yankee Workshop**, **Shaker Shops West**, and **Shaker Workshop**. (For more complete furniture descriptions, see *Solid Wood Furniture* above.)

Great care should be taken when you finish your unfinished or assembled kit furniture pieces so they'll not only have a professional look, but also be healthy, too. With any kit or unfinished furniture item, first lightly sand it. Then thoroughly vacuum it using a soft dusting attachment wearing a cartridge-type respirator mask. Next, apply the finish. Of course, you'll only want to use personally tested, tolerable brands. As an alternative, consider not using a stain. That way, the natural beauty of the wood shows through and you don't have to worry whether the stain will be tolerable or not.

It's important to remember that whenever you are coating a piece of furniture with any type of finish, you need to have adequate ventilation and wear a cartridge-type respirator mask. (This work may not be appropriate for sensitive persons to do themselves.) When you're done, let the furniture air out in dry, uncontaminated surroundings. This could be outdoors, or indoors in an unused room that is well-ventilated—until the piece becomes tolerable.

CUSTOM FURNITURE

Despite the fact that most furniture is now both mass-produced and mass-marketed, you can still purchase custom-made furniture. You should be aware that the cost range of such pieces can be great. For example, there are artist/cabinetmakers whose finished work sells for thousands of dollars, and then there are local cabinet shops who will make exactly what you want at affordable prices. No matter who makes your furniture, you'll want to make sure they'll use tolerable materials and products you have specified. (See *Solid Wood Cabinets* above for more information on finding the right woodworker.)

Many people are worried that they have to come up with their own furniture designs, but that isn't necessarily so. You can create your own designs if you like, or you can purchase published plans and patterns. For example, complete instructions for slatted futon frame/couches are sold by **Nontoxic Environments**. Other furniture plans are offered for sale in woodworking magazines and also in how-to books that are usually available at lumberyards. Of course, many furniture-makers will draw designs and plans specifically for your project. However, the more work he (or she) does on your job, including designing, the more your furniture will ultimately cost.

When it comes time for you to choose a hardwood species, it's often best to pick one that's naturally low in odor (maple, tulip poplar, beech, or birch), if you're a sensitive person. While softwoods such as white or yellow pine are less expensive, the natural terpenes they give off could be bothersome. It should also be noted that oak, although a very popular furniture hardwood, can release natural tannin compounds. These, too, may be irritating for long periods of time to susceptible persons (see *Testing Woods* and *Solid Wood* in *Chapter 12: Home Workshop and Garage*). Naturally, it's important that only tolerable glues and finishes be used.

If webbing is required for your custom furniture, 100%-cotton webbing (also known as *chair tape*) can be purchased from **Shaker Workshop** and **Shaker Shops West** in a variety of colors. This webbing can be woven to make very attractive chair backs and seats. If your furniture will need stuffing, organic cotton and untreated wool batting can be purchased from a number of sources, including **Nontoxic Environments**.

If you decide to actually build your custom furniture yourself, you'll want to work in as safe a manner as possible. This means having plenty of ventilation and wearing necessary protective gear. However, no matter who makes your custom furniture, sensitive individuals should be aware that it'll likely be intolerable for some time, primarily due to the recently applied finishes. Therefore, ideally, put the new furniture outside to air, or place it in a little-used room that can be well-ventilated—at least for a few weeks. Whatever place you choose, it should be dry and free of contaminating odors.

To find a capable local furniture-maker, you can check your classified phone directory under Cabinet Makers, etc. You can also ask for suggestions at local interior-decorator studios and lumberyards handling hardwoods. (For more on finding the right woodworker, see *Solid Wood Cabinets* above.) One mail-order firm you may want to contact to make custom furniture is **Pompanoosuc Mills**. This company welcomes sensitive clients and will make items especially for you, if they're similar to what they normally build. Also, an interior-decorating company that will make custom upholstered pieces using organic materials is **Organic Interiors.**

ANTIQUE FURNITURE

Antique furniture is often made of solid wood or a combination of solid and *veneered wood* (a thin layer of a valuable hardwood glued over a lesser quality wood base). Usually, the glues used in antique pieces are natural, as well as the fabrics and battings; that is, unless the furniture has been redone at some point using synthetic materials.

Antique pieces can lend warmth and charm to your home, but they can have drawbacks. Unfortunately, perfume, tobacco, and musty odors are fairly common in old pieces. Anther possible problem is mold or mildew contamination either in the past or ongoing. Therefore, you should check all antique furniture for personal tolerance before placing it in your house. If you can detect only mild odor problems, it may be that airing the furniture outside for a time will make it acceptable. Make sure to choose a location that is both dry and uncontaminated with other odors.

However, sometimes objectionable odors will have permeated the wood of your antique furniture. If that's happened, you may have to strip the finish off, sand the piece, and then refinish it before the furniture will become tolerable for you. This job should probably be left to a professional, if you are a sensitive individual. If you decide to do furniture stripping yourself, you'll want to do it outdoors if at all possible. If you have to do it indoors, you must have very good ventilation. Using a water-based less-toxic stripping product such as Safest Stripper (**3-M Do-It-Yourself Division**) is suggested over using typical solvent-based brands. Water-based strippers should be available at your local paint and hardware stores (see *Paint Strippers* in *Chapter 12: Home Workshop and Garage*). Whenever you're stripping paint, be sure to wear protective eyewear, rubber or neoprene gloves, and a cartridge-type respirator mask.

After the antique piece has been stripped, you'll need to lightly sand and vacuum it. Then, if necessary, you can stain the furniture using a tolerable water-based product. Finally, you'll want to coat the piece with a pretested tolerable clear finish. When you're all done, it's usually best to place the refinished antique furniture outdoors, or perhaps in a well-ventilated room, until the newly applied finishes are no longer bothersome. As always, the place you choose for airing should be dry and free of contaminating odors. If you're very chemically sensitive, this work would best be done by someone else who isn't sensitive.

If your antique furniture must be reupholstered, good choices for replacement materials are natural-fiber fabrics and stuffing (see *Natural Fibers* and *Natural Stuffing*, as well as *Finding Fabrics and Notions* in *Chapter 3: Clothing*). You can also supplement natural battings with metal springs, if necessary, for items requiring firmer support. It should be noted that the cloth yardage used as fabric covering should be laundered to remove any intolerable new-fabric odors before the actual upholstery work is done. This is especially important for sensitive persons (see *Removing New Clothing Odors* in *Chapter 7: Cleaning*).

One very important cautionary note for sensitive individuals when furniture is upholstered is: Be sure that whoever does the work does not smoke, wear perfume, or work in an area where others do. Otherwise, your newly reupholstered pieces could pick up these odors and be intolerable to you. While airing could dissipate these odors, there is, of course, no guarantee this would be absolutely successful.

MAKING USED FURNITURE TOLERABLE

Sometimes individuals own bothersome furniture they don't want to, or simply can't afford to, replace at the moment. For example, a person may own a sofa covered and stuffed in odorous synthetic materials, but it's only a few years old and he (or she) can't afford to buy a new one made of healthier materials. What do you do? Some sensitive people choose not to have a sofa, rather than one that could pose health problems for them. However, for those who are less sensitive and want to try a less-drastic approach, there are options. For example, the sofa could be put outdoors to air for several days (or weeks) in dry, uncontaminated surroundings. This might cause enough chemical, perfume, and/or tobacco odors to be released so that the sofa becomes tolerable enough to be placed back indoors. However, if airing doesn't help enough, the sofa could be draped with *barrier cloth* yardage. Barrier cloth is a white, densely woven, untreated, 100%-cotton that can help block many odors. Two mail-order sources for barrier cloth are **The Cotton Place** and **Janice Corp.** Unfortunately, from an aesthetic viewpoint, barrier cloth isn't very attractive. However, it can be dyed (for less-toxic dyes, see *Finding Fabrics and Notions* in *Chapter 3: Clothing*).

If you decide to refinish or reupholster a contemporary piece of furniture, most of the section about antique pieces will apply to it as well (see *Antique Furniture* above). If you have the choice, you'll want to have the seats made with *removable* cushions stuffed with natural stuffing and covered in washable all-natural fiber fabrics. (Non-removable cushioning can be more difficult to clean.) In fact, all upholstery and slipcovers fabrics ideally should be made of washable natural-fiber material (see *Natural Fibers* and *Finding Fabrics and Notions* in *Chapter 3: Clothing*).

Ready-made natural-fiber slipcovers are sometimes available in local department stores, upholstery shops, and interior design studios. Through catalogs, **Ballard Design** offers 100%-cotton slipcovers in several sizes, and **Pottery Barn** sells 100%-cotton and cotton/linen slipcovers. Also, you can contact **Organic Interiors**, an interior-decorating company, or a local upholstery shop, to make custom organic-fabric slipcovers for you.

WINDOW TREATMENTS

Originally, windows (derived from *wind eyes*) were just open holes in walls. They let in light and air, and in some cases allowed smoke to leave. As architecture advanced, windows also became important from an aesthetic viewpoint. In time, complex windowpane designs and elaborate interior-decorating treatments became fairly common, at least in the residences of the upperclass. Today, more people than ever have window treatments that are more decorative than they are functional. However, for certain windows, privacy and energy savings are still important considerations.

Unfortunately, most modern interior window treatments have real problems that few people seem to recognize. For example, many decorative treatments can't be easily dusted or thoroughly cleaned. Also, the fabrics used to make typical curtains and draperies are usually synthetic. These can release bothersome chemical odors from the compounds making up the fabric fibers. Then, too, most fabrics, especially certain natural-fiber fabrics, will break down over time from having been exposed to ultraviolet (UV) radiation from the sun. Unfortunately, deteriorating fabric creates loose fiber parts that become airborne dust. It also means that nearly all fabric curtains and draperies must periodically be replaced.

The good news is that there are more practical and healthier choices for interior window treatments than many of the typical ones now being used. Ideally, a healthy window treatment should be attractive, functional, made of all-natural materials, be easy to maintain, and not be subject to rapid deterioration by ultraviolet rays from sunlight. This section will discuss some of the better window treatment options to consider for your home.

METAL BLINDS

From a health standpoint, metal mini-blinds are an excellent window-treatment choice, and they're usually quite tolerable for sensitive individuals. Generally, metal blinds are made of either aluminum or steel painted with baked-on enamel. Because they're metal, they hold-up well even in strong sunlight. Another advantage is that all-metal blinds are adjustable; by raising or lowering the blinds and altering the angle of the slats, they can easily adapt to different natural lighting needs and conditions.

Today's metal mini-blinds can be purchased in a wide selection of colors and slat widths. In addition, you can buy them in either horizontal or vertical slat designs. Vertical mini-blinds look more like draperies, and they don't collect dust easily. However, horizontal blinds tend to be less expensive and are usually available with more options. For example, some horizontal blinds can be purchased with a special privacy feature that allows them to be closed much more tightly than standard blinds.

Metal blinds can be purchased either ready-made or custom-made. Ready-made blinds are usually sold in only a few standard sizes and colors, but you can get them right away and they're very economical. To find them locally, check department stores, building centers, and discount stores. On the other hand, custom-made blinds are each manufactured to fit a specific window, so they must be specially ordered. Of course, their price is higher than for standard ready-made blinds, but you can get them in the exact color, size, and style you want. While your local department stores and drapery shops should be able to order custom-made metal blinds, there are a number of discount mail-order companies that sell custom metal blinds directly to the public at very affordable prices. You can often find their advertisements in home remodeling and decorating magazines. Two such companies are **Baron's Window Coverings** and **National Blind Factory**.

One of the advantages to metal mini-blinds is that they're easy to maintain. They can be simply swept free of dust by using your vacuum cleaner's soft dusting attachment on both sides. (Special mini-blind vacuum attachments are available. A mail-order source is **Lillian Vernon**.) Occasionally, you may want to wash your metal mini-blinds. To do so, use a soft sponge or cloth that has been dipped in a tolerable dishwashing detergent and water solution (see *Hand Dishwashing Products* in *Chapter 7: Cleaning*). Next, wring out the sponge and gently go over the slats. Then, rinse the slats using the sponge and clear water. To prevent spotting gently dry the slats using a soft towel.

Sensitive individuals should be aware that the new paint on their metal blinds could outgas bothersome odors. However, washing the blinds (as described above) and then hanging them outdoors, or in a well-ventilated unused room, usually eliminates these odors after a few days or so. (Blinds with baked-on finishes are oftem quite inert.) Be sure the place you choose for airing is uncontaminated by other potentially polluting odors.

WOOD, REED, AND BAMBOO BLINDS

Wood, reed, and bamboo blinds are all-natural, attractive choices for window treatments. Depending on the material and whether or not it's been split, the slats could be less than 1/4" (sometimes known as *matchstick*) up to 1" wide. These types of blinds can be rolled up or down, but there's no way to adjust the angle of the slats. To purchase wood, reed, or bamboo blinds, check your local department stores, drapery shops, and import stores. Usually they're sold as uncoated (natural), stained, or painted in a few standard sizes. All are usually inexpensive or moderately priced. More expensive custom sizes may be available at some department stores and drapery shops.

You should be aware that any new wood, reed, or bamboo blind that has been stained or painted may need to air for some time before it becomes tolerable, if you are a sensitive person. To do this, simply hang them outdoors where precipitation and contaminating odors can't reach them, or in a well-ventilated, unused room, until they lose their odor.

There are still other concerns with wood, reed, and bamboo blinds you might want to consider before purchasing them. First, natural materials will eventually deteriorate from exposure to ultraviolet radiation from the sun, so they'll probably have to be replaced at some point. Fortunately, this could be many years from when you first hang them. Another possible concern is how you maintain natural blinds. Actually, you can remove most dust by using a vacuum cleaner's soft dusting attachment. Of course, if you do need to wash them, it's best to read the manufacturers' tags first for their recommended cleaning instructions. However, simply sponging the blinds with clear water often works well. Make certain they're able to dry quickly, to prevent mold or mildew.

FABRIC ROMAN SHADES

Roman shades often make an interesting window treatment. They're actually a special type of fabric blind made to fold up into continuous uniform horizontal layers when raised. If you decide on Roman shades, consider buying those made with untreated natural-fiber fabrics. Linen is an especially good choice because it doesn't deteriorate from sunlight exposure.

However, you should be aware of certain drawbacks with Roman shades. First of all, shades of this type can sometimes be difficult to clean. While you can gently vacuum any Roman shade with a dusting attachment, certain shades may not be able to be washed. Also, most of the materials used (except linen) will eventually break down from the ultraviolet rays of sunlight.

To purchase Roman shades, first check local department stores and drapery shops. These retail outlets can usually custom-make them for you. By mail order, a source for ready-made 100%-cotton Roman blinds is **Pottery Barn**. Also, **Holland Corp.** makes 100%-organic versions that can be taken apart and washed. They come in one standard size (33"w x 67"h) and custom sizes.

FABRIC ROLLERS

Fabric rollers as window treatments have been around for decades. They're simply rods equipped with a metal spring that have a length of fabric attached to them. Today, fabric rollers are generally inexpensive and made with synthetic materials such as vinyl. However, custom drapery departments and shops can often make fabric rollers in any materials and dimensions you choose. You can purchase ready-made 100%-cotton canvas and linen/cotton fabric rollers through the mail from **Pottery Barn**.

Unfortunately, fabric rollers will eventually deteriorate when exposed to the sun's ultraviolet radiation; that is, unless you choose linen. Also, because most fabric rollers can't be laundered, you'll want to occasionally take them down and thoroughly vacuum them. To do this, lay them on a clean, smooth surface and completely unroll them. Then very carefully vacuum one side at a time using a soft dusting attachment. You may find you'll need someone to hold the fabric down securely while you're vacuuming.

CURTAINS AND DRAPERIES

Washable, untreated 100%-natural-fiber curtains can usually provide a softer appearance for your windows than blinds, shades, or rollers. Sometimes all-cotton curtains are available in ready-made sizes, styles, and colors at local department stores and drapery shops. Through the **Ballard Designs** catalog, you can buy pre-made full-length 100%-cotton-duck curtains. Also, **Pottery Barn** has natural-fiber curtains in several short and full-length styles. Unfortunately, both mail-order companies recommend that these curtains be dry-cleaned, not machine washed (see *Is Dry Cleaning a Problem?* in *Chapter 3: Clothing*). However, **The Seventh Generation** offers washable 86" green-cotton curtains. They come in 39" widths with fabric tabs for hanging. These particular curtains can be machine-laundered in cold water, but you should expect 6 to 8% shrinkage. Several attractive styles of brass curtain rods and tiebacks are also available from the same company.

Of course, natural-fabric curtains can also be custom-made. Local department stores, upholstery shops, and drapery specialty shops should be able to provide this service for you. Also, **Organic Interiors** can make custom, organic-fiber curtains by mail order. Another option is to make the curtains yourself. To do this, check your local fabric stores for appropriate patterns and materials (see *Custom-Made Clothing* in *Chapter 3: Clothing*). Remember, however, that fabric curtains will eventually deteriorate from exposure to sunlight, unless you choose linen. Therefore, fabric curtains often have to be replaced every several years.

Another popular window-treatment option is lined draperies. Linings help protect the decorative room-facing fabric from damaging sun exposure. Generally, lined draperies are much heavier than curtains and provide more privacy, but they're usually fairly expensive. This is because most lined draperies are custom-made, requiring the labor and skill of a professional seamstress to construct them, and they require two layers of fabric. To buy lined draperies, you'll want to check with local department stores and drapery shops. One mail-order source is **Organic Interiors**. This particular interior-decorating firm will custom make draperies using organically raised materials.

Unfortunately, virtually all lined draperies must be dry-cleaned in order to maintain their shape. Not only can this be expensive, but it means your draperies will acquire harmful solvent odors. If professional cleaning must be done, hang the newly dry-cleaned draperies outdoors so the solvent odors can dissipate before rehanging them. Between cleanings, it's best to regularly vacuum both sides of your lined draperies using a soft dusting attachment.

SWAGS

A popular window treatment is using a *swag* (sometimes also called a valance). A swag is actually defined as a wreath or short section of decoratively folded or gathered curtain fabric suspended over a window. These days, some swags are quite ornate and complicated; others are quite simple. In an ideal healthy household, swags should be made of washable, untreated, 100%-natural fiber fabric, and be designed so that they can be easily taken down and laundered (see *Finding Fabrics and Notions* in *Chapter 3: Clothing*).

In the last few years, special swag hardware has become available so that nearly anyone can create attractive swags themselves. Doing it yourself is much less expensive than hiring a professional decorator to do the job, and more rewarding and fun. While most local department stores and drapery shops sell these do-it-yourself supplies, the hardware is often made of plastic. Sometimes plastic pieces can easily bend or break, and in some cases they can emit odors that certain sensitive persons may find bothersome.

Fortunately, all-metal enamel-coated ladder-type tracks for making swags are manufactured and sold by **Kurtain Kraft**. Metal hardware is preferred because retains its shape and does not release synthetic odors. To create a swag using **Kurtain Kraft** parts, simply pull a piece of fabric through the metal tracking; no sewing or special tools are required. At any time later, the fabric can be quickly removed for cleaning, or replaced to create an entirely different look.

Another swag option is to install either a large metal rod or wooden dowel across your window top, then, simply drape fabric over it. Surprisingly, this can make for a very stylish window. Wrought-iron rods, as well as those made of hardwood, are sold by **Pottery Barn**. They also sell metal holdback hardware which is designed to hold back long draping fabric to the sides of the window frame. By the way, an usual swag can be created using corbel-style plaster swag rod holders from **Pottery Barn**.

SHUTTERS

Wood shutters can provide an all-natural, homey window treatment that can also provide a great deal of privacy. Unfortunately, wood shutters are commonly made of softwood pine. When new, many softwoods can give off terpene odors that can be irritating to certain persons (see *Solid Wood* in *Chapter 12: Home Workshop and Garage*). To purchase wood shutters, check your local department stores, drapery shops, building centers, or unfinished-furniture stores.

Actually, a number of wood shutter styles are available, including those with adjustable slats and fabric inserts. Generally, however, only certain standard sizes are offered, and these are often sold prefinished, with either a paint or stain with clear finish. However, they are also usually available in an unfinished, natural state. Sensitive individuals should be aware that any stain or paint can be intolerable for some time when it's new. If you personally find a stain or paint bothersome on your new shutters, place them outside in an area protected from the weather and polluting odors, or put them in a well-ventilated, unused room until they become acceptable.

Of course, if you decide you'd like to paint, stain or apply a clear finish to the wood shutters yourself, you'll want to use only tolerable products (see *Chapter 12: Home Workshop and Garage*). It's also important that this work be done only with good ventilation while wearing a cartridge-type respirator mask and other appropriate protective gear. After the finishes have been applied, the shutters will need to air in a dry, uncontaminated area until they become odor-free. Note that, coating with finishes is usually work that shouldn't be done by very sensitive persons.

For those wood shutters designed to have fabric panel inserts, it's best to choose untreated, washable, 100%-natural-fiber fabrics. After purchasing the cloth, it's best to launder it first before cutting it to size. That way, the fabric will be both preshrunk—and tolerable.

As a rule, wood shutters are relatively easy to maintain. They can be easily vacuumed regularly with a soft dusting attachment. Those shutters with fabric panels can have the fabric occasionally removed and washed in a tolerable laundry product.

DECORATIVE GLASS

Decorative glass can be used to create beautiful and unexpected window treatments. *Stained glass* (generally, glass colored with metallic oxides fused through the entire depth), *enameled glass* (glass that's been permanently surface-decorated using baked-on translucent or opaque glazes), and *beveled glass* (thick glass with angled edges) can be used by craftspeople/artists to meet your specific window needs. To find such a skilled glass worker, check your telephone book classified section under Stained Glass or Windows. Of course, when you find a prospective artisan, you'll want to see examples of his (or her) work before you agree to any commission, and make sure to get price and time estimates. You should be aware ahead of time that any one-of-a-kind creation will likely be expensive. As a rule, the larger and more complicated the design and the more renowned the reputation of the glass worker, the higher the finished price will be. In addition, the cost will also depend on the types of glass actually used.

If you can't afford an entire custom-made window, you might consider hanging just a small *roundel* (circular disk) or rectangular decorative glass panel. Many museum shops, art fairs, and catalogs sell these at reasonable prices. Another option is to simply buy a single sheet, or an antique panel, of stained glass and frame it with metal or wood. Once framed, you can securely hang it by a chain in front of your window. Not only can this provide your room with interest, it can increase your privacy as well. To find sheets of stained glass, you'll want to check at local glass stores and craft shops. Note that, these stores may also be able to cut the glass sheets to size for you.

Another relatively inexpensive option is to actually replace the clear glass in your window with a single sheet of opalescent or textured glass. Of course, this will involve some installation work using window putty. For this job, **Nontoxic Environments** sells less-toxic alternative putties you may want to try. Unfortunately, these putties may still prove bothersome to some sensitive individuals. Therefore, testing beforehand is important. However, most newly applied putty is not a significant problem because it is used primarily on the exterior of the window.

Some stained, enameled, or beveled glass panels and roundels are held together with brass or copper foil or *cames* (grooved metal ribbons) and non-lead solder. However, a great many decorative glass items are created with lead came and lead solder. Unfortunately, lead is a toxic heavy metal. It can cause a variety of negative health effects if swallowed or inhaled. Yet it needs to be said that lead came and solder that is already in place is very unlikely to cause problems for adults because it doesn't outgas. However, if children handle it or put their mouths on it, the lead would be harmful to them. If you are concerned about this, you should only buy decorative-glass pieces held together with copper or brass and using lead-free solder.

SHOWER CURTAINS AND DOORS

An ideal shower curtain or shower door should protect your bathroom from water damage, and not be a cause of potential health problems for you and your family. While most people don't consider the potential negative health consequences when they buy a shower curtain or door, it's something that is wise to take into account.

SHOWER CURTAINS

For several decades now, shower curtains have become more decorative and elaborate. Some now consist of several layers of lace and fabric panels. However, virtually all shower curtains have an inner layer of waterproof vinyl. Unfortunately, vinyl can pose certain problems. New vinyl can outgas chemical odors that can be bothersome, especially for sensitive people. While not usually a health concern, older vinyl can easily crack and tear.

A relatively recent innovation in shower curtains is a treatment that enables them to be advertised as "unable to support mold growth." It's likely that such curtains have been treated with chemical fungicides to resist mildew contamination. While resisting fungus is an admirable trait, a shower curtain's relatively large surface area would expose someone to a considerable amount of potentially intolerable compounds. Of course, certain sensitive persons would be more susceptible to these negative effects than others.

A healthier shower curtain choice would be an untreated 100%-cotton-duck canvas shower curtain These curtains are made of heavy, plain-weave, white fabric that can be regularly machine-washed and dried. Cotton-duck shower curtains are available from several mail-order companies including **Janice Corp.** and **The Cotton Place**. Also, green-cotton-duck shower curtains are sold by **The Seventh Generation**. If you like color in your bathroom, you can easily dye cotton curtains. **Richman Cotton Company** offers a wide selection of less-toxic dyes for use on cotton.

SHOWER DOORS

A very good alternative to shower curtains is glass shower doors. These are attractive, inert, and permanent. An ideal style is one that has glass doors with polished edges rather than glass panels set into metal frames, as well as a free-draining lower tub molding rather than a water-blocking lipped track. Without conventional frames and lower tracking, water is able to drain away quickly and there are fewer places for mold to grow. One manufacturer of glass shower doors of this type is **Alumax, Magnolia Division**. Call the company for a nearby dealer. Your local building centers and plumbing supply stores often handle similar brands.

Keep in mind that new glass shower doors will require some installation work. This obviously will add to their expense if you can't do the work yourself. Also, shower-door installation always requires caulking, which generally has a strong odor when newly applied. One brand of caulk you may want to try for this is Kwik Seal tub and tile caulk (**Dap Products, Inc.**). While this product does contain a mildew preventive, it's often well tolerated by sensitive individuals within a relatively short period of time. Unfortunately, if a caulk doesn't contain any fungicides, it can become contaminated with mold or mildew very quickly, so it'll need to be replaced over and over again. Of course, no matter what type of caulk you use, it's best to apply it with good ventilation and while wearing a cartridge-type respirator mask. As might be expected, this isn't a job for sensitive persons to tackle themselves.

LIGHTING

Good lighting is important for both safety and aesthetics. Sunlight from windows and skylights can provide a certain amount of light, but it may not be enough, or, for privacy reasons, you can't take advantage of it. Of course at night, windows and skylights offer no help in illuminating your home's interior, so artificial lighting is necessary, either from electric lamps or from flames.

Most people don't think of the health ramifications of the lamps and fixtures they use daily in their homes, except perhaps whether the light given off is bright enough to do an intended job. However, when you buy bulbs and tubes, you may want to consider the light spectrum they emit (and also their energy efficiency and life expectancy). When you buy lighting fixtures and decorative lamps, you might also consider how easy they'll be to clean and what materials were used in their construction. As always, everything you put in your home has a potential effect on your well-being—even what you choose for lighting.

SOME ARTIFICIAL LIGHT BASICS

The first artificial illumination was undoubtedly campfires and bundled torches of dried grasses or wood. Eventually, stone lamps were developed. These contained liquefied fat or oil and a wick. These were followed by the creation of candles made of beeswax or hardened animal fat. Lamps (later using kerosene with glass chimneys) and candles remained the major interior illumination sources until gas lighting began being used in cities and towns in the 1800s. With the invention of electric lighting in the late 19th century, lighting with gas became passé. Today, except for emergencies, in places where the occupants choose not to use electricity, and when a special mood is sought using flames, virtually all artificial lighting in American homes is with electric bulbs and fluorescent tubes.

Many people want to know, "How much artificial light do I need in my home?" Actually over the years, lighting engineers have changed the recommended lighting requirements from time to time. As a rule though, in most situations there needs to be overall *general illumination* sufficient enough to see clearly when there's no other sources of light. Extra *task lighting* is required over kitchen countertops or in reading areas, for example. Remember, it's usually best to err on the side of having too much light than not having enough for safety's sake, and yet *glare* (harsh, piercing light coming directly from a lighting source) and *reflected glare* (glare that has bounced off objects) can sometimes pose safety problems.

If you want to be absolutely certain of the ideal lighting requirements for your home (locations for certain illumination, types of fixtures needed, etc.), you should contact a professional lighting engineer. (Check in the phone directory under Lighting.) While, his (or her) services are very desirable, they could be fairly costly, too. As an alternative, local lighting stores may have lighting consultants who will come to your home at a reasonable cost. These people usually don't have an engineering background, but are familiar with typical home-lighting needs and popular new lighting trends. However, you should keep in mind that consultants who are connected with lighting stores may tend to suggest more fixtures and costlier ones than you may truly need. Remember, nearly every fixture permanently mounted into ceilings or walls will require installation by an electrician, and every bulb or tube that is turned on means a higher utility bill. Therefore, it's important to combine suggestions from others with your own common sense.

Whenever you buy a bulb or tube for a fixture or lamp, be sure to get the correct wattage. For example, some fixtures come with a label stating, "Don't use a bulb greater than 60 watts." These warnings are issued because bulbs of greater-than-recommended wattage could easily create too much heat for the fixture to operate safely. Therefore, always check to see if a fixture or decorative lamp has a recommended wattage label. Also, when replacing a bulb or tube, be certain that the electricity to the fixture or decorative lamp is turned off in order to prevent accidental electrocution.

BULBS AND TUBES (LAMPS)

The two major categories of lamps are: incandescent bulbs and fluorescent tubes. In the lighting industry the word *lamp* refers to both types. Admittedly, this can be confusing inasmuch as most people think of a lamp as a base unit with a shade, that sits on a table or the floor. However in this section, the word lamp will follow the industry standard and apply to both incandescent bulbs and fluorescent tubes.

TYPICAL LAMPS

For decades, both incandescent lamps and fluorescent tubes have been commonly used in homes. Each type has its advantages and drawbacks. The following sections will discuss some of these.

Typical Incandescent Lamps

The oldest type of electric lamp type is the incandescent bulb, the first practical one having been created in 1879 by Thomas Edison. With the construction of electric generating stations, incandescent lamps soon became commonplace. Today, they remain the most popular kind of lamp used in American homes.

By definition, an *incandescent lamp* is a clear or frosted glass bulb having a looped filament and a metal screw base. Inside the bulb, the air (with its relatively high level of oxygen) has been removed so that combustion can't occur. Generally, an inert gas (from a combustion standpoint) such as nitrogen, or a mixture of inert gases, is then pumped in at about a third of the normal atmospheric pressure. These inert gases are added to slow down the filament's *sublimation* (evaporation from a solid directly to a gaseous state). Sublimation results in the black discoloration seen in old bulbs. When too much of a filament has sublimated, the bulb will burn out. Because of the inevitable process of sublimation, typical incandescent lamps generally don't last as long as typical fluorescent lamps.

In many incandescent bulbs, the looped filaments are made of *tungsten*, a rare metallic element. When an incandescent bulb is on, the electric current enters through the metal screw base and flows into the tungsten filament. The filament temperature then rises rapidly, up to several thousand degrees Fahrenheit. This causes the tungsten to glow. In reality, several forms of radiation are actually emitted. These include visible light, some ultraviolet rays, and a great deal of infrared radiation (heat). In fact, a fairly large percentage of all the electricity used by typical incandescent bulbs goes, not to producing light, but to generating unwanted infrared heat.

Traditionally, incandescent bulbs have been chosen over other lamp types for most residential applications: table and floor lamps as well as bedroom, hall, and bath ceiling fixtures. This is because incandescent bulbs are able to be manufactured, at low cost, in virtually any size or shape to fit in nearly all types and sizes of fixtures. Also, their yellowish-white glow is considered by many to be warm and friendly.

Typical Fluorescent Lamps

The other relatively common type of lamp used in homes is the fluorescent tube. Actually, fluorescent tubes are a much more recent invention, having been first shown to the public in 1933. However, by the 1950s they had nearly replaced incandescent lamps in public institutions, offices, and commercial buildings. They also began to be used more frequently for certain residential applications.

By definition, a fluorescent lamp is a glass tube with an interior phosphor coating and a special gas (usually a combination of argon and mercury) filling the interior. The ends of the tube are sealed with metal caps having one or two prongs. When a fluorescent tube is turned on, the electricity passes from one end of the tube to the other. As the electricity travels through the gas-filled interior, ultraviolet radiation is created. It's actually the ultraviolet rays that cause the phosphor coating on the tube walls to glow, creating visible light—usually a white or bluish-white light. Because of the blue/white color, some people feel typical fluorescent lamps make a room look cold.

As mentioned previously, fluorescent lamps have been the lighting choice for decades for nonresidential uses. This is because they've been commonly manufactured as very long tubes (4'–8') that are able to emit a great deal of light, produce little heat, and use less electricity than incandescent bulbs. However, they do have their drawbacks. For example, typical fluorescent lamps have been limited in their shape to some form of long narrow tube. They also require *ballasts* (transformers) in their fixtures to convert 110-volt electricity into the much higher voltage needed to cause the phosphor coating to glow. Unfortunately, at one time, highly-toxic *polychlorinated biphenyls (PCBs)* were used in some of these ballasts. Even though the ballasts created today no longer contain PCBs, older ballasts filled with PCBs still exist in many fluorescent fixtures, and these have the potential to leak this poisonous liquid as they wear out.

Another problem with typical fluorescent lamps is that they create potentially problematic electromagnetic fields (EMFs) (see *Chapter 11: Electromagnetic Fields*). In some cases, these fields can actually be fairly strong. In addition, typical fluorescent fixtures emit low levels of X-rays. Finally, some fluorescent lamps tend to produce a rapidly flickering light that goes on an off 60 times a second—light which some people find disturbing.

LAMP INNOVATIONS

In recent years, a number of lamp manufacturers have devised variations on the typical incandescent bulb and fluorescent tube in order to overcome their limitations.

Incandescent Lamp Innovations

Incandescent lamps are now available that are designed for longer life or the capacity to emit a full spectrum that mimics natural-light.

One interesting innovation is the use of special *diodes* that are attached to the tips of the metal screw bases of certain incandescent bulbs. Diodes are tiny electronic devices that only permit electric current to pass through them in one direction. Home electric lines carry *alternating current (AC)* in which the flow of electricity repeatedly switches directions 60 times a second. Because a diode-equipped bulb uses only electricity flowing in one direction, it is only on half the time. This creates a continuous on/off light pattern. However, it's so rapid that most people can't perceive it, so they just see continuous light. By having the bulb on only half the time, the bulb's life expectancy is greatly extended.

The Enterpriser line of light bulbs (**Carysbrook Mfg.**) encompasses a very large selection of diode-equipped incandescent bulbs. Beside having diodes, these bulbs have other special features. For example, the filaments have additional built-in support to help them resist damage from vibrations. Also, the bulbs are filled with an 85% krypton-gas mixture to better stop filament sublimation (see *Typical Incandescent Lamps* above). Finally, the bulbs' screw bases are made of brass, which is corrosion-resistant. Because of these innovations, Enterpriser bulbs are sold with a lifetime-replacement guarantee. If you are interested in buying them, they can be ordered directly from the manufacturer.

Another incandescent innovation is the *color-corrected bulb*. Lamps of this type are designed to more closely mimic the spectrum of natural sunlight, rather than the yellowish glow of typical incandescent bulbs. This is important because there is some evidence that humans benefit by being exposed to light indoors that is more similar to sunlight. One brand of color-corrected incandescent bulbs is Chromalux (**Lumiram Electric Corporation**), which are imported from Finland. They achieve a more-natural light using *neodymium*-tinted glass. (Neodymium is a rare, rosy/violet-colored earth element.) Chromalux bulbs are available only from dealers including **Baubiologie Hardware**, **N.E.E.D.S.**, and **Ott Light Systems**.

Fluorescent Lamp Innovations

As with incandescent lamps, fluorescent lamps with improved design features are now available. One popular innovation is the *warm-white* fluorescent tube that emits less light from the blue and green portions of the visible light spectrum. As a result, the light from warm-white fluorescent lamps appears less harsh than the light given off by typical fluorescent lamps. To purchase warm-white fluorescent lamps, check your local lighting centers and hardware stores.

Another development is the *full-spectrum* fluorescent tube, which gives off light that more closely duplicates the spectrum of natural sunlight. Researchers have found there are positive health benefits from using full-spectrum lighting instead of conventional indoor lighting. This is particularly true for those individuals with *Seasonal Affective Disorder (SAD)*. SAD is a form of depression that reoccurs every winter. It affects certain susceptible individuals because, for them, the decreased amount of sunlight during the shorter winter days triggers a biochemical imbalance in their bodies. Interestingly, individuals with SAD generally improve remarkably if they sit in front of several bright full-spectrum fluorescent tubes for a few hours a day during the winter.

Vita-Lite full-spectrum fluorescent tubes (**Duro-Lite Lamps, Inc.**) are available in sizes ranging from 15" to 96". They can be ordered directly from the company. Also, **Ott Light Systems** offers full-spectrum fluorescent tubes as well as special fixtures to mount them in. The Ott Neo-Radiation Guarded (NRG) Systems have grounded, lead-shielded *cathodes*. (Cathodes are the metal ends of the tubes where electricity enters and leaves the lamps.) Lead shields are placed over the cathodes to reduce emissions of both electromagnetic fields and X-rays.

One very popular fluorescent lamp innovation is the *compact* fluorescent. These fluorescent lamps have smaller diameter tubes (in a variety of shapes, some quite complex), built-in *ballasts* (transformers), and screw bases. Therefore, compact fluorescent lamps can be used in many of the same fixtures and decorative table lamps as incandescent bulbs. While they're more expensive to purchase, they're very long-lasting and quite energy-efficient so that over time they can save you a considerable amount of money. Unfortunately, some designs are just too large to fit in fixtures and table lamps that were originally designed for smaller incandescent bulbs. To find compact fluorescent lamps, you'll want to check your local hardware stores, building-supply outlets, and lighting centers. Also, your electric-power utility may offer them at discounted prices. By mail order, you can purchase them from **Real Goods**.

By the way, the built-in ballasts used in compact fluorescent lamps come in two types: magnetic and electronic. The electronic ballasts cost a little more but they don't cause the light to flicker, and they give off lower-intensity electromagnetic fields (EMFs) (see *Chapter 11: Electromagnetic Fields*).

CHOOSING THE RIGHT LAMP

Because of all the varieties available, it's important to know what you really want before purchasing a lamp for a specific application. Some considerations to keep in mind are the fixture's recommended lamp wattage, the desired brightness, the type of socket the fixture has, the size of the bulb compared to the size of the fixture, the lamp's energy efficiency, the type of light spectrum emitted by the lamp, the lamp's initial cost, the lamp's lifetime operating cost, and whether the lamp has a flickering on/off quality or gives off a steady uniform light.

Admittedly, it can be confusing to compare different types of bulbs and tubes in order to figure out the best lighting option. Often, personnel working at local electrical supply companies and lighting centers can be helpful. In addition, one mail-order company that can assist you is **Real Goods**. This firm offers a fine selection of compact-fluorescent lamps and its catalog allows you to compare the features of various lamps.

FIXTURES AND DECORATIVE LAMPS

The following sections will discuss the different mounting devices available for bulbs and tubes, or in other words fixtures and decorative lamps.

CEILING AND WALL FIXTURES

Ceiling and wall fixtures can be attractive lighting additions to your home. However, ideally, you might want to avoid those made of plastic, especially if you are a sensitive person. Plastic fixtures can emit unpleasant "plasticky" odors when they're hot, which some people find bothersome. Also, you might want to avoid fixtures with open-bowl shades, if possible. The open bowls tend to become dust and insect accumulators. While intricate chandeliers may be attractive, you should keep in mind that they'll probably be very difficult to clean. This is particularly true for most crystal-glass chandeliers.

It's not difficult to find healthfully designed ceiling and wall fixtures; most department stores, lighting stores, and building centers now carry good selections. You can also mail-order fixtures as well. For example, metal and glass ceiling fixtures are available from **Home Decorators Collection**. The company also handles stained-glass ceiling fixtures. In addition, **Pottery Barn** sells simple wrought-iron chandeliers.

FLOOR AND TABLE LAMPS

It's best to choose lamps that are innately healthy. From an air-quality standpoint, floor and table lamps having metal, wood, glass, or ceramic bases with glass shades are ideal. Shades that are made of natural fabric or paper are good second choices, but generally these can't be washed. If possible, avoid lampshades made of synthetic fabrics or plastics, especially if you are a sensitive person. The heat generated by hot bulbs can cause these shades to release potentially intolerable odors.

It should be fairly easy to find healthier types of lamps by checking your local furniture stores and lighting centers. Some very good selections can also be mail-ordered. For example, **Pottery Barn** sells attractive wrought-iron table and floor lamps with Kraft-paper shades. They also offer table lamps made of pottery, metal, and solid wood. The shades used are either paper or linen. **Shaker Workshop** handles stoneware table lamps, while solid-maple table lamps, as well as metal ones, can be purchased from **Crate and Barrel**. In addition, **Home Decorators Collection** sells metal floor and table lamps. The company's lamps with metal bases and stained-glass shades are particularly good looking.

One option is making your own lamp shades. Some craft stores offer wire frames that you can cover with any type of fabric you want, such as organically raised cotton.

You should remember that floor and table lamps need to be routinely cleaned. Lamp bases can be regularly dusted with a soft, all-cotton flannel cloth. It's also best to remove any glass shades from time to time and wash them with a tolerable dish detergent. On the other hand, fabric shades can be occasionally removed and carefully vacuumed using a soft dusting attachment. Of course, you'll want to be especially gentle when you vacuum paper shades because they can be easily damaged.

It's also important to occasionally dust the tops of the light bulbs used in open-shade lamps. This is necessary, especially for sensitive individuals, because accumulated dust particles on the bulbs can burn and give off odors when the bulbs are lit and become hot. In order to safely dust bulbs, you'll first need to unplug your lamps. Then, you can go over the bulbs using a dry, soft 100%-cotton flannel cloth. It's best to never use a dampened cloth or a vacuum attachment for dusting light bulbs because of the possibilities of breaking the bulb and causing electrocution.

FLAMES

Ideally, it's wise to avoid burning kerosene, vegetable oil, bottled gas, Sterno (trademark brand of canned, flammable, hydrocarbon jelly), alcohol, and other fuels for lighting indoors. This is especially true for sensitive individuals and those with asthma or other breathing problems. This advice also applies to all types of candles, even those made of natural materials such as beeswax or animal and vegetable *tallow* (hard fat). In addition, you should avoid all fireplaces and wood stoves, except those with well-sealed glass doors and outside-air supplies. Some gas fireplaces now have sealed combustion chambers.

The reason for avoiding these items is that they can give off polluting combustion gases and smoke when they're lit. Both smoke and combustion gases can cause serious negative health effects, including respiratory inflammation. See also *Combustion Gases* and *Smoke* in *Chapter 9: Indoor Air.*

ACCENT PIECES

Accent pieces can give your home personality, but it's probably best to pick only those that are nontoxic and natural. Of course, this is especially important if you are a sensitive person. Also, you should probably put more thought into choosing each accent piece than superficial reasons such as picking "a color that would go with the carpeting." After all, you don't have to fill each empty nook and space of an entire room or house all at once. Instead, you may want to try acquiring only very special things, ones that are truly meaningful to you and your family. These special pieces would be added to your home slowly, perhaps over many years. Whatever you decide to do, keep in mind that too many knickknacks can create a confusing and cluttered appearance, and they can become hard-to-clean dust accumulators.

What could possibly be attractive, healthy, low-outgassing collectibles? Actually, good choices are ceramic figurines, plates, porcelain dolls, bronzes, pewter items, tin ware, crystal, glassware, shells, and rocks and minerals, to name a just a few. To find items for a special collection, you might check museum shops, galleries, and art/craft fairs, as well as shell and rock shops, among other places.

Other healthful home accents include wooden pieces (carvings, etc.) and baskets. Round, cherry, Shaker-style boxes are available from **Shaker Workshop. Shaker Shops West** has them in both cherry and walnut. Both companies also have a nice selection of natural-material Shaker baskets and hardwood bowls. In addition, good-looking wood-framed mirrors are sold by **Pottery Barn**.

Then, too, special accent metal or glass furnishing pieces can add visual interest to your home's interior, and local furniture stores generally offer a variety of these. Brass hall trees, umbrella stands, and metal wastebaskets are also available by mail order from the **Home Decorators Collection**. In addition, you might consider buying metal picture frames. These are available in a range of colors and styles that are attractive, virtually inert, and easy to clean. **Graphic Dimensions Ltd.** is one popular mail-order source. (Lacquered or painted items amy require an airing period in uncontaminated surroundings before they become tolerable.) Glass vases can make beautiful decorating additions. Two catalogs that often handle these are **Crate & Barrel** and **Pottery Barn**.

A good suggestion for your collections are solid-wood display units with glass doors, which you might purchase or have specially built (see *Custom Furniture* above). These can be used to show off your small, delicate pieces to their best advantage. They are available as hanging wall cabinets or glass-topped tables. In such a display case, your collectibles will be protected from airborne dust.

To give your home a cozy feel, you can add natural-fiber afghans, quilts, hangings, and pillows. These are not only charming, but also practical. One interesting choice is Japanese buckwheat-hull pillows covered in 100%-cotton, which are sold by **Nontoxic Environments**. They also offer all-cotton cases to fit them. In addition, **Nontoxic Environments** handles square, kapok-filled pillows with removable, 100%-cotton cases in 18", 24", and 28" square sizes. Of course, you might decide to create your own afghans and pillows (see *Knitting and Crocheting*, *Natural Stuffing*, and *Finding Fabrics and Notions* is *Chapter 3: Clothing*). If you'll need feather and down pillow inserts, they're sold by **Pottery Barn** in several sizes.

PLANTS

Live plants inside your home can provide you with a sense of unity with nature. Many Americans also believe that their house plants will clean their home of air pollution. Actually, some early studies by the National Aeronautics and Space Administration (NASA) did indicate that living plants could provide dramatically reduced formaldehyde levels in houses. In their initial research, NASA scientists placed plants inside a sealed chamber, injected a certain amount of formaldehyde into the chamber, then measured the concentration of formaldehyde after a certain amount of time had passed. After a while, the formaldehyde had, in fact, disappeared. What happened was the plants (actually, bacteria on the plant's roots) metabolized the formaldehyde and used it as food.

However, NASA's early findings have since been challenged. More-thorough research at Ball State University and other laboratories has concluded that house plants simply cannot substantially reduce formaldehyde (or other contaminants) present in indoor air. In this research, plants were again placed in a sealed chamber, but a continuously outgassing source of formaldehyde, such as particleboard, was also placed in the chamber. (Houses often contain particleboard and other continuously outgassing sources of formaldehyde, so these new experiments were designed to mimic a real-world situation.) The result was a slightly lower level of formaldehyde, but not a significant reduction. When there is a continuously outgassing source of formaldehyde, the plants do, indeed, start consuming the formaldehyde, but they usually can't metabolize it as fast as it is released.

In reality, having very many plants in a house results in a higher indoor relative humidity (from watering), and formaldehyde outgasses at a faster rate as the humidity goes up. While house plants will create a certain amount of oxygen, they simply aren't effective air filters.

Even though they aren't going to substantially improve the air in your home, you'll probably still like to have a few live house plants around. If so, you might consider choosing either cacti or *succulents* (plants with thick waxy leaves). Cacti and succulents require little maintenance and only occasional watering and misting. Without the need for a great deal of water, these plants rarely become contaminated with mold, mildew, or insect infestations. In addition, fertilizer applications are kept to a minimum.

With any live plant, it's always best to choose containers with drainage pans to prevent overwatering and rot. Usually, flower shops, craft galleries, and import stores sell many attractive and appropriate plant pots. For displaying your plants, **Ballard Designs** offers unusual designer steel plant stands. They also sell plaster and ceramic plant pot pedestals. You'll also want to check **Home Decorators Collection** for other attractive plant stands.

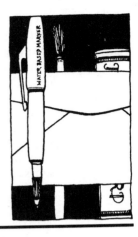

CHAPTER 6
LIFESTYLE

It's often hard to believe, but everything from stationery to pencils to exercise equipment can affect your home's indoor air quality. Even though such items may seem of minor consequence, choosing the least offensive types available can sometimes make a real and noticeable difference in your health and that of your family. Of course, this is especially true for sensitive individuals.

STATIONERY

Many sensitive individuals find typical paper bothersome or intolerable. Often this is because of the chemicals manufacturers use to transform logs into paper. Fortunately, there are a few less-bothersome paper choices available.

PAPER

Paper is defined as sheets of *felted* (interlaced) plant fibers. Traditionally, to make paper, plant matter or used natural-fiber fabric is chopped and mashed until the individual fibers separate, creating paper pulp. The pulp is then added to water in a vat and the mixture is thoroughly stirred. Then, a framed screen is placed in the vat and lifted out. The water drains through the screen leaving a thin layer of pulp that has formed uniformly on the screen's top surface. The wet sheet is then removed from the screen and allowed to dry.

This basic papermaking process was actually invented in China at the beginning of the second century AD, using silk and rice as the major plant fiber sources. The Chinese government successfully kept papermaking a secret for five hundred years, until the Japanese and Arabs (through clandestine means) eventually learned what paper actually consisted of and how it was made. During the Middle Ages, Arab papermaking methods (using flax and hemp) spread across Europe. Up until then, that part of the world used only *papyrus* (crisscrossed strips of papyrus-plant pith beaten flat) and *parchment* (stretched and polished goat, sheep, or calf skin) for sheets of writing material. Paper quickly replaced these because it was cheaper, easier, and faster to produce. However, papyrus and especially parchment were still reserved for special documents.

While paper was quicker to produce than papyrus or parchment, papermaking was still a relatively slow process. After all, the individual sheets had to be made one at a time. However, by the industrial revolution in the nineteenth century, papermaking at last became mechanized. With time, more advanced machinery—coupled with the innovation of using wood for the fiber source in paper pulp—created a major industry. As a result, inexpensive papers became increasing available.

TYPICAL WOOD-PULP PAPER

Most typical wood-pulp paper today originates from pine and fir trees. Transforming softwood logs into thin paper sheets requires a great deal of technology—and many noxious chemicals. As a result, some of this country's worst toxic sites have been found surrounding certain paper mills. Fortunately, laws are now targeted toward greatly reducing the environmental-pollution problems created by paper production.

THE THREE BASIC PAPER GRADES

Today, modern paper mills use wood pulp created in one of three ways, each of which produces a different type of paper. Mechanically ground wood is used to make wood pulp generally for the cheapest paper grades such as newsprint. This method is fast and inexpensive to achieve. However, it leaves undesirable plant residues in the pulp and in the resulting paper. As a result, low-grade papers often appear somewhat coarse and may yellow or discolor fairly quickly.

Machine-ground wood combined with chemicals and then cooked for a brief time creates the wood pulp used in most middle-grade papers. These papers still have some unwanted plant residues, but they are less coarse-looking than the lowest-grade papers. Finally, the best papers come from wood pulp that was created by having the raw wood mechanically chipped, combined with chemicals, and then cooked for a very long period of time. This is the costliest and most time-consuming method to create paper pulp, but this pulp produces smooth and attractive paper without unwanted residues.

HOW TYPICAL BEST-GRADE PAPERS ARE MADE

The actual steps to get from wood log to finished paper are many. This is especially true when making higher-grade papers. Therefore, a brief explanation of this particular method will be discussed to enable you to better understand how the paper you come into contact with is made.

To create the best papers, wood chips and certain chemicals (sulfite salts or a solution of caustic soda and sodium sulfide) are placed in a special tank known as a *digester*. Once filled, the digester is operated for half a day at a very high heat. These conditions, along with the chemicals, cause the *lignin* within the wood chips to break down. Because the natural lignin holds the plant cell walls together, its deterioration allows the cellulose fibers to separate and form pulp. After the pulp is formed, it is then thoroughly cleaned and the chemicals are washed away and any debris removed. Bleach is then sometimes added for whitening. Unfortunately, if chlorine bleaches are used, toxic *dioxins* may be created as by-products. (Dioxins are a family of chlorinated hydrocarbons that have been shown to be carcinogenic and able to cause fetal abnormalities in certain animals.)

Next, the pulp undergoes a beating process to make it less rigid and more flexible. It may also be colored (usually with synthetic dyes) and have materials known as *fillers* added. Fillers such as white chalk, clay, and titanium dioxide give paper a better appearance. Certain gluey plant secretions (rosin, starch, and/or various gums) referred to as *sizings* are also commonly added. They increase a paper's resistance to the water of water-based inks. As it turns out, many sizings are acidic. Therefore, eventually they'll cause cellulose fibers to disintegrate. Fortunately, alkaline sizing agents are now in use but acidic types remain the norm.

Once the pulp has undergone all these processes, it's finally ready for the paper-forming machines. While there are two basic equipment types, both use screening to capture a thin pulp layer, followed by several steps to remove the water. The dried paper is next wound onto reels. Rolled paper is then cut into sheets.

It should be mentioned that some papers may undergo still further finishing operations. For example in *calendering*, particular finishes are added to the paper as it passes through a series of steel rollers. Pigment, glaze, and/or glue mixtures may be applied to one or both sides of the sheets to add glossiness and/or increase opacity. As a result of all the treatments undergone in its creation, it's little wonder that most typical wood pulp papers are bothersome to many sensitive individuals. Even low-grade papers such as newsprint, which have far fewer production steps, are usually as bothersome as high-grade papers—sometimes more so. This is due to a combination of the mill treatments and the greater amounts of softwood residues present in lower-grade papers.

RECYCLED PAPER

A growing number of paper companies are now producing recycled papers. Ideally, this lessens the quantity of trees needed for the mills. In reality though, paper labeled "recycled" may contain a only a small portion of truly recycled material. Often, the recycled material is leftover scrap from the mill's own manufacturing process and not paper that consumers have taken to recycling centers. To brighten most recycled paper's otherwise muddy tinge, additional bleaching processes are often used. If chlorine is the bleaching agent, dangerous dioxins may be created. Therefore, when you purchase paper labeled "recycled," you might want to determine the actual percentage of recycled material, how much of it is post-consumer paper, and whether dioxin-forming bleaches were used.

One mail-order company that offers unbleached recycled paper—as well as a wide range of other recycled home and office stationery—is **Earth Care Paper. Paper Direct** has a selection of recycled office papers as well. Also, you'll want to check **The Seventh Generation** and **Nontoxic Environments**. Unfortunately, it should be noted that many sensitive people are bothered by *any* wood pulp paper—recycled or not. Therefore, while obviously better environmentally, recycled paper may not be any more tolerable for many sensitive individuals than typical wood pulp papers. By the way, you should generally expect to pay more for recycled paper than for typical papers. This is probably due to lower production runs and perhaps the industry sensing that the environmental consumer market will likely pay the extra cost.

ALTERNATIVE PAPERS

A number of alternative papers are now available to consumers. Of them, 100%-cotton papers are often a good choice. Fortunately, many office-supply stores carry at least one line of standard 8½" x 11" cotton paper with matching envelopes. In particular, **Southworth Company** manufactures parchment-deed résumé-quality cotton paper and envelopes you may wish to try. You'll need to check your local stores for its availability. If you are unable to locate it, you can contact the company for the nearest dealer.

Another option is rice paper. Rice paper has been used for centuries in the Far East. In fact, it may have been the first type of paper (see *Paper* above). In the U.S., rice-paper stationery may sometimes be found in Oriental import stores. Other alternative papers you may find acceptable are 100%-linen, linen/cotton blends, and various papers made of other plant materials. For example, office paper and envelopes made of waste jute plant material are available from **World Fibre**. Note, alternative-plant papers can often cost more than typical wood-pulp papers.

You might also consider buying papers that were made by hand. Happily, handmade papers are becoming more available all the time. In most cases, such papers are produced by small specialty companies or individual artists. The papers they create are often both unique and attractive. A wide variety of materials can be used to create the paper pulp for homemade papers—sometimes even old cotton blue jeans. Fortunately, the pulps, emulsions, and additives used in the production of handmade papers are more likely to be less toxic than those used by large papermaking firms. As a result, many handmade papers are tolerable for even very sensitive persons. However, you can expect handmade papers to be relatively expensive. In fact, they are often sold by the individual sheet because of their high price. To find handmade papers locally, check art-supply stores. Note that, local bookstores and libraries often have books on do-it-yourself papermaking. Creating your own paper can save you money and be fun all at the same time.

WRAPPING PAPER

Wrapping paper is often colorful, attractive—and intolerable for some sensitive persons. This is probably due to both the paper itself, as well as to the added dyes and printed inks. Unfortunately, this remains true for recycled wrapping paper as well. For those who would still prefer to use wrapping papers made from recycled paper, **Earth Care Paper, Inc.** offers a number of styles. By the way, of all the manufactured wrapping paper generally available, foil papers without printing are often the least bothersome. Foil papers should be available in your local stationery shops, department stores, and discount stores.

Of course, other more tenable options are available to wrap gifts. One is to use a sheet of handmade paper available from some art stores. A very simple wrapping paper can be made from brown Kraft paper (from a grocery bag perhaps) or several layers of white tissue paper. Another option for wrapping material is heavy-duty aluminum foil. You may also want to wrap small packages in leftover natural-fabric cloth. By the way, a very unusual wrap is a gift bag made of 100% waste jute plant material available from **World Fibre**.

WRITING IMPLEMENTS

Today, many pens contain inks that are bothersome to sensitive persons. This section will explore a few of the more tolerable options you may want to try, as well as information on pencils, erasers, etc.

PENS AND MARKERS

In its broadest definition, a pen is any hand-held tool used to transfer ink to a flat writing surface. As early as ancient Egypt, scribes used reeds and hollow bamboo sections as pens. Pens didn't change much until 6th century AD Europe when the *quill* (split feather shafts) became the common pen. Quills remained in popular use up through the 19th century until steel-point pens gradually replaced them. Inks up to this time were usually made of *lampblack* (finely ground carbon pigment dispersed in water or oil and sometimes stabilized by plant gums or glues), indigo, crushed *galls* (abnormal lumpy growths) from oak and other trees, or from the dark fluids of octopus, squid, and cuttlefish. Many of these inks, especially lampblack, produced writing fluids that were very long-lasting and weren't affected by light or moisture after they had been applied. By the way, India ink is a lampblack ink still used today, but mainly for artwork and *calligraphy* (decorative hand lettering).

By 1884, the fountain pen was invented. Generally, these used (and most still do) inks that were water-soluble dyes. These inks were designed to be more free-flowing and less likely to clog the pen's ink reservoir or writing *nib* (pen tip). Unfortunately, these inks had relatively poor light- and moisture-resisting qualities. In 1888, the ball-point pen was introduced. Ball-points required their own type of ink—one that was thick and viscous, so it wouldn't drip out around the ball-bearing tip and yet not clog. Interestingly, it wasn't until the mid-1940s that ball-points with the appropriate inks were perfected and actually began replacing fountain pens. (Modern ball-points use an ink made of a combination of oils, solvents, and synthetic polymers and dyes.) By 1964, the soft-tip pen (marker) was introduced from Japan. Until the last few years, all soft-tip markers used inks that were synthetic dyes dissolved in alcohol. These inks were designed to prevent the tips from drying up or clogging. Now, some soft-tip markers use water combined with water-soluble synthetic dyes as ink. In the last ten years, a variety of other pens types have become available in the U.S., some with their own new forms of ink.

Unfortunately, however, today's ball-point, roller-ball, fountain, and cartridge pens as well as markers, especially solvent-based markers, can be sources of intolerance for some sensitive individuals. Of all the pens available, water-based fine-line felt-tip markers seem to be one of the better choices. (As a general rule, water-based products are nearly always better tolerated, healthier options than odorous solvent versions.) Also, you should keep in mind that if you choose a fine-point pen, you'll greatly limit the ink flow as compared to a regular or wide-nib pen, thus, minimizing your ink exposure.

If you are sensitive, it would be best to experiment with several brands of water-based fine-line felt-tip markers. That way, you can determine for yourself which ones will be the most benign to you. To find water-based marker pens, check both your local office-supply and art-supply stores, which usually carry very large selections. Also, most drugstores and discount houses carry at least a few brands. Incidentally, two brands you may want to try are Expresso and Pilot.

PENCILS

It's often surprising, even to sensitive people, that a common pencil could be bothersome. But the truth is, it often can. This can be better understood if you analyze how pencils are actually made. Typical pencils contain a "lead" core of *graphite*, a composite carbon compound. Graphite lead is actually made by combining powdered mineral graphite, clay, and water, then extruding the mixture to create very small diameter rods. The wet rods are dried, then kiln-fired at nearly 2,000°F. Afterwards, the baked rods are impregnated with wax to give them a smooth quality. Next, the graphite (in common pencils) is encased by two precut wood sections that are held together with glue. It should be noted that the wood used for pencils is nearly always *incense cedar*, a very aromatic softwood species. Finally, the wood is coated with paint and an eraser is attached with a metal ring.

As a result, the aromatic cedar woods, glues, paints, and/or erasers may sometimes pose intolerance problems to certain sensitive individuals. In some cases, even the graphite may be a problem, probably because of the wax. Fortunately, a metal mechanical pencil (with replaceable "lead" and covered eraser) is usually a more acceptable option for anyone who finds conventional pencils too bothersome. Metal mechanical pencils are sold at most stationery, office supply, and drafting-supply stores. Two popular brands you may want to try are Cross and Pentel.

By the way, pencil lead is sold in several hardnesses. (The more clay in the graphite, the harder it is.) The most common pencil type is B grade. However, B and softer leads can smear easily on your hands and paper. To avoid this, try using harder HB lead. It generally provides clean and legible writing, without excess smearing problems. While H and HH grades are also available, they're often so hard that they produce lines too fine and light for easy reading.

ERASERS AND WHITE-OUT FLUIDS

Erasers are substances that are able to remove pencil or ink from paper. Unfortunately, many erasers are surprisingly odorous. This is understandable because most are made of natural rubber, an innately aromatic material. Probably one of more bothersome types of erasers (for sensitive people) are tan gum erasers, which are made of a gummy, yet crumbly, rubber compound. Kneaded erasers, which are soft and pliable, are usually somewhat better tolerated, as are hard pink erasers.

Interestingly, erasers made of vinyl rather than rubber can often be quite acceptable eraser choices for many sensitive individuals. Generally, vinyl isn't a material suggested for an ideal healthy household. However in this case, vinyl is preferred over natural rubber because it outgasses less over time. These days, white vinyl erasers are often used on acetate or plastic film, but they can work well on paper, too. By the way, vinyl erasers come in a variety of shapes, from small rectangles to spiral paper-wrapped pencil shapes. One popular brand of vinyl erasers is FaberCastell whose vinyl-eraser pencils are sold under the name of Vinyl Peel-Off Magic Rubs. To find vinyl erasers locally, check drafting-supply, office-supply, and art-supply stores.

While many erasers can pose certain tolerance problems, typical *white-out fluids* (also known as correction fluids) are usually far worse. (White-out fluids are opaque, quick-drying substances that are applied with a brush to unwanted ink or print on paper to cover over and create a new white surface that can be written on.) So hazardous can white-out fluids be that they're undoubtedly some of the most odorous and potentially dangerous pollutant sources in home offices. Bottles of white-out fluid generally have warnings against inhaling them and stressing the need for adequate ventilation when applying them. This is because they often contain noxious petroleum-based solvents and other chemicals as ingredients.

Recently, some "enviro-friendly" white-outs have been marketed. Two are Bic Wite-Out For Everything, which "contains no chemicals able to damage the ozone layer," and Liquid Paper Multi Fluid, which "complies with California's strict Proposition 65 Environmental Guidelines." Remember, however, these may still be intolerable products for sensitive individuals. Therefore, when you find it necessary, you might consider using *white-out tape* (correction tape) instead of white-out fluid. This simple opaque white gummed ribbon is a far safer, less odorous alternative. White-out tape is available at most local office-supply stores. 3M Post-It Correction Tape, which is removable, is one brand you may want to try. Other brands are available that can provide permanent adhesion.

TELEPHONES

Telephones have come a long way since Alexander Graham Bell's 1876 original patent. However, they all still have one thing in common: Telephones convert the vibrations of speech into transportable electric signals able to be reconverted back into audible sound. Today, telephones have become an essential component of daily life. They can be used to shop, bank, and run a home office, besides their social function in talking with friends and family. Unfortunately, some sensitive individuals are unable to use their phone because they find it intolerable. The good news is, there are solutions so that nearly everyone who wants to use their phone can, without jeopardizing his or her health.

PROBLEMS WITH TYPICAL TELEPHONES

Why are many phones intolerable to certain sensitive individuals? One of the major reasons is that modern telephones are usually made of one or more types of synthetic plastic. New telephones can release odors outgassed by these materials for months—or even years in some cases. Fortunately though, just placing untreated 100%-cotton over the mouth and ear pieces often helps seal in these emissions. By mail order, **The Cotton Place** offers ready-made untreated 100%-cotton telephone covers. A simple homemade alternative is to use clean cotton handkerchiefs held in place by strings or rubber bands.

Remember, you'll want to launder cotton telephone covers frequently to minimize bacterial growth.

Some telephones may also be a problem because they have a biocide-saturated paper inside their mouthpieces. Biocides are chemicals designed to kill life, in this case bacteria and fungus. If you suspect you are reacting to a biocide hidden within the mouthpiece, you may be able to remove it. Some telephone mouthpieces unscrew or snap apart. If yours does, you should be able to pull out any chemically laden paper that may be inside and simply put the mouthpiece back together again.

POSSIBLE ACCEPTABLE ALTERNATIVE TELEPHONES

If you want to replace a bothersome plastic phone, more tolerable alternatives are available. The following sections will discuss some of these.

ALTERNATIVE-MATERIAL TELEPHONES

Telephones likely to be acceptable to sensitive persons are often those not made of plastic. Surprisingly, a number of such phones are now available. For example, new metal telephones, usually in brass or brass plate, can be found in some department stores and phone centers. In addition, **Billard's Old Telephones** and **Phoneco, Inc.** are two mail-order sources selling restored metal telephones, as well as ones made of wood. In addition, both companies offer older *Bakelite* models.

What is Bakelite? First invented by Leo Bakeland in 1909, bakelite was actually the second synthetic plastic ever created. (*Celluloid* was the first.) Although it's the end product of heated phenol (also known as *carbolic acid*) and formaldehyde, it's far more tolerable than its ingredients would suggest. Physically, Bakelite is a very hard and durable material, one that's much less susceptible to outgassing than many softer modern plastic compounds. As a result, bakelite is quite often tolerable for even very sensitive individuals.

SPEAKER TELEPHONES

Another telephone option that sensitive individuals might want to try is a speaker phone. Speaker phones are usually plastic; therefore, the units themselves could be bothersome. However, because these phones allow their users to avoid direct physical contact with the receiver (in fact, a listener can actually be some distance from the telephone), the chances for adverse health reactions are greatly reduced.

These days, speaker phones are manufactured by a number of companies and the models and features they offer constantly change. Therefore, to know which speaker phone is currently rated best, check a recent issue of a consumer guidebook or magazine. These should be available at your local library or bookstore. Generally, you'll find that speaker phones are handled by department and discount stores, as well as phone centers. One mail-order source for several brands is **Hello Direct**.

You may be happy to learn that you may qualify to receive a *free* speaker telephone (see *Telephone Company Assistance* in *Appendix 2: Utility and Governmental Help* for information on acquiring a free speaker phone) and/ or free directory assistance from your telephone company due to a valid physical disability or health problem.

ELECTRONIC EQUIPMENT

Electronic equipment has revolutionized the American life-style. Sadly, problems with bothersome odors and EMFs (electromagnetic fields) from many of these devices have posed difficulties for certain sensitive persons. However, these problems can often be lessened or even overcome.

ELECTRONIC-EQUIPMENT ODOR PROBLEMS

Some sensitive individuals are finding that their new electronic equipment—televisions, stereos, video cassette recorders, and computers—are intolerable for them to use. This is often due to both outgassing of the plastic housings and the electronic workings inside. In particular, some transformers give off fairly strong, objectionable odors.

AIRING PROBLEM ELECTRONIC EQUIPMENT

Running intolerable electronic equipment unattended in a seldom-used room with open windows can often be helpful in reducing bothersome odors. You could also run the equipment in a garage, if there's no possibility of contamination by gasoline, oil, or combustion gases. Operating new electronics on a sheltered porch also can work well. However, keep in mind that very cold or very hot temperatures, as well as moisture, can cause damage.

How long should your new electronic equipment run before it loses its objectionable "new" odor? A few days may be enough, but more likely it'll take several weeks—or more. (In fact, a few devices never seem to lose their odor.) While some electronic equipment can safely remain turned on and unattended for extended airing periods, other items should be turned off from time to time. You'll have to use your best judgment and read your owner's manual thoroughly. You may also want to contact the manufacturer for assistance in determining the best approach.

ELECTRONIC-EQUIPMENT CONTAINMENT BOXES

Sometimes, particular electronic items never seem to become acceptable, despite lengthy airings. In those situations, special *containment boxes* can be a good solution. These specially designed boxes help isolate or contain odors released by electronic equipment so they can't reach the room's air and be inhaled by sensitive persons. Containment boxes are generally built of glass or Plexiglas with metal or solid-wood frames. Ideally, a containment box should be vented directly to the outdoors with a small fan, or attached to a portable indoor air filter. By the way, containment boxes used for electronic equipment should always have air passing through them. This is because the heat generated by the electronic components needs to be dissipated or damage could result.

At least two mail-order companies sell ready-made containment boxes. The reading boxes (See *Reading Boxes* below) made and sold by **Allermed Corp.** can actually be used to hold certain electronic devices. These boxes can be ordered with either Plexiglas or tempered glass (glass unable to easily shatter into sharp shards.) **Allermed Corp.**'s boxes are designed to work with its Ultra-Safe air filter (see *Portable Room Air Filters* in *Chapter 9: Indoor Air*). Also, **The Safe Computer and Reading Box Company** makes and sells glass containment units with aluminum corners. These computer boxes come equipped with fans designed for outdoor venting. You can order them directly from the company.

While some computers and monitors (the TV-like viewing devices of computers) can release odors that make them intolerable, some sensitive individuals find that the printer for their computer is often even more troublesome. It doesn't seem to matter what brand it is or whether it's a *dot matrix printer* (printer that creates letters and designs with tiny dots of mechanically stamped ink), an *ink-jet printer* (printer in which droplets of ink are applied with nozzles at high speed), or a *laser printer* (printer that uses a laser to quickly create a pattern on which metallic particles are electrostatically adhered). Printers are just plain odorous. Many sensitive people think that having a laser printer would obviously be the best choice because it doesn't actually use ink—something that's often bothersome. However, laser printers give off ozone (O_3). Unfortunately, ozone is a reactive, harmful gas with an unpleasant odor.

To use any bothersome printer, you might consider placing it in a separate vented or filtered containment box. Unfortunately, this is often too costly or impractical to do. Another possible solution is to use a very long computer-to-printer cable. The printer can then be placed in a room other than where the computer is located—perhaps in a closet. It is hoped that the new site for the printer will be one that can either be vented outdoors or, at the very least, is a space that is otherwise seldom used by the sensitive individual.

ELECTRONIC EQUIPMENT EMF CONCERNS

Virtually all electronic equipment creates *electromagnetic fields (EMFs)* when it's running. EMFs consist of electrical and magnetic energy and these fields originate wherever electricity is found: wires, motors, and electronic components. Unfortunately, sometimes the strengths of these fields can be at levels that are potentially harmful to people, if exposed to them for too long (see *Chapter 11: Electromagnetic Fields*). Actually, until fairly recently, EMFs were not considered something to be concerned about. As a result, electronic-equipment manufacturers didn't purposely create products designed to minimize EMFs. However, because of recent research linking EMF exposures to certain negative health effects, many of the newest electronic components have reduced emission levels compared to earlier models. Therefore, a newly purchased computer monitor or television may emit EMF levels much lower than an older unit.

What's a safe EMF level? At this time it's believed by many experts that a long-term exposure to EMFs below a level of 1–3 milligauss is acceptable. (A gauss is a measurement of magnetic-field strength; a milligauss is $1/1000$th of a gauss.) However, it should be noted that others argue that a long-term exposure to only 1 milligauss or less is truly safe. Because there's no clear-cut agreement on this point, you must ultimately decide for yourself what you consider allowable. To find out what EMF levels your particular equipment is actually giving off, the levels can be measured with special equipment. **Baubiologie Hardware** offers gauss meters. Another good source for gauss meters is **Befit Enterprises, Ltd.**'s Cutting Edge Catalog.

You should be aware of certain simple practices that can improve your margin of safety when you feel EMF levels are too high. EMF levels generally decrease rapidly with distance from their generating source. Therefore, just positioning yourself several feet from your stereo or television can often offer sufficient protection. Also, both **Baubiologie Hardware** and **Befit Enterprises, Ltd.**'s Cutting Edge Catalog sell EMF-reducing products that you can install directly on the equipment at issue.

To reduce exposure to EMFs from your computer, try placing the keyboard two or three feet away from the monitor and the computer itself. As a rule, computers and monitors create the more intense EMF fields—not keyboards. In addition, you might want to purchase a special computer EMF-blocking screen that can be attached to your monitor. Such screens are available from **Safe Technologies**, from some monitor manufacturers, and from other computer-product companies. Also, check local computer stores and mail-order businesses advertising in computer magazines. In addition, **Nontoxic Environments** sells electromagnetic computer shields as well as special backlit computer monitors specially designed to reduce a user's exposure to EMFs.

PRINTED MATTER

Many people assume that reading is a benign activity. It would seem as if it would be, at least at first. However, books, magazines, and newspapers can be some of the more bothersome things brought into any home. This section explains why and what you can do to make reading safer—if you're a sensitive person.

PROBLEMS WITH PRINTED MATERIAL

New books commonly cause tolerance problems for many sensitive persons. This is usually due to the paper, the glues used in binding, and the ink. Once, printing inks were made of varnish, linseed oil, and *lampblack* (finely ground carbon pigment). Now most modern printing inks consist of synthetic film-forming resins, pigments, and solvents that can be very odorous. However, some new inks use natural resins derived from soybeans. These soy-based inks tend to be less bothersome—unless you have a particular intolerance to soy.

Newspapers are commonly intolerable to sensitive persons because of the low-grade newsprint used, as well as the ink. Because many newspapers are printed daily, the inks are both extremely fresh and odorous. In addition, if newspapers, books, magazines, or other printed items are purchased in drugstores or other retail outlets, they easily could have absorbed perfume and other potentially objectionable odors from the store. Because of their porous nature, newspapers are also very susceptible to mildew and dust accumulation in storage.

Of special concern are older books. While old books will have lost most of their new paper, glue, and ink odors, they can be very bothersome overall. This is because they usually have picked up tobacco smoke and perfume odors over many years of use. In addition, they can sometimes be contaminated with dust, insects, mildew, or just plain mustiness.

STORING PRINTED MATERIAL

Ideally, in a healthy household all the printed materials should be stored so they can't negatively affect the indoor air, especially if there are sensitive persons in the family. One safe way to store books is in *lawyer's bookcases*.

These are actually nothing more than wooden cabinets with shelving, but with glass doors in front. One mail-order source of solid-wood and glass lawyer's bookcases finished with beeswax is **Dona Designs**.

Of course, magazines and newspapers can also be placed in lawyer's bookcases. However, infrequently used closets, metal boxes, trunks, or cabinets, can be useful for storing periodicals as well (see *Metal Containers* in *Chapter 8: Housekeeping*). To find suitable metal cabinets, you'll want to check local department stores, office-supply stores, and hardware stores.

SIMPLE ALTERNATIVE READING STRATEGIES

Without a doubt, there's unmistakable appeal to reading in your bed or curled up on the living-room couch. However, for those bothered by books, newspapers, and magazines, reading outside, or near an open window indoors, are generally much healthier choices. Plenty of fresh air and ventilation ensures that odors from bothersome printed material are diluted and dissipated.

Another simple, safer reading approach is to make the printed matter itself less bothersome. It seems that some sensitive persons are able to read indoors if the printed material has been sufficiently aired outdoors first. Airing actually can be done using a clothesline and clothespins. Correspondence, newspapers, and small magazines can all be hung on a line until they become tolerable. Of course, it's important to make sure the surroundings are dry and free of contaminating odors, pollen, etc.

Some sensitive people actually *bake* their printed matter before they read it. This can be accomplished several ways. For example, you can put books in a mesh laundry bag, open your clothes dryer door, drape the bag's strings over the door, and then close the door on the strings so that the laundry bag is held in place inside the dryer. This will hold the book in place so it won't tumble around. At that point, turn the dryer on medium heat for 30 minutes. (It'll be necessary to experiment beforehand with temperature settings and running times.) A variation of this method is to place a book on a heat-resistant open-mesh tray that can be attached to the inside of the dryer door. Such a tray must be made with care so it will suspend the book in the center of the dryer's drum without the tray or the book falling to the bottom of the drum.

Another "bake-out" procedure is to warm your books or other printed materials in your electric oven or portable toaster/oven on a very low setting. If you try this, be sure the range-hood fan is running on high speed and a window is open. Unfortunately, bake-outs done in clothes dryers and kitchen ovens often prove less than satisfactory because of the danger of fire, problems with contaminating the appliance itself, and the possibility of odors entering the living space.

For some very sensitive persons, no amount of fresh air or "baking" of books etc. is adequate to make reading tolerable. For these individuals, wearing a 100%-cotton mask containing an activated charcoal insert can be very helpful. The activated charcoal can adsorb a great deal of the bothersome odors before they reach the wearer's nasal passages. Several mail-order sources for all-cotton filtering masks including **The Living Source, The American Environmental Health Foundation**, and **Nontoxic Environments.** Some of these companies also offer 100%-silk masks as well (see *Personal Facial Filters* in *Chapter 9: Indoor Air*).

READING BOXES

Some extremely sensitive persons find that even wearing filter masks just don't provide enough protection from the outgassing chemicals and other odors emanating from printed material. For such people, *reading boxes* are often ideal solutions. Reading boxes are actually specially designed cases made with glass or Plexiglas tops (and sometimes sides as well) in a wood or metal frame. Printed material is placed inside and the reader looks through the clear glass or Plexiglas to read.

You should be aware that some reading boxes are unvented. These are usually very simply constructed, small, and fairly inexpensive. However, those that can be vented to the outdoors or into an air-filtering unit are much better, healthier choices. This is because vented and filtered models can actually *remove* bothersome contaminants so they won't enter the living space to cause problems. Unvented units will accumulate odors that can seep out when a page is turned (in certain types) or when a book is placed inside or removed from the enclosed chamber. Vented units will cost more and generally lack portability.

There are at least two mail-order sources for reading boxes. Reading boxes manufactured and sold by **Allermed Corp.** come with either Plexiglas or tempered glass and are designed to work with the company's Ultra-Safe air filter (see *Portable Room Air Filters* in *Chapter 9: Indoor Air)*. **The Safe Computer and Reading Box Company** makes and sells glass units with aluminum corner frames. These boxes are supplied with a fan and are designed to be vented to the outdoors. They can be ordered directly from the company.

If a reading box does not seem affordable, but you still need a barrier between you and the printed page, you might try using large-sized cellophane bags. These work fairly well for small catalogs, paperback books, and letters (see *Cellophane* in *Chapter 8: Housekeeping)*. Unfortunately, cellophane is quite brittle. Therefore, your cellophane reading bags probably will have to be replaced often. Cellophane bags can be ordered from both **The Living Source** and **Janice Corp.** As an alternative, zip-sealing plastic bags are even more effective at isolating ink and paper odors than cellophane bags. They're also much sturdier. However, the plastic itself can be bothersome. Fortunately, airing zip-sealing plastic bags outside in dry uncontaminated surroundings for several days often makes them tolerable.

RECORDED PRINTED MATERIAL

Books and magazines are now available on audiocassette, CD ROM, and audio CD. Because of this, sensitive persons who can't tolerate ink and paper can often enjoy reading again by becoming "electronically literate."

BOOKS AND MAGAZINES ON AUDIO TAPE

An alternative to actually reading is listening to books and magazines recorded on four-track audio tapes. The major supplier of four-track books in our country is the National Library of Congress, which has a program available for those with physical disabilities that prevent the normal use of printed materials. The physical conditions generally recognized for admittance into the program are blindness, stroke, amputation, etc. Interestingly, those with MCS (Multiple Chemical Sensitivity) (see *MCS, A New Medical Condition* in

Chapter 1: Getting Started) may also qualify—that is, if their physician signs the application confirming that their illness prevents them from being able to read. For information on the program and an application form, ask your local librarian or write or phone **The Library of Congress**, Washington DC 20542; (202) 707-5104.

Once your application has been approved, a tape player will be assigned to you on a loan basis. You can request new or used equipment. You'll also receive a list of available books and magazines in a variety of categories. Your tape machine and book and magazine selections are always sent and returned by mail. If you would prefer to purchase your own machine, **LS & S Group** offers a catalog featuring a large selection. Models, brands, features, and prices vary. The company also has recorded tapes you may want to purchase for your very own.

At least two other organizations offer books on tape you might want to contact. **The Jewish Guild For the Blind** has popular fiction and nonfiction books on regular audiocassettes. The books are read by volunteers, so the quality isn't always up to professional standards. However, the service is free to all adults of any faith. Only a statement from your doctor or social-service worker is required, confirming that you are unable to read books or magazines. **Recordings for the Blind** is a nonprofit organization with over 60,000 titles available. To enter their program, a small initial registration fee is required. After that, the services are free. The books from this foundation are on four-track tapes. If you don't already have a four-track tape machine, the foundation has some for sale.

Of course, not only the disabled are using tape-recorded books. Today, major companies are producing and marketing audiocassette books for the general public. As a matter of fact, because books on audiocassette are becoming so popular, new titles are constantly being released. Many local libraries—probably including yours, too—now have them available for check-out by anyone. There are also several mail-order companies that specialize in selling books on audio cassette. Two such catalogs are **The Mind's Eye** and **Audio Editions**. Also, **Books On Tape** offers cassettes for both purchase or rental.

BOOKS ON CD

Another electronic reading option is purchasing and using *CD-ROM* books. (CD-ROMs are **c**ompact **d**isks with **r**ead **o**nly **m**emory, so they're complete in and of themselves and at the same time they can't be recorded over.) CD-ROMs allow the printed words to appear on your computer monitor's screen. Therefore, you actually get the pleasure of seeing printed words, but without the need for paper or ink. This can be ideal for sensitive people who can't normally tolerate books but can tolerate their computer.

The books now available on CD-ROM can be used on either PCs (IBM-compatible units) or Macintosh products (Apple computers), or both. Dictionaries, encyclopedias, and other reference books are now particularly popular. The classics of literature are also widely available. To find books on CD-ROM, check local computer software stores and mail-order catalogs.

One exciting CD-ROM alternative is Dr. Tomorrow's Electric Bookstore (**Polar 7 Enterprises**). This is actually a CD-ROM containing an entire "locked" book collection. Descriptions of the individual books appear on your monitor when you use the disk. When you find a book you'd like to read, you simply call the company. After they charge your credit card for your chosen selection, they'll issue you a "key." This is your private number that will immediately "unlock" the book. Afterwards, the printed words of the unlocked book can be read at any time on your screen.

If you'd rather listen rather than read from your computer monitor, **The Jewish Guild for the Blind** and **Recordings for the Blind** both have recorded books on compact audio discs. These are loaned at no charge to those who qualify. (See *Books and Magazines on Audio Tape* above for how to qualify.)

HOBBIES

Since World War II, there has been a surge of interest in crafts and in-home hobbies. Americans now spend millions of hours—and millions of dollars—on their personal leisure-time activities. In most cases, indoor hobbies provide enjoyment and satisfaction. However, the health consequences of these pastimes are rarely considered. Your health and well-being dictate otherwise. Certain hobby activities use toxic and/or very odorous materials that can pollute the indoor air, causing symptoms ranging from respiratory problems to cancer in some cases.

HOBBIES IN GENERAL

Most people love their hobbies. Why wouldn't they? After all, hobbies are outward expressions of inner personalities. Fortunately, many hobbies are actually quite benign from a health standpoint: They don't pollute your home or cause any physical harm. For example, sewing is generally considered a safe hobby. For the general public this is usually true, and it can be for even sensitive people, too—with a few modifications. These might include using only pre-washed, natural-fiber fabrics, and/or only operating the sewing machine with a nearby open window (for more on sewing, see *Custom-Made Clothes* in *Chapter 3: Clothing*).

However, a number of pastime activities are fairly dangerous. Plastic model making, which often uses toxic glues and paints, is just one of these. If possible, such hobbies should not be done indoors without adequate ventilation and personal protective equipment, such as a chemical respirator mask. This is true even for healthy individuals.

Actually, it's wise to really examine all the hobbies in which you and your family engage. Of what are the materials made that you currently use? What warnings are on the packages and containers? What potential negative effects do these materials have on you and the environment? Taking the necessary steps to make your hobbies both enjoyable and healthy is just plain common sense.

ARTS AND CRAFTS

If you enjoy doing arts or crafts, finding acceptable and safe materials can be rather frustrating. It's now becoming evident that many products that were used for years—and only assumed to be harmless—may not be so innocent. The truth is many art materials contain potentially harmful solvents and other ingredients. Other hobby-related materials can create dangerous airborne dust that could cause respiratory problems.

As a general rule for safer arts and crafts, use water-based products whenever possible. Products using water, rather than alcohol, oil, or solvents as their base ingredient, nearly always are less odorous, toxic, and volatile. Also, it's important to read and follow all label directions and project instructions carefully, to wear correct protective gear (see *Protective Gear* in *Chapter 12: Home Workshop and Garage*), and to always have plenty of ventilation. Remember, too, it's best to store art materials so they can't affect the indoor air. To do this, metal cabinets with doors, such as those available at most office supply stores and some hardware departments, are often ideal (see *Metal Containers* in *Chapter 8: Housekeeping*).

To help you choose healthier art and craft supplies, read *The Artist's Complete Health & Safety Guide* by Monona Rossol. Also, check your local library and bookstores for other books dealing with nontoxic or less-toxic art materials and projects. In addition, you can join **ACTS (Arts, Crafts & Theater Safety)**. Membership includes a monthly newsletter and free telephone consultations. *The Natural Choice* catalog from **Eco Design Co.** offers several natural art materials by mail order.

EXERCISE EQUIPMENT

Home exercise equipment is geared to make you healthier. However, some pieces are made with odorous synthetic foam grips and other plastic parts. Also, it's not uncommon for some equipment to have chains, hydraulic shocks, or other parts requiring lubrication using smelly petroleum-based products. In addition, if there are natural or synthetic rubber cords, foot grips, belts, etc., these too can outgas odors. It is little wonder that much home exercise equipment is just too bothersome for many sensitive individuals to use, especially when it's new. (And remember, never begin any exercise program without your physician's approval.)

TOLERABLE MANUFACTURED EXERCISE EQUIPMENT

The best home exercise equipment—at least from an odor standpoint—are those pieces which are all, or mostly, metal. If possible, you'll also want to choose equipment that won't require any lubrication. However, if lubrication is necessary, you might consider using E-Z-1 Lubricant available from **E.L. Foust Co., Inc.** (see *Lubricants* for other choices in *Chapter 12: Home Workshop and Garage*). This is a low-odor liquid synthetic product that's especially good for stopping squeaky metal-to-metal noises. Unfortunately, it may not be adequate for certain applications such as chain drives, etc.

You may find that certain pieces of equipment may not be tolerable when first purchased, but can become tolerable if aired outside for some time in dry, uncontaminated surroundings. Bungee-type stretching cords are one such example. Sometimes equipment can become acceptable simply by removing the foam handlebar grips and/or placing a tightly fitting 100%-cotton cover over the rubber or vinyl seat. It should be noted that some alterations could make the equipment's product warranty or guarantee invalid. Remember never to do any modifications that result in potential safety problems.

TOLERABLE HOMEMADE EXERCISE EQUIPMENT

As an alternative to manufactured devices, you might consider making homemade exercise equipment to suit your own physical and tolerance requirements. For example, you could buy sections of cotton or nylon rope to use as nontoxic jump ropes. Hand-held bags of strong 100% cotton with Velcro covers are ideal for weight lifting. The bags can be filled with steel shot (avoid lead) that is available at most gun shops and discount store hunting departments. These easily opened bags can be emptied and laundered when necessary, or have more or less shot added as needed. You can even make small bags with Velcro straps to attach to wrists or ankles.

Also, a ready-made at-home stepper could be simply the bottom step of your stairway. A sturdily constructed wooden box 2", 4", 6", or 8" high could also be used, if set on a slip-resistant surface. The higher the box, the more difficult the workout will be. You should know, however, that wood—and especially concrete—steppers won't have the give (resiliency) of plastic steppers. Therefore, if you have back, leg, or foot problems, these alternatives might not be as appropriate.

It should be pointed out that many exercises don't require any equipment. In this age of health clubs and exercise-equipment "infomericals," that can be easily forgotten. Actually, some very healthful exercises require only knowledge of the technique, as gained from an instruction video or book, some comfortable clothing, and perhaps a soft mat. Walking around your home, stretching exercises, yoga and other Eastern practices, isometrics, and the old-fashioned exercises you did in physical-education classes in school are just a few examples of low-tech exercising methods. To find what appeals to you, check bookstores and libraries for appropriate books and tapes.

TOLERABLE EXERCISE CLOTHING AND MATS

Finding exercise clothing and mats that are tolerable to sensitive people can sometimes be difficult but there are some mail-order sources from which you can order. For example, **The Richman Cotton Company** sells 100%-cotton sweat wear. Also, **Janice Corp.** sells all-cotton women's leotards. In addition, **Janice Corp.** offers untreated all-cotton exercise mats in a 26" x 66" size with 100%-cotton covers. Both **Jantz Designs** and **Sinan Co.** handle 27" x 60" organic cotton-filled exercise mats and matching carrying cases.

SAUNAS

Recently, saunas have become more common among Americans, particularly in new upscale homes. While most of the people who purchase saunas aren't as a rule, sensitive, some individuals with MCS (Multiple Chemical Sensitivity) are buying them as a means to detoxify themselves after experiencing bothersome chemical exposures. Therefore, this section will introduce you to what saunas are, how they work, and what's available in the marketplace.

TRADITIONAL SCANDINAVIAN SAUNAS

Traditionally, *saunas* are small, separate wooden bathhouses used in Finland and other Scandinavian countries. Generally, they have two interior seating levels and a vented ceiling. These small structures are heated to relatively high temperatures (170–200°F), using small heating stoves. The warmth is transferred directly to fracture-resistant stones. The rocks then radiate their acquired heat into the room. If desired, steam is created by ladling water onto the hot rocks. High temperatures inside the sauna causes users to perspire. After sweating for a time within the hot confined space, sauna users traditionally open the doors to the outside, run out, and take a dip in a lake or stream—or jump into a snow bank if it's wintertime. The whole procedure is considered cleansing and invigorating.

MODERN AMERICAN SAUNAS

Today in America, most saunas are built into houses rather than being separate structures. These indoor saunas customarily are one of three basic types: custom-built, or constructed from a prefab kit or a precut kit. Each has its advantages and disadvantages.

Whether they are custom-made or derived from a kit, nearly all saunas have insulated walls covered with cedar or other softwood paneling. Often there are one or two benches. The doors of the sauna may have glass panels to prevent claustrophobia. The stoves are often either electric or gas heaters.

THE THREE BASIC SAUNA TYPES

A *custom-made* sauna has the advantages of fitting just the space you have and having the exact features you want. Of course, the relatively high labor costs, plus the time, trouble, and expense to find the appropriate materials has to be considered if you opt for a custom-built sauna rather than going with a prefab kit with everything included in one package. You'll probably also want to hire only skilled, knowledgeable individuals to do the work, from designing to actual construction. (To find a designer, talk with local architects. They may be able to draw the plans themselves or recommend someone.)

On the other hand, *prefab* (prefabricated) *sauna kits* are modular systems. Each prefab sauna company offers several models in different sizes. Generally, the sauna's insulated walls are built at the factory and then shipped to your site. The manufacturer's labor, materials, and design costs are all included in the initial prefab kit price. It should be pointed out that prefabs are often separate, freestanding chambers designed to be assembled on hard-surfaced floors such as concrete. Often they're placed in basements. If you are capable enough and not a very sensitive person, you may be able to do most of the installation work yourself.

A sauna option that's lies between custom and prefab saunas in cost and labor is a *precut sauna package*. These usually contain tongue-and-groove wood paneling already cut to fit inside a framework built by the homeowner, or a contractor. Insulation and exterior wood siding are usually not provided. Kits may include heaters and other equipment, depending on the model and options chosen.

Note that, all saunas require electrical wires for lights as well as heaters (if the heaters aren't gas-fired). Therefore, having the necessary permits and professional expertise is essential. If you do the work yourself, you'll want to wear appropriate protective gear when necessary.

CHOOSING TOLERABLE SAUNA MATERIALS AND EQUIPMENT

If you're a sensitive person, it's critical to choose an appropriate wood species for your sauna walls—especially the sauna's interior. The wood should be a type that can withstand heat and moisture, yet be tolerable (see *Testing Woods* in *Chapter 12: Home Workshop and Garage*). Remember that virtually any wood will release far more odors when hot, damp, or both.

Sauna manufacturers often offer a selection of several wood species from which to choose. These may include western red cedar, white cedar, white pine, aspen, sugar pine, ponderosa pine, Sitka spruce, hemlock spruce, cypress, and/or redwood. No wood species is absolutely perfect and certainly no one type is right for everyone. However, one species you might seriously consider if you're a sensitive individual is redwood, which is often fairly well tolerated. Although redwood is a softwood, it is less odorous, especially over time, than cedar, pine, and fir. Also, redwood has an attractive smooth grain and is naturally rot-resistant. However, you should be aware that like all wood, redwood has a fairly strong odor when it's been freshly cut. In addition, any water or sweat that gets on the redwood can cause darkening.

For the floor of your sauna, ideally you'll choose concrete, masonry (brick or stone), or ceramic tile (see *Ceramic Floors* in *Chapter 5: Interior Decorating*). These choices are good because of their ability to easily handle the moisture created by perspiration and steam and never need replacing. It's also wise to choose an electric over a gas heater so potentially harmful combustion gases aren't created (see *Combustion Gases* in *Chapter 9: Indoor Air*). Also remember to have protective guardrails installed around your sauna's heater.

It's important, too, to seriously consider proper ventilation for your new sauna. Unfortunately, some American saunas are built with no provisions for ventilation whatsoever. This can easily create stale and stuffy conditions, yet it's always preferable to have adequate fresh air. (You might read *Understanding Ventilation* by John Bower for more insights and information on ventilation. This book is available from **The Healthy House Institute**.)

Finally, don't forget to insulate in a way that is permanent and will minimize potentially bothersome odors. You should be aware that when the walls of your sauna become hot, the insulation within them will likely release more odors than when the walls are cool. (For more on insulation, read *The Healthy House* and *Healthy House Building,* both by John Bower and available from **The Healthy House Institute**.)

CHOOSING THE RIGHT SAUNA KIT

All in all, installing a sauna in your home is a major investment. Therefore, take the time to do the necessary informational research, material testing, and acquisition of any building permits, etc. If your friends have saunas, ask them for their experiences, suggestions, and recommendations. Also, ask your physician or other health-care professional for his (or her) ideas. If you want to purchase a kit, make sure to contact several manufacturers. A few you might write or call for literature are **Almost Heaven Hot Tub, Inc.**, **Amerec Products**, **Finnleo Saunas**, **McCoy, Inc.**, and **Cedarbrook Sauna**.

For each company you contact, compare their costs for the wood, the heaters, etc., as well as for shipping. Find out what features are standard and which ones are optional. Also, make sure you know what materials and degree of site readiness are expected to be provided by the homeowner, you. In addition, learn what's covered in the sauna's guarantees and warranties and for how long. By the way, don't forget to inquire how long you should expect to wait from the time you place your order until your sauna kit reaches your door. Finally, ask the company for the names of several clients who have already bought their saunas. Hearing what owners have to say can often be very enlightening.

PORTABLE SAUNA

Recently, a Basic One Person Sauna has become available from **The Safe Reading Box and Computer Co.** This low cost sauna consists of a 72" x 25" x 25" folding aluminum frame covered with prewashed, untreated, 100%-organic cotton cloth. This sauna was designed especially for individuals with MCS. It has a heater housed in a separate metal chamber that has been precleaned and run at 275°F for 72 hours to burn off any residual odors. This sauna can be used either horizontally or vertically. A larger (96" x 36" x 36") model is also available. (**The Safe Reading Box and Computer Co.** can also custom make saunas in a variety of sizes with either thermal-glass or ceramic-tile walls.) This company's saunas are shipped with a manual describing the L. Ron Hubbard sauna/detoxification program in detail.

LUGGAGE

Most people take their luggage for granted. However, that's often not true for many sensitive persons. Finding tolerable luggage for these people can actually be a very real and very serious problem. The following sections will explain why, and offer some less bothersome luggage suggestions.

TYPICAL LUGGAGE CONCERNS

Most of the typical luggage being made today is either *hardside* (the exterior retains it's original shape) and often made of hard plastic, or *softside* (the exterior is pliable) and made of a synthetic fabric treated with water and/or stain-resistant chemical compounds. Luggage interiors are usually treated synthetic fabrics, soft vinyl, or made with a combination of these materials. Consequentially, it should be of little wonder that many sensitive people find new luggage intolerable.

The answer might seem to be that sensitive individuals use older suitcases and bags—ones that have lost most of their "new" odors. However, old luggage can pose its own problems. For example, older pieces will have likely absorbed perfume, tobacco, as well as musty and other undesirable odors over the years.

Even if tolerable luggage is found, once it's taken on a trip, it inevitably will absorb ambient perfume and tobacco odors. Therefore, once-acceptable luggage will have quickly become unacceptable. Unfortunately, trying to make bothersome luggage tolerable again can be difficult. After all, most luggage pieces can't be completely washed or laundered; generally, the only cleaning possible is a surface sponging, something that may not be particularly effective. Airing contaminated luggage outdoors for an extended period in dry, uncontaminated surroundings can help, but it may not be enough.

ALTERNATIVE LUGGAGE SUGGESTIONS

Although it's doubtful that there's a set of matched luggage available that's made of tolerable materials, is completely washable, and at the same time is affordable, sensitive persons might consider a few luggage options. One is using untreated, 100%-cotton or untreated nylon athletic bags. These are sometimes still available at local department stores and sporting-goods stores. Surprisingly, some of these bags are hand- or even machine-washable. You might also check the **Mother Hart** catalog. This mail-order company offers all-cotton athletic bags from time to time. One very attractive option is a 36" long, 21" diameter duffel bag made of heavy, hand-woven cotton cloth from Guatemala. These washable bags are sold by **Pueblo to People**.

Another more tolerable luggage option is to use untreated 100%-cotton garment bags. These are occasionally sold in luggage and department stores. You might also consider sewing your own athletic, duffel, or garment bags. Patterns for these are sometimes available at local fabric shops. When choosing a fabric, ideally you may pick a washable, heavy-duty, tolerable natural-fiber cloth. Cotton canvas, cotton duck, and barrier cloth are good. You also might choose a sturdy rip-proof untreated nylon.

No matter your final choice, if you're a sensitive person it's a good idea to also take along an extra bag to hold the clothing that has been worn. That way, soiled clothes that have picked up potentially bothersome odors won't need to be directly adjacent to your uncontaminated fresh clothing. For your worn-clothing bag, you might simply use a pillowcase or you could make a drawstring *barrier-cloth* bag. Barrier cloth is a special tightly-woven untreated cotton that can act as a relatively effective odor barrier. It's available by the yard from **The Cotton Place** and **Janice Corp**. You also might use an unscented plastic garbage bag for your worn, contaminated clothing. And remember not to put the worn-clothes bag in your main luggage piece until you are actually ready to leave. Odors coming from the worn clothing will permeate through a standard cotton bag to some degree, and through barrier cloth and plastic.

PETS

A pet is defined as any domesticated or tamed animal that is cared for with kindness and considered a companion. Actually, a pet of any species can be a source of entertainment, enjoyment—and even love. However, it could also be a source of unwelcome mess, pests, potential infestation, and allergens. At the very least, all pets require your personal time, money, and emotional input. Therefore, before you acquire any pet, it's wise to evaluate what the pros and cons of pet ownership will mean for you and your family. This is especially important for sensitive or allergic persons.

If you decide to go ahead and get a pet, choose the appropriate animal(s). For some people, the special closeness of a dog or cat is essential and worth any possible drawbacks: high food bills, required vaccinations, licenses, etc. Other individuals may decide that a chameleon—needing only marginal attention, having no shedding fur or *dander* (loose animal skin or feather flakes), requiring no veterinary checkups, little food, only a few dollars for initial purchase, and a small terrarium—is all they realistically feel comfortable with. Of course, still others may decide that having an outdoor bird feeder is as much animal-human interaction as they're able to responsibly handle at this point in their lives. Whatever the decision, if it works for you and the animal(s), then it's the right choice.

PET CARE IN GENERAL

Of course, there are some basic health guidelines for owning any pet. One of these is to keep all pet bedding clean. As a result, you'll want to choose only dog and cat beds that have washable covers for easy laundering. Also, you'll want to regularly vacuum the floors around your pet's sleeping area or cage. (Repeated vacuuming will minimize flea infestations as well as eliminate excess fur, feathers, dander, and dirt that could aggravate allergies.)

Also, with any pet, it's best to take special care of their food and water. Therefore, washing your pet's food and water dishes daily is a good practice. You'll also want to store open pet-food packages in nontoxic containers with tight-fitting lids, and refrigerate them if it's necessary. In the case of large dry-food bags, you might use clean, new galvanized garbage cans for convenient, sealed storage.

CATS

It's been estimated that as long ago as 8,000 BC, cats were already present in prehistoric villages. In ancient Egypt, people not only appreciated the presence of cats, but also revered them because they kept homes and granaries relatively rodent-free. About that time domesticated cats first became differentiated from wild cats. In time, cats were kept by growing numbers of families as settlements and urbanization spread. However, after the Christianization of Europe, cats in some places were considered links to the pagan past, thus, losing much of their former favor.

Eventually, keeping cats as pets became more popular again. But surprisingly, it wasn't until the late 19th century that cat breeds became established. (Interestingly, some experts believe there's still no such thing as a specific, true, domestic cat breed.) Recently in the U.S., cats have replaced dogs as America's most common household pet, most likely because cats can live indoors comfortably, require less attention, and cost less to keep than dogs.

What type of cat is best for a healthy household? Naturally, there's no real answer to that question. However, long-haired cats will shed more hair than other types. Therefore, if you choose a cat(s) with long fur, it will require extra grooming than a short-haired cat. Whether with long or short hair, cats should be brushed regularly to eliminate as much loose fur as possible. This not only will make your housekeeping easier, but it'll also reduce the number of hair balls formed. To find cat brushes, check local pet stores. By mail order, cat brushes, combs, and even brush attachments for vacuums are sold by **Pedigree.**

It's also a good idea that any long- or short-haired cat, especially if it's allowed to go outdoors, should be combed regularly with a *flea comb.* This is a specially designed comb with very close teeth that are able to remove tiny fleas. To use a flea comb, simply comb through the fur. Taking your fingernail, push off any accumulated fleas into a bowl of water to drown. If you'd like to buy a flea comb, they're available from **Save Our ecoSystem (SOS).** **Pedigree** also has them, as well as herbal and other all-natural anti-flea and ear-mite products, hair-ball remedies, and shampoos (for other less-toxic flea remedies, see *Fleas* in *Chapter 8: Housekeeping*). Also check with your veterinarian and local pet-supply stores for less-toxic anti-flea products. Important note: All topical preparations (compounds applied locally to the skin and fur), will impart their particular odors to your cat. Therefore, before using them (if you're a sensitive person), make certain these products will be tolerable to you. This is particularly necessary if you normally have close contact with your pet.

It should be mentioned that if you are allergic to cat fur but want a cat anyway, you might consider owning one of the nearly hairless breeds, such as Sphinx. Nearly hairless cats are also likely to have fewer flea problems. However, any nearly hairless cat will need extra vigilance on your part so that it is kept warm and draft-free. If the cat goes outside, it must be shielded from too much sun exposure. After all, it doesn't have much of a fur coat to act as protection.

As with all pets, keep your cat's sleeping area clean and properly store and serve its food. With cats it's also necessary to ensure that they're free of round-worms, ear mites, and that their vaccinations are up-to-date. In addition, place your cat's litter box in a location where young children can't get into it. For a litter-box filler, you might consider using old-fashioned clay litter rather than one of the typical new fillers now available that often contain synthetic dyes and scents. Fortunately, simple clay litter is still handled by some pet-supply stores, and it can be ordered from **Natural Animal**. Another option is to use an alfalfa-pellet litter fill that contains *chlorophyll*, the green compound in plant leaves that can act as a natural deodorizer. This type of filler is usually available at most pet stores. However, you could find the chlorophyll's odor a bit strong, if you're a very sensitive person. If so, you might want to mix clay and alfalfa fill together or use alternate layers of them to make your litter-box filler more tolerable.

As a rule, it's a good idea to remove any soiled litter daily and completely empty and wash the litter box weekly. One very good method to help minimize litter-box odors no matter what filler you use is to pour a large box of baking soda into the bottom of the box before you pour in replacement filler. You'll also want to keep the area around the litter box clean. This means, vacuuming the site regularly and/or washing the floor, depending on the type of floor. Remember also to wash the room walls next to the litter box frequently. This is especially important if you own a male cat that has not been neutered. These cats in particular may spray when urinating. To find an appropriate cleaner that will have germicidal and deodorizing properties and yet be safe for your walls and cat, ask your veterinarian for his (or her) recommendations. If you are a sensitive person, you'll also want to test the product to make sure you find it tolerable.

It must be said at this point that, *if you're a pregnant women, you shouldn't be involved with litter-box maintenance whatsoever.* This is because there's a risk of becoming infected with *toxoplasmosis*. While this parasitic infection usually only causes mild symptoms in children and adults, it can damage developing fetuses. (Even if you don't personally handle the litter-box job, there is apparently some risk in just having a cat. Therefore, check with your obstetrician recommendations concerning your pregnancy and pet cats.)

When you're in the market to buy less-toxic cat items, check with your veterinarian, pet shop, and alternative grocery stores. Also, you might look through cat magazines. One mail-order company offering many healthier cat items is **Pedigree**. This catalog sells stainless-steel water and feed bowls, folding epoxy-coated wire cages with handles, nylon and leather collars, as well as catnip kits complete with wood planting boxes and organic soil. They also have *sisal* (natural grass/straw) catnip-filled toys and scratching posts. Other catalogs likely to be of interest to cat owners are **Non-toxic Environments, The Seventh Generation, Body Elements/TerrEssentials**, and **The Vermont Country Store**.

Veterinarians, pet shops, libraries, and local bookstores should be able to supply you with all-around information on cat care. In addition, the **Pedigree** catalog handles a few cat-care guides. One is *Natural Healing for Dogs & Cats* by Diane Stein, a 186-page book suggesting pet remedies such as vitamins, herbs, and massage.

DOGS

Researchers have concluded that about 10,000 years ago early domesticated dogs (descendants of wolflike animals) first began living in human company. Soon afterwards, individuals began creating different physical forms of dogs to better suit certain tasks (for example, hunting badgers, hunting birds, hunting rats, protecting sheep, etc.) through selective breeding. Over time, the sizes, shapes, and fur qualities became further exaggerated. As a result, today's dog-certification organizations have come to recognize certain distinctly different breeds. Interestingly, the American Kennel Club lists 130 breeds, the British Kennel Club lists about 170, and the Federation Cynologique, Internationale recognizes 335 dog breeds. However, most dogs are actually mongrels (mixed breeds). In the U.S., the dog population, both purebred and mixed, is thought to be as high as 50 million.

No matter what the breed, or "non-breed," it's important that your pet be groomed regularly. This means routine bathing and brushing, especially if it has long hair. If you're a sensitive person, you'll want to wash your dog using a mild, low-odor pet shampoo. Your veterinarian, alternative grocery store, or pet-supply center may have these for sale. One catalog source is **Pedigree**. Frequent brushings will help minimize coat matting, shedding of loose fur onto floors and furnishings, as well as reduce the amount of allergens (allergy-provoking substances), such as hair and dander, in the air. Dog brushes, including brush/vacuum attachment types, are generally available in local pet stores. By mail order, they're available from **Pedigree**. You also might use a *flea comb* frequently on your dog. A flea comb is a nontoxic way to eliminate fleas, so it's safer for you and your dog. To use one of these closely toothed combs, simply pull it through the fur. Then, using a fingernail, push off any accumulated fleas into a bowl of water to drown them. Local pet stores or veterinarians may have these combs for sale. If not, they can be ordered from **Save Our ecoSystem (SOS)** and **Pedigree**.

By the way, **Pedigree** also sells some herbal and other all-natural types of anti-flea products (for other less-toxic flea remedies, see *Fleas* in *Chapter 8: Housekeeping*). Other similar remedies are probably available from your veterinarian and local pet-supply stores. However, remember that your pet will take on the odor of herbs or any other *topical preparation* (compound locally applied to skin, etc.), so make sure this will be acceptable to you before you use them if you're a sensitive person. For those people who want to avoid shedding and most flea problems, consider a nearly furless dog. However, these dogs, such as the Mexican Hairless, will be more susceptible to sunburn, cold temperatures, and drafts. Therefore, as the pet's owner, you'll have to be more diligent in providing preventive care.

Of course, if you plan to own any type of dog, it's important to keep your pet's indoor sleeping and eating areas clean and to store all pet food safely. If your pet has an outdoor doghouse, the bedding should be clean and regularly changed as well. Also, backyard fecal droppings from your dog should be scooped up and properly disposed of on a regular basis. In addition, make sure that roundworms, tapeworms, and heartworms are not now affecting your dog, and that all vaccinations are current, especially those for rabies.

Naturally, you'll want to provide your dog with good-quality equipment and toys, ones you'll also be able to tolerate if you're a sensitive individual. Local pet stores will undoubtedly carry some of these. By mail order, **Pedigree** offers nylon and leather collars and leashes, stainless-steel feed and water bowls, epoxy-covered folding metal cages with handles, and natural rawhide chews. In addition, **Non-toxic Environment**, **Natural Animal**, **The Seventh Generation**, **Body Elements/TerrEssentials** and **The Vermont Country Store** handle some less-toxic dog items you may find interesting.

For dog-care books, check your veterinarian's office, local pet stores, book shops, and library. Through its catalog, **Pedigree** sells a few dog-care guides including *Natural Healing for Dogs & Cats* by Diane Stein. This particular book suggests herb, vitamin, and therapeutic-massage remedies for common dog ailments.

BIRDS

Birds of many species have been kept as pets for centuries. This has been particularly true in the Orient where small singing birds are highly treasured. Today in the U.S., birds in the parrot family (parrots, macaws, parakeets, cockatoos, cockatiels, etc.), canaries, and various finches are probably the most common. Most very small pet birds have a life span of only a very few years. However, some large birds in the parrot family can live 70–80 years, definitely creating a long-term owner/pet commitment.

While pet birds are colorful, perky, and cute, they do have their drawbacks. One big negative is that they're often noisy a great deal of the time, which can get tiring even with a vocalizing canary. But perhaps worse is how surprisingly messy most birds can be. Feathers, dander (loose skin flakes), droppings, and food are usually on their cages, in the air, or on your nearby furnishings, floors, and walls. To help minimize these potential *allergens* (allergy-provoking substances) it's best to clean your bird's cage and surroundings daily, if at all possible. For some years people were afraid to keep parrots out of fear of getting *psittacosis* (parrot fever). This is actually a bacterial infection that can be transmitted by feathers, dander, and droppings. Human symptoms vary from none to a severe form of pneumonia. However, it's now known that many other bird species carry the bacteria and that certain antibiotics work well as an effective treatment for the condition.

Many owners are concerned that their pet bird will get *mites* (a type of microscopic parasite). A common remedy for this external parasitic infection has been to hang a chemically saturated anti-mite repellent on the bird's cage. These are purposely designed to continually release harmful mite-killing airborne compounds. Unfortunately, many such repellents are actually nothing more than mothballs disguised in special packaging. Obviously, these mothball chemicals are not healthy for mites. Sadly, in most cases, they also aren't healthy for birds or humans either.

Finally, if you routinely cover your bird's cage at night, you might consider an untreated, washable 100%-cotton pillowcase for the job. If it doesn't fit properly, you may want to custom make a cover. Of course, be sure to wash the cover regularly using a tolerable product.

FISH

Probably the first pet fish (varieties of goldfish) were kept centuries ago in the Orient. Today, keeping pet fish is extremely popular in many areas of the world, especially in the U.S. In fact, it's estimated that 350 million aquarium fish are sold in America annually. Many of these are tropical fish, coming originally from fresh and salt water in warm climates. Others are actually from temperate regions. Of course, the goldfish remains a favorite pet fish.

While fish are low-care pets, they certainly require some care. Their tanks, water, and even filtering equipment can become contaminated with mold and other microbial growth, if not properly cared for. In addition, the chemical composition of the tank water must be kept compatible for the types of fish living in it. The fish themselves must be monitored to see if they've acquired any types of infection. If they have, appropriate medications usually have to be added to the water and/or other measures taken.

If you decide on fish as pets, make sure that the aquarium, water, and filters are always clean. If your setup requires you to wash the tank and equipment periodically, check with your local pet-supply store for safe, low-odor products that will clean, but not cause any harm to your fish—or to you. Of course, having a good tropical fish guide on hand is always a good idea. These should be available at pet stores and bookstores.

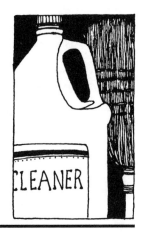

CHAPTER 7
CLEANING

A major way to keep your household healthy is to use less-toxic, low-odor cleaning products. Fortunately, quite a few are now available to choose from, and by using them, you'll definitely help create better indoor air for you and your family. The following sections provide basic information to help you make more knowledgeable cleaning decisions. It also gives specific product suggestions for floor cleaners, safer dish soaps, laundry products, etc.

CLEANING PRODUCTS

What exactly is soap? What is detergent? What's in typical cleaning products and alternative cleaning products? These questions are addressed below, along with some general information to help you decide what types of cleaning products to use in your own home.

SOAPS VS. DETERGENTS

Many home cleaning products are classified as either soaps or detergents. Interestingly, many people really don't know what these everyday words mean. However, it's a good idea to take the time to learn so you can understand their basic similarities and differences. That way, you can better judge what types of products will meet your personal cleaning preferences.

SOAPS

Soaps have a long history. They've been used to clean for thousands of years—at least in certain parts of the world. However, it wasn't until the ancient Greek era and then the Roman age that soap making techniques were better understood and the product became somewhat more consistent. Later during the Middle Ages, a number of towns in Spain, England, and France became well known as important soap-making centers. Yet, producing soap still remained a relatively slow and difficult process that usually yielded soaps of low or varying quality.

It was not until the 1800s that soap and soap-making changed much. At that time with the emergence of modern chemistry and the industrial revolution, exact formulas, processes, and machinery were finally developed. As a result, soap manufacturing finally began to take place on a large scale. That trend continued so that today in the U.S., there are literally hundreds of different types and brands of soap available. Despite other alternatives in the marketplace, soap remains the most popular skin-cleaning product. However, since the development of detergents, soaps are no longer commonly used for washing hair, dishes, laundry, or general housework.

By definition, soaps consist of natural animal fats and/or plant oils combined with some form of lye, usually *sodium hydroxide* ($NaOH_3$, which is a white, water-soluble, solid, caustic compound sometimes known as *caustic soda*). Soap comes in bars, liquids, flakes, and granular forms. Unfortunately, soaps used in *hard water* (water with a high calcium and magnesium content) create a scum known as *soap curd* (see *High Concentrations of Common Minerals and Metals* as well as *Water Softeners* in *Chapter 10: Home Water*). Soap curd is an insoluble white solid matter formed by the dissolved calcium and magnesium actually reacting with the fats and oils making up the soap. Soap curd reduces the effectiveness of any soap to clean well and, at the same time, creates a scum on sinks, tubs, etc. that can be difficult to remove.

Soaps are actually able to clean because they contain natural *surfactants* (**surf**ace **act**ing compounds). Surfactants are necessary because they counter the effects of normally occurring *surface tension* in wash water. In water droplets that do not contain surfactants, the water molecules are much more attracted to each other than they are to the surrounding air molecules. This causes the droplets to pull in (or tense) on themselves, creating comparatively large, rubbery-surfaced spheres.

However, water containing surfactants behaves quite differently. This is because all surfactant molecules have one end which attracts water molecules (a *hydrophilic polar end*) and an opposite end that doesn't (a *hydrophobic nonpolar end*). Therefore, the presence of these "strangely" behaving surfactant molecules alters the usual attraction patterns in water droplets, which would otherwise cause them to pull tightly inward. The lowered surface tension results in relatively small water droplets having surfaces that are less rubbery. These smaller droplets can more easily form very thin sheets of water, as in soap bubbles, therefore more suds are possible. Smaller droplets are also better able to penetrate and lift up dirt particles as well as keep them in suspension. Finally, smaller droplets permit more thorough rinsing. All of these factors contribute to better cleaning.

DETERGENTS

Because the fats and oils in soaps create problems with soap scum, detergents were developed. This actually occurred fairly recently, during the 1930s, when very simple *unbuilt detergents* were first created. These early granular products consisted simply of one or more naturally derived surfactant compounds. Although they did reduce the water's surface tension and didn't form as much scum, they didn't clean as effectively as was expected. As a result, after World War II the first modern *built detergents* were created and marketed. Generally, these detergent formulas contained synthetically derived surfactants originating ultimately from crude oil and additional builder ingredients. These included substances such as phosphates, carbonates, silicates, amines, zeolites, sodium EDTA, and sodium sulfates. (Minute quantities of metals such as cadmium, lead, mercury, and arsenic were also frequently present as contaminants.) These builder compounds further controlled the minerals in hard water, increased the alkalinity, and enhanced the surfactants' capacity to lower the water's surface tension. Eventually, other ingredients were added to certain detergent formulas, including compounds to prevent dirt particles that are suspended in the water from redepositing themselves, *oil emulsifiers* (compounds able to stabilize oil in water), *optical brighteners* (compounds able to give cleaned items the appearance of being whiter), bleaching agents, suds-controlling compounds, perfumes, and/or dyes.

Despite their cleaning advantages, detergents over the years have had certain problems. For example, virtually all the early detergents used surfactants that couldn't biodegrade easily. Because of this, huge quantities of foamy suds began forming and accumulating in American sewers and waterways in the 1950s and early 1960s. Another major concern has been with certain phosphate-containing ingredients. As it turns out, when these phosphate compounds dissolve in water they release phosphorus. When the phosphorus reaches lakes and streams, it acts as a fertilizer, causing algae and other aquatic plants to proliferate much too rapidly. The resulting overgrowth, or *blooms*, can create unbalanced ecosystems in which algae and plants clog the surface of the water.

Fortunately, since 1965, all laundry detergents in the U.S. are now voluntarily made to be biodegradable. Also, the amount of phosphate content has been either lowered or eliminated. (Certain states and localities have completely banned all phosphate-containing detergents.) To compensate for the cleaning effectiveness that has been lost through phosphate reduction or removal, a number of other ingredients such as the optical brighteners mentioned earlier are now commonly added.

Today, you can buy detergents in granular, gel, and liquid forms. Although most detergents contain totally synthetic formulas, a few are being made with naturally derived compounds. Because of their effectiveness, detergents are now used for most cleaning jobs. That is, except washing skin, although there are some detergents designed to do that as well.

SHOULD YOU USE SOAP OR DETERGENT?

Both soaps and detergents contain surfactants that are able to lower wash water's surface tension. Therefore, both have the capacity to lift soil and suspend it in the water in order to clean. However, detergents have been specially designed to have these qualities enhanced—and to minimize soap scum. On the other hand, soaps tend to be made of mostly natural ingredients, while detergents generally are not. Also, soaps usually have simple formulas while most detergents contain a complex variety of ingredients.

Of course, whether to use a soap or detergent is ultimately your own personal decision. However, for sensitive individuals, using any typically available soap and detergent brands may prove too bothersome. For such people, alternative unscented products with basic formulations in either category are often far more tolerable.

TYPICAL CLEANING PRODUCTS

As everyone knows, grocery aisles are filled with a huge variety of cleaning products. Nearly all of them claim to work better, act faster, and smell fresher than all the others, including previous versions of the same product. A portion of these products are now also labeled "safer to the environment." Generally, such cleaning products claim to be "eco-friendly" because they are biodegradable, are concentrated (requiring smaller plastic packages), have refills available, have packages made of recycled material, and/or have packages capable of being recycled. Surprisingly, the ability of the products to directly affect human health usually isn't an "eco-consideration." As a result, only a few national brand items are unscented or simply formulated. Even fewer are all-natural.

In reality, most typical modern cleaners are made with complex synthetic ingredient formulas, artificial colors, and artificial fragrances (see *Problems with Scents* in *Chapter 2: Personal Care*). Some products also contain powerful solvents and/or strong disinfectants. Therefore, many common cleaning products have label warnings for their proper use and storage, as well as suggestions for antidotes. Unfortunately, most consumers buy and use a product without much forethought, assuming that if it's on the shelves, it *must* be safe. Therefore, printed warnings are often ignored or briefly scanned because it's thought they are somewhat overprotective advice. The reality is, they aren't.

In America, where over ninety percent of all poisonings occur at home, the leading cause of reported cases is from cleaning products. Generally, these poisonings are distinct, singular, acute events. Commonly, they involve the swallowing of some type of cleaner by a toddler. However, how children (as well as adults) fair from exposure to such products over a period of years when they're used as intended is far less clearly understood. Interestingly, some individuals who have acquired MCS (Multiple Chemical Sensitivity) believe that typical cleaning products were a contributing factor, sometimes a major factor, to their acquiring the illness in the first place (see *MCS, A New Medical Condition* in *Chapter 1: Getting Started*). Yet, no matter how they initially did get the condition, many people with MCS eventually become unable to tolerate most typically available cleaners.

ALTERNATIVE CLEANING PRODUCTS

Fortunately, a growing number of alternative cleaning products are becoming available. Many of these have formulas that most very-sensitive people can tolerate. The following sections introduce you to some of these alternative products.

ALTERNATIVE CLEANING PRODUCTS IN GENERAL

Even major manufacturers and retailers know of the environmentally conscious "green market" and want to tap into it as much as they can. Therefore, consumers wanting less-toxic or more natural products shouldn't be lulled into complacency by product labels that simply proclaim they're "eco-safe." Often these types of terms and phrases are not legally regulated. Anyway, "environmentally friendly" claims may simply be based on the packaging—not the contents itself.

The truth is, it will usually take some effort on your part to determine if an alternative product is really healthier for you to use. Of course, a complete and thorough reading of a product's label is a good first step. By doing this, you can eliminate certain prospective cleaners simply by reading the fine print. Unfortunately, labels may not reveal all. For example, the word *non-toxic* doesn't legally mean the product has no hazardous ingredients or is safe if ingested (see *Healthy Definitions* in *Chapter 1: Getting Started*). Also, apparently some toxic substances legally don't have to be listed as ingredients, if they're in small-enough quantities.

As a result, many people who want to find truly safer cleaning products often end up bypassing conventional stores. After all, there are now a number of outlets that are more likely to offer acceptable alternatives. Some even specialize in them. Health-food shops, food co-ops, alternative grocery stores, and alternative catalogs are some of these sources.

SOME SUGGESTED ALTERNATIVE CLEANING PRODUCTS

You may want to become familiar with several brands of safer cleaning products. These are ones that have been well tolerated by many sensitive individuals. While there are certainly many other very good options on the market, these particular products are good starting points in your personal quest for developing a healthy household. Remember, to test any new product for personal tolerability before using it, especially if you're a sensitive person (see *Testing* in *Chapter 1: Getting Started*).

Note that, cleaning-product suggestions for specific cleaning tasks are listed under their appropriate headings in the following sections of this chapter: *Household Cleaning Jobs, Bathroom Cleaning Jobs, Kitchen Cleaning Jobs,* and *The Laundry.*

Alternative Product-Line Suggestions

One alternative line of cleaning products you'll probably want to become acquainted with is Allens Naturally (**Allens Naturally**). This brand is sold in many alternative groceries and health-food stores, and can be ordered directly from the company. The line includes a glass cleaner, several household cleaners, an automatic-dishwasher detergent, a dishwashing liquid, and a few laundry products. All the various cleaners are biodegradable, highly concentrated, contain no dyes or perfumes, and they're very economical.

Another fine alternative cleaning product line is Seventh Generation (**The Seventh Generation**). These products include bathroom, laundry, dish, and household cleaners. All of these are biodegradable, dye-free, perfume-free, and phosphate-free. Seventh Generation products can be ordered through its catalog. Some alternative groceries and health-food stores carry them as well.

Interestingly, Ecover (**Ecover**) natural detergent cleaners use coconut oil rather than *surfactants* derived from crude oil. Ecover products are biodegradable and contain no phosphates, chlorine, enzymes, or synthetic perfumes. However, you should be aware that certain of their cleaners do contain aromatic essential oils and, therefore will have a scent (see *Natural Essential Oils and Perfumes* as well as *Problems with Scents* in *Chapter 2: Personal Care*). Their line includes laundry products, household cleaners, toilet cleaners, and dish soaps. They're sold through some alternative retail outlets and by mail order from **Simmons Handcrafts**.

You should also be aware that Neo-Life (**Neo-Life Company of America**) makes a line of liquid, concentrated, biodegradable cleaners that many sensitive people have been able to use successfully, including an automatic dishwasher powder and a laundry detergent. Neo-Life products are offered through mail order by **The Foundation for Environmental Health, Inc.**, among others.

In addition, Granny's Old-Fashioned Products (**Granny's Old-Fashioned Products**) manufactures highly concentrated, biodegradable, dye-free, perfume-free, inexpensive cleaners. These include laundry products, carpet cleaners, and dishwashing liquids. Most of Granny's cleaners come in a range of package sizes. You can purchase these products through catalogs such as **N.E.E.D.S.** and **The Living Source**.

Multipurpose Cleaning-Product Suggestions

You'll undoubtedly find some alternative multiuse cleaning products of interest. After all, multipurpose products can make shopping, storage, and cleaning easier because just one cleaner can do so many jobs. One such multipurpose cleaner is SafeChoice Super Clean (**American Formulating and Manufacturing (AFM)**) sold by **N.E.E.D.S.**, **The Living Source**, and other AFM dealers. This is a concentrated, synthetic, liquid cleaner containing no dyes, perfumes, or phosphates. It's also non-caustic, non-acidic, and biodegradable. Super Clean is designed to be diluted with water into various concentrations in order to do specific cleaning tasks.

Today there are several concentrated, natural, citrus-solvent cleaners you might find acceptable. However, they do have a natural citrusy odor that some sensitive individuals find bothersome. These particular cleaners are meant to be diluted with water into different concentrations, like the Super Clean. Two brands of concentrated citrus cleaner are De-Solv-it (**Orange-Sol, Inc.**) and Citra-Solv (**Chempoint Products, Inc.**) and both are sold in some local groceries and retail outlets. In addition, Citra-Solv is available through mail order from **The Seventh Generation** and **Simmons Handcrafts**.

Two products that most sensitive persons find they can tolerate well are Bon Ami Cleaning Powder and Bon Ami Cleaning Cake (**Faultless Starch/Bon Ami Company**). Both are unscented, undyed soaps combined with finely powdered mineral feldspar. They can be used to clean everything from pots to window glass. These Bon Ami products are sold at some groceries and through **The Living Source**. Note, Bon-Ami offers two powdered cleaning products; the material in a cylindrical can contains a synthetic detergent, while the material in a rectangular can contains soap.

Another multiuse product you might like is Safe-Suds (**Ar-Ex, Ltd.**). This is a concentrated (many users dilute it with three parts of water), mild, liquid, synthetic detergent containing no lanolin, perfumes, fillers, water softeners, or bleaches. It's biodegradable and non-alkaline. It can be used for washing dishes by hand, household cleaning, and hand-washable laundry.

One unusual multipurpose product is San-O-Zon, which is handled by **Cottontails OrganicWear**. It's an unscented, undyed, natural, sodium and borax powder combined with "activated oxygen." It can be used as a laundry aid and for a number of household cleaning jobs. This particular product has natural deodorizing and disinfecting properties.

Suggested Catalog Sources for Alternative Cleaning Products

There are a number of catalogs you may want to obtain if you're interested in mail-ordering alternative, less-toxic, cleaning products. One of the best is **enviro-clean**, which actually specializes in alternative cleaning products. Every product in the catalog has a written description, as well as a chart that let's you know whether it's natural, biodegradable, organic, etc. Note, a number of their products are not scent-free; therefore, you'll want to order carefully if unscented products are important for you. A few other good catalog sources handling several alternative cleaners are **The Living Source, N.E.E.D.S., Non-toxic Environments**, **Natural Lifestyles Supply**, among many others.

HOMEMADE ALTERNATIVE CLEANING PRODUCTS

Often, you don't need to buy prepackaged alternative cleaning products. Some of the simple, common, natural ingredients you probably already have on hand can often clean surprisingly well. One excellent example is baking soda. Baking soda and water can cleanse and deodorize everything from clothing to bathtubs. Also, white vinegar with water can clean hard-surface floors, remove calcium buildup, and make windows sparkle.

Combining two or more household substances can accomplish still other cleaning jobs, such as mixing salt and lemon juice to clean brass. However, it's probably best not to create your own multi-ingredient cleaning products, unless you're using time-tested, well-researched recipes. After all, there's the possibility you could inadvertently create something harmful—both to what you're cleaning as well as to you. For many excellent suggestions, read *Clean and Green* by Annie Berthold-Bond. This book contains hundreds of home-made cleaning-solution formulas that are relatively easy to make, effective, inexpensive, and above all, safe. This book also suggests a number of "eco-friendly," manufactured cleaning products. Other similar books should be available at your local library or bookstore.

HOUSEHOLD CLEANING

The following sections offer suggestions for specific healthier cleaning products and practices for the most common household jobs. While many possible alternative cleaners are now available, only a few are mentioned below. For the most part, these are ones that have worked successfully for a number of sensitive individuals. They're generally effective and affordable, and are of the undyed and unscented variety.

As you'll also notice, certain products are listed under many headings because of their ability to do a number of household jobs very well. The truth is, only a few products are necessary to safely clean your entire home. Many other cleaning product manufacturers and mail-order sources are listed under *Product Sources* in *Appendix 3: Resources for a Healthy Household*.

DUSTING

As the saying goes, dusting seems to be an endless job. However, certain dusting methods are more effective than others. One rather ineffective method is using a feather duster. These simply whisk dust into the air only to have it resettle within a few hours. Then, too, some feather dusters are made so they can't be easily cleaned. A better approach would be to dust using a lightly dampened, untreated, washable, 100%-cotton flannel cloth. You can use a scrap piece of flannel fabric for this or purchase pre-made cotton flannel dusting cloths with bound edges. Packs of these can be mail-ordered from **Colonial Garden Kitchens**. Also, the **Back to Basics** catalog offers Knit Wipes, sections of white 100%-cotton knit fabric that can be used for dusting. In addition, reusable, unbleached, 100%-cotton cloths are sold in packs of twenty by **The Seventh Generation**.

For dusting hard-surface floors, washable 100%-cotton-cord floor mops lightly misted with water often work very well. They often are still sold at hardware and grocery stores. Also, Fuller Brush Floor Dusters (**Fuller Brush**), made of hand-washable, 90%-cotton cording, can be ordered from most Fuller Brush dealers including **enviro-clean**.

Another good dusting approach is to use a natural-wool duster. Interestingly, dust particles initially cling to the wool because of static electricity. Then, the wool's natural *lanolin* (sheep skin oils) causes the dust to adhere to the wool fibers—until you shake the duster out. You might be able to find wool dusters locally. If you can't, **Colonial Garden Kitchens** offers a hand-washable, natural-wool-fleece dusting mitt with an attachable four-foot wooden handle. With the long handle in place, your ceilings or wooden floors can also be easily dusted. In addition, **The Seventh Generation** sells 100%-wool dusters with 32" wood handles. The company also sells wool dust mops. Both products are made of scraps from wool-carpet manufacturers, which can be washed.

(For more on what actually makes up dust, see *Dust* in *Chapter 9: Indoor Air*. Also, for information on dusting lamps and bulbs, see *Floor and Table Lamps* in *Chapter 5: Interior Decorating*.)

POLISHING

Polishing is defined as bringing a luster to any material, usually by rubbing or buffing. It's generally one of those jobs to which few people seem to look forward—not only because of the elbow grease required, but also because many typical polishes are extremely odorous, and, thus, can't be used by sensitive individuals.

The following sections offer a few safe and effective polishing suggestions you might want to try. For other specific polishing needs, check *Clean & Green* by Annie Berthold-Bond. It also should be noted that many alternative polishes for a variety of uses are sold by **enviro-clean**.

(Note: For polishing linoleum see *Linoleum* below, and for polishing shoes see *Leather* in *Chapter 3: Clothing*.)

POLISHING METALS

Polishing brass or copper can be accomplished using a simple solution made of equal parts of fresh lemon juice and table salt. White vinegar can be substituted for the lemon juice. When you're ready to polish, be sure to use a sponge or soft cotton cloth to prevent scratching. Cotton flannel dusting cloths that can be used for this are sold in packs from **Colonial Garden Kitchens**.

Bar Keepers Friend (**Servaas Laboratories, Inc.**) also works well on copper and brass, as well as on stainless steel. It's commonly sold in grocery stores and in some hardware stores. To use it, just sprinkle a small amount of the powder on a wet soft cotton cloth or sponge. Then, gently rub the cloth across the metal. Once clean, rinse any residue off the metal with clear water and towel dry.

In addition, Bon Ami Cleaning Powder (**Faultless Starch/ Bon Ami Company**) does a good job cleaning chrome and stainless steel. It can be found in some local grocery stores and hardware stores. You can also order it from **The Living Source**. To use it, you'll want to follow the same directions as for Bar Keepers Friend cited above. Be sure to test these powdered products first on a small inconspicuous area before using them on highly lustrous surfaces.

One very effective metal polishing product you might want to try is Maas Polishing Cream, often available in local grocery stores. If you want to mail-order it, **The Vermont Country Store** is one catalog source. Maas is actually an imported European white cream, which comes packaged in tubes. It works quickly on most metals to create a brilliant sheen. Unlike most other manufactured cream-type polishes, Maas is both low-odor and nonflammable. To use it, just dab a small amount of the cream onto a soft cotton flannel cloth. Then gently rub the metal surface. Finish up by lightly buffing with another clean cotton flannel cloth.

POLISHING WOODS

For polishing woods, you might try using a solution containing equal parts of lemon juice and a rancid-resistant vegetable oil such as virgin olive oil. To actually use this type of polish, just dab a soft cotton flannel cloth into the mixture and rub the wood's surface in the direction of the grain. Cotton flannel dusting cloths that you can use for polishing wood are sold in packs from **Colonial Garden Kitchens**.

Scratches can be easily concealed on some medium- or dark-wood furniture pieces by rubbing the nicked areas with a piece of walnut or pecan nut meat. Then, buff the area lightly with a soft cotton flannel cloth. On clear finished, light, unstained wood, you might try using a cotton swab dipped in a tiny amount of virgin olive oil. Then, carefully apply the oil just to scratches and lightly buff the area with a soft cotton flannel cloth.

SWEEPING

For routine sweeping jobs, hardwood-handled *broomcorn-bristle* brooms have done a good job for centuries. Broomcorn is actually a particular type of sorghum plant specially cultivated for producing stiff bristles. However, because it's a natural material, it's important to keep broomcorn-bristle brooms dry to prevent rot or mildew. Broomcorn, or other natural bristle brooms, are still usually available at grocery stores, discount stores, and hardware stores.

Another fairly effective sweeping method is to use a lightweight nonelectric carpet sweeper. These require no electricity, yet can pick up surface dust and some loose dirt and debris as well. Carpet sweepers are designed to work on low-nap carpets and rugs and smooth surfaces such as wood, linoleum, and tile floors. One brand you might try is the Fuller Brush Electrostatic Carpet Sweeper (**Fuller Brush**). This particular sweeper has a metal case, a replaceable boar-bristle rotor brush, and can fold flat for easy storage. These sweepers are available from most Fuller Brush dealers including **enviro-clean**. Of course, several other similar sweepers are also available. One is the very popular Bissel Carpet Sweeper, sold in many local discount and department stores. One mail-order supplier is **The Seventh Generation**.

An alternative approach to using a bristle-brush sweeper is to try the Hoky Carpet Sweeper. The Hoky utilizes rotating rubberized spiral blades, which are said to provide superior pickup action compared to bristles. However, if rubber odors are bothersome to you, these machines may not be appropriate. Hoky sweepers can be found in some local department and discount stores, or mail-ordered from the **Colonial Garden Kitchens** catalog.

VACUUMING

Vacuuming can be an excellent and healthy method to remove dust and debris from your floors, walls, and furniture. That is, if the vacuum is not only powerful enough but properly filtered or vented to the outdoors. Most vacuums currently being used don't have very efficient filters and, as a result, aren't very healthy to use.

Of course, vacuum cleaners have been around for some time now. The first one actually was invented in the mid-nineteenth century. On early models, a suction was created by manually operating fans or bellows while pushing the unit back and forth. Not surprisingly, users found that this was complicated, tiring, and inefficient. It wasn't until small, reliable, electric motors became available sometime after the turn of the century that vacuum cleaners became more commonly used in homes. Unfortunately, many portable electric vacuums haven't advanced all that much since that time. This section explains how vacuum cleaners work and suggests some healthier vacuum cleaner brands.

HOW VACUUM CLEANERS WORK

Many people vacuum one or more days a week. But, how many of them actually understand how these familiar machines work? Some vacuums contain rotating brushes or beating agitators which first loosen the surface dirt on the floor. At the same time, a high-speed fan whirls inside the motor's housing to create a powerful suctioning action. As the air is pulled into the vacuum, it brings along the freed debris, which is deposited into a paper or cloth filter bag or sometimes a special self-contained receptacle. The air then flows through the bag or receptacle and quickly back into the room, supposedly leaving the dirt behind.

Unfortunately, many conventional portable vacuum cleaners are ineffective in separating the dirt from the air that returns to the room. As a result, a fairly large percentage of particulate matter is often blown back into air of the room you have just cleaned. (The precise percentage depends on the vacuum model, as well as how full the collection bag or permanent receptacle is.)

It should be noted that particulate matter is made up not only of soil grains, but also lint, human and pet hair, human and pet *dander* (skin flakes), mold spores, pollen grains, and dust mite fragments and feces, among other unpleasant contaminants (see *Mold, Pollen*, as well as *Dust Mite Body Parts and Feces* in *Chapter 9: Indoor Air*). If you operate an inefficient vacuum,

200

you'll end up breathing this delightful concoction continually as it passes through the filter into the room. It should not then be surprising to learn that many susceptible persons find that vacuuming actually provokes allergic and asthmatic symptoms rather than preventing them.

ALTERNATIVE PORTABLE VACUUM CLEANERS

Because most typical portable vacuums blow large quantities of what they pick up back into the air, alternative models are now available for those who want healthier vacuums. These units have filters designed to more effectively trap dirt. The following sections introduce you to some of these.

HEPA and HEPA-Type Filtered Vacuum Cleaners

There are now several vacuums available that use *HEPA* filters. HEPA is an acronym for **h**igh **e**fficiency **p**articulate **a**rresting (or sometimes **a**ccumulator or **a**ir). HEPA filters are generally made of a specially constructed synthetic material such as fiberglass. The spaces in this filtering fabric are so tiny that most minute particles can't pass through it.

In many of the HEPA-equipped consumer vacuum cleaners, almost all the particles larger than 0.3 microns are trapped. Therefore, bacteria (0.3–30 microns) and pollen (10–100 microns) are usually stopped. Interestingly, certain specialized commercial-grade HEPA filters are even more efficient. Some are even able to filter out the infinitesimally small particles making up tobacco smoke. It's no wonder then that HEPA-equipped vacuums are used by professional asbestos and lead paint-removal contractors who must thoroughly and safely remove hazardous material. Note that, when comparing filter efficiencies, several different efficiency tests can be used (see also *HEPA Filters* in *Chapter 9: Indoor Air*).

If you're interested in a consumer-quality, portable, HEPA vacuum, several merit your consideration. Vita-Vac (**Vita-Mix Corporation**) is a small metal-canister unit sold directly by the company. Dealers such as **N.E.E.D.S.** also handle it. Vit-a-Vac has a 4-stage filtering system. The first is a hygienically sealed bag that inhibits fungal growth. Next is a 14-layer cellulose bag filter to remove visible dust. Then there's an activated charcoal filter to adsorb odors (see *Activated Charcoal and Activated Alumina* in *Chapter 9: Indoor Air*). Finally, there's a "HEPA-type" filter that is said to be 99% efficient in eliminating particles larger than 0.3 micron in size.

Allervac UZ 932 HEPA (**Euroclean**), which can be ordered from dealers such as **Nontoxic Environments**, is a 14-pound polypropylene HEPA-equipped vacuum. It has been designed with a triple-filtration system. This consists of a multilayer paper bag, a prefilter to eliminate large particles, and a 99.97%-efficient HEPA filter that will remove particles down to 0.3 microns. Euroclean also makes a number of other HEPA models.

In addition, Miele (**Miele Appliances, Inc.**) offers several vacuums featuring HEPA filters that are sold through their dealers such as **earthsake**. One model is claimed to trap particles as tiny as viruses. Miele vacuums are made of ABS plastic (a hard synthetic material made of **a**crylonitrile, **b**utadiene, and **s**tyrene), the same type of plastic used in making football helmets. The Miele units have three filters, including an *electrostatic* type that uses an electrical charge to attract particles (see *Electrostatic Filters* in *Chapter 9: Indoor Air*).

Finally, Nilfisk (**Nilfisk of America, Inc.**) manufactures several plastic HEPA-equipped vacuums, as well as ones having aluminum canisters. These are sold by dealers such as **Nontoxic Environments** and **Ozark Water Service and Environmental Services**. Nilfisk vacuums work in four stages. First there is *cyclonic action* (a centrifugal air pattern) that's capable of removing heavy particles. Next, there are two filters, including one called a "felt microfilter," that are designed to eliminate most of the larger-sized particles. Lastly, there's a HEPA filter. In the Nilfisk GS 90 model, 99.97% of particles 0.3 microns or larger are said to become trapped. In addition, an optional ultra-efficient HEPA filter is available that is claimed to be 99.999% efficient down to a very minute 0.12 microns.

Some negative points of buying a HEPA vacuum should be considered. First, all HEPA-equipped units are, no doubt, going to be more costly than conventional models; some are, in fact, quite expensive. Many of the manufactures also won't have dealers in your hometown, so that, if repairs become necessary, you may have to ship your machine to a faraway designated repair center. You also should remember that the bags and filtering materials will have to be replaced periodically. Another important consideration if you're a sensitive person is that many HEPA filters can outgas odors from the resins and other synthetic materials making up the filtering fabrics. These can be bothersome to certain susceptible individuals.

Water-Filtered Vacuum Cleaners

An unusual alternative portable vacuum approach is water filtering. Rainbow SE (**Rexair, Inc.**) is one brand that uses this method. (To locate a nearby dealer, call the manufacturer.) The Rainbow SE works by creating a powerful air flow that pulls dirt and debris into a water reservoir. Ideally, most of the dirt is left in the water as the air bubbles its way though. Incidentally, Rainbow SE vacuums can also be adapted for washing carpets.

Unfortunately, it seems that water filter-equipped vacuums may not work particularly well on certain types of particulates. Also, there is some concern that water-reservoir units could become potential havens for mold and mildew growth. At any rate, these vacuums are somewhat cumbersome to maneuver and expensive to purchase.

More Efficient Filter Bags for Typical Portable Vacuum Cleaners

If you don't care to—or can't at the moment—replace your present conventional portable vacuum cleaner, you might consider buying more efficient vacuum cleaner replacement bags for the model you currently own. Such bags are designed to more effectively trap and retain small particles than standard vacuum bags.

More efficient filtering bags are available at some local vacuum-cleaner shops and other outlets where vacuum cleaners are sold. By mail order, **The Vermont Country Store** offers these types of bags to fit most popular vacuum cleaner models. Note that, more efficient replacement vacuum bags may still not be effective enough for those with certain allergic conditions.

CENTRAL VACUUMS

Many persons find that for them, the easiest and most efficient home vacuums are *central vacuum systems*. Central vacuum systems have large, permanently mounted canisters with a motor attached. These are usually placed near or on an exterior wall in a utility room or basement. Most of these units are vented to the outdoors, although some models are designed to vent indoors. Of the two, the exterior-venting types are generally considered healthier. With outdoor-venting units, the air that's pulled into the vacuum isn't sent back into the living space after it passes through the filter, but to the outdoors instead. This eliminates most concerns over the filter's efficiency.

However, no matter which model you purchase, all central vacuums require special tubing that is permanently installed within the walls of the house. To access these, special vacuum hose outlets are mounted strategically around the home's interior. To operate the vacuum, you simply plug in the hose (usually 20' or 30' long) into one of the outlets, which automatically turns the vacuum motor on. A variety of cleaning attachments are available, including an agitating head. With only the hose to maneuver, these vacuums are easy to use throughout the house.

There are many central vacuum manufacturers. Two you might consider are **Beam Industries** and **Nutone/Scovill**. To purchase their products, contact the companies for their nearest dealers. And don't forget to check your local phone book for other brands and retailers.

Be aware that there are a few drawbacks to owning a central vacuum unit. First, central vacuums are rather expensive to buy and to have installed. Because they require interior-wall piping installations, they also can be difficult to incorporate into some existing homes, although manufacturers generally have a number of tips in their product literature. Also, it's important that sticks, Christmas-tree needles, toothpicks, etc., don't get sucked into the vacuum's piping within the walls. If such items should become lodged, they could trap debris that could begin to clog the pipe. Finally, as with nearly all vacuums, the receptacle's collection bag must be replaced periodically for maximum suctioning efficiency. For models without a bag, the receptacle must be emptied regularly.

COPING WITH VACUUM HOSE ODORS

Whether a conventional vacuum cleaner, an alternative portable model, or a central system, some sensitive individuals may find the vacuum hose very bothersome to them. This is likely due to the odors given off by the vinyl or other plastic materials, of which the hoses are made. To rectify this situation, you can try washing your hose with diluted (1^1/$_2$–2 cups in 1 gallon water) SafeChoice Super Clean (**American Formulating and Manufacturing (AFM)**) and then rinsing. This product is sold by most AFM dealers including **N.E.E.D.S.** and **The Living Source**. It's likely you'll have to wash a vacuum's hose several times. You might even need to increase the concentration of Super Clean to water, if necessary.

Sometimes hanging odorous hoses outdoors for several weeks in dry uncontaminated surroundings will make them more tolerable. If you can't hang them outside, you might suspend them in a room that's seldom used, but well-ventilated. If the hose remains too odorous, even after cleaning and airing, you should consider using untreated 100%-cotton barrier cloth to make a long tube that can be used as a hose cover. (For more on sewing, see *Custom-Made Clothing* in *Chapter 3: Clothing*.) Barrier cloth is a special tightly woven cotton that often seals in many odors. It's available from **The Cotton Place** and **Janice Corp.** When the covers are completed, simply pull the vacuum hoses through the cloth tubes. The ends can be held in place using strings or rubber bands. Of course, you'll, no doubt, want to remove the covers from time to time to wash them using a tolerable laundry product.

CLEANING HARD-SURFACE FLOORING

Sometimes various hard-surface flooring materials require their own particular cleaners and care products. Generally, however, all hard-surface floors can be cleaned with the same equipment. For example, to pick up dust and dirt, all-cotton dust mops lightly misted with water, or dry all-wool dust mops work well on all hard floors. Simple carpet sweepers are another good choice for light pick-ups. For vacuuming, a soft brush attachment is a good option.

For washing hard-surface floors, ideally you should choose floor-cleaning equipment that will be kind to your floors, the environment—and you. Two examples of safer floor-washing tools are the Fuller Brush cellulose sponge mop (**Fuller Brush**) and the Fuller Brush 100%-cotton-string wet mop (**Fuller Brush**). Both of these can be purchased from most Fuller Brush dealers including **enviro-care**. Of course, similar products are sold in many local hardware, grocery, and discount stores.

CERAMIC TILE AND VINYL FLOORS

Ceramic tile and vinyl floors are relatively easy to care for. Here are some healthier cleaning solution options.

Washing Ceramic Tile and Vinyl Floors

Ceramic tile and vinyl flooring can be safely washed using a mop with a simple dilute solution of 1 cup white vinegar in 2 gallons of water. No rinsing is necessary with this solution. One-eighth cup of liquid soap mixed in 2 gallons of water can also be used to wash ceramic and vinyl floors. However, rinsing will be necessary. Heavenly Horsetail All-Purpose Cleaner (**Infinity Herbal Products**), which is sold at some health-food stores, is one liquid-soap product you might want to try for this job. However, this particular soap has a herbal formula whose natural scent may be bothersome to some sensitive individuals.

Another liquid-soap option is to use an unscented Castile soap such as Dr. Erlander's Jubilee Liquid Castile Soap (**Erlander's Natural Products**). This product can be ordered directly from the company. Dr. Bronner's Baby Liquid Castile Soap (**Dr. Bronner**) is another unscented Castile product, and it's often sold by local health-food stores. However, if you're unable to locate this, it can be ordered from the company. Note: If you add 1 tablespoon of San-O-Zon to any soap/water solution, it will help disinfect and deodorize. San-O-Zon is a patented sodium-borax unscented powder. It can be ordered from **Cottontails OrganicWear**.

Safe-Suds (**Ar-Ex, Ltd.**) is yet another type of product that can be used to wash ceramic or vinyl floors. It's a concentrated unscented, liquid, synthetic detergent that can be bought at some local pharmacies or ordered directly from the manufacturer. To use it, mix 1 teaspoon in 2 gallons of water and then mop. You'll find that rinsing is necessary. SafeChoice Super Clean (**Ameri-**

can Formulating and Manufacturing), which is available from **N.E.E.D.S.** and **The Living Source**, is also a good unscented liquid detergent option. To use this product, mix 1 cup of it in 1 gallon of water and mop; afterwards, rinse. You might also try Rugged Red (**Neo-Life Co. of America**) in a weak solution. Again, you'll need to mop and then rinse with clear water. Rugged Red is available from **The American Environmental Health Foundation, Inc.**

Still another alternative for washing your ceramic or vinyl floors is Citra-Solv (**Chempoint Products, Inc.**). This product is sold in many health-food stores and by mail order through **The Seventh Generation** and **Simmons Handcrafts**, among others. To use it, dilute it at a ratio of 1 oz. to 2 cups water, or even a weaker solution. After mopping, rinse the floor with clear water. As you might expect, Citra-Solv has a natural citrusy odor.

As a final note, several other very good alternative cleaners for washing ceramic and vinyl floors are available from **enviro-clean**.

Cleaning Oily Grout Stains

To remove oil and grease stains from unsealed ceramic tile grout joints, use *fuller's earth*. Simply mix the fuller's earth and water to create a paste. Then, apply the gray, wet, plaster-like mixture to the stain and leave it overnight. The next day you can either wash it off or brush it off with a stiff brush or broom, then vacuum up the dusty residue. Be aware, though, that this entire procedure might have to be repeated in order to remove some stubborn stains.

Fuller's earth is actually a type of powdered, natural clay. However, it does have a somewhat earthy pungent odor when wet. Fuller's earth can be purchased or ordered through some drugstores and hardware stores. One distributor of fuller's earth is Humco Laboratory.

Filling Small Nicks in Glazed Ceramic Tile

If you drop a sharp or heavy object on a glazed ceramic floor tile, the tile may chip. When this happens, the tile surface color will be missing and the base ceramic itself (often off-white) will show through. To repair these little nicks, simply fill them using a crayon that closely matches the color of the glazed tile. Surprisingly, the wax in the crayon creates a filler that is usually fairly durable. Note: Sealants or shiny-finish products probably won't adhere to waxy crayon. However, most glazed ceramic-tile floors don't require sealants or finishes.

LINOLEUM FLOORS

If you have a natural linoleum floor, it's important to care for it properly to ensure it has a long, attractive life. The following sections will tell you how to do just that.

Washing Linoleum Floors

Linoleum floors can usually be washed safely with 1/8 cup Dr. Erlander's Jubilee Liquid Castile Soap (**Erlander's Natural Products**) mixed in 2 gallons of water. To use it, mop with the solution and then rinse. Dr. Erlander's products can be ordered directly from the company. As an alternative soap, you can use Heavenly Horsetail All-Purpose Cleaner (**Infinity Herbal Products**) instead. This liquid herbal product is available at some local health-food stores. If you can't find it, call the company for the nearest dealer. To use it, follow the same directions as for Castile soap. (Note: This particular product's natural herbal odors may prove to be too bothersome to some sensitive persons.) By the way, if you add 1 tablespoon of San-O-Zon to either the Castile soap or herbal soap and water solution, it'll add disinfecting and deodorizing properties. San-O-Zon is a sodium-borax unscented powder handled by **Cottontails OrganicWear**.

You might also try Citra-Solv (**Chempoint Products, Inc.**) to wash your linoleum floors. This concentrated cleaner is often available in local health-food stores and can be mail-ordered from **The Seventh Generation** and **Simmons Handcrafts**. For general cleaning, use a dilution at a ratio of 1 oz. (or less) to 2 cups water. To remove heel marks, use a much more concentrated solution. If you choose to use Citra-Solv on your floors, it's a good idea to rinse afterwards with clear water. (Note that, this product has a citrusy odor.) Other linoleum cleaners are handled by **enviro-clean** and **Nontoxic Interiors**.

Linoleum Polishes, Wax Removers, and Other Care Products

An easy homemade linoleum polish is simply using 6 tablespoons of cornstarch dissolved in 1 cup water. Apply with a soft cotton flannel cloth in a sweeping buffing motion. Those with corn allergies should probably avoid using this.

To remove wax, you'll want to use a heavy concentration of *washing soda* and water. You can apply the solution with a sponge or sponge mop, allow it to dry, then rinse with clear water. If you choose to do this, using an unscented washing soda is probably best, if you're a sensitive person. Dr. Erlander's Jubilee Washing Compound (**Erlander's Natural Products**) is one washing soda brand, which can be ordered directly from the company. Scented washing soda is generally available in grocery stores.

Another wax-removing option is to use Citra-Solv (**Chempoint Products, Inc.**) This product is now often available in local health-food stores. It can also be ordered from **The Seventh Generation** and **Simmons Handcrafts**, among others. To use it, mix 1 cup with 10 cups water. You'll need to scrub the floor using a floor brush, then rinse with water. (If the wax doesn't seem to be coming off, a stronger concentration may be necessary.)

Other linoleum-care products are available from **enviro-clean** and **Nontoxic Interiors**. You might also talk with your linoleum dealer for his or her suggestions. Remember that, natural, unsealed linoleum can be negatively affected by water. Therefore, you'll want to make certain your linoleum's surface is effectively protected. If you're a sensitive person, make sure the products you use are tolerable to you (see *Testing* in *Chapter 1: Getting Started*).

HARDWOOD FLOORS

Ecover Liquid Floor Soap (**Ecover**), available from **Simmons Handcrafts**, is a possibility for cleaning hardwood floors. However, this biodegradable, vegetable oil-based soap does contain essential oils of rosemary, eucalyptus, and citronella that are aromatic and will linger. These can sometimes be bothersome to sensitive individuals (see *Problems with Scents* in *Chapter 2: Personal Care*). Use 1 capful in 1 gallon of water. Unfortunately, the highly advertised Murphy's Oil Soap contains pine-oil extracts that can be too bothersome to many sensitive people.

Another option is to use unscented, liquid Castile soap. Dr. Erlander's Jubilee Liquid Castile Soap (**Erlander's Natural Products**) is one such product. It may be ordered directly from the company. Dr. Bronner's Baby Liquid Castile Soap (**Dr. Bronner**) is another brand. It's commonly available at health-food stores. If you are unable to find it locally, it may be ordered from the company. To use these products, pour $1/8$ cup liquid Castile soap plus $1/2$ cup white vinegar into 2 gallons of water. After washing, rinse your floor with clear water.

Another liquid natural-soap product you might try is Heavenly Horsetail All-Purpose Cleaner (**Infinity Herbal Products**.) However, it does contains aromatic herbs. This may be bothersome to some sensitive individuals. Heavenly Horsetail is sold in some health-food stores. If you can't find it, call the company for the nearest dealer. To use it, simply follow the same cleaning directions for using liquid Castile soap.

Some people may want to try using a mild, unscented dish detergent with water, followed by rinsing. However, using detergents may not be as good for wood floors as soap products that contain oils and/or fats. If your floor needs to be disinfected and/or deodorized, add 1 tablespoon of San-O-Zon to your floor cleaning solution. This unscented sodium-borax powder is sold by **Cottontails OrganicWear**.

For other appropriate hard floor-surface cleaners, check in the **enviro-clean** catalog. Note: Avoid using too much water on your hardwood floors. Even if they're sealed, small breaks or cracks in the hard protective surface will permit water to become absorbed by the wood. Excess moisture may easily cause damage, either discoloration or warping. Therefore, always wring sponges or mops thoroughly before using them on wood floors.

CLEANING RUGS AND CARPETS

Rugs and carpets require special care to keep them clean and looking good. Ideally, only tolerable, less-toxic, lower-odor products should be used, especially if you're a sensitive person.

REMOVING RUG AND CARPET DUST

If small, 100%-cotton rugs have only surface dust on them, it can be removed by vigorously shaking the rugs outdoors. Of course, you'll want to hold your breath when you do this so as not to inhale the airborne dust particles. Another easy method of removing dust is to put small cotton rugs in the clothes dryer for about fifteen minutes. Using the "heat" rather than the "air" setting will help tighten the yarns that may have stretched out of shape in *dhurrie* rugs (flat, heavy, woven, cotton rugs).

A very old rug cleaning method that is able to remove deeply imbedded dust and debris is to beat your rugs while they hang securely on an outdoor line. Unfortunately, finding a rug-beating tool anymore can be a problem. However, heavy, looped-wire, wood-handled beaters might still be found in a few local antique shops. If you can't find a real rug beater, you might try using an old tennis racket instead. If you use a racket, make sure that there are no protruding string knots or other rough areas that could snag the rug's fibers. Because beating a rug can take some time, it's a good idea to wear a protective dust mask. These are sold in most hardware stores and they can be mail-ordered from **E.L. Foust Co., Inc.** (see also *Protective Gear* in *Chapter 12: Home Workshop and Garage*).

Of course, large rugs and carpets that can't be removed should be vacuumed regularly, ideally with a specially filtered portable vacuum or a central vacuum system vented to the outdoors. Vacuuming can reduce the accumulated dirt that can be abrasive to your carpet's fibers. Frequent vacuuming also can help reduce dust mite and flea problems.

REMOVING RUG AND CARPET STAINS

Most people who use rugs and carpeting invariably have to deal with stains that get on them. While there are a number of highly-odorous, solvent-type, carpet stain removers on the market, these can be very bothersome, especially to sensitive persons. Fortunately, there are some less noxious alternatives. Actually, many small spots can be safely removed using a solution of club soda, which often works well with small, fresh stains. Simply pour a small amount of the club soda on the affected area. Then, blot the dampness away using a clean sponge or a clean 100%-cotton towel. You might find you'll have to repeat the procedure, if necessary.

For removing greasy stains from carpet, try using 1 oz. Citra-Solv (**Chempoint Products, Inc.**) dissolved in 2 cups of water. Citra-Solv is a highly concentrated cleaner that is often available at local heath-food stores. It can also be ordered from **The Seventh Generation** and **Simmons Handcrafts**. Apply the solution to the stain with a clean sponge and then alternately brush and blot the area with a clean damp cotton cloth. Finish up by rinsing with clear water and blotting. Note that, this cleaner is citrus-based, so it does have a citrusy odor.

Another product you might try to remove carpet stains is White Wizard Spot Remover and All-Purpose Cleaner. This is an odorless, nontoxic, eco-friendly product in a paste-like consistency. The manufacturer claims the product is able to get out many grease, blood, ink, and other stains. It is sold in 10 oz. plastic tubs in some local grocery and hardware stores. It's also available by mail order from **The Seventh Generation** and **Colonial Garden Kitchens**, among others. To use it, carefully follow the package's directions.

If your carpet has pet stains, special cleaners, available from **Pedigree**, are sold to remove these. For various types of other carpet stains, **enviro-clean** offers several alternative spot cleaners. Also, check *Clean & Green* by Annie Berthold-Bond for still other specific stain-removal suggestions. It's important to note that whatever you use to clean your carpet, it's wise to test it first to make sure it won't bleach or damage the carpet fibers, and that it'll be tolerable to you.

THOROUGH CLEANING OF RUGS AND CARPETS

Of course, from time to time your rugs and carpets will have to be thoroughly cleaned—not just vacuumed or spot cleaned. This section discusses some methods that can be used to accomplish this. As you'll see, in some cases the problems associated with cleaning carpets both thoroughly and safely can be great. In fact, one medical condition, *Kawasaki Syndrome*, has been linked to newly cleaned carpets. It seems that in some instances, 16 to 25 days after a carpet's been cleaned, the condition manifests itself in certain children.

The symptoms are systemic and generally include a high fever. That's one of the major reasons why hard-surface flooring options are often suggested for ideal healthy houses.

It should be pointed out that it is erroneous to think that sprinkling baking soda on a carpet, and then vacuuming it, will actually clean the carpet. This simply is not true. All that baking soda can do is absorb some of the carpet odors without adding any additional ones. Note that, any baking soda that isn't completely vacuumed up will tend to accumulate in your carpets.

Simple Rug Washing

Many small 100%-cotton rugs can be safely laundered in your washing machine, then dried in an automatic dryer or hung on a line. However, you should realize that in many cases there will be some shrinkage, especially after the initial washing and drying.

Surprisingly, some wool Oriental rugs can actually be laid flat outdoors in a clean area and gently scrubbed with mild bar soap and water. The lathered rugs should then be thoroughly rinsed with clear water and allowed to completely dry while flat. However, this cleaning method should only be undertaken after talking with the dealer from whom you bought the rugs.

Check with Oriental-rug dealers to see if they can recommend a rug-cleaning company that will use less-toxic cleaning products. Some rug dealers offer such a service, and will pick up your rugs, clean them in their shop, then return them to your home.

Solvent Cleaning Rugs and Carpets

Some manufacturers recommend that their natural-fiber rugs be dry-cleaned only. As it turns out, dry-cleaning uses petroleum-derived solvents rather than water as the cleaning fluid. For certain rugs, this may be necessary in order to prevent the dyes from running or the fibers from deteriorating. When you bring your rugs to a dry-cleaning establishment, ask that no added scents, deodorizers, or moth-preventive chemicals be used on your rugs. This is especially important for sensitive persons. Once your newly cleaned rugs are home, it's a very good idea to air them outdoors in shaded, dry, uncontaminated surroundings until the chemical odors have dissipated.

If you can't (or don't care to) take your large rugs to a dry-cleaner, there are now companies that use milder dry-cleaning solutions to clean them right in your house. (This method is also used on wall-to-wall carpeting.) The companies that do this promote the fact that they don't use water, and, thus, their cleaning methods won't promote the growth of microorganisms.

With home dry-cleaning, solvents are first sprayed directly onto your rugs or carpeting. They then enter the fibers causing the dirt to be pushed toward the surface. Next, the freed dirt has to be removed. To do this, some companies use a second solution containing *ionizers*. These provide charged ions that attach themselves to the dirt particles. The solution also usually contains *optical brighteners* (to make the newly cleaned carpets appear brighter-looking) and perhaps deodorizers and other additives as well.

After an ionizing solution has been applied, a special machine is used that has a whirling oppositely charged (as compared to the ionized dirt particles) nylon pad that is able to pick up the dirt particles *electostatically*. (This is the natural force that causes opposite charges to attract.) The pads are repeatedly rinsed or replaced until they no longer get dirty—meaning they aren't able to pick up any more dirt particles, and the rug or carpet is considered clean.

Note that, solvent-based rug/carpet cleaning solutions nearly always contain scents, either natural or synthetic. These scents may linger for a long time after the cleaning is done. Also, the solvents can be bothersome to sensitive persons. If you absolutely must have this type of cleaning done in your home, it's wise to have good ventilation and to be out of the house while the actual cleaning is taking place. In fact, if you're very sensitive, you may have to stay elsewhere for some time until the odors are tolerable.

Using powdered-solvent cleaners rather than wet-solvent sprays is another in-home dry-cleaning approach for cleaning your rugs and carpets. With this method, rugs and carpets are often first lightly dampened with water. Then, the powdered solvent is sprinkled on them. In some cases, this material is actually composed of cellulose (a natural material derived from plants) saturated with solvents, detergents, and other additives. After it's been applied, it remains there for a predetermined length of time to absorb the dirt.

Next, using some type of extraction equipment or very powerful vacuum, the powdered solvent is removed. However, in reality it's impossible to remove all of it; some will remain imbedded in the rugs and carpets. As you routinely vacuum though, more and more of the powdered solvent will eventually come out. Fortunately, these powders are designed to be nonabrasive to fibers. Note that, the same concerns and prudent measures suggested earlier in connection with the wet-solvent cleaners apply to the powdered solvent cleaners as well.

Rug and Carpet Shampooing and Wet-Extraction Cleaning

Many people choose to avoid solvent rug cleaners altogether because of the odors they generate and, thus, opt for rug and carpet cleaning methods that use water. However, it should be noted that using water solutions can create damp fibers, backing, and padding, which could easily accelerate mold and bacterial growth.

Water-solution rug and carpet cleaning can be done using either a rotating head shampoo machine or a special application/extraction machine (sometimes incorrectly called a *steam cleaner*). Application/extraction machines provide both a spraying action and a suctioning action that occur simultaneously. If you have your home professionally cleaned using a water solution, it's likely that this type of equipment will be used.

Unlike shampooing machines, application/extraction machines are able to remove a great deal of the detergents and moisture they put in the carpet. This is important because any remaining detergent can leave a gummy coating on the carpet fibers that will act as a glue to hold dirt particles in the future. Therefore, recently-cleaned rugs or carpets with detergent residues may have to be cleaned again rather quickly. In addition, excess moisture left in your carpet will require more time to evaporate, it could potentially damage certain carpet fibers and backing materials, and it can greatly encourage microbial growth. Another distinct advantage to extraction machines over shampooing machines is that their vacuuming effect is able to pull up deeply imbedded dirt—not just surface dirt.

No matter which type of machine you choose, you should be aware that typical carpet shampoos generally contain a complex mixture of synthetic ingredients, including colorants and fragrances. Therefore, these products are often not very well tolerated by sensitive people. Fortunately, there are now several alternative rug and carpet cleaning products that have more simple formulas; some are even unscented.

One of these you might want to try is SafeChoice Carpet Shampoo (**American Formulating and Manufacturing (AFM)**). It's sold by most AFM dealers including **enviro-clean**, **N.E.E.D.S.**, and **The Living Source**. This product is an unscented, water-based, synthetic emulsion designed to be low-odor. It can be used in shampooing machines or application/extraction machines. Be sure to follow the package directions carefully to get the best results.

Another alternative carpet shampoo is Karpet Kleen (**Granny's Old Fashioned Products**). This can be purchased from dealers such as **N.E.E.D.S.** and **The Living Source**. Karpet Kleen contains no dyes, fragrances, phosphates, or preservatives. It's recommended to be used in an application/extraction-type carpet cleaning machine. Follow the package directions carefully for proper dilution. Other alternative carpet cleaning products for shampooing machines and/or application/extraction machines are available through **Nontoxic Interiors** and **enviro-clean**.

Important note: If you purposely choose an unscented carpet shampoo, be sure to consider the condition of the cleaning equipment in which you plan to use it. After all, rented units will have absorbed odors from perhaps hundreds of cleanings with typical carpet-cleaning solutions containing perfumes, natural lemon scents, disinfectants, deodorizers, etc. Therefore, it may be wise to own your machine if at all possible, especially if you're a sensitive person. Carpet-cleaning machines are sold in most department stores, vacuum shops, and discount stores.

CLEANING WINDOWS

Most common window cleaners are extremely odorous. This is because many of them contain ammonia, perfumes, alcohol, or other powerful ingredients. Generally, these products can't be safely used by sensitive persons. However, there are more tolerable window-cleaning solutions available.

For example, a very weak dilution of SafeChoice Super Clean (**American Formulating and Manufacturing (AFM)**) in water works quite well to clean windows. You need to use only 5 eye dropper drops of this unscented, synthetic liquid in a spray bottle filled with 16 ounces of water. Then, you simply shake the bottle well, spray the window, and clean it using tolerable paper towels. Non-linty cotton cloth such as flannel can be used, either fabric scraps or cloths with bound edges such as those sold by **Colonial Garden Kitchens**. Super Clean can be purchased from most AFM dealers, including **N.E.E.D.S.** and **The Living Source**.

Another alternative window-cleaning option is to use Bon Ami Cleaning Powder or Bon Ami Cleaning Cake (**Faultless Starch/Bon Ami Company**). Both are available in some local grocery stores and can be mail-ordered from **The Living Source**. To use them, either sprinkle a small amount of the white unscented powder on a wet sponge or gently rub a wet sponge across the cleaning cake. Then, apply a thin even coating to the dirty windows. Finally, you'll have to completely buff away the film before it dries, using a clean, dry, soft non-linty cotton cloth.

Of course, a white vinegar in water solution is a favorite old-time window cleaner. It has many advantages, too; it's nontoxic, all-natural, inexpensive, and effective. However, certain sensitive persons might find the vinegar odor somewhat bothersome. To use vinegar to clean your windows, mix $1/4$ cup white vinegar with 1 pint of water and pour it into a spray bottle. Then mist the glass with the solution and clean it off with tolerable paper towels or non-linty cotton cloth. A few other alternative window cleaners are available from **enviro-clean.**

CLEANING WALLS

In most cases you usually don't have to clean your home's painted interior walls very often. But when you do, you'll want to choose less-toxic, low-odor products to do the job, especially if you're a very sensitive individual.

Most painted walls can be safely washed with a solution of SafeChoice Super Clean (**American Formulating and Manufacturing**) and water. This unscented liquid cleaner can be ordered from AFM dealers including **N.E.E.D.S.** and **The Living Source.** To clean your walls, mix 1 cup Super Clean in 1 gallon of water. Then dip a sponge or soft cotton cloth into the solution, lightly wring it, and very gently scrub the walls. Finish by rinsing with clear water.

You might also try Citra-Solv (**Chempoint Products, Inc.**) to clean your painted walls. This concentrated cleaner is sold in some local health-food stores or it can be ordered from **The Seventh Generation** and **Simmons Handcrafts.** To use Citra-Solv, mix 1 cup in 1 gallon of water. Then apply and rinse as with the Super Clean/water solution. Note that, this cleaner has a citrusy odor.

Another option is to use TSP (trisodium phosphate) and water in a very weak solution. TSP is a crystalline material that can be used as a powerful, un-scented cleaner. At least one brand of TSP—Red Devil TSP/90 Heavy Duty Cleaner (**Red Devil, Inc.**)—has a modified trisodium phosphate formula that is phosphate-free. It's usually sold in paint and hardware stores. To use Red Devil TSP, mix 2 teaspoons of it in 1 gallon of warm water. Then, dip your sponge in the solution and wring it nearly dry. Next, you can gently scrub the walls starting from the wall bottom up to avoid creating streaks. You'll find that cleaning just a small area at a time usually works best. In most cases, rinsing isn't necessary. By the way, whenever you use TSP, wearing rubber gloves is a good idea to prevent any skin irritation from arising.

Before using any cleaning solution on your walls, it's best to test a small inconspicuous spot first. That way you ensure that your painted surfaces won't be harmed before you proceed any further. (For greasy walls, see *Greasy Problems* below.)

KITCHEN CLEANING

Practically every day, your kitchen requires several cleanups. Ideally, you'll choose products for this job that are effective, low-odor, and well-tolerated by you. This means avoiding most of the typical kitchen cleaning products available in your local grocery store. Fortunately, the sections below offer some safer kitchen cleaning product alternatives.

SPONGES AND BRUSHES

Bright, synthetically dyed cellulose (a natural material derived from plants) sponges are sold in nearly every grocery store. However, you should be aware that certain cellulose sponges are now modified to have antimicrobial properties. Such sponges are designed to prevent the sour odor (mostly from bacterial contamination) that many sponges develop. Unfortunately, this special treatment itself gives antimicrobial sponges an objectionable odor. Therefore, many sensitive individuals may not be able to tolerate them. Certain very sensitive persons also may not even be able tolerate the dyes used in either the treated or untreated sponges.

If you want to use sponges but don't find typical cellulose sponges acceptable, you might try undyed cellulose sponges sold by **Simmons Handcrafts** and **The Seventh Generation**. You might also opt for natural sea sponges (*porifera*) sold by **Simmons Handcrafts**. However, you should know that these alternative sponges can be rather expensive, especially the sea sponges.

No matter what type of sponge you choose, it's a good idea to rinse them out thoroughly after each use, then wring them out, allowing them to dry. In addition, you might occasionally boil your cellulose sponges in water a few minutes to freshen them. Another freshening approach is to soak your sponges in $1/2$ teaspoon San-O-Zon dissolved in 1 of cup warm water for about twenty minutes. (A baking soda-and-water solution can also be used.) After soaking, you'll need to rinse the sponges completely with water. San-O-Zon is a white, unscented borax-sodium compound available from **Cottontails OrganicWear**. Two other very simple ways to clean your cellulose sponges are to wash them in your automatic dishwasher or your clothes washer.

If you like to use brushes in your kitchen, natural-bristle, wood-handle, vegetable brushes are available from **Simmons Handcrafts**. Check your local health-food stores for others. After you use your natural-fiber brushes, they should be completely dry before being stored. In addition, you might want to clean the brush heads occasionally with a San-O-Zon-and-water solution as was described above for sponges. However, it's probably best to test before soaking any brushes in a cleaning solution to see if the natural bristles are affected. Although it is unlikely the bristles could be damaged, it could occur. To test, simply place a similar old brush or a few bristles from a new one in the solution and see what happens.

SCOURING

Many typical cleansers and scouring products contain chlorine bleach and synthetic colorants and dyes, all of which can be bothersome to sensitive persons. However, a number of alternative products are readily available that are really quite safe to use.

Probably the most benign of all cleansers is baking soda sprinkled on a sponge or soft cloth. It can be used to gently scour pots, pans, countertops, and stove tops. Also, the family of mild, unscented Bon Ami products (**Faultless Starch/ Bon Ami Company**) work well. Bon Ami Cleaning Powder (in the rectangular container) is very tolerable to most very sensitive persons. It consists only of powdered soap and finely ground feldspar (a natural mineral). Bon Ami Cleaning Cake has the same formula, but in a compressed bar form. In addition,

Bon Ami Cleanser (in the round can) is a powdered synthetic detergent combined with finely ground feldspar. Bon Ami products, especially the cleanser, are available in some local grocery and hardware stores. They can also be ordered from **The Living Source**. Other alternative scouring cleansers, including a cream type, can be bought from **enviro-clean**.

Unfortunately, most brand-name soap pads usually contain detergents, fragrances, and dyes that can be bothersome for sensitive individuals. For these people, stainless steel pads without soap or detergent can be a better choice. These types of pads can be used over and over again with your own tolerable soap, cleanser, or detergent choice—and the pads will never rust. Fuller Brush Stainless Steel Sponges (**Fuller Brush**) is one available brand you might try. They're sold by Fuller Brush dealers including **enviro-clean**. Also, bronze scouring pads are available under the Chore Boy name in many grocery stores. Copper pads and those made of 100% nylon are other good options. Usually, a variety of metal and nylon scouring pads made without soap or detergent are handled by local grocery and hardware stores.

RUST AND CALCIUM REMOVAL

If your tap water has high levels of iron and calcium minerals, it can cause your sink, faucet, and glasses to become discolored and/or crusty-looking. Unfortunately, removing rust and calcium buildup can be a difficult job, but some products can effectively clean it off.

For removing rust stains (and calcium), Bar Keeper's Friend (**Servaas Laboratories, Inc.**) is often very effective. This product is a finely powdered, unscented cleanser containing *oxalic acid* as its active ingredient. In this concentration and form, the oxalic acid is relatively safe. In fact, it's considered safe enough to use in your automatic dishwasher to clean rust stains and lime scale that have built up there. However, any oxalic acid-containing product, because it's poisonous, should always be stored safely away from children and pets. Bar Keeper's Friend is often sold in grocery stores. Another similar product is Zud, which is sold in some grocery and hardware stores.

To remove *lime scale* (the crusty white hard-water buildup made mostly of calcium compounds), you might try full-strength white vinegar. The encrusted object or area should be soaked with the vinegar for 5–30 minutes. (Exactly how long will depend on how thick the scale is.) Then, you can clean the scale off with a non-scratching scrubber.

For stubborn calcium deposits and rust spots, try CLR (**Jamie Industries**). This clear, almost odorless fluid is basically a phosphoric and glycolic acid combination. While these particular products are usually nonpoisonous, they can cause inflammation. Therefore, wearing rubber gloves is a good idea when using CLR. Also, be sure it's stored so that children and pets can't obtain access. When using CLR, carefully follow the label instructions. This product is sold by many drug, grocery, and hardware stores. Other calcium and/or rust cleaners are available through **enviro-clean**.

CLEANING GREASY PROBLEMS

Of course, a number of pine-solvent and petroleum-derived solvent cleaners can be found on grocery-store shelves. While most of them are very effective at cleaning grease, the solvents and other ingredients (dyes, fragrances, and other cleaning agents) are often intolerable for sensitive persons. Below are some alternative products that such people might want to try.

For greasy areas on painted walls or finished cabinet doors, a solution of diluted Safe Suds (**Ar-Ex Ltd.**) often works well. This concentrated, unscented, undyed detergent is sometimes available at local pharmacies. It can also be ordered directly from the company. To use it, try squeezing about 2 table-spoons into a gallon of warm water. (You'll probably want to experiment with the concentration.) Then, dip a sponge or cotton cloth into the solution and wring it out. Scrub the greasy areas and then rinse them. While Safe Suds isn't as heavy-duty as some other products, it's very mild and gentle to use.

One very good product for removing grease is SafeChoice Super Clean (**American Formulating and Manufacturing (AFM)**) which can be mail-ordered from many catalogs including **N.E.E.D.S.**, **The Living Source**, and **enviro-clean**. To use this particular heavy-duty, unscented, undyed, synthetic liquid, use about 1 cup in 1 gallon of warm water. (You may need to increase the concentration up to perhaps 2 cups in 1 gallon water if the area is particularly greasy.) Then proceed as with the Safe Suds solution. Some greasy objects can be soaked in the solution for 15 minutes, then scrubbed and rinsed.

Yet another grease-cutting product you might try is a concentrated citrus solvent cleaner that has been properly diluted in water. One such cleaner is Citra-Solv (**Chempoint Products, Inc.**), which is available at some local retail outlets such as grocery and hardware stores. Citra-Solv can also be mail-ordered from **The Seventh Generation** and **Simmons Handcrafts**. To use it, mix 1 oz. in 2 cups of water and again proceed as with the Safe Suds mentioned above. If the grease isn't totally removed, try using the product at nearly full-strength. You can also soak certain greasy objects, then scrub and rinse them. Note that, this product is citrus-based and has a citrusy odor. Therefore, very sensitive persons and those allergic to citrus should take care.

Yet another grease-cutting alternative is TSP (trisodium phosphate). TSP is a white or clear crystalline substance that acts as a powerful, unscented cleaner. It is often tolerable for even sensitive persons. One phosphate-free brand is Red Devil TSP/90 Heavy Duty Cleaner (**Red Devil, Inc.**), commonly sold in paint and hardware stores. To use TSP to remove grease, try using 2 level tablespoons dissolved in 1 gallon of warm water. As with the other cleaners, follow the directions given with Safe Suds above. However, with this product in particular, it would be a good idea to also wear rubber gloves to prevent skin irritation.

Several catalogs, including that by **enviro-clean**, offer other alternative cleaners you might try as well. It's important that, if you want to clean grease from painted walls or finished cabinets, you should test a small inconspicuous area first with the solution of your choice. This is to find out for certain if the solution could cause damage before using it over a large area.

(For cleaning greasy stains from grout, see *Cleaning Oily Grout Stains* under *Cleaning Ceramic and Vinyl Floors* above.)

WASHING DISHES

As with most types of cleaning products, commonly available dish soaps and automatic dishwasher compounds usually contain fillers, colorants, and fragrances—among other potentially bothersome ingredients. No wonder many sensitive people find they just can't use them.

The following two sections suggest a few of the alternative dishwashing products now marketed that tend to be better tolerated. Some of these are made with all-natural ingredients, while others are unscented, synthetic detergents. Of course, you'll want to choose the products that best suit your own personal needs. **Enviro-clean** and other catalogs, carry other brands you might like to try.

HAND DISHWASHING PRODUCTS

One synthetic product that's both mild and effective for hand-washing your dishes is Safe-Suds (**Ar-Ex, Ltd.**), which is available at some pharmacies or can be ordered directly from the manufacturer. This concentrated liquid is biodegradable and non-alkaline. It contains no enzymes, phosphates, fillers, perfumes, or dyes. Because it's so concentrated, one bottle will last three times as long as a conventional dishwashing liquid.

Another dishwashing liquid you may want to try is Allens Naturally Biodegradable Dishwashing Liquid (**Allens Naturally**). This product is sometimes sold in alternative grocery stores and can be easily ordered from the company. It contains no dyes, harsh chemicals, or perfumes. It is sold in a large one-quart size container.

Still another option is Ecover Dishwashing Liquid (**Ecover**). Ecover products are sold through dealers such as **Simmons Handcrafts**. This product happens to be a natural, biodegradable detergent with no enzymes or synthetic perfumes. However, it's scented with natural herbs, thus, it may prove bothersome to some very sensitive individuals.

In addition, Mellow Yellow (**Neo-Life Co. of America**) is a liquid cleaner that can be used for dishwashing. This particular product is non-alkaline and non-acidic, but it does have a lemon-oil scent. Mellow Yellow is sold through dealers such as **The American Environmental Health Foundation, Inc.**

A good choice is Aloe Care Dishwashing Liquid (**Granny's Old Fashioned Products**). This inexpensive, gentle, dishwashing liquid is often tolerated by sensitive people. It's sold by **N.E.E.D.S.**, **The Living Source** and others.

Finally, you might consider Seventh Generation Dish Liquid (**The Seventh Generation**). This is a natural detergent with no artificial dyes or fragrances. However, it's scented with citrus oils, which could pose some tolerance problems for certain susceptible people. This product comes in both 32 oz. and 1-gallon sizes, which can be ordered directly from the company catalog.

AUTOMATIC DISHWASHER COMPOUNDS

One alternative powdered dishwashing detergent you might try is Allens Naturally Automatic Dishwasher Detergent (**Allens Naturally**). This is a concentrated, unscented product that is sometimes found in alternative grocery stores. It can also be mail-ordered from the company.

Another brand you might consider is Seventh Generation Automatic Dishwasher Detergent (**The Seventh Generation**). This detergent is free of phosphate, chlorine, and synthetic fragrances and can be ordered directly from the company catalog. Note that, this product isn't recommended by the manufacturer for use with hard water (water with high concentrations of calcium and magnesium). Still another option is Neo-Life Automatic Dishwashing Powder (**Neo-Life Co. of America**). It contains no artificial colors or synthetic perfumes. Call the company for a mail-order source or a nearby dealer.

Finally, Earth Tools Automatic Dishwasher Detergent (**Earth Tools**) is also an alternative dishwasher detergent you may find acceptable. It can be ordered through the company catalog.

On a side note, to help eliminate lime scale (calcium buildup) and/or iron stains inside your automatic dishwasher, fill the machine's dispenser from time to time with 1 heaping tablespoon of Bar Keeper's Friend (**Servaas Laboratories, Inc.**). Then, run the dishwasher empty with no dishes through a normal cycle. This unscented powdered product contains oxalic acid as it's active ingredient. Because of this, make sure this product is stored in such a way that children and pets can't obtain ready access to it. It is usually available at local grocery stores.

CLEANING DRAINS

A number of alternative drain cleaners are now available. One of these is Drain Klear, described as a nontoxic product that contains no lye (an extremely caustic and dangerous substance). Instead, Drain Klear works by "enzyme action." It's available as a powder in 16-ounce containers. One mail-order source is **Colonial Garden Kitchens**. Other alternative drain cleaning products are handled by **enviro-clean**.

A simple homemade drain-cleaning solution, which works best if the drain isn't completely blocked, is to pour $1/2$ cup of baking soda down the drain, followed by $1/2$ cup of white vinegar. After letting it work for five minutes, pour down 2 quarts of boiling water into the drain. If you do this as a preventive measure every few months, you'll probably never develop severe clogs.

CLEANING OVENS AND STOVETOPS

Practically everybody knows how odorous and harmful many typical oven cleaners are. Some are among the most dangerous kitchen products currently available. Fortunately, the following sections discuss some safer alternatives.

CONVENTIONAL OVENS

Let's face it, a full-scale oven-cleaning job is unpleasant no matter what you use. Therefore, preventive measures are a good idea to minimize the necessity for doing it at all. For example, if your oven owner's manual allows it, place a sheet of heavy-duty aluminum foil on the bottom of your oven to capture any spills. Also, to prevent burned-on splatters from building up on your oven's interior walls, scrub them occasionally with baking soda, using it as a mild scouring powder. To do this, just sprinkle some baking soda on a wet sponge or cotton dish cloth and go over the walls. Afterwards, rinse them thoroughly.

If you need a heavy-duty oven cleaner, Nature's Choice Spotless Oven, which is sold by **enviro-clean**, is one alternative oven-cleaning product you might try. This particular cleaner is phosphate-free and contains no chlorine, caustic ingredients, or petroleum solvents.

217

SELF-CLEANING OVENS

Naturally, cleaning a self-cleaning oven is much different that cleaning a conventional oven. While it doesn't require manual labor, you'll need to follow the proper procedure as laid out in your oven owner's manual for the best results.

Generally however, the first step is to remove all the oven racks. This is because if they're left in the oven during the cleaning cycle, the high heat will likely discolor their chrome finish. Therefore, you'll want to clean the racks separately in the sink. After the racks have been removed, you can activate the cleaning cycle.

However, you should realize that it's very important to have good ventilation when the cleaning cycle is in operation, as well as afterwards while it's cooling off. After all, the incineration of greasy substances can be very odorous. It's often a good idea to close off your kitchen from the rest of the house, if possible. Then, you'll want to open a kitchen window and put the range-hood fan on high. (Note: Range hoods that aren't vented to the outdoors are virtually useless.)

GLASSTOP STOVES

For cleaning your glass stovetop, you might try Bon Ami Cleaning Powder (**Faultless Starch/ Bon Ami Company**) as a gentle, non-scratching scouring powder. It's available in some grocery stores and can be ordered from **The Living Source**. To use it, simply sprinkle the powder on a wet sponge or soft wet cotton cloth, then gently rub across the glass. After that, rinse the stovetop. For stubborn spots, make a paste of the powder and water, then, leave the damp mixture on the affected areas for at least five minutes (you may find you need to leave it on longer). When the burned-on drips are softened, gently scrub them off and then rinse the glasstop. As an alternative to Bon Ami Cleaning Powder, try baking soda.

Other alternative cleaning products, including a gentle cream cleanser, are available from **enviro-clean**. For the very worst burned-on spots, try scraping them off carefully using a single-edged razor blade.

BATHROOM CLEANING

Bathroom cleaning is another one of those humbling, repetitious household jobs that no one seems to look forward to doing. But by using less-toxic, low-odor products, the job is at least a healthier one.

MOLD AND MILDEW

As most people know, mold and mildew are not only unsightly, they also can provoke allergic and asthmatic attacks in susceptible persons. Unfortunately, mold and mildew can be a common problem in bathrooms.

MOLD AND MILDEW PREVENTION

A logical method for minimizing mold growth in your bath area is to squeegee the shower walls after you've taken your shower. Standard squeegees are often available at local auto-supply and janitorial-supply outlets. However, many will probably be fairly large and unattractive.

Fortunately, squeegees designed specifically for use in bathrooms are often available in bath stores and bath departments. One mail-order source is **Lillian Vernon**. Bathroom squeegees tend to be small and generally made with molded plastic handles. Interestingly, some of these squeegees have a built-in hook so they can be hung over your shower head when not in use. Of course, if you don't want to squeegee, you can simply sponge off the shower walls, although it'll probably take longer.

In addition, another very effective anti-mold strategy is to have good ventilation in your bathroom. After all, mold and mildew thrive in moist surroundings. Therefore, anything you can do to lower the relative humidity of the bathroom's air is a good idea—and ventilation is one way to do that. If your bathroom doesn't have a window or you simply don't want to open it, you might consider installing a bathroom exhaust fan. Once it's installed, you'll have to remember to use it regularly unless it works in conjunction with the room's light. Another option is to have the ventilation fan wired to a *dehumidistat*. This is a special device that can measure and monitor the air's relative humidity. It can be set to automatically turn on the ventilation fan when the humidity reaches a predetermined level. (For more on relative humidity, dehumidistats, and ventilating fans, see *High Relative Humidity* in *Chapter 9: Indoor Air*.)

SOLVING MOLD AND MILDEW PROBLEMS

If, despite your best efforts, mold or mildew becomes a problem in your bathroom, some less-toxic solutions are available for combating it other than the typical mildew-removal spray products sold in grocery stores. For example, hydrogen peroxide (H_2O_2) is one highly effective mold killer. (Use the 3% dilution that is sold in pharmacies for use as an antiseptic.) To use this clear, odorless liquid, simply pour the hydrogen peroxide into a spray bottle and thoroughly spritz the affected areas: the bathroom fixtures, tile, and/or grout. Wearing protective eyewear is probably a good idea whenever you do this (see *Protective Gear* in *Chapter 12: Home Workshop and Garage*). Because hydrogen peroxide is a bleaching agent, you should avoid spraying it on colored fabric shower curtains.

Another mold-fighting option is full-strength white vinegar. Just apply it to the moldy areas, either with a sponge or a sprayer. Then leave it there a few minutes and rinse it off. (Some very sensitive persons might find the vinegar odor bothersome.)

Yet another natural alternative is a solution of unscented borax and water which can be used to sponge the affected areas. Try 1 tablespoon in 2 cups warm water; if that doesn't remedy the situation, experiment with other dilutions. Afterwards, be sure to rinse. It should also be mentioned that borax has a mild bleaching effect. (For more on unscented borax, see *Borax* below.)

In addition, some individuals have used medicinal antiseptics, such as Zephiran (**Withrop Pharmaceuticals**), to deal with their mold and mildew problems. This particular product contains a *benzalkonium chloride* solution. Zephiran is available in your drugstore, although you may have to special-order it. It can be mail-ordered from **The American Environmental Health Foundation, Inc.** Suggested use is one part of the antiseptic to ten parts water. Then, mix it and apply the solution to the mold or mildew problem area.

Rinsing it off is probably a good idea. It should be pointed out that products such as Zephiran are relatively expensive and they tend to have a somewhat medicinal odor. Yet, many sensitive persons have found that they tolerate this product very well.

Citrus-seed extract has also been shown to be an effective antifungal agent. One highly concentrated version is marketed as ParaMicrocidin Liquid (**Nutricology, Inc.**) in a hypoallergenic, vegetable-glycerin base. This particular product can be mail-ordered directly from the manufacturer. ParaMicrocidin comes in a small 1 fluid-ounce bottle. Originally it was designed to be a nutritional supplement and to be greatly diluted—2–5 drops in 8 ounces of water. Some sensitive individuals, however, have found it effective in killing mold and mildew. To use it, mix the citrus-seed extract with water and apply the solution to the affected areas; then rinse it off. Caution: This product is extremely concentrated; in its full-strength form, it can irritate eyes and skin. Therefore, take care in preparing your diluted solution.

To remove some mildew and mold stains, try SafeChoice Super Clean (**American Formulating and Manufacturing (AFM)**), which is sold by AFM dealers such as **The Living Source** and **N.E.E.D.S.** To use this concentrated, synthetic liquid, mix it at the ratio of 1 part to 1 part water. Then, apply it to the stained areas with a sponge and rinse with clear water.

Other effective alternative mold and mildew cleaners you might consider are sold by **enviro-clean.** (For cleaning mold from air-conditioners, etc. see *Mold* in *Chapter 9: Indoor Air*.) Note: Very sensitive persons or those with mold allergies should not do mold and mildew cleanup work themselves.

CLEANING SINKS, TUBS, AND TILE

Ideally, for cleaning your bathroom's sink, tub, and ceramic tile, you'll want to use products that can do the job, yet are tolerable to you. Two such products you might try are baking soda or Bon Ami Cleaning Powder (**Faultless Starch/Bon Ami Company**). To use them, simply sprinkle one of the powders on your sponge or soft cotton cloth and scrub. Because these products can leave white streaks, be sure to rinse thoroughly. Bon Ami products are sold in some grocery and hardware stores, and can be ordered from **The Living Source.**

Other alternative bathroom cleaners and cleansers are available from **enviro-clean** (see *Scouring* above for other possible products you can use in your bathroom). Important note: If you have an acrylic or fiberglass tub, be sure to first carefully test the cleaning product you plan to use on them on a small, inconspicuous spot to make sure it won't leave abrasive marks. (For suggestions on removing calcium scale or rust stains, see *Rust and Calcium Removal* above.)

CLEANING TOILETS

Finding an effective, quick-acting, unscented, less-toxic, toilet-bowl cleaner is surprisingly difficult. Both the alternative toilet-bowl cleaners from **Ecover** (available from dealers such as **Simmons Handicrafts**) and **Seventh Generation** (which can be ordered directly from **The Seventh Generation**), as well as others sold by **enviro-clean**, generally take several hours to work, if not overnight. This is because these "enviro-friendly" products use enzymes as their active ingredients rather than the extremely caustic substances used in typical fast-acting toilet-bowl cleaners. It should also be noted that most of the alternative products often contain naturally derived scents.

Therefore, if you're a sensitive person who needs to clean the toilet quickly and you also don't want to smell a deodorizing scent, you might try $^1/_8$ cup of full-strength SafeChoice Super Clean (**American Formulating and Manufacturing (AFM)**), which is sold by AFM distributors such as **N.E.E.D.S.** To use this liquid synthetic cleaner, just pour a small amount around the inside of the bowl and scrub thoroughly with a toilet brush. Then, flush to rinse the bowl. It should be noted that this product doesn't claim to be sanitizing or *germicidal* (the ability to kill microorganisms).

Another option is using powdered, unscented borax to clean your toilet quickly. A real plus for borax is that it does have some germicidal properties and can act as a natural deodorizer. To use borax, just sprinkle a small amount ($^1/_8$ cup or less) around the interior of the toilet bowl. Then, scrub *at once* with a toilet brush and flush to rinse. Important note: If borax powder is allowed to sit for even a few moments, it'll form a hard crystalline crust. This is not only extremely difficult to scrub-off, but once it's freed this crust could possibly lead to a clogged toilet drain. By the way, powdered borax can be used along with Super Clean. To use it this way, pour the Super Clean in the toilet first, then the borax. Scented borax (such as the Twenty Mule Team Borax brand) is readily available in boxes in most grocery stores. Unscented borax can be purchased at a chemical-supply company in a 50- or 100-pound bag. To find a chemical-supply company near you, check your local classified phone directory. (To store bulk unscented borax, see *Metal Containers* in *Chapter 8: Housekeeping*.)

Another sanitizing option is to use San-O- Zon, which is sold by **Cottontails OrganicWear**. This is an unscented, undyed, sodium-borax powder. To use San-O-Zon, sprinkle it directly from its small can around the inside of your toilet bowl. Then, brush and flush to rinse it off. You should be aware that this is an fairly expensive product, so this may not be option some people will want to try.

If your toilet bowl interior has rust stains, sprinkle Bar Keeper's Friend (**Servaas Laboratories, Inc.**) inside it. Then, let sit for a few minutes. After that, scrub the bowl with a toilet brush and then flush to rinse. Bar Keeper's Friend is a white, unscented, finely powdered cleaner containing *oxalic acid*. Therefore, this isn't a nontoxic product, although it's relatively safe in this particular form and concentration. However, you'll want to store it so that children and pets can't get access to it. Bar Keeper's Friend is sold through many local grocery stores. A similar product is Zud, which is also sold in some grocery and hardware stores.

CLEANING MIRRORS

(See *Cleaning Windows* above.)

LAUNDRY

It's important to use laundry products that will properly clean your clothes both and still be a healthy choice for you. Of course, this is of primary importance for sensitive people who often find that typical laundry products can make their clothes intolerable for them to wear. To help these people and others, the following sections will offer suggestions for alternative laundry products and methods. As always, choose those that best suit your own particular needs.

LAUNDRY BASICS

When you're ready to wash your clothes and other washable fabric household items, certain laundry basics are worth keeping in mind. First, try using the least amount of soap or detergent necessary to do the job. This will make rinsing more effective and will save you money. Note that, thorough rinsing is necessary so that cleaning-product residues don't remain on fabric fibers. This gummy residue can act as a glue, attracting dirt particles, and it can abrade the fibers as well.

It's also a good practice to wash each load on the shortest and gentlest cycle of your washing machine that still offers effective cleaning. By doing this, you subject your machine washables to the least amount of wear and tear from the rotating agitator. Of course, it's always best to sort your laundry items carefully to create loads that are similar in color, fiber, and fabric weight. Finally, it's often wise to use the lowest water levels at the coolest temperature settings (that will still permit effective washing) in order to minimize problems with color fading and fabric shrinkage, and to save on energy costs.

LAUNDRY PRODUCTS

If you're a person who goes to the trouble and expense of purchasing washable, all-natural clothing and household fabric items, you'll probably want to take special care in selecting your laundry products. As everyone knows who has been in a supermarket, dozens of laundry products are available. However, it's wise to consciously decide what product qualities and ingredients are truly desirable or essential for you and your family, rather than using what's on sale, what's been recently advertised on TV, what your mother uses, or even what you've used in the past.

Some determining factors you might want take into account when choosing a laundry product are the naturalness of the formula, whether or not it's biodegradable, whether it contains *phosphates* (which release phosphorus that can cause ecological problems in waterways and streams), whether the product is liquid or powder, and of course, whether it works well and is cost effective. However, for many sensitive individuals and all those interested in minimizing indoor odors, knowing whether a laundry product is scented or not will also likely be a top priority (see *Testing* in *Chapter 1: Getting Started* and *Problems with Scents* in *Chapter 2: Personal Care*).

TYPICAL LAUNDRY PRODUCTS

As has been mentioned, many sensitive individuals find that, for them, typical laundry products are intolerable. This shouldn't be too surprising when you consider that most conventional laundry detergents contain bleaches, enzymes, whiteners, softeners, and many other potentially bothersome ingredients, as well as synthetic dyes and fragrances.

However, it's not just people with MCS (Multiple Chemical Sensitivity) who have found that typical laundry products are unacceptable to them. The ingredients in most modern laundry products often account for tolerability problems in a certain segment of the general public outside those identified as chemically sensitive. Often, for these people, it's the synthetic dyes and fragrances that cause them to experience skin irritation or allergic symptoms.

Yet, even if the added scents in laundry products are naturally derived, they can still be intolerable or just plain unwelcome for some persons. If you plan to use scented laundry products, remember that the fabric fibers of your clothing, etc. will tend to absorb ever-greater amounts of "citrus lemon," "pleasantly herbal," or "outdoors fresh." These scents can be difficult to remove if you ever decide you don't want them in your clothes anymore. Even with extended airings or washing in unscented alternative products, certain scent-saturated items may never be completely free of scented, laundry-product odors again.

In order to reach the sizable market of those who are opposed to scented laundry products for whatever reason, some major manufacturers are now marketing versions of their popular scented detergents as "scent-free." In a number of cases, these are not simply the same products made *without* scents. Instead, they are often products actually made with the original scents *plus* added *masking fragrances*. Synthetic masking fragrances are added because they're capable of countering or masking the odors of the original scents. As a result, "scent-free" becomes a complex chemical mishmash.

Therefore, in a strange twist of chemistry as well as popular definition, some unscented products actually contain *more* synthetic fragrances than the scented products. For those individuals who find that the odor of these scents is simply undesirable, masking fragrances may make a popular name-brand laundry product acceptable to them. However, for others who react to synthetic fragrances because of their chemical make-up, scent-free laundry products with masking fragrances can be bad options.

ALTERNATIVE LAUNDRY PRODUCTS

Fortunately, for those people who want to use laundry products that have uncomplicated formulas without a lot of extra additives, a growing number of alternative products are now available. The following sections will discuss some of them you might want to try.

Powdered Alternative Laundry Products

Many powdered alternative laundry products are very simple compounds that can be purchased in bulk at very low prices. If you decide to go ahead and buy in bulk, be aware that wholesalers usually deal in very large quantities (see *Buying in Quantity* in *Chapter 1: Getting Started*). Therefore, one bag purchased from a chemical-supply company could weigh 50–100 lbs.

If you buy that much of a compound, be sure you'll have the proper storage container on hand so it can be kept dry and not spill out (see *Metal Containers* in *Chapter 8: Housekeeping*). To find a chemical-supply company near you, you'll want to check in your classified telephone directory.

Sodium Hexametaphosphate

For some time now, unscented *sodium hexametaphosphate (SHP)* has been recommended by some people as an alternative laundry cleaning product for sensitive persons. (Calgon is the brand name of a scented version that is often available in grocery stores.) SHP is actually a powdered natural sodium-phosphate compound that is soluble in water.

Once, SHP was commonly used as a water-softening agent to enable soaps and detergents to create suds easier. However, because of its phosphate content, its use has diminished. As it turns out, phosphates were found to disrupt normal water ecology and cause overabundant algae growth. Because of this, phosphate laundry products have become illegal in some states and local jurisdictions. SHP laundry products would fall under such regulations.

However, if phosphates haven't been banned in your state or locale, you might try SHP. Suggested use is about $1/4$ cup per wash load. To buy a relatively small quantity of unscented SHP, order from **Nigra Enterprises**. It also can be purchased in bulk from area chemical-supply houses.

Washing Soda

Another natural alternative to conventional laundry detergent is old-fashioned *washing soda*. Also known as *sal soda*, it's actually a form of sodium carbonate. For your washing machine, $1/4$ cup per load is often suggested.

By the way, Arm & Hammer Washing Soda is a brand of washing soda with a synthetic scent that is often sold in grocery stores. An unscented washing soda under the name Dr. Erlander's Jubilee Washing Compound (**Erlander's Natural Products**) can be mail-ordered directly from the company. In addition, some local chemical-supply companies handle the FMC Sesqui brand. If so, it is often sold under its chemical name, sodium sesquicarbonate, in 100-pound bags.

Baking Soda

A few extremely sensitive persons have used as little as $1/2$ cup of baking soda (sodium bicarbonate) in their washing machine—without any other laundry product—to clean their clothes and other fabric washables. This may work well for you, too, and it's certainly a very mild substance.

Of course, there's usually no problem finding baking soda in your local grocery store. But if you plan to use large quantities, you might consider purchasing it in bulk from a chemical-supply company to save money.

Borax

Borax is actually hydrated sodium borate, a mined, water-soluble mineral. It's been used as a laundry soap or detergent supplement for many years. One reason for this is that it can help soften the wash water so that soaps and detergents will clean better. However, another big advantage of using borax in your washing machine is that it helps remove odors in your laundry. Interestingly, some sensitive individuals use unscented borax as a substitute for conventional laundry detergents; in other words, they use it strictly by itself. If you plan to do this, $1/4$ cup per load generally works effectively, although you might choose to use more (perhaps up to $1/2$ cup). Note: Borax has a mild bleaching action.

You may have noticed that Twenty Mule Team Borax is often available in grocery stores. Unfortunately, this is a scented product. If you don't care to use laundry products containing fragrance, you can buy unscented borax in bulk from a local chemical-supply company.

Other Alternative Powdered Products

Actually, a number of alternative powdered laundry products are now being manufactured. However, a number of these contain natural scents such as lemon oil or another natural essential oil. Therefore, if you're very sensitive, have citrus allergies, or just don't want to use products with scents of any kind, you'll want to carefully experiment before using these products with a full load of wash.

One alternative laundry powder you might like to try is Allens Naturally Ultra Concentrated Powder Laundry Detergent (**Allens Naturally**), which can be ordered directly from the manufacturer. It's also sometimes sold in alternative grocery and health-food stores. This particular product is biodegradable, undyed, and perfume-free. Just 3 tablespoons per load is all that's needed.

Another good product is Ecover Concentrated Laundry Powder (**Ecover**). It's available through dealers such as **Simmons Handcrafts** and is also sometimes sold in alternative grocery stores. This particular powder is an all-natural, biodegradable detergent that's both enzyme- and phosphate-free. Because it's highly concentrated, a special measuring scoop is included to enable you to use the right amount. Generally, $3/4$ scoop per load is effective.

You might also try Neo-Life Super Plus (**Neo-Life of America, Inc.**). To buy it, call the company for the nearest dealer. The manufacturer suggests using $1/4$ cup of this undyed, biodegradable detergent per load. For other alternative powdered cleaning products, check the **enviro-clean** catalog, among others.

To help sanitize your laundry, use San-O-Zon, which is sold by **Cottontails OrganicWear**. Using $1/2$ cup per load has been suggested. San-O-Zon is a sodium-borax compound that is unscented and undyed. However, it should be noted that it has a slight bleaching effect.

Liquid Alternative Laundry Products

Some individuals prefer liquid laundry products over powder types. With liquids, they point out, there are no problems with powders not completely dissolving, and thus, there's never any white streaks on clothing or hardened lumps in the washing machine's soap/detergent dispenser. The following sections offer some liquid product suggestions you might try.

Vinegar

Some sensitive persons simply use white, distilled vinegar without any other products in their washing machines to clean to their clothes and household fabric washables. Using vinegar in your washer has several advantages. It's natural, nontoxic, biodegradable, relatively inexpensive, and can help remove many odors. It can also help fabrics retain their original color. Interestingly, most of the distilled vinegar available in grocery stores is actually made of fermented grain (alcohol) that has undergone a distillation process to produce purified acetic acid. This acid is then diluted with water. Therefore, full-strength kitchen-use white vinegar is actually only 3–6% acetic acid and the rest is water.

To use white vinegar, try $1/2$–2 cups in your washing machine per load, depending on the size of your load (You should probably experiment with a whole range of dilutions to see what works best for you.). It should be noted that certain individuals may find vinegar odors unpleasant or bothersome. If you do, you might want to open a nearby window and/or activate a ventilation fan. Fortunately, vinegar odors in wet items will virtually disappear after they're hung outside to dry or they're dried in the automatic dryer. However, you should be very cautious about soaking items overnight in your washing machine using vinegar; it can cause certain metal parts to rust.

If you plan to use white vinegar regularly in your washing machine, it's a good idea to buy gallon-size jugs of a generic store brand. That way, you'll save a lot of money, compared to buying several small bottles.

Other Alternative Liquid Products

There are actually a number of manufactured liquid alternative laundry products you may want to try. One that many sensitive persons have used successfully is Power Plus/Laundry Concentrate (**Granny's Old Fashioned Products**). It's sold through dealers such as **N.E.E.D.S.** and **The Living Source**. By the way, Power Plus is one of the few alternative laundry products that's completely unscented. In addition, it's undyed, biodegradable, extremely concentrated, and very affordable. The manufacturer recommends you use just I tablespoon per wash load.

Another product you might want to use is Ecover Liquid Wash (**Ecover**), which is sold by Ecover dealers, one being **Simmons Handcrafts** (it's also sometimes found in some alternative grocery stores). This liquid detergent is natural, biodegradable, and undyed. However, it does contain citrus oils, giving it a mild citrusy odor. To use Ecover Liquid Wash, the manufacturer suggests you try just 1½ capfuls per load.

You might also want to try Seventh Generation Laundry Liquid (**The Seventh Generation**). It's sold through the company catalog, and you can sometimes find it in alternative grocery stores as well. This product contains natural coconut-oil surfactants (compounds that lower the water surface tension) and citrus oils. It has no added artificially-derived scents, is undyed, and is biodegradable. To use this liquid, the manufacturer recommends you use ¼ cup per washing load. You'll find that the Seventh Generation Liquid has a mild citrusy odor. For some other alternative liquid laundry cleaning products, check the **enviro-clean** catalog, among others.

ALTERNATIVE BLEACHES

Most natural soaps, washing compounds, and alternative-formula detergents—let alone vinegar, or baking soda—don't contain additives such as optical brighteners (compounds that make fabrics appear brighter), enzymes, and bleaches, all of which are found in typical laundry products. As a result, after using alternative products awhile, you may find that your clothes don't look quite as bright as they did before you started using these types of cleaners. Therefore, you might decide you need to use something extra in your wash.

For a number of people, bleach is that "something extra." If you also decide to use a bleach, you should seriously consider using an oxygen-type bleaching agent such as hydrogen peroxide rather than chlorine. While both are unstable and reactive, hydrogen peroxide has virtually no odor and is much safer to handle. To use common liquid hydrogen peroxide (the 3% dilution sold in drugstores), fill your washer with water first and then pour in ⅓–½ cup of the hydrogen peroxide. After that, you can add your washables and run the washing cycle through as usual.

Another bleaching option is to use Ecover Non-Chlorine Bleach (**Ecover**). This bleach is basically a prepackaged, super-concentrated hydrogen peroxide-and-water product. In fact, it is so concentrated that just 2 oz. per load is recommended. Ecover Non-Chlorine Bleach is available through Ecover dealers, including **Simmons Handcrafts**. It's also sometimes sold in alternative grocery stores.

One other alternative bleach you might try is Seventh Generation Non-Chlorine Powdered Bleach (**The Seventh Generation**). This is a biodegradable, oxygen-based, powdered product using sodium percarbonate as the active bleaching agent. It also contains soda ash, sea salt, and enzymes, but no dyes or scents. To use it, the manufacturer suggests you try $1/4$ cup per load. By the way, a liquid alternative bleach is also available from the same company. Seventh Generation Bleach is available directly from the company and sometimes at local alternative grocery stores as well. For other alternative bleach choices, look in **enviro-clean's** catalog and others.

Although they're not considered by most people as bleaches, sodium hexametaphosphate (see *Sodium Hexametaphosphate* above), San-O-Zon (a sodium-borax product available through **Cottontails OrganicWear**), and borax (see *Borax* above) do have a mild bleaching effect on fabrics. However, for the most effective alternative bleaching, you're encouraged to use one of the alternative bleaching products discussed above.

STAIN-REMOVAL PRODUCTS

Typical fabric stain-removal products usually contain certain ingredients that can be very bothersome to sensitive individuals, namely synthetic solvents or perhaps synthetic colorants and fragrances. Therefore, these individuals sometimes have difficulty locating products to remove spots and stains from clothing items. Fortunately, there are now a number of alternative products that work fairly well and that should be less bothersome to them.

One alternative stain-removing product is White Wizard Spot Remover and All Purpose Cleaner. This white, jellylike product is sold in 10 oz. plastic tubs in some local grocery and hardware stores. It can also be mail-ordered from **The Seventh Generation** or **Colonial Garden Kitchens**. White Wizard is nontoxic and low-odor, but is strong enough in many instances to remove blood, ink, and grease stains from fabrics. For the best results, carefully follow the package directions.

Another alternative stain remover is Citra-Solv (**Chempoint Products, Inc.**), which can be used on a variety of stains including oil and grease spots. Citra-Solv is a highly concentrated liquid citrus solvent and sold in some health-food stores. It can also be ordered from **The Seventh Generation** and **Simmons Handcrafts**. To use it, try a dilution of 1 oz. in 2 cups of water. Then, simply apply the solution to the stained area and gently brush it. Afterwards, you'll need to blot the area with a damp cloth until the stain is gone. Because it's made from citrus, Citra-Solv has a prominent citrusy odor.

For a prespotter on laundry day, SafeChoice Super Clean (**American Formulating and Manufacturing (AFM)**) used in a 1-to-1 dilution with water often works well. (For certain stubborn stains, you might even use it full-strength.) Super Clean is an unscented, undyed synthetic liquid cleaner that is especially effective on many grease and oil stains. You can purchase this product through AFM dealers such as **N.E.E.D.S.** and **The Living Source.** To use Super Clean, dab the solution onto the spot, rub the cloth, and then let it sit there a few minutes before you put the item in the washing machine for laundering.

Yet another alternative fabric stain remover is Soil Away (**Granny's Old Fashioned Products**). This is an unscented, biodegradable, stain and soil remover that has been specially formulated to remove many ink, blood, crayon and other stains. To use Soil Away, follow the package directions carefully for the most successful results. Granny's products, including this one, can be mailordered from **N.E.E.D.S.** and **The Living Source**, among others.

To remove rust stains from fabrics, you might try moistening the affected areas with water and sprinkling them with enough Bar Keepers Friend (**Servaas Laboratories, Inc.**) to make a paste. Then let this set for 5–10 minutes. After that, rinse the fabric thoroughly with clear water. In addition, to remove an orangish coloring from items that have been repeatedly washed in water having a high iron content, add to your washer 3–4 tablespoons of Bar Keeper's Friend for each 2 gallons of water. Then simply run the load through as usual. This product is actually an unscented, undyed, fine powder that's commonly sold in grocery and hardware stores. Because the active ingredient is oxalic acid, which is toxic, Bar Keepers Friend should definitely be stored in a place where it's inaccessible to children and pets.

For more alternative stain-removal products, check the **enviro-care** catalog, along with others. For a great number of alternative stain-removal remedies, read *Clean and Green* by Annie Berthold-Bond. Important note: No matter what stain-removal product or homemade recipe you decide upon, it's always best to first carefully test it on an inconspicuous spot to see whether the fabric's color will fade or the fibers will in some way be damaged from using the product.

FABRIC SOFTENERS

Many sensitive persons are bothered by typical fabric softeners that can leave intolerable residues on fabric fibers. What do typical fabric softeners contain? Liquid types of fabric softeners contain water, synthetic surfactants (compounds able to lower the water surface tension), emulsifiers (compounds able to suspend oil molecules in water), and synthetic fragrance. Fabric softener dryer sheets are sections of nonwoven rayon (see *Rayon* in *Chapter 3: Clothing*) saturated with surfactants and synthetic perfume. What fabric softeners actually do is make cloth fibers more porous to water. It's been said that, they actually act as moisturizers for fabric.

If you find typical fabric softeners bothersome, you might try using ¹/₄ cup white vinegar or ¹/₄ cup baking soda, which you can add to the wash water of each load. While neither of these will be quite as effective as typical fabric softeners, they can help make your clothes feel less scratchy and stiff.

An alternative manufactured fabric softer you might try is Allens Naturally Anti-Static Fabric Softener (**Allens Naturally**). It can be ordered directly from the company or bought in some alternative grocery stores. This particular product is water- and soybean-based. It's also unscented, alcohol-free—and it's biodegradable. The manufacturer suggests you add 1 to 2 oz. to the final rinse water.

One more alternative fabric softener worth considering is Ecover Concentrated Fabric Softener (**Ecover**). This is a biodegradable, natural-ingredient liquid. However, Ecover Fabric Softener does have a mild odor because it includes essential oils (concentrated scents) among its ingredients. Therefore, people who want to avoid even naturally derived scents should probably try another alternative product. To use it, you simply pour 1 capful per load in the final rinse water. This product is available from dealers such as **Simmons Handcrafts** and is sometimes sold in alternative groceries as well.

REMOVING NEW CLOTHING ODORS

Unfortunately, brand-new garments, even if they're made of untreated 100%-cotton, can often release strong odors that will require special cleaning techniques to remove them. Otherwise, these bothersome odors can make new clothes unwearable for many sensitive people, even after one or more normal washings.

Why is this so? These new-clothing odors are actually due to the chemicals (many of which are not water-soluble) applied during the fiber plant's cultivation, and later during the milling or dying process. They may also include absorbed perfume and tobacco odors picked up at manufacturing plants, warehouses, transport vehicles, or at retail outlets. However, it should also be noted that even pristine organic cotton fabric can be bothersome—just because of cotton's innate fairly strong grainy smell.

If you're a person who finds new clothing odors objectionable, some sensitive people have found that adding $1/2$–1 cup of powdered milk per wash load will help remove these smells. Also, unscented borax (about $1/3$–$1/2$ cup per load) will often help. However, be careful when using borax with dark fabrics because of its mild bleaching effect. In addition, baking soda can help make your new clothes more tolerable. In this case, you might try using $1/2$–1 cup per load. Many sensitive people find that in order to sufficiently get out the odors using one of these natural powders, they often have to repeat the wash cycle over and over again—perhaps as many as ten times—depending on how sensitive they are.

Another simple new-odor reducer is white vinegar. Vinegar has the added benefit of helping fabric retain its color—something that the powders mentioned above can't do. To use white vinegar, pour 1 cup to 1 quart into the washer—the exact amount depends on the load size. By the way, a number of sensitive individuals find that if they alternately wash with vinegar and then baking soda, their new clothes seem to become tolerable sooner.

Still another possibility to remove unwanted odors in new clothing is to use about $1/8$–$1/4$ cup SafeChoice Super Clean (**American Formulating and Manufacturing**) for each wash load. This unscented, undyed, biodegradable, synthetic, liquid detergent is sold by most AFM dealers including **N.E.E.D.S.** and **The Living Source**. However, be aware that Super Clean can bleach some colors slightly.

One product that seems particularly effective at removing most new clothing odors is San-O-Zon, which can be purchased from **Cottontails OrganicWear**.

To use this unscented, undyed, sodium-borax powder, one procedure you might try is to fill a basin or plastic bucket (something that's non-reactive) with warm water and add 1–4 tablespoons of San-O-Zon. Then stir the water to dissolve the granules completely. After that, add a new garment and soak it for 24 hours. The next day, place the soaked item in your washer and pour in the San-O-Zon/water solution. Then run the garment through a complete wash/rinse/spin cycle. Of course, you can repeat the entire regimen from the beginning if you find it necessary. By the way, San-O-Zon does have a mild bleaching effect.

It should be mentioned that it's not uncommon for some sensitive individuals to want to soak their problem clothing overnight in the washing machine in order to reduce unwanted odors. And if you're using baking soda, that may be fine. However, soaking overnight with vinegar, products containing bleach, or other fairly reactive compounds can be potentially corrosive to metal washer interiors. Therefore, rust formation could easily result which in turn could discolor fabrics. To soak clothing for more than an hour or two, use a plastic bucket or some other type of container incapable of reacting, as described with the San-O-Zon above.

It should be pointed out, that no matter what you use to remove new clothing odors, extended airing may also be necessary. However, be sure to hang your clothing outdoors only in dry, uncontaminated surroundings. Some individuals have actually had to air certain items daily for a week or more. In fact, airing for months is not that uncommon for those persons who are extremely sensitive.

HAND-LAUNDERING

Often, knits, delicate fabrics, woolens, and embellished articles should be hand-laundered only. Ideally, for this job you want to choose a mild, unscented cleaning product. Of course, this is especially important for very sensitive persons.

For hand-laundering, alternative hand-washing dish detergents often work very well. One you might try is Safe Suds (**Ar-Ex, Ltd.**). Safe Suds is a mild, unscented, undyed, biodegradable, synthetic detergent that can be ordered directly from the manufacturer or purchased through a local pharmacy. (For other possible products, see *Hand Dishwashing Products* above.)

To use Safe Suds or a similar product for hand-laundering, simply add a small amount to a sink or basin which is half-filled with water. (Cooler water will minimize shrinkage and maximize color retention.) Then, swish the water to create suds. Next, place your garment in the basin and gently squeeze the sudsy water through the fibers. (Another option is to simply allow the item to soak for a few minutes.) Then, rinse the garment several times in cool, clear water. After that, remove the item and gently squeeze out the water. You may also want to lay the item on a large, clean towel and roll it up to absorb any excess water. Finally, the garment can be hung to dry or laid flat on a clean, dry towel or special sweater drying rack.

DRYING

Most people automatically think of drying their clothes in a dryer but, surprisingly, there are more options to drying wet washable items than you might first think. Of course, you'll want to choose the method most appropriate for each particular article.

AIR-DRYING

The two main methods of air-drying are hang-drying and flat-drying. Each has a number of possible approaches and methods. Some of these will be discussed below.

Hang-Drying

Hanging clothes and other washable items outdoors to dry is not only an inexpensive way to dry them, but it also can give them a renewed freshness. This is because the air blowing through fabric fibers helps lift out odors, while at the same time the ultraviolet rays from the sun will act as a mild bleach and disinfectant.

However, if you plan to dry your items outside, be alert to the presence of unwanted outdoor odors, especially if you're sensitive. This is because smoke from burning leaves, barbecues, and fireplaces as well as traffic exhaust can quickly become absorbed by fabric fibers. You should also be alert to days with a high pollen count if you're an allergic person, not hanging your clothing outside on those days either. In addition, everyone should make certain that his or her clothesline and clothespins are clean and in good repair so they won't soil or damage hanging items.

For drying small, hand washables indoors, you might want to purchase a solid-wood, folding, drying rack. These are made with a number of dowel rods in alternating positions so that many of your small items can be dried at the same time. Such racks are often sold in hardware stores. You can also buy them from the **Vermont Country Store**. Enameled steel-wire drying racks are handled by **Taylor Gifts**.

Also, certain damp clothing items can be hung to dry over the tub or outdoors on heavy anodized aluminum hangers. (Anodized aluminum has a protective coating.) Such hangers won't rust or bend out of shape. These may be purchased at some department stores, and they can be mail-ordered from **Colonial Garden Kitchens** and other catalog suppliers.

For drying slacks, you might try using special pants stretchers which were once fairly common. Slacks dried on these metal frame devices don't have to be ironed—often a real plus. Fortunately, pants stretchers are now becoming available again. Some mail-order sources are **Harriet Carter, Taylor Gifts**, and **Walter Drake & Sons**.

Flat-Drying

A number of washable items in your home, including most sweaters, are best dried by flat-drying. Of course, one very common way to do this is to lay out your damp sweater or other item on a thick 100%-cotton terry towel that's completely colorfast. This is fine, but sweater drying racks have real advantages over using towels.

Sweater drying racks are often constructed of a nylon-mesh fabric stretched across a folding metal frame that is formed in such a way that it's able to hold the mesh several inches from the floor. This open-weave mesh and raised rack design allows the air to flow freely around and through the yarns of a damp sweater that has been laid out on top of the mesh to dry. Therefore, the sweater dries much faster so that musty odors, which can develop if a sweater remains damp for too long, are avoided. You can buy sweater drying racks in some local department and discount stores. They can also be mail-ordered from **Harriet Carter** and **Walter Drake & Sons**.

Whenever you need to flat-dry an item, it's often a good idea to use a pattern as a layout guide, to make sure it'll retain its prewashed size and shape. To make a drying pattern, simply lay the dry clothing item on a piece of heavy, plain, undyed paper. Then, draw a line around the garment with a pencil. Next, remove the item, cut the paper along the drawn line, and label the pattern as to the garment for which it was created. After your garment has been washed and placed on the drying towel or rack, you can then place the pattern on top of it and shape the clothing to match it. Finally, you'll want to remove the pattern, allow it to dry, and save it for reuse. Instead of paper patterns, some people make fabric patterns, which are not as easily damaged by moisture or repeated use.

MACHINE-DRYING

Of course, most of your washable items can be put in an automatic clothes dryer to dry them. Certainly, automatic dryers are quick and convenient. However, if your dryer operates on natural gas or propane, there may be some concerns of which you might not have been aware.

Some sensitive individuals using gas dryers have reported they can't tolerate items dried in them. Apparently their clothes seem to have absorbed natural gas odors or the byproducts of combustion. (Unfortunately, modifying gas dryers so that absolutely no gas odors ever reach what's being dried inside them can be difficult, if not impossible.) It must be pointed out that, sensitive persons can be affected by extremely minute quantities of pollutants. Therefore, if you are a very sensitive person, it is generally best to use only electric dryers. (See *Clothes Dryers* in *Chapter 8: Housekeeping*.)

If you are sensitive, it would also be wise to never use any typical fabric-softener sheets in your automatic dryer. Sometimes their synthetic fragrances and other potentially bothersome ingredients can make your dryer intolerable for some time.

IRONING

It's doubtful many people like to iron. However, if it has to be done, you might as well do it in the most healthful manner possible. This section offers some suggestions to do just that.

IRONS

In bygone days, irons were made of heavy, cast iron with ground and polished bases and handles attached on top. These irons had to be repeatedly heated over a fire or hot stove after they had released their absorbed heat. Therefore, people often owned two of them to use alternately. Today, electric irons heat themselves, and many create their own steam. Note: Steam irons should only have distilled water used in them so that their small steam vent openings don't become clogged with hard water buildup (see *Distilled Water* in *Chapter 10: Home Water*).

Many irons now available in the U.S. are made with nonstick *soleplates* (the flat ironing surfaces). In some cases, this is achieved by applying or bonding certain synthetic chemical compounds to the metal's surface (see *Nonstick Coatings* in *Chapter 8: Housekeeping*). While permitting a smoother, gliding ironing action, some of these synthetic nonstick surfaces could have the potential to outgas synthetic odors when they are heated. These can be bothersome to some sensitive persons. In addition, some of these coatings are not exceptionally durable, although most are more scratch-resistant than they were a few years ago.

A healthier nonstick iron is one with a stainless steel soleplate. Stainless steel is inherently non-sticking, without the need for synthetic chemical compounds. Unfortunately, because synthetic, nonstick irons are now more durable (as well as cheaper) new irons with stainless steel soleplates are often difficult to find. However, you can sometimes find used ones in secondhand stores or at garage sales. If you do find a used one, check to see if it's cord and plug are damaged and then plug in the iron to see if it heats properly. Remember, you might not be able to return used merchandise. Note: Some very sensitive individuals will have to carefully clean and air outdoors a recently purchased, used iron to remove absorbed perfume, tobacco, and laundry-product odors, etc. Unfortunately, in some cases the irons will remain intolerable.

However, if you don't want an iron with a nonstick soleplate, irons are often available with a polished-aluminum soleplate. One manufacturer of these is Black & Decker. However, some persons may find such irons have a tendency to "drag" on certain fabrics, especially if the soleplate has any residue on it. Therefore, it's important to keep a polished aluminum soleplate as clean as possible.

IRONING-BOARD PADS AND COVERS

For sensitive individuals in particular, ironing pads and covers should be washable, untreated 100%-cotton. Teflon-coated, or other similar ironing-board covers, and those containing flame-retardant compounds can be bothersome. Despite their real and obvious advantages of easier ironing and fire prevention, the chemicals used in them can be released into the air by your heated iron. If you'd like to buy untreated, undyed 100%-cotton ironing board covers, they can be ordered from **Janice Corp**. and **The Cotton Place**.

For ironing-board padding, you might try using a folded, untreated, 100%-cotton, flannel blanket. Ready-made, untreated, all-cotton, ironing-board pads are sold by **Janice Corp.** Ironing-board cover fasteners that can hold your cover and pad securely in place are handled by **Walter Drake & Sons**.

SPRAY STARCHES

Most of the typical spray starches sold in grocery stores contain a variety of substances, including corn starch, silicone, propellants, and sometimes *proprietary ingredients* (compounds that are company secrets) such as certain corrosion inhibitors. Some products might also contain scents. These spray starches are designed to not only give your soft, limp fabrics firmness, they're also formulated to allow your iron to glide across them more easily.

If you want to avoid typical spray starches, you can make a simple homemade version by dissolving 2 teaspoons of cornstarch in 1 cup of water. Then, pour the mixture into a spray bottle and spray the solution on your clothes as needed while ironing.

Because cornstarch can sometimes leave a noticeable whiteness on dark fabrics, you might want to spray dark items using cold black tea instead of the cornstarch/water mixture. Cold black tea can also act as an ironing starch for fabric. (However, refrain from spraying black tea on light-colored items.) Of course, if you use tea bags to make the tea, no tea leaf particles will get on your clothes. If you use regular black tea, you can effectively strain it by pouring it through a coffee filter.

MAKING IRONING TOLERABLE

Many sensitive persons find that ironing is something that—quite literally—makes them sick. This is because some clothing that seems odor-free at room temperature can emit bothersome odors when it's ironed. The high heat actually causes the release of perfume and other odors that had been deeply embedded in the fabric fibers.

Therefore, if you are a sensitive individual, it's important for you to iron with good ventilation. Simply opening the windows in the room where you are ironing can often help. However, also operating a window fan will work even better. You might also want to wear an activated charcoal-filled mask (see *Personal Facial Air Filters* in *Chapter 9: Indoor Air*).

DRY CLEANING

(See *Is Dry Cleaning a Problem?* in *Chapter 2: Clothing.*)

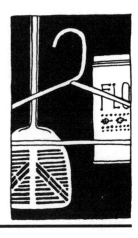

CHAPTER 8
HOUSEKEEPING

This chapter covers a broad array of housekeeping topics, from choosing appliances to coping with pests. Each section suggests healthier alternatives to typically used products and procedures.

APPLIANCES

Very few of us would like to give up our modern household appliances. There's no argument that these devices make our lives much easier at home. However, many new appliances release chemical compounds into the air that can be bothersome to sensitive people.

Fortunately, you can sometimes find healthier appliance models. The following sections offer information on what features you might look for and what features to avoid when you're ready to buy a new appliance. Of course special options, size, color, energy efficiency, and cost are also important, but in this book, an appliance's potential health effects has top priority. By the way, appliance models offered by manufacturers change fairly frequently, sometimes annually. Therefore, while the information supplied here on specific brands and/or models was accurate at the time it was written, it may not be by the time you read it. However, the general guidelines should still be valid.

SMALL APPLIANCES

Small electric appliances are great for getting certain household jobs done quickly, but they can have drawbacks. Nearly all of them have plastic housings and fast whirring motors that can give off bothersome odors. Those with heating elements can be particularly offensive because the elements are sometimes made of materials that emit offensive odors when they're heated up.

It's not surprising then that some sensitive people find they become ill when they use their small appliances, especially if they're new ones. If you are bothered by your small appliances, having good ventilation you when you're operating them can help reduce odors. One obvious way of doing this is to open nearby windows. If you're using an appliance in the kitchen, you can also turn on a range-hood fan that is vented to the outdoors. In addition, you might wear a charcoal-filled mask to act as a simple air filter (see *Personal Facial Filters* in *Chapter 9: Indoor Air*).

Another common problem with portable electric appliances is that their electric motors tend to create rather powerful *electromagnetic fields (EMFs)*. These are areas in which electric and magnetic effects are fairly intense (see *Chapter 11: Electromagnetic Fields*). If you are exposed to high levels of these fields for long periods of time, you could experience a number of negative heath effects. Fortunately, as a rule, small-appliance use is brief. Therefore, exposure time to their EMFs is short as well. However, those who are hypersensitive to electromagnetic fields should consider avoiding small appliances whenever possible.

Actually, it would probably be wise for everyone to reevaluate his or her small appliance needs. After all, it's easy to let your kitchen counters and cabinets become packed with electric gadgets, many of which you've sometimes forgotten you even had. The truth is, some small appliances are designed to do jobs that could just as easily be done by hand, such as an electric knife. Others are too limiting in what they can do, such as an electric hot-dog cooker. As an alternative, you might seriously consider owning just a few multipurpose devices. You could sell or give the extraneous electric gadgets away. In doing this, your kitchen cleaning and organizing would inevitably become simpler.

The appliances you decide to keep could be stored easily inside your emptier cabinets. If you prefer, you could keep your appliances out on the countertop, but covered with washable natural-fabric covers in order to keep them clean and dust-free. If you wanted to, you could even make the covers yourself (see *Custom-Made Clothing* in *Chapter 3: Clothing*).

As a safety precaution, it's important to never keep most small appliances continually plugged in. Many electrical fires have resulted from this practice. Therefore, you'll always want to read your appliances' owner manuals for proper safe operation.

(For information on vacuums, see *Vacuuming* in *Chapter 7: Cleaning*.)

MAJOR APPLIANCES

Major appliances are an investment; they're expensive and generally designed to last at least 10 years. Therefore, it's extremely important to take the necessary time and energy to choose them wisely.

BUYING MAJOR APPLIANCES IN GENERAL

Because of the cost involved, buying a major appliance is often considered a frightening and risky venture by sensitive people. They may fear they will buy something they can't tolerate but will have to live with for many years. If you are a sensitive person, when you're ready to purchase a major appliance the first step is to ask other sensitive friends for their experiences and appliance-model recommendations. If you belong to a support group, it's a good idea to ask such things at meetings or through the group's newsletters. However, you must keep in mind that appliance models change frequently. Therefore, particular ones on which you have had favorable reports could have since been "improved" with potentially bothersome modifications. In some cases, you may find that some of the suggested models have been completely discontinued. Despite this, asking other sensitive individuals often remains your best initial new-appliance information source.

Of course, buying new is not always the only way to acquire needed appliances; you can buy used models. Actually, a few sensitive persons have purchased stoves, refrigerators, etc. that they found tolerable and that were currently being used in the homes of friends or family members. In some cases, a sensitive person has traded a brand-new appliance for a used one.

However, a word of caution is in order if you plan to purchase any pre-owned major appliance. If you buy one that's too old, it could soon need costly and potentially odorous repair work. In fact, in the worst-case scenario, the appliance may not be fixable at all. There are also special concerns if you buy a used appliance from a dealer or stranger that you believe should be tolerable. For example, you won't know the specific history of that particular appliance. The back or bottom could have been sprayed with insecticides or it could have been repaired with parts that could now make the unit bothersome to you. Therefore, if it's at all possible, arrange a several-day trial period with the seller. If he or she agrees, get the agreement in writing. During the trial period, you'll be better able to judge whether you'll have tolerance problems before being committed to purchasing the appliance. You might also try to get such an arrangement when buying a brand-new appliance. A few sensitive persons have been able to do this. However, realistically, getting a trial-period arrangement with a seller on any new or used major appliance is often difficult to obtain.

DISHWASHERS

Although they had been invented earlier, it wasn't until after World War II that many American kitchens have had automatic dishwashers. These days, it's a rare home that it built without one. However, while they certainly can minimize the drudgery of hand-dishwashing, as a rule, most new dishwashers are bothersome to sensitive people. This is often due to several factors. One is the odors given off by the rubber hoses, belts, insulation, and gaskets. Another is the release of petroleum compounds from oils on the motors, and yet another is the outgassing of plastic liners and vinyl-covered wire trays on the interior.

Although you can't eliminate rubber parts or the motor and mechanical components, you can buy automatic dishwashers without plastic liners. Therefore, if you're a sensitive person, you'll want to think about purchasing a model with a porcelain-on-steel or all-stainless interior. You should be aware though that some vinyl will be present in nearly all models no matter what the interior walls are made of. This is because vinyl protector caps are usually used on the tips of the wire racks.

While there are certainly others worth considering, two dishwasher brands you'll want to check out are Bosch (**Robert Bosch Corp.**) and Asko (**Asko, Inc.**). Bosch models are imported from Germany and Asko units from Sweden. Both of these models have stainless-steel interior walls as well as special energy- and water-saving features. They're also designed to generate a minimum of noise. To purchase them, you'll need to contact the respective companies for their nearest dealers.

Not only are new dishwashers often suspect, but sensitive individuals are sometimes unable to tolerate even older dishwashers. If you find that a running dishwasher makes you feel ill, try running the unit only after you've closed the kitchen off from the rest of the house and have opened one or more kitchen windows. You might also want to turn on the range hood too (make sure it is vented to the outdoors), if your stove is equipped with one. Then, be sure to stay out of the kitchen until the dishwasher has cooled off.

Of course, if you own a dishwasher, you'll want to use a low-odor, tolerable automatic dishwashing compound in it, especially if you're a sensitive person. Unfortunately, most typical brands contain synthetic fragrances whose odors can easily fill your kitchen whenever your dishwasher is operating. Even some of the alternative brands contain natural scents—such as lemon oil, which certain individuals may find unacceptable (see *Automatic Dishwasher Compounds* in *Chapter 7: Cleaning*).

On a critical note, a few very sensitive individuals have found they simply can't tolerate an automatic dishwasher, no matter what brand, how old it is, whether they are personally out of the room while it's operating, or what cleaning compound is used in them. Naturally, in those situations doing the dishes by hand, using a tolerable dishwashing liquid, may be the only satisfactory solution.

STOVES

The earliest stoves designed exclusively for cooking were cast-iron models with holes in the top for pans to sit on. By the middle of the eighteenth century, cast-iron stoves with baking chambers were introduced. Then in the 1840s, natural-gas cast-iron cooking ranges were invented, and for the first time an "automatic" energy source had replaced hand-stoked wood, charcoal, and coal fires. Finally, in 1914, the electric range made its debut.

Today, stoves are no longer simple cast-oven behemoths. In fact, few other modern major appliances offer as many choices and options as stoves. The following sections discuss some of the more popular types of stoves found in today's marketplace. Ultimately, it's up to you to choose which type will be most appropriate for your own particular needs.

Gas Ranges and Cooktops

Natural-gas and propane ranges have long been popular stove choices, but they can pose problems of which you might not be aware.

Problems with Gas Ranges and Cooktops

Generally, gas ranges are not suggested for use in healthy households. The major reason for this is that they produce polluting combustion by-products. These include carbon dioxide, nitrogen dioxide, small amounts of formaldehyde, and potentially deadly carbon monoxide (see *Combustion Gases* as well as *Formaldehyde* and *Carbon Monoxide* in *Chapter 9: Indoor Air*). Older models that are equipped with perpetually-burning pilot lights can be particularly troublesome in this regard. Their small, but constantly burning flames release combustion by-products continuously. A carbon-monoxide detector is highly suggested for all homes equipped with natural-gas appliances.

Another gas-appliance concern is the possibility of gas-line leaks developing. In a few situations, leaks from interior gas lines have led to sufficient natural-gas concentrations to cause explosions. However, leaks need not release large amounts of natural gas in order to become a problem. Unfortunately, some sensitive individuals have detected leaks and become ill as a result of natural gas escaping from extremely tiny gas-line leaks. Apparently, a few such persons can detect leaks that are barely detectable on typical gas-company testing equipment. Natural gas, thus, is one substance that a great many persons with sensitivities simply can't tolerate breathing, no matter how small the percentage present in the air.

To many "normal" people, it seems somewhat puzzling that exposure to very small amounts of natural gas could be detected or cause problems. However, just consider of what natural gas is comprised. Methane makes up 88% to 95% of the total volume and the remainder consists of gaseous ethane, propane, butane, pentane, along with less noxious carbon dioxide, nitrogen, and helium. Besides these, a "marker" chemical (methyl mercaptan) is also added to provide the strong, distinctive odor associated with gas so that leaks will be more noticeable to everyone. Is it any wonder then that those with hypersensitivities to petrochemicals could be so susceptible?

Making Gas-Range Operation More Tolerable

Despite the potential problems associated with gas ranges, some sensitive individuals may be unwilling or unable to give up their present gas ranges. If that's your situation, it's important that you at least use adequate kitchen ventilation when using your stove. Ideally, a powerful range hood vented to the outdoors should be installed and always used. Broan (**Broan Manufacturing Co.**) and Nutone (**Nutone/Scovill**) are two well-known range-hood manufacturers. You can call the companies for their nearest dealers. Other brands may also be available at your local appliance dealers. (Note: A powerful fan may require a window to be slightly opened so that air can easily come in to replace the air forced outside by the fan.) If you do plan to buy a new gas range, choose one with an electronic ignition so that no pilot light is always burning in it.

Carbon monoxide is produced during the incomplete combustion of natural gas. When natural gas is not burned completely, it has a yellow flame. If your gas stove is adjusted properly, it will have a blue flame and produce much less carbon monoxide.

Whenever you're using your gas range, you might consider wearing a charcoal-filled mask to act as a filter. However, admittedly, this could be awkward and uncomfortably warm to wear while cooking (see *Personal Facial Filters* in *Chapter 9: Indoor Air*).

Possible Problems with Electronically Controlled Models

If you're a sensitive person and decide to go ahead and purchase a new gas range, you should be aware of the possible implications posed by some of the models fitted with electronic touch buttons and clocks. Because these particular electronics can be damaged by high heat, many of the gas stoves equipped with them have special built-in thermostats inside their control panels. When the thermostat detects a certain temperature (around 140°F in some brands), it triggers a fan to run. The fan blows air across the electronic components and then back into the room. Even if the oven has been turned off, the fan will stay running until the thermostat senses that the temperature in the panel has gone below the triggering temperature.

Unfortunately, in some cases, the noise from these fans has proven to be irritatingly loud. Also, these fans could blow electronic odors (plastic-like smells, etc.) into the kitchen air. Therefore, if you're a sensitive individual, you may want to ask the appliance dealer to turn on, as a demonstration, a stove you are considering before you purchase it. That way, you can better decide whether the fan will likely cause problems for you. If you think it will, you might consider purchasing a model with an analog (non-digital) clock and controls.

Electric Stoves

Of course, besides gas, the other major type of stove is electric. While usually more healthful than gas models, electric cooktops and ovens do have potential sources of intolerance of which you should be aware.

Electric Cooktops

Electric cooktops, either combined with an electric oven or as separate countertop units, now come in several basic types. These include porcelain-on-steel or stainless-steel construction with traditional spiral elements or European plate-type elements. Another popular type is the smooth-surface, radiant, glass cooktop.

Over the years, spiral elements have been the style typically used on electric cooktops. Unfortunately, many new stovetops using traditional spiral elements are often intolerable for sensitive individuals when the elements are turned on. Because these elements are made of composite metal/ceramic formulations whose ingredients are considered trade secrets, knowing exactly what's in them is impossible. However, whatever these elements are made of, they seem to many sensitive persons to be less tolerable than those made ten years or so ago.

Whether today's electric elements are essentially different or not, if you're bothered by those in your new cooktop, there's a procedure you can follow that might alleviate the situation. That is to operate the spiral elements on high heat for thirty minutes or so, allow them to cool, and repeat the cycle over and over again for several days. This may burn off whatever is bothersome, especially if it's just a surface coating, without causing damage. Of course you'll want to do this only if children can't get to the cooktop, and you can monitor the procedure. Also, you'll want to have the kitchen closed off from the rest of the house to prevent odors from dissipating to other rooms, the kitchen windows opened, and a range-hood exhaust fan (one that is vented to the outdoors) turned on high speed.

Sadly, for some sensitive people new elements seem to remain intolerable after they've undergone a burning-off procedure, even after they've been used for several months. In those particular situations, the best solution might be to trade your stove's new elements for older, used ones. Perhaps you have a non-sensitive friend with tolerable elements of the same size. Many times, other people are happy to give you their old elements for a set of relatively new ones. You might also consider buying used elements from a local appliance-repair shop.

The newer-style European plate-type elements have a definite cleaning advantage over the traditional spiral elements. Because they are in a solid plate shape, there are no reflector pans used with them to accumulate debris or become discolored. They also provide more stable surfaces that are able to heat more uniformly.

However, some sensitive individuals have found that certain plate-type heating elements pose the same intolerance problems as many of the new spiral elements. This is probably because they're made of the same, or very similar materials. To make plate-type elements more tolerable, try the same burning-off procedure discussed previously with spiral elements. However, if you decide you want to trade elements or replace them with used ones, this can sometimes be difficult because this is a relatively new style and used ones may be difficult to find.

Fortunately, most radiant, glass cooktops are usually tolerable for sensitive individuals. These models have their elements underneath a one-piece, smooth, glass layer. However, if you decide on this type of cooktop, you must use pans with very flat bottoms. This is because pans without flat bottoms won't heat up properly. It's also important that you clean the glass surface thoroughly after every use. Any drips that are allowed to remain can become burned on and very difficult to remove (see *Glasstop Stoves* in *Chapter 7: Cleaning*).

No matter what type of electric cooktop you ultimately choose, it's best to have a range hood that is vented to the outdoors. This will eliminate potentially bothersome food odors, excess steam, and other cooking odors from your kitchen's air. Range hoods with *activated charcoal filters* that are designed to blow filtered air back into the kitchen are very poor ventilation choices. These are often called *recirculating range hoods.* They can't eliminate steam and they're only slightly effective at removing some cooking odors. (For more on range hoods that vent to the outdoors, see *Making Gas Range Operation More Tolerable* above.)

By the way, certain electric cooktop models using electronic controls and electronic clocks can also be equipped with a fan to prevent the electronic components from overheating. (For possible problems with these, see *Possible Problems with Electronically Controlled Models* above.)

Electric Ovens

Electric ovens now come as conventional, continuous-cleaning, and self-cleaning units. The conventional models are the traditional standard type that have the smooth porcelain-on-steel interiors that require periodic manual cleaning. Typically, highly odorous, and dangerous cleaning products are used to dissolve the buildup of grease splatters in such ovens. (For cleaning conventional ovens with less-toxic cleaners, see *Conventional Ovens* in *Chapter 7: Cleaning.*) Conventional ovens are the least expensive electric ovens because they utilize the oldest and most basic materials.

Continuous-cleaning ovens differ from conventional ovens because their porcelain-on-steel interiors don't have a smooth finish; instead they have a porous, matte finish. This special surface is designed to prevent minute grease particles from clumping together and adhering to the oven walls. (In conventional ovens, these clumps usually remain on the walls, grow larger, and must eventually be removed by manual and/or chemical means.) Because the separate, tiny grease molecules remain as they are, they can quickly incinerate during the oven's normal operation and never build up. By the way, incineration is especially efficient when the oven's temperature is at least 400°F. Unfortunately, some sensitive individuals find that this continual incineration process produces bothersome odors.

The third electric oven type is the self-cleaning model. These particular ovens have steel linings that have been treated with a special oil. Extra insulation (usually fiberglass) is also placed within the ovens' side walls. Both of these measures permit very high temperatures to be used during the self-cleaning cycle and yet not create damage to either the oven or the adjacent kitchen cabinets. Unfortunately, both the oil coating and the insulation can be quite bothersome to sensitive persons, especially on new units. Sometimes the owner's manuals will actually recommend that you run your new self-cleaning oven once through the cleaning cycle before you use it for normal cooking. This initial operation of the cleaning cycle is meant to reduce odors released from the special oil treatment. However, even after this has been done, some sensitive individuals may still find that their self-cleaning oven remains intolerable to them. In that case, you may have to repeat the cleaning cycle several more times.

Whenever you use the cleaning cycle, you probably should close off the kitchen from the rest of the house, open the kitchen windows, and have the range-hood exhaust fan turned on high speed. Even several hours after the cycle has been completed, the windows should remain open, with the exhaust fan operating. Note: Be sure to always remove all interior racks before using the cleaning cycle. This will prevent permanent chrome discoloration.

Some sensitive people have installed an appropriate electrical outlet in their garage and temporarily placed their new electric range there until it has become tolerable. When the range is in the garage and the overhead door is open, the oven can be run through the high-temperature cleaning cycle several times a day. Doing so for a week is usually enough to make a new oven tolerable. Once tolerable,the stove can safely be placed in the kitchen. (Note: Make sure children and pets can't get access to an operating stove.)

Many sensitive people have found that conventional or continuously-cleaning electric ovens can be intolerable because of the hot baking and broiling elements. This shouldn't be surprising when you realize these oven elements are often made of the same or similar ceramic/metal composite material of which commonly bothersome cooktop elements are made. However, some sensitive individuals have found that if they heat their electric oven on high (or broil) for a period of time (perhaps 1–2 hours), shut it off, and repeat this process many times over several days, the intolerance problems subside without damaging the elements. As in the case of running a self-cleaning cycle, it's best to do this procedure only with proper ventilation (or in a garage). Of course, the elements in self-cleaning ovens will automatically go through this baking-out process during the self-cleaning cycle.

It should be noted that some electric ovens with electronic touch controls and electronic clocks may pose concerns to some sensitive individuals. (For more information, see *Possible Problems with Electronically Controlled Models* under *Gas Ranges* above.)

Microwave Ovens

As everyone knows, microwave ovens can streamline the cooking process. In the last two decades, their popularity in houses has skyrocketed. As a result, few American kitchens are now without one. However, there are drawbacks and concerns associated with microwave ovens with which you should become familiar.

How Microwave Ovens Work

Many healthy persons cook with microwaves because they can heat up prepackaged microwave dinners, reheat leftovers, make hot water almost instantly for coffee, and pop popcorn without oil, but these people still use their electric or gas stove for other types of cooking. On the other hand, some sensitive persons who find that they simply can't tolerate their stove turn to microwave ovens as their main (sometimes only) method of cooking. Interestingly, few people—no matter why they use a microwave oven—actually know how they work.

As it turns out, microwave ovens are equipped with a special electron tube known as a *magnetron*. This device emits a narrow stream of *microwave radiation* (radar). At the same time, a small fan scatters the rays around the walls of the oven to produce more even distribution.

But how do radar waves cook? It seems that radar is powerful enough to pass through paper, glass, and china easily. However, it has a far more difficult time passing through liquid, including the tiny liquid molecules within foods. In fact, in liquid, the radar-wave energy becomes trapped and this causes the liquid molecules to begin to vibrate rapidly. Soon, the vibrating liquid molecules collide into each other, creating friction. It's the heat produced by friction that actually cooks the food. Because microwave ovens create internal friction almost immediately, they don't require preheating or lengthy cooking times. Conventional ovens, on the other hand, slowly heat foods from the outside surfaces inward.

Unfortunately, complex foods (with areas of varying moisture content and/or density within them) or fairly dry foods don't often cook particularly well in microwave ovens. In addition, browning is not possible unless special devices and/or sprinkled substances are used. Therefore, some foods cooked in microwaves can have a poorer appearance, blander taste, and less-even doneness than if they had been cooked in regular electric or gas ovens.

Microwave Oven Concerns

From a health standpoint, everyone should be aware that many microwave ovens sooner or later can emit potentially harmful microwave radiation (radar). (Currently, the U.S. Bureau of Radiological Health has set a permissible leakage level of 5 milliwatts per each square centimeter of near-surface area.) While apparently no direct correlation between using microwave ovens and ill health has yet to be documented, there are concerns that ongoing research is beginning to address. What is now known is that microwave exposure from other sources besides microwave ovens has led to certain health problems including cataracts and perhaps even cancer.

If you're in the market to purchase a microwave oven, it would be wise to choose a sturdily constructed model with a tight-sealing door. One very good idea before purchasing a unit would be to check the current consumer guidebooks and magazines at your local library or bookstore for the models with the highest safety ratings. If possible, you'll want to buy only the safest unit you can afford in your size, feature, and price range.

When your microwave oven is actually at home and operating, it's been recommended by some experts that you try to stand at least three feet away from it as a safety measure. This is because microwave emission levels drop off quickly just a short distance from their source. In addition, you might seriously consider purchasing a *microwave detector*. These radar monitors will permit you to personally measure your oven's emissions frequently. These devices can be ordered from **Nontoxic Environments** and **Baubiologie Hardware**. If a problem is detected, it would be best to have the machine repaired by a trained repairperson as soon as possible, or have it replaced.

As many people are aware, the cookware you place your food in when you're microwaving is also important. When possible, use glass or ceramic cookware rather than plastic because they are more stable when subjected to cooking temperatures. Heated plastic can give off bothersome odors that can give a "plastic" taste to the cooking food.

Portable Turbo-Convection Ovens

Portable turbo-convection ovens have been gaining in popularity the last few years. This is not surprising. These small units have many advantages over other oven types.

How Portable Turbo-Convection Ovens Work

Fairly new to American kitchens are countertop *turbo-convection ovens*. Actually, although the small, portable consumer models have only become available relatively recently, large commercial convection ovens have been used for some time. (Some regular residential electric stoves also have had a built-in convection-oven feature.) However, because many people still aren't familiar with these appliances, an explanation is in order. By definition, a portable turbo-convection oven is a small, easily-movable oven unit equipped with a fan and capable of circulating heat in a spinning, tornado-like fashion.

In actual construction, these ovens (often 12–14" in diameter) consist of a pot/container with feet and a snugly sealing lid. Most units come equipped with two or more chromed-wire cooking racks. The oven controls generally include a temperature adjustment knob and a timer, which are on the top of the lid. Underneath the lid, there's a spiral electric heating element and a multi-vaned fan. When the oven is turned on, the element heats up and the fan blows simultaneously. This dual action inside a small sealed space exposes the food (which is on one or more of the racks inside the pot) to both the immediate and continuously intense hot air. With a turbo-convection oven, no warm-up time is required and, ideally, this results in a relatively quick cooking time and lower energy use. Fortunately, many sensitive persons seem to tolerate these ovens very well.

Interestingly, most foods cook as well in these ovens as in regular full-size ovens. In fact, some foods actually seem to cook better, such as meats, which generally come out brown and crispy with most of the fat dripping down into the convection oven's bottom (a big plus over microwave ovens). Therefore, some people find that portable turbo-convection ovens are a more healthful way to prepare meats. These ovens are also fairly easy to clean and they produce very little smoke. And, because they're small, you and your kitchen remain cooler while cooking, compared to using a large oven.

However, portable turbo-convection ovens do have drawbacks. One is that a few foods, such as 9"-round cake layers, can't be cooked evenly. This is because the center isn't fully exposed to the hot blowing air. One manufacturer's manual suggests solving this problem by baking in Bundt-style cake pans that have a hole in the center. Another problem is that some very large items, such as turkeys or strudels for example, just won't fit into most of these ovens. In addition, it can sometimes be difficult to get your cooked food off the lower rack without your hands getting burned on the pot's hot walls.

Choosing the Right Portable Turbo-Oven

Various turbo-convection oven models are constructed differently from each other. For example, some have lids and pots made of a special translucent heat-resistant plastic. However, it is generally better for sensitive individuals to choose units made with non-synthetic materials. These would include all-glass models or those made with enameled-metal pots and glass lids.

Actually, the models with enameled-metal pots and glass lids are especially good for several reasons; the base is unbreakable, lightweight, and maintains its original appearance very well over time. However, because the finish is an applied porcelain-enamel coating and not a high temperature-fired, glazed finish, it's a good idea to heat-cure the finish to make it hard, durable, and odor-free before you use it to cook food. To accomplish this, you can cock the glass lid (to let odors escape easily) and run the unit on high heat for an hour. Then, shut it off, let it cool down, and repeat the process until the finish no longer releases bothersome odors when its heated up. Doing this procedure outdoors or on an open porch is a good idea to prevent any odors from contaminating your house. However, if you have to do it indoors, you'll want to run the portable turbo-convection oven directly beneath your exhausting range hood. Also, you'll want to close off your kitchen from the rest of the house, open the kitchen windows, and turn the range hood on high speed. (Note: As a safety precaution, don't leave an operating oven unattended where children or pets can get access to it.)

It's relatively easy to find small turbo-convection ovens locally. And because they are becoming more commonplace, their prices are coming down substantially. You can often find these ovens in kitchen departments, gourmet shops, and even discount stores. One brand, Aroma Aeromatic Oven (**Aroma Manufacturing Co. of America**), is available as either an all-glass model, or with a glass lid and a porcelain-enameled metal pot. To purchase this particular brand in your area, call the company for the dealer nearest you.

If at all possible, turbo-convection ovens should be operated under a range hood that is vented to the outdoors. That usually means setting it directly on your cooktop, so be sure it sits level and is not near a hot cooktop element.

REFRIGERATORS

Artificial refrigeration (cooling that doesn't use ice or snow to cool) is based on the principle that a liquid that is volatile (able to rapidly evaporate) will absorb heat when it evaporates and, as a result, will cool its surroundings. The first artificial refrigeration was actually developed in 1748 in Scotland. Eventually, various cooling methods and *refrigerants* (the volatile liquids used to cool) were introduced and used for commercial applications. By the 1920s, many American homes began to be equipped with refrigerators rather than iceboxes. And, by the end of World War II, the majority of all U.S. households had refrigerators.

In home units, *Freon* became the primary refrigerant after it was created by a team of DuPont researchers in 1930. Freon is actually a trademarked family of refrigerants that are made of chlorine and fluorine specially positioned in certain hydrocarbon compounds (usually methane or ethane). These resulting *halogenated hydrocarbons* (*halogenated* refers to the presence of chlorine and fluorine) or *halocarbons* are considered nontoxic to humans and are nonflammable. However, it's now known that escaping Freon can release chlorine atoms that can damage the ozone layer in the upper atmosphere. Because the ozone layer acts as a buffer, protecting us from too much ultraviolet radiation from the sun, scientists are now developing refrigerants that are less damaging to the ozone layer.

Today, modern refrigerators still operate on the same basic artificial refrigeration principles and still use refrigerants. The major differences between refrigerators from the early 1950s and today include cosmetic changes (shape and color), the use of plastic materials for interior panels and inner-wall insulation, special features (self-defrosting models, ice makers, ice-water dispensers, etc.), and improved energy efficiency.

New Refrigerator Problems

Because nearly all new domestic model refrigerators are made with plastic interiors, they can give off odors that can be bothersome to sensitive people. If you find that your new refrigerator is intolerable because of this, you might want to wash the interior and let it air it out for an extended period before actually using the refrigerator in your kitchen. To do this, if possible, place your new refrigerator in a screened porch or garage. Of course, you'll need to make sure the area is dry and free of objectionable odors. Then, remove the refrigerator's doors or simply prop them open. However, if the doors are not removed, the porch or garage must be securely locked to prevent children from entering and getting inside the refrigerator. (Note: Some jurisdictions may legally require that such a refrigerator have its doors removed.)

Next, you can wash the new refrigerator's interior with a tolerable, unscented cleaner. One you might try is SafeChoice Super Clean (**American Formulating and Manufacturing (AFM)**), which is a light amber-colored, concentrated synthetic detergent available from **The Living Source, N.E.E.D.S.**, and other AFM dealers. To use it, mix 1 cup into 1 gallon of water. Then dip a clean sponge into the solution, wring it out, and go over all the plastic in the interior. You also might try a baking soda-and-water solution as an alternative. However, whatever you use to clean and eliminate odors, rinse it off with clear water and a sponge. Afterwards, simply leave the refrigerator alone to air for several days or weeks before permanently placing the unit in your kitchen. In most cases, once the refrigerator is operating, the cold temperatures will dramatically reduce any synthetic odors released by the plastic interior. This is because outgassing decreases at lower temperatures.

However, besides a plastic interior, a new refrigerator's motor can also be troublesome in some cases. This is because the oils on the new motor can give off fairly strong odors that can be blown into the kitchen area by the refrigerator's fan. In addition, bothersome odors from the new insulation (either a foam insulation or fiberglass) may also be wafted into the air at the same time. Fortunately, all these odors generally diminish over time.

It has been suggested by some persons that you should consider purchasing a refrigerator equipped with wire shelves rather than those featuring solid glass shelves. The theory behind this is that wire shelves will allow for better cold air circulation inside the refrigerator. Solid glass shelves, on the other hand, can act as a barrier to good internal airflow. Better circulation means that the refrigerator's motor will need to run less to keep the refrigerator cool. If you want to follow this buying suggestion, as of this writing, White-Westinghouse (**White Consolidated Industries, Inc.**) and Kenmore (**Sears Roebuck and Co.**) both have a few models equipped with enameled, wire shelves. It should be mentioned that another approach might be simply to purchase a very efficient model such as units with their freezer compartment on the bottom.

Unfortunately, some very sensitive individuals have simply not been able to handle their new refrigerator so they have completely removed it from their kitchen. These people have found that placing the refrigerator elsewhere, such as a seldom-used room, the garage, or the basement is, for them, worth the inconvenience. By the way, as an alternative, a few persons have actually had a special containment compartment constructed within their kitchen in which to place their bothersome refrigerator. This can be built like a small closet so that only the front of the refrigerator is exposed to the room. A small, continuously running exhaust fan in the back of the compartment keeps air flowing from the kitchen, past the refrigerator, and to the outdoors. This approach can work well, but it should be remembered that a certain amount of outdoor air will continually be entering the house whenever the fan is running—air that might be polluted. A containment compartment requires not only the necessary space, but also the extra money to build it.

Commercial Refrigerators

Some very sensitive individuals have opted to buy a commercial refrigerator rather than a residential model. The reason for this is that commercial models are generally made of stainless steel, both outside and inside. Therefore, they don't have the odor problems associated with plastic interiors.

However, there are drawbacks to owning a commercial refrigerator. A major problem is that many of them are only refrigerators; they have no frozen-food compartment. This means you end up having to purchase and find space for a second unit, a freezer. Also, commercial refrigerators tend to be quite large, so they may jut out unattractively into your kitchen's floor space. You might even have to take out adjoining cabinets to make room for it. In addition, commercial units are generally not designed for especially quiet operation.

As a result, their noise can be quite annoying. Furthermore, these units can be quite expensive. Finally, these refrigerators may have motors that could emit bothersome odors like residential refrigerators. However, some models have a motor that can be mounted in a remote location. In other words, you can have the refrigerator in the kitchen and the motor (with its odors and noise) in an adjacent garage.

If, despite all the negatives you're still interested in a restaurant-quality refrigerator, check your classified phone directory under Commercial Kitchen Supplies or a similar heading for a nearby dealer. However, a better approach to owning a stainless-steel refrigerator might be to buy one of the elite brands sold for use in very upscale kitchens. To purchase one of these refrigerators, consult with a certified kitchen designer. To find such an individual, check your local telephone classified directory. Such a person should be familiar with current models that might be suitable for use in your home.

Routine Refrigerator Maintenance

No matter what type of refrigerator you end up buying, it's important that it be properly maintained. Besides the usual interior cleaning, you should remember to dust the cooling coils (either behind or underneath your refrigerator) every other month or so. By doing this, your refrigerator will be able to work more efficiently. In turn, this means the motor won't have to operate as often. Therefore, potentially bothersome motor and insulation odors won't be blown into your kitchen as frequently. Also, regularly dusting of the coils will prevent dust from being dispersed throughout your kitchen as well. In addition, it eliminates a haven for dust mites or other microorganisms.

To make dusting your refrigerator's coils easier, use a specially designed cleaning tool. These long wands with short spiral bristles are particularly useful for dusting coils that are underneath refrigerators. To buy one, check in your local discount, hardware, and department stores. One brand, Fuller Brush Refrigerator Coil Brush (**Fuller Brush**), is handled by most Fuller Brush dealers, including **enviro-clean**.

Another ongoing maintenance job is to clean your automatic-defrosting refrigerator's drip pan. Unfortunately, many people aren't even aware that their refrigerator has such a drip pan. Actually, these are located under the refrigerator to catch the melting frost from the freezer compartment during the defrosting cycle. If you regularly remove and clean the drip pan, it'll discourage mold growth. Actually, it's a good idea to simply clean it every time you clean your refrigerator's coils.

If you find that mold has, indeed, colonized your refrigerator's drip pan, you can pour 3% hydrogen peroxide (this is the dilution commonly sold in drugstores) directly into the pan, scrub it, and rinse it off. Then wash the pan using a tolerable dish detergent, rinse it, towel dry it, and finally put it back under the refrigerator. (For more mold-cleaning options, see *Mold and Mildew* in *Chapter 7: Cleaning*.)

WASHING MACHINES

A number of home washing devices have been invented over the years, especially in the late 19th century. Some consisted of covered, wooden, barrel-like tubs that were manually operated to paddle or agitate the clothing inside.

Whether these actually saved any labor or got the clothing clean is debatable. Finally, in 1911, Frederick Maytag developed the electric washing machine. By 1922, he began marketing washers with aluminum tubs.

New washing machines appear, at first glance, not to have changed very much since the mid-1950s. They're nearly all porcelain-enamel steel boxes with control panels on top and tubs inside equipped with agitators. But in the last few years, one change that sensitive persons should be aware of is that many manufacturers are now building their washers with plastic tubs rather than metal (either porcelain-on-steel or stainless steel) ones.

If you've recently bought a washer with a plastic tub and found it bothersome, try running several complete washing cycles (without clothes or other washable items) using hot water and a tolerable laundry washing compound, unscented borax, baking soda, or perhaps white vinegar (see *Alternative Laundry Products* in *Chapter 7: Cleaning*). After enough cycles, one would hope that any odors from the plastic tub will have dissipated enough that they won't be absorbed by fabric fibers. By the way, even some new porcelain-on-steel tubs can be odorous because of the recently applied finishes. To counter this, follow the same regimen as for new plastic-tub washers.

When you're ready to buy a new washer and want to avoid one with a plastic tub, Hotpoint (**General Electric Co.**) and GE (**General Electric Co.**) models are still made with porcelain-on-steel tubs, as of this writing. For other brands still equipped with porcelainized-steel or stainless-steel tubs, check your local appliance dealers.

However, no matter what model you end up with, all new washers have rubber belts, lubricated gears, and oily-smelling motors—all of which can be quite bothersome for at least several months for many sensitive people. To minimize any intolerance problems, be sure to have good ventilation in your laundry area. Of course, opening the windows will help, but if this becomes tiresome or there are no windows, you might consider installing an exhaust fan that is vented to the outdoors like the ones commonly used in bathrooms. Two well-known manufacturers of vented fans are Nutone (**Nutone-Scovill**) and Broan (**Broan Manufacturing Co.**) These, and similar ones, should be available in your local building centers.

It should be pointed out that having a vented fan in your laundry area is actually a good idea for other reasons besides just expelling new washer odors. For example, vented fans can remove bothersome odors from dirty clothes and laundry products as well. In addition, they're usually able to remove much of the excess moisture that builds up in the laundry room area on wash days. This is important because drier air will provide a less favorable climate for mold or mildew growth.

CLOTHES DRYERS

Although the first electric washing machine was marketed in 1911, it wasn't until a number of years later that the home dryer was brought out. This was because hanging the wash to dry was perfectly acceptable to most people. Even after they were introduced, residential automatic dryers were initially seen as frivolous luxuries. Therefore, it took some time before the American public commonly bought both an automatic washer *and* a dryer.

Today of course, there are two basic types of dryers: those that dry using heated electric elements and those that dry by burning natural gas. From a health standpoint, the healthiest dryers are the electric models, especially for sensitive persons. This is because natural gas (or bottled *propane* gas) has the potential to cause several problems. These include the creation of polluting combustion by-products that might not be completely vented outside, the potential for seepage from small gas-line leaks, and an occasional slight, but detectable, odor of natural-gas or combustion by-products that is absorbed by the drying clothes. (For a more complete discussion of potential gas appliance problems, see *Problems with Gas Ranges* above.) Unfortunately, in some areas of the country, the cost of operating an electric dryer is much higher than one fueled by natural or bottled gas. However, for extremely sensitive individuals, the added cost of using an electric dryer may be well worth it.

If you are ready to purchase a new electric dryer, you should be aware that many are now equipped with plastic drums. If you want one with a porcelain-on-steel drum, as of this writing all Hotpoint (**General Electric Co.**) models, as well as all GE (**General Electric Co.**) models except its Extra Large Capacity R Series have them. (The Extra Large Capacity R Series dryers are fitted with steel drums coated with a synthetic material.) Unless the owner's manual prohibits it, you should run your new electric drier on the hottest temperature for the longest cycle several times until any odors (either from the new plastic or from the new porcelain-on-steel coating) are no longer bothersome to you.

It's very important that your dryer be vented to the outdoors. While you might think that all clothes dryers are hooked up this way, sometimes they are vented to the indoors. While the purpose of venting a dryer to the indoors is to keep the warm air inside the home to help reduce heating bills, serious problems can result with this approach. Vent filters will almost never adequately remove the tiny lint particles, so they enter the living space. This could lead to allergic reactions and/or the creation of respiratory problems. Then too, any perfume or other odors in your clothing that have been released into the dryer by the high heat will also get blown into the living space. This situation is particularly unacceptable for sensitive individuals. Finally, the air from an operating dryer contains a fairly large amount of water vapor. The introduction of this additional moisture could easily lead to mold or mildew problems in the laundry room. (See *High Relative Humidity in Chapter 9: Improving Indoor Air.*)

COOKWARE

As most Americans now know, it's important to eat healthy foods. That often means fewer synthetic ingredients, less refined sugar, less fat, less sodium, etc. Others, of course, want to be vegetarians or eat only organic foods. In addition, many sensitive and allergic persons want to choose only those foods which they can personally tolerate. Furthermore, there are certain people who can't eat sugar or are on a special weight-reduction diet. Still others follow a healthful diet based on a specific religious belief or codified cooking philosophy. Because cooking "healthy" can have so many definitions, this book doesn't even attempt to cover such a broad subject. These days, many cookbooks are available in local libraries and bookstores that can guide you. Also, organizations and support groups can offer pertinent advise, buying sources, and recipes. (Of course, you'll always want to follow the advice of your personal physician.)

What this book does discuss is cookware, so that no matter how you define *healthy food*, you'll be able to cook it in healthful pots, pans, baking dishes, and other utensils.

NONSTICK COATINGS

Anymore, most new cookware comes with interiors lined with some type of nonstick coating. These coatings often allow burnt food to be easily wiped away from the pan's bottom and sides. They also allow you to cook with little or no oil. However, nonstick coatings do have drawbacks. For example, most of them are synthetically derived compounds that some sensitive persons and those interested in all-natural living might want to avoid.

One of the earliest and most well-known nonstick coating is *Teflon*. Teflon is actually a type of *polytetrafluoroethylene* that is a trademark of DuPont. It was originally developed in 1938. However, it wasn't until 1954 in France that it first began to be used on cookware. By the late 1960s and 1970s, Teflon-coated pans became increasingly popular in America. However, some early Teflon formulations proved to be somewhat fragile and fairly easy to scratch or peel.

Since Teflon's introduction onto cookware, other nonstick pan coatings have also been developed. Each new generation of nonstick coating has tried to retain Teflon's slipperiness, and at the same time be more durable. Today, some of the newer, tougher, synthetic, nonstick coatings are more or less permanently bonded to cookware interiors. However, while these are less likely to become damaged or peel, they still often require the use of plastic, rather metal, utensils.

For very sensitive persons in particular, unless a pan comes with a label specifically stating that the nonstick finish or treatment is all-natural, it might be wise to consider buying something else. This is because most of these coatings are still vulnerable to slight deterioration as a result of normal wear and tear, so there's the possibility that minute particles of the coating could flake off into your food and be swallowed. There's also the possibility that certain synthetic coatings could begin to *sublimate* (evaporate from a solid state into a gaseous state) at very high temperatures. This can happen when an empty pot is accidentally left on a heated burner. Once in the air, the synthetic compounds released from the overheated coating could be inhaled.

METAL POTS AND PANS

Of course, metal pots and pans have been used for cooking for hundreds of years. Today, one of the most popular metals used in modern cookware is aluminum. The three main reasons for this are that aluminum heats up quickly, doesn't rust, and is relatively inexpensive. However, aluminum can react with many acidic foods. As a result, there's the possibility that aluminum-containing compounds can be absorbed by food and become ingested. This may be a significant concern. Recent research has shown that there is a relationship between aluminum deposits found in the brain, and Alzheimer's disease. While aluminum cookware has not specifically been implicated, it might be wise to consider using other alternatives. That is, until studies definitely show cooking with aluminum cookware is not a contributing factor to this debilitating condition.

Acceptable metals for pans also include cast iron, tin-lined copper, porcelain-on-steel, and stainless steel. By the way, stainless steel-lined aluminum cookware would also be fine because the stainless-steel layer forms an impenetrable protective barrier between the cooking food and the aluminum itself. However, if the stainless steel layer should become severely worn or sustain deep, penetrating scratches, these pans could no longer completely prevent aluminum from interacting with the food.

It's usually not difficult to find appropriate metal pans locally. Most kitchen shops, department stores, discount outlets, and restaurant-supply stores generally carry them. One popular brand you might try is Revere stainless-steel pans (**Corning, Inc.**). If you can't find these stainless-steel/copper-bottom pans in your area, they can be ordered directly from the manufacturer.

Mail-order companies that specialize in kitchenware often carry several metal-pan lines without nonstick coatings (for information on nonstick coating concerns, see *Nonstick Coatings* above). Three such companies are **Colonial Garden Kitchens**, **The Wooden Spoon**, and **Williams-Sonoma**. A number of alternative health catalogs also carry similar metal cookware. These include **Natural Lifestyle Supplies** and **Nontoxic Environments**, among others.

GLASS, GLASS-CERAMIC, AND POTTERY COOKWARE

Probably the least reactive cookware is made of glass. Actually, glass could only be used as a cookware material after scientists at Corning Glass Works formulated a type of glass that could withstand temperature extremes and chemical exposures, and yet be easy and inexpensive to manufacture. (Typical window glass, known as *soda-lime glass*, is relatively cheap and easy to make. However, it's fairly fragile.) Between 1912 and 1915, Corning researchers created *borosilicate glasses* that could meet their demanding criteria. *Pyrex* became the trademark for this glass. Interestingly, Pyrex apparently acquired it's name because it was the first glass in which pie could be baked.

One very good glass cookware line available today is the original version of Vision cookware (**Corning, Inc.**). This line is often sold by local kitchen shops, department stores, and discount stores. (These outlets may handle similar brands as well.) If you can't find it, Vision cookware can also be ordered directly from the company. This particular cookware is made of thick Pyrex glass with molded handles. Its translucent color allows you to see easily inside a pot or pan without raising the lid.

However, it should be mentioned that some Vision pots are made with molded pouring spouts. These will permit steam to continually escape while you're cooking because they can't be sealed completely. Therefore, you might prefer to choose pots without the pouring-spout feature. In addition, within the last few years, a new modified Vision line has become available, one using an interior synthetic nonstick coating. Many sensitive persons in particular might choose to avoid these. Fortunately, you can order Vision cookware without nonstick surfaces directly from the company.

The familiar white Corningware (**Corning, Inc.**) and other similar *Pyroceram* ceramic pots and pans make excellent cookware. Often the pots, pans, and baking dishes made with these glass/ceramics can be used in the microwave, on a cooktop, in the oven, and, once it has cooled down, in the freezer. All these attributes shouldn't be surprising when you learn that Pyrocerams were originally created to encase missile nose cones. However, to be certain what your particular glass ceramic cookware is safely designed to do, carefully read the label instructions for the manufacturers' very specific recommendations. To buy Pyroceram cookware, check in local kitchen departments and gourmet cooking stores. Also, kitchen specialty catalogs such as **Colonial Garden Kitchens**, **The Wooden Spoon**, and **Williams-Sonoma** generally carry the product. In addition, the Corningware brand of glass ceramic cookware can be purchased directly from the company (**Corning, Inc.**).

Especially attractive casserole and baking dishes can be made of pottery (fired or baked clay). Commonly, local kitchen specialty stores, as well as artisan potters, offer them for sale. However, to ensure your safety before using these pieces, it's a good idea to make sure that the glazes on them are lead-free. This is a particularly necessary step before cooking with imported and/or handmade items. Two brands of lead test kits that work quickly and easily on cookware are Lead Check Swabs (**HybriVet Systems, Inc.**) and Lead Alert (**Frandon Enterprises**). Lead-testing kits are often available in local hardware stores and both of the above-mentioned brands can be ordered by mail directly from the manufacturer.

CUTTING BOARDS

For a number of years, consumers have been strongly advised to use plastic rather than wood cutting boards. Experts believed that the solid, uniform surfaces of polyethylene or other synthetic materials would minimize the sites for food debris to accumulate and so lessen the possibility for contamination by microbes. However, in a reversal of expectations, recent tests at the University of Wisconsin-Madison revealed that wood cutting boards actually appear to inhibit microbial growth. It's theorized that some natural compound in wood may have an antibacterial quality. Of course, it's still advised to wash all cutting boards frequently, no matter what they're made of. This is especially important after cutting foods such as raw meat or hard boiled eggs because they can be quite attractive to certain harmful bacteria.

If you opt for a wood cutting board, you might consider a close-grained, low-odor hardwood such as maple, especially if you're a very sensitive person. Fortunately, maple cutting boards are often sold in most local kitchenware departments and kitchen/gourmet cooking stores. It should be mentioned that most new wood cutting boards, even maple ones, can have a bothersome wood odor. If you find the odor of your new cutting board objectionable, you can wash it several times with a tolerable dish soap and/or with baking soda and water. Then rinse it completely, towel it dry, and place it outdoors in the sun to air for a few days. (Be sure the surroundings are dry and uncontaminated.) When the cutting board is no longer bothersome, bring it inside, wash and rinse it thoroughly, let it dry, and begin using it.

PAPER GOODS

Toilet tissue, facial tissue, paper napkins, and paper towels have more or less become indispensable items since they were introduced to American consumers one by one, mostly since World War I and some since World War II. The eventual widespread acceptance and use of disposable paper items reflected a buying public that now had more income and who were less willing to spend the time and energy to launder cloth counterparts such as handkerchiefs and dish towels.

Unfortunately, for many sensitive individuals, finding truly low-odor, tolerable toilet paper, paper towels, paper napkins, and facial tissue is often a real challenge. To help you in this, the following sections offer a number of suggestions. (For more information on papers and paper production, see *Paper* in *Chapter 6: Lifestyle*.)

LOCALLY PURCHASED PAPER GOODS

Of course, most people like to buy their paper goods locally. However, there are certain advantages to ordering them through the mail, especially if you're a sensitive person.

ODOR ABSORPTION PROBLEMS

Some of the major paper-product manufacturers now market unscented, undyed products. Just two examples of these are Charmin Free toilet paper and Original Kleenex white facial tissue. However, keep in mind that these unscented versions are manufactured in the same plants, stored in the same warehouses, transported in the same vehicles, and stacked on the same shelves as the far-more-numerous synthetically dyed and scented products. Unfortunately, paper by its very nature is extremely absorbent. Therefore, because of the collective handling, it's not that uncommon for some sensitive persons to purchase packages of unscented white toilet paper and not to be able to clearly distinguish it from scented rolls.

To make your recently purchased paper goods more tolerable, you might try storing them on a screened porch to air out, if possible. When you do this, make certain that the surroundings are dry and that the air is relatively uncontaminated. During this airing out period you might decide to unwrap certain plastic-wrapped items, such as paper towels, so that they can more easily lose their absorbed odors. The length of the airing time will depend on how sensitive you are and how odorous the paper goods were when you brought them home. Therefore, sufficient airing could take as little as a few hours or as long as several days.

When your paper goods have become acceptable to you, you can then bring them in, remove and dispose of the first few sheets of the unwrapped items, and finally store them. At this point, proper storage is essential to keep your now-tolerable paper goods from becoming contaminated and, thus, intolerable. Having a storage area that is clean, dry, and free from objectionable odors is best.

One side note worthy of mention is that buying foil-wrapped boxes of facial tissue, such as Original Kleenex, will have at least two advantages for sensitive people. First, the foil exteriors generally protect the contents from airborne odors. Second, the boxes themselves will have perfume and other unacceptable odor molecules adhering only to the metal foil's surface rather than deeply absorbed into the cardboard. Therefore, the foil-wrapped boxes often become more odor-free fairly quickly.

OTHER CONCERNS WITH TYPICAL PAPER GOODS

Unfortunately, added perfumes and dyes are not the only ingredients of paper goods that sensitive persons can find objectionable. This is because most paper products are subjected to a variety of chemicals in the transformation from pine logs to finished items. For example, chlorine compounds are often used to bleach typical papers white. In the process, toxic dioxins are also created as by-products. In addition, formaldehyde may also be added during production to increase a paper's absorbency. (See *How Typical Best Grade Papers are Made* in *Chapter 6: Lifestyle*.)

BUYING ALTERNATIVE PAPER GOODS LOCALLY

The good news for those people who find they can't tolerate typical paper goods is that some alternative grocery and health-food stores now carry alternative paper products. These are often unbleached, made of recycled paper, and free of perfume, dye, and other potentially bothersome additives. However, despite these laudable qualities, it's likely these paper goods will still have absorbed surrounding store odors, which originated from customers wearing perfumes and other scented personal-care items, as well as from products actually used to clean the store. All these odors have the possibility of proving bothersome to sensitive persons.

One method you can use to prevent locally purchased paper goods from absorbing unwanted odors is to simply special-order them through the store. That way your paper goods will arrive in unopened cases. You should realize that case orders will mean a lot of packages to store properly at home, requiring advance preparation (see *Buying in Quantity* and *Storage Concerns* in *Chapter 1: Getting Started*).

DIRECT MAIL-ORDERED PAPER GOODS

Actually, a very good method of buying tolerable paper goods for sensitive people is to order paper items directly from specialty environmental/ecology catalogs. Such catalogs generally handle paper products that are undyed, unscented, dioxin-free, and made of recycled paper. Some of the paper goods offered are made of 100%-recycled materials, often with a high proportion of post-consumer paper. Many are unbleached as well. Besides getting paper goods with many desirable qualities, mail-ordering avoids all the concerns over your paper products absorbing grocery-store odors (see *Odor Absorption Problems* and also *Buying Alternative Paper Goods Locally* above). Besides this point, direct mail-ordering is also very convenient. You can order whenever you want (often with your own telephone) and the items are delivered straight to your home.

As a rule, the paper goods that you can mail-order can be purchased in either small quantities or by the case. Keep in mind that purchasing in bulk will usually save you money (see *Buying in Quantity* in *Chapter 1: Getting Started*). If you do buy by the case, you have the added assurance that your paper goods haven't been exposed to any warehouse odors. However, even if they have been, it's likely that products ordered from the ecology/environmental catalog company will be less intense and less of a problem, having been stored in a warehouse, than the perfume and cleaning-product odors that would have been absorbed if they had been on retail store shelves.

Which catalog should you choose to order your paper goods from? One you might consider is **The Seventh Generation**. Besides handing a wide variety of alternative paper goods, the company offers an optional automatic shipping program. If you request this, you decide the products you want , the quantity, and how often you want them delivered. Then the items are delivered automatically at the intervals you requested (revisions from your initial plan can be made along the way). Another catalog you may want to check for alternative household paper goods is **Eco-Source**, but there are others. (Note: A few other mail-order companies also offer automatic shipping programs.)

CLOTH ALTERNATIVES TO PAPER GOODS

Despite the ample availability of alternative paper goods, some individuals may still find them unacceptable. This may be for philosophical reasons (not wanting to exploit trees, for example) or perhaps because all paper, alternative or not, causes certain individuals to experience unhealthy reactions. For these people, substituting cloth for paper products is suggested wherever possible. For example, washable, 100%-natural fiber handkerchiefs, napkins, dish cloths, and dish towels can easily, and often, very satisfactorily, eliminate the need to purchase and use paper napkins and paper towels (see *Tablecloths, Placemats, and Napkins* as well as *Kitchen Towels* and *Potholders* in *Chapter 4: Linens*).

(Note: If you're interested in washable 100%-cotton feminine napkins, see *Feminine Hygiene* in *Chapter 2: Personal Care*.)

PLASTIC AND CELLOPHANE GOODS

Most Americans now use a variety of plastic goods (plastic bags, plastic wrap, plastic storage containers etc.) in their homes. Before Word War II, most of these consumer products didn't exist. Today, many people could not imagine running a household without them.

It's easy to understand why plastic goods have become so popular. Generally, they're relatively inexpensive, fairly durable, and water-resistant. However, there's a downside. Plastics are usually not biodegradable (see *Biodegradable* under "Healthy" Definitions in *Chapter 1: Getting Started*), they're usually made of nonrenewable petroleum derivatives, and they can give off chemical odors that can be bothersome, especially to sensitive people. Therefore, for a variety of reasons, some individuals have decided to minimize, or completely eliminate, the use of plastic goods in their homes.

PLASTIC

What exactly are plastics? By definition, plastics are natural or synthetic materials that become moldable (plastic) when they're heated. Some plastics become flexible every time they are reheated (they are called *thermoplastic*); others are only flexible the first time they are heated (they are called *thermosetting*). Today's plastics are generally man-made *polymers* whose chemical structures consist of very long chains of carbon atoms that wouldn't normally occur in nature. The basic building-block components for these polymer chains are commonly derived from petroleum or natural gas.

Actually, the number of plastic types now being manufactured has become large, and continues to grow. Interestingly, *celluloid*, made from cellulose nitrate and camphor, is considered the first synthetic plastic. It was created as long ago as 1856 as an ivory substitute. It wasn't until after the turn of the century that the second synthetic plastic, *Bakelite*, was introduced. This plastic material was particularly popular. It was commonly used for many decades in a variety of products including telephones (see *Telephones* in *Chapter 6: Lifestyle*). Eventually, just prior to World War II, modern synthetic polymer plastics were developed, including nylon, polyester, and vinyl, among others. Of all the synthetic plastics, the softer types are generally less tolerable for sensitive persons. This is because chemical ingredients called *plasticizers* are added to these products to give them greater flexibility, and these ingredients are often particularly odorous and bothersome.

If you find that typical plastic goods are unacceptable to you, in many cases you can still find satisfactory substitutes available. For example, plastic food-storage containers can be replaced with glass containers. Also, typical plastic wrap can often be replaced by cellophane. In addition, you might find that using plastic garbage bags is unnecessary, if you use brown grocery bags instead. The list goes on.

However, if you find that you really do need to use plastic garbage bags in your home, you might consider purchasing only those brands that are unscented, especially if you're a sensitive person. (Surprising to many people, some brands of garbage bags are now being manufactured with synthetic scents that are quite odorous.) You might also consider buying brands made with at least some recycled plastic. Fortunately, recycled and unscented plastic garbage bags are often available at your local supermarkets, alternative grocery stores, discount stores, and hardware stores. One mail-order source is **The Seventh Generation**.

Incidentally, concern over plastic bags' biodegradability may be overblown in many cases. For example, if the bags wind up in landfills, very little of anything can be expected to biodegrade in such situations.

CELLOPHANE

Often *cellophane* is suggested for sensitive individuals as a substitute for plastic wrap. But what is cellophane? Cellophane is actually a transparent film that is derived primarily from wood and cotton fibers. The fibers are softened in a solution of *caustic soda* and *carbon bisulfide* that breaks down *cellulose* (the tough resilient material making up the walls of the plant cells). The resulting gluey substance is then formed into clear, filmy sheets. Interestingly, the word cellophane was created by combining the word cellulose with *diaphanes* (Greek for transparent).

First developed back in 1892, cellophane was the first clear packaging film ever made. Today, it remains the only packaging film that will not soften when exposed to heat. However, cellophane has other pluses as well. Fortunately, it's produced from renewable natural materials, is biodegradable, and has virtually no odor. Unfortunately, cellophane also has certain negatives associated with it. It tears relatively easily, can't cling or be molded easily around what is being wrapped, and becomes brittle and yellow with age. Because of these drawbacks, plastic films, such as vinyl (polyvinyl chloride or PVC) and polypropylene, have nearly replaced cellophane since the 1960s, except in a few applications.

Although cellophane is no longer common, it's still possible for consumers to find and use cellophane products. For example, cellophane bags (which come in a variety of sizes and can be sealed shut using standard paper-covered wire twisties), as well as cellophane wrap sold on rolls, can be bought from **Janice Corp.** and **The Living Source.**

(Note: For information on cellophane tape, see *Tapes* in *Chapter 12: Home Workshop and Garage.*)

FIRE EXTINGUISHERS

Since the human race discovered fire, people have been afraid of uncontrolled blazes. Virtually all of us still are—and with good reason. Fires can quickly destroy our belongings and wreck our lives. Therefore, it behooves every household to be equipped with appropriate fire extinguishers that are handy, effective, and in good working order. Because quite a few models are now available to choose from, this section will acquaint you with the basic types and where they are best used.

WHAT IS FIRE?

To best know how to combat fire, it's a good idea to understand what exactly fire is. By simple definition, fire is a form of combustion that occurs when a material is ignited in the presence of oxygen, producing light, heat, and flames. Oxygen is required both to initially ignite the fire and to sustain it, even though the oxygen doesn't burn itself. On a molecular level, fires are actually rapidly occurring chain reactions. Without oxygen, the chain reaction stops. Therefore, depriving fires of their chief oxygen source—air (air contains 21% oxygen)—is one of the most basic firefighting approaches.

The other basic firefighting method is to introduce *fire-retardant chemicals.* Fire-retardant chemicals are designed to stop the fire's chain reactions by "mopping up" the extremely reactive *free radicals* (the unstable atoms or molecules having unpaired electrons) that actually perpetuate a fire. (In a fire, reactive free radicals grab electrons from stable molecules, making these donor molecules into reactive free radicals, and so on. However, if fire-retardant chemicals "mop up" the free radicals, the chain reaction stops and the fire goes out.)

While the explanation of what fire is may sound somewhat benign, everyone knows the potential destruction fires can bring about. Every year thousands of in-home fires burn furnishings, the homes themselves, and the occupants. However, fires also produce extremely dangerous invisible *combustion gases,* as well as smoke. In many cases, the smoke and combustion gases, from even an extremely small short-lived fire with just a few flames, can quickly spread throughout an entire house and become absorbed into virtually everything. Unfortunately, smoky odors are very difficult to remove. However, *ozone* (O_3, a very reactive unstable form of oxygen) produced by ozone-generating machines is sometimes helpful in eliminating smoky smells (see *Ozone Generators* in *Chapter 9: Indoor Air*).

Yet, while the damage from smoke (and combustion gases) to a home's interior can be bad, the potential effects on the occupants from exposure to these airborne substances can be even worse. Interestingly, although it's dangerous to breathe the smoke and gases created by burning natural materials, it's far more devastating to inhale the extremely toxic substances produced by many synthetic materials as they burn. For example, certain man-made plastics, when they're on fire, can create the extremely toxic gas *phosgene*, which has been used as a chemical warfare agent. It should be little wonder then that the results of inhaling smoke and combustion gases from an in-home fire can include respiratory distress, severe lung damage, suffocation, and/or poisoning. Not surprisingly, far more people are harmed and killed by these combustion by-products than by burning.

HOME FIRE-PREVENTION BASICS

Remember: When it comes to home fires, you should be well-informed and prepared. Post the fire department's emergency phone number by every telephone, along with your own address and phone number. Often in a panic situation, remembering something as simple as your own street number becomes difficult. Have appropriate fire extinguishers and smoke detectors strategically placed in your home and garage (see *Smoke Detectors* in *Chapter 9: Indoor Air*). Also, have an escape plan. Your local fire department should have informational materials available on appropriate strategies for preventing and dealing with home fires.

SIMPLE FIREFIGHTING STRATEGIES

At the moment they start, many types of very small fires can often be extinguished quickly by smothering. Of course, this is simple oxygen deprivation. In practice, a pot lid can often quickly put out a grease fire in a pan. Also, a boot or shoe can effectively stifle an escaped fireplace ember that has landed on the carpet.

Of course, many people believe water is the best and simplest means to put out a fire. However, water has its limitations. With some types of fire, it can actually make a bad situation worse. For instance, water should never be used on grease fires because it can cause dangerous splattering. Also, water should never be used to douse fires involving electric wires or appliances because the risk of electrocution is far too high.

Baking soda is another substance often considered an easy, universal fire stopper. Baking soda works effectively on grease fires and on electrical fires, but it's not very effective on burning plastic, paper, fabric, or wood. If you plan to rely on a box of baking soda for firefighting, it's necessary to actually have at least one full box (or better yet, more) conveniently on hand specifically for that purpose.

PORTABLE FIRE EXTINGUISHERS

For effective firefighting, peace of mind, and sometimes to meet legal requirements or to lower your insurance premiums, it's important to have portable fire extinguishers handy and available for quick use throughout your home. Quick use is imperative because these portable devices work best on small fires; they aren't intended to be capable of much more than that. Many experts believe that, ideally, you should have a portable fire extinguisher placed in at least your kitchen, your garage, and your home workshop, as well as having one unit located in the central portion of your house. It's also suggested that if your home has several levels, you should have at least one extinguisher on each floor.

It's also extremely important to have the right kind of fire extinguisher in a particular area. An extinguisher should be designed to cope with the specific types of fires likely to occur in the locations they are to serve. After you've purchased and conveniently placed all your fire extinguishers, it's then important to make sure that you and all your family members know how to actually operate them. It's vital that each of you read the label directions thoroughly before the panic of a fire situation occurs. (Don't test-spray them, however; you only need to understand how to use them.)

Commonly, modern portable fire extinguishers consist of a canister filled with an *extinguishing agent*, a pressure-producing device, and a nozzle or hose for dispersal. To work properly, many extinguishers must have adequate internal pressure. Therefore, you'll want to check all your extinguishers' pressure gauges at least once a year. If you find the pressures inadequate, call your local fire department for advice on where to get your fire extinguishers recharged. Sometimes, the fire department itself will recharge your extinguishers free or at a minimal charge.

FIRE TYPE CLASSIFICATIONS

Although virtually all home fires are rapid molecular chain reactions requiring oxygen, there are certain differences in fires, based on exactly what is being burned. Actually, however, research has shown there are only three basic in-home fire classifications to which virtually *every* combustible material and substance found in a house belong. It's also been determined which firefighting methods work best against each of these three fire types.

The three fire classifications are known as *Type A, Type B,* and *Type C.* Type A fires involve the burning of common combustible materials such as wood, paper, fabric, many plastics, and rubber. Type B fires are burning flammable fluids including gasoline, oil, kitchen grease, tar, oil-based paints, and also natural gas. Type C involve burning electrical equipment such as wiring, electronic devices, and electric appliances.

It should be noted that fire extinguishers capable of handling the A and B classifications are also rated for the relative fire sizes they can adequately handle. In other words, a extinguisher designated 2A has double the fire-extinguishing capacity of a 1A model. When a fire extinguisher is labeled for Type C fires, it simply means the *extinguishing agent* can't conduct electricity. There are no numerical prefixes used to rate Type C extinguishers. Often, fire-prevention specialists advise that your kitchen fire extinguisher be a BC type, while the others in your home be multipurpose ABC units. Of course, buying an extinguisher with a higher AB numerical prefix (such as 2A40BC) has more firefighting capacity than one with a lower numerical prefix (such as 1A10BC).

FIRE EXTINGUISHER TYPES

The first truly modern portable extinguishers were *soda-acid extinguishers.* These were designed with a sodium bicarbonate/water solution-filled container under another container holding sulfuric acid. When the extinguisher was turned over, the contents of the two canisters mixed and formed carbon dioxide gas. This pressurized gas then forced a liquid out through the hose to extinguish the fire.

Today, soda-acid extinguishers are still found in some older buildings. However, for the most part, they've been gradually replaced by other types of extinguishers. The following sections will discuss the models that are now commonly available for home use.

Ammonium Phosphate (Dry Chemical)

Ammonium-phosphate dry-chemical fire extinguishers are generally called *multipurpose extinguishers*. They have ABC ratings, and therefore will work against all home fire classifications. (Numerical prefixes, if present, depend on the particular model.

With these extinguishers, *monammonium phosphate* is the extinguishing agent. When it's dispersed, it's a fine powder. Therefore, you should keep the dispersal spray away from your face to avoid inhaling these dusty chemicals. Because this fine chemical powder can be broadly distributed, cleanup can sometimes be tedious after spraying it. A dry-chemical ammonium phosphate extinguisher will put out an electrical fire but it will most likely ruin electronic equipment.

Sodium Bicarbonate

Sodium bicarbonate fire extinguishers simply use baking soda powder as their *extinguishing agent*. These units are rated BC to counter grease, oil, and electrical fires. (Numerical prefixes, if present, depend on the model.) Sodium bicarbonate extinguishers create no odor and clean up problems are minimal. As stated earlier, baking soda doesn't work against Type A fires: wood, paper, fabric, or plastic fires.

Carbon Dioxide

Carbon dioxide fire extinguishers work only against Type C electrical fires. When carbon dioxide units are activated, they release extremely cold, snow-like carbon dioxide particles. These smother the fire and then immediately vaporize. Carbon dioxide extinguishers pose little odor or cleanup problems. However, because they are not recommended for other fire types, their effectiveness is limited.

Halon

Halon fire extinguishers work well against Type C electrical fires. Unlike multipurpose dry-chemical extinguishers, halon does not damage electronics. However, these extinguishers contain *liquefied halocarbon gases* (carbon compounds with chlorine or fluorine, etc.), which have been shown to damage the Earth's protective ozone layer. As a result, after 1994, halon fire extinguishers will no longer be sold.

SUGGESTED HOME FIRE EXTINGUISHERS

For your kitchen, the sodium bicarbonate fire extinguisher, First Alert Kitchen KFE2 (**BRK Electronics Corp.**), has been highly recommended in several consumer magazines. These units come in white canisters with a convenient mounting bracket. They are available at many local hardware and discount stores. If you're unable to locate them, call the company for the nearest dealer.

For other areas in your home and garage, dry-chemical ammonium phosphate extinguishers having ABC ratings are probably the best choice. First

Alert Multi-Purpose FEA10 (**BRK Electronics Corp.**) has been cited as a particularly good unit. This model is rated as 1A10BC. Another very similar extinguisher is the Kidde Fire Away 110 (**Walter Kidde**). Both of these are generally sold in hardware and discount stores. If necessary, call the manufacturers for their nearest dealers. While chemically sensitive people might be bothered by the powder dispensed by these extinguishers, combustion by-products, smoke, and a fire itself would be of much greater concern.

HOUSEHOLD STORAGE

From ancient times, people have used baskets, bags made from animal skins, clay pots, hollow gourds, and many other things, to hold their belongings. And today, it's just as important to properly store items you want to keep. This usually means finding cabinets and containers that will keep your possessions free of dust, pests, and moisture.

However, before storing any item, it's best to honestly assess whether you really need to save it. Too often people go to the trouble and expense of storing things they'll never, or at best, rarely ever use again. Therefore, you might consider simplifying your housekeeping by thinning out unnecessary (but stored anyway) knickknacks, clothing, reading material, and household furnishings. You can often sell them, give them away, or simply throw them out. A good way to start is to dispose of stored items that haven't been used for at least five years.

CLOSETS

Closets are commonly the first place to store items you want to keep. Unfortunately, closets quickly become haphazardly stuffed. As a result, what's inside can become nearly inaccessible, lost, forgotten, or even damaged. To counter this tendency, the following sections offer some closet-organization ideas and products.

CLOSET RACKS AND SHELVING SYSTEMS

A good storage approach for nearly all homes is to logically utilize the available closet space. When you do this, the goal is to create closets that contain the maximum amount of items and still be user-friendly—that is, easy to keep clean and easy to keep organized.

One method for accomplishing all this is to install wire-mesh closet-shelving systems and racks. With wire-mesh units, you can custom design your closet interior to suit specific needs. You may want to do the actual design and installation work yourself or hire a remodeling contractor or a professional closet designer. To find a qualified professional, check your local classified telephone directory under appropriate listings. Before agreeing for them to do the work however, be sure to get a price estimate, estimated completion date, information on guarantees or warranties, and an idea of what specific materials will be used.

It should be noted that much of the wire-mesh shelving available today is vinyl-coated steel. This material has certain drawbacks. Vinyl has the capacity to emit chemical odors when it's new, which are often especially bothersome to certain sensitive people. Also, as vinyl ages it has a tendency to crack and become unsightly.

Perhaps a better alternative would be to buy baked-on epoxy-finished wire shelving. One company that manufactures this type of shelving is **Lee/Rowan** and their units are available in a wide variety of shapes and sizes. Especially convenient are their freestanding racks that come with wire-mesh drawers. To find the nearest dealer, contact the company. Another possible shelving-system option you might consider are the good-quality, heavy-duty metal units that can be mail-ordered from **Hold Everything**.

COAT HANGERS

For many years, common coat hangers were made of thin steel wire, often painted or coated. Today, many household coat hangers are made of molded plastic. However, to avoid rust problems, bending, breaking, and/or synthetic materials, consider purchasing heavyweight anodized-aluminum hangers. (Anodizing is a protective coating on aluminum to prevent it from pitting and acquiring a dark discoloration due to oxidation.) Because these hangers are ruggedly constructed and can't rust, you can even hang wet articles on them to dry. Heavyweight anodized-aluminum hangers are often available in local department and discount stores. One mail-order source is **Colonial Garden Kitchens**. It should be noted that these hangers are more costly than their steel wire or plastic counterparts, but they're practically indestructible, so they'll never need to be replaced.

Another good hanger option is to use traditional wood/steel hangers. Like the heavy-duty anodized-aluminum hangers, these hangers are strong, made of natural materials, and rather expensive. However, if they become wet, the steel parts can rust (if they aren't painted or coated). Wood/steel hangers can still be purchased in some local department stores. You can also mail-order them from **The Vermont Country Store**. All-wood hangers with metal hooks are available from **Hold Everything**.

If you're a sensitive person who can't tolerate plastic but can't afford expensive wood or aluminum hangers either, the best solution is to use thin, coated-steel, wire hangers. You can still sometimes buy thin, steel-wire hangers in some department and discount stores, and from local dry cleaners. If you must buy your steel coat hangers from a dry cleaner, if at all possible, choose new hangers rather than used ones that could have absorbed dry-cleaning solvent odors. However, some dry cleaners only offer used ones for sale.

Sometimes, but not always, used, dry-cleaner coat hangers can be made tolerable. One method to accomplish this is to first gently wash them in a solution of baking soda and warm water. Then rinse them off with clear water and carefully dry them with a soft towel. (Gentle handling and towel drying are important so that the painted surfaces aren't damaged. Chips and scratches could eventually become rusty.) Next, hang the coat hangers outside in the sun for several days in dry, uncontaminated surroundings. When they no longer seem bothersome to you, bring them inside. You can then place one of the cleaned hangers on your nightstand near your pillow. If you're able to sleep well throughout the night, they're probably safe for use.

METAL CONTAINERS

Especially for sensitive persons, metal cabinets, trunks, and containers make excellent storage units. Often, objects with odors you personally find intolerable can be kept safely inside metal containers. Metal acts as an effective barrier in isolating unwanted smells released by stored items so they don't reach the room air. However, at the same time, you should be aware that just one odorous item stored in a closed metal container can contaminate the entire contents with the odor. This point extends to the interior walls of the container itself. Therefore, carefully consider what you plan to store together inside any metal container. The following sections, offer suggestions on using metal containers and some sources of where to get them.

METAL CABINETS

Large metal cabinets with doors can be used to store just about anything. This includes out-of-season clothing, food, books, tools, etc. Sometimes the purchase of one or more of these relatively inexpensive cabinets can solve most of your storage needs.

These days, metal storage units are available in several sizes and colors, with varying interior configurations. Some cabinets have interiors with permanently mounted shelves. Other models have adjustable shelves or wardrobe-style clothing rods. In addition, certain units are made with key locks or are designed to accept padlocks. When you're ready to buy a metal cabinet, check your local office-supply stores, as well as discount stores and hardware stores. In addition, department stores, such as **Sears, Roebuck and Co.**, often stock them.

METAL TRUNKS

Another metal storage option you might consider are metal trunks. These are particularly good for storing toys, scrapbooks, sweaters, out-of-season clothing, and/or blankets. However, if you decide on a metal trunk, check to see if it's really all-metal.

Unfortunately these days, many metal trunks are actually lined with particleboard, strandboard, hardboard, plywood, or even cardboard. Formaldehyde released by these materials, especially the man-made wood components, can accumulate inside these trunks and be absorbed by everything stored in them. Formaldehyde can be irritating to the mucous membranes of most people who breath it, and it can be an intolerable substance for sensitive persons. All-metal trunks might be found at department stores, army/navy surplus stores, and luggage shops.

METAL BOXES

Metal boxes can work well for storing smaller items such as stamps, pens and pencils, crayons, and sewing supplies. Of course, one popular type of metal box is the *tinware* used for holiday candy and baked goods. (Actually, these are not really made of tin, but nowadays are made of steel, although many do have an interior tin coating.) In addition to these seasonal metal boxes, small, colorful knickknack metal boxes are usually available throughout the year in kitchen departments, gift shops, and discount stores.

Another clever storage option is to use tinware canisters. Flours, grains, coffee, and baked goods store well in these—that is, if the tops seal tightly. Often you'll find you can purchase tinware canisters in the kitchenware department of local stores. However, an even better choice would be to buy stainless-steel canisters, which are much more durable. One mail-order source for these is **Williams-Sonoma**. In addition, other kitchenware catalogs such as **Colonial Garden Kitchens** and **The Wooden Spoon** usually carry them from time to time.

Large metal tinware-style bread boxes are sometimes sold with tightly fitting lids, but are generally harder to find than smaller metal boxes. These look somewhat like giant shoe boxes and are perfect for storing note cards, art supplies, wrapping paper, cleaning products, etc. If you can buy several, label them on the outside so you will know what they contain and stack them in a closet. To find tinware-style bread boxes, check your local department and discount stores.

An interesting metal storage container worth considering is a hinged, unfolding metal box with interior storage trays. Boxes like these are good for holding spools of thread or other sewing notions. They also make good jewelry boxes—if they have divided compartments, and you line the trays with soft fabric. These metal unfolding boxes are available at stores that sell hand tools, especially mechanics' tools. Also, check sports departments for metal fishing-tackle boxes. These are becoming harder to find now that plastic versions are available, but they can still be found in a few stores.

METAL GARBAGE CANS

Small (2' and under) *galvanized* garbage cans often work surprisingly well as storage containers, especially for sensitive people. (Galvanized garbage cans are actually made of steel with a protective zinc coating that helps prevent rusting.) For example, they can hold bulk quantities of laundry powders such as unscented borax or washing soda. They can also be used for dry storage of cereal, wild bird seed, cat food, dog food, or cat litter-box filler. Small metal garbage cans can also be used to hold magazines, video tapes, and toys.

One special job for metal garbage cans is serving as a clothing hamper for sensitive people. Often, metal garbage cans are good for this function because the metal doesn't allow often-bothersome soiled clothing, perfume, tobacco, and perspiration odors from dissipating into the surrounding air. However, it should be pointed out that any dirty clothing should be laundered fairly quickly and not kept for extended periods in a sealed metal container because the moisture can't evaporate. If damp clothing is left inside a can too long, musty odors or mildew could result. Important note: Metal garbage cans used as hampers should be routinely washed with an unscented, tolerable cleaner, rinsed with clear water, and placed in the sun for airing. To buy a small galvanized metal garbage can, check your local hardware , department, and discount stores.

GLASS CONTAINERS

Glass storage containers have many advantages over their more popular plastic counterparts. Because of its transparency, glass offers a totally clear view of what's stored inside it. Also, glass is made from common natural ingredients and is completely recyclable. For sensitive individuals, perhaps the best trait is the fact that it's chemically inert and odorless. Therefore, it won't react with stored food and give it a plastic taste or odor. Furthermore, properly sealed glass containers isolate the odors of what's stored in them.

Of course, the biggest drawback to glass is that it's breakable. Therefore, it's important to take care when you handle and store glass containers in order to prevent them from cracking or shattering. After all, broken glass not only means the damage or loss of your stored contents, but it also can cause you personal injury. This is one of the primary reasons plastic has steadily replaced glass containers since World War II.

RECYCLED GLASS CONTAINERS

Despite widespread use of plastic containers these days, many grocery items are still sold in glass bottles and jars. Once these have been emptied, washed, and dried, they can be easily used for storage purposes. For example, you can use glass jars with screw lids (such as those used for mayonnaise or nut butter) to store screws, bolts, and/or washers. In the bathroom, glass jars can be used to store cotton balls and cotton swabs. In the kitchen, they can hold spices, tea, and leftovers, etc.

NEW GLASS CONTAINERS

Of course, you can buy new glass containers that have actually been designed for home storage needs. One type, glass canning jars with wire clamps and rubber-ringed glass lids, are a very good choice for holding a variety of food items from grains to leftovers. This is because their tightly sealing tops help prevent air, mold, insects, and other undesirables from getting into the stored contents. You'll find that these glass storage containers are usually available in several sizes. If you're interested in buying them, check your local kitchenware departments, gourmet cooking shops, discount stores, hardware stores, and wherever else you would expect home-canning supplies to be sold. In addition, one mail-order source is **Colonial Garden Kitchens**.

Rectangular, heavy, molded-glass food-storage sets with glass lids were once common in American homes. However, for the most part, they virtually disappeared when lightweight plastic storage containers began being marketed. However, somewhat surprisingly, these are still being sold by **Williams-Sonoma**. For other glass-container possibilities, check local kitchen departments and gourmet shops, as well as specialty kitchen catalogs such as **Colonial Garden Kitchens** and **The Wooden Spoon**. (For even more possibilities, see *Glass, Glass-Ceramic, and Pottery Cookware* above.)

WOODEN CONTAINERS

Early storage containers were often made of wood. Today, they remain attractive, natural, and useful storage choices.

WOODEN WARDROBES AND CABINETS

(See *Solid Wood Furniture, Unfinished and Kit Furniture*, and also *Antique Furniture* in *Chapter 5: Interior Decoration*.)

WOODEN TRUNKS

In many furniture stores, hope chests or storage chests can be found in a number of styles and with a variety of wood finishes. However, many of these are lined with cedar wood, which is extremely aromatic. Of course, the cedar lining is meant protect stored items from clothing moths. Unfortunately, it's been shown that cedar apparently does little to deter moths. However, the cedar odors will be absorbed by virtually everything stored in these chests. For sensitive persons in particular, this would be a very unacceptable situation because they often react negatively to cedar's natural terpene odors.

Instead of buying a new, cedar-lined chest, consider acquiring an old wooden trunk. These can be used for storing out-of-season clothing, linens, scrapbooks, or games. (You absolutely should not use one of these as a toy chest for small children because an open hinged lid could easily fall shut on a child.) Sometimes you can find wooden trunks in antique stores, flea markets, and garage sales. If the one you're interested in has already been restored, you'll want to consider whether the finishes and interior lining (often fabric or wallpaper) will be tolerable for you, if you're a sensitive individual.

On the other hand, if you come across an unrestored wooden trunk, check to see if it's moldy or very musty. If it is, you may never get all the mildew smells out of it, so it would probably be best not to buy it. However, if it appears in good condition, it's advisable to go ahead and buy it and either strip the paint and finish off it yourself or have the work professionally done. Once it's been stripped, it should be sanded, coated with tolerable finishes, and fitted with tolerable interior materials. (For more on refinishing, see *Antique Furniture* in *Chapter 5: Interior Decoration*. See also *Wallpaper* in *Chapter 5: Interior Decorating*, as well as *Testing Paints and Finishes* and other appropriate headings in *Chapter 10: Home Workshop and Garage*.) Of course, when doing any refinishing work, be sure to wear the appropriate protective gear and not actually use the trunk until the new finish odors have dissipated. If you are very sensitive, it would be wise to have someone else do all the refinishing work for you.

WOODEN BOXES

Small wooden boxes can be not only decorative accessories but they also can be practical storage units. They can hold sewing notions, coins and other small collectibles, stationery, pens and pencils, and clothing accessories such as scarves, handkerchiefs, and belts.

Fortunately, new wooden boxes, such as Shaker hardwood round boxes with lids, are now becoming popular again. You might be able to find them in local craft stores or furniture stores. By mail order, you can buy them in either cherry or walnut from **Shaker Shops West. Shaker Workshop** handles only the cherry Shaker-style boxes. Of the two woods, cherry is often less odorous and better tolerated by sensitive individuals than walnut.

If you find serviceable antique wooden boxes, the odds are they've absorbed perfume, tobacco, and other odors over the years. If they don't seem too bothersome, you might go ahead and purchase the boxes and let them air outside in dry, uncontaminated surroundings for a few days to several weeks. This often helps. However, if it doesn't help enough, you might want to refinish your wooden boxes. (For more on refinishing, see *Wooden Trunks* above.)

INDOOR PEST CONTROL

Let's face it, coping with household pests is unpleasant. Quite frankly, it's often also frustrating and upsetting. No one likes to think they actually have unwanted creatures in their house or go through the actual procedures of getting rid of them. However, instead of using typical toxic chemicals to control pests, try using safer alternative approaches, so at least you yourself won't be harmed in the process. To help you do this, the following sections suggest less-toxic, but still effective, pest-preventive and exterminating methods.

SIMPLE PEST-PREVENTIVE MEASURES

Unfortunately, certain pests are not only unsightly but also can be destructive or carry diseases. And, of course, virtually no one willingly chooses them as housemates. Yet, perhaps unknowingly, many homes almost seem to put out pest "welcome mats."

If you don't want pests sharing your home, the first line of defense is to do everything possible not to attract them. This means there should be no conveniently accessible sources of pest meals in your house. Therefore, all your tables, countertops, and floors should be kept free of crumbs and spilled liquids. Also, all your food should be stored in tightly sealed containers inside closed cabinets. Furthermore, to deter clothing moths, that can devour wool and other fabrics, store your clean, natural-fiber clothing in tightly sealed bags, etc. So as not to readily invite termites, keep dead shrubs and woody debris away from your house foundation.

You should also keep in mind that your home should not have appealing habitats for pests to live and nest in. Therefore, clean all the excess clutter from your home and dust and vacuum frequently. One very important thing to do is to be sure to eliminate any moisture problems in your home. This is because many household pests are extremely fond of taking up residence in damp environments. Therefore, be sure to fix any leaky pipes, wet basements, dank crawl spaces, and overly humid rooms. (For information on high humidity and ventilation fans, see *High Humidity* in *Chapter 9: Indoor Air*.)

Finally, your house should be as completely sealed from the outside as is practicable. This should make most pest entry extremely difficult, if not impossible. To do this, make sure any cracks in the foundations, walls, and attic spaces are sealed (see *Caulks* in *Chapter 10: Home Workshop and Garage*). Also check to see that all the exterior doors close completely when shut. If they don't, you'll need to add weather-stripping or perhaps do other repair measures. In addition, you'll want to check that your window screens are in good condition and repair or replace them if necessary.

COPING WITH PESTS

If, despite your best efforts, pests still find their way into your home, the next step is deciding whether or not you can tolerate their presence. Actually, some creatures are classified as pests even though they may be quite beneficial. This is certainly true for certain small, non-dangerous spiders. Other pests such as silverfish, which admittedly look rather disgusting, are apparently harmless. At their worst, its seems silverfish usually only eat some paper or glue.

However, while a nonpoisonous spider or a few silverfish may be acceptable, if large populations develop you may decide they all have to go. Swarms of anything in your home are not a tolerable situation. Of course, other pests, such as rats, wouldn't be welcome even if only one found its way into your home. When pests must be removed from residences, they're usually either taken outside or killed. Using methods and chemical compounds to stop reproduction or maturation of the next generation is a third option. For the most part, this approach isn't yet commonly used, although methods against certain pests are now available.

In most pest-control situations, extermination is the management method chosen. This may involve recruiting the pest's natural biological enemy, such as obtaining a cat to control mice. More often though, something deadly to the pest is used. This could be benign to humans and the environment, such as sticky fly paper, or a potentially dangerous, but legal, synthetic organic chemical, such as the termiticide dursban.

TYPICAL PESTICIDES

Chemical pesticides derived from nature have been popular for centuries against many types of household pests. In this century, scores of petroleum-derived substances toxic to pests were introduced. Unfortunately, it was not until fairly recently that the effects of most of these newer pesticides on non-targeted creatures was more completely understood.

EARLY PESTICIDES

These days, most Americans commonly use chemical applications to solve their household pest problems. Actually, this is not a new concept. In the first century AD, the ancient Greeks had already recognized that *arsenic* (a toxic mineral element) would exterminate many pest populations. In the Orient, the Chinese were also using arsenic compounds as well as various natural-oil extracts. By the 1700s in Europe, both tobacco juice (whose nicotine is poisonous) and *pyrethrum* (chrysanthemum flower heads) were found to be effective pesticides.

Because of great advancements in chemistry, the 1800s saw the introduction of pesticides created from copper oxide and a combination of copper and arsenic salts. Later during the 1930s, pesticides based on *inorganic heavy metals*, such as lead and mercury, were developed. However, these heavy-metal compounds were usually not used around homes but only on growing crops in the fields. In any case, because they accumulated in the soil and were only effective at levels that were found to be toxic to non-pest species, they have since been virtually abandoned.

MODERN ORGANIC PESTICIDES

The so-called modern pesticide era began with the creation of *synthetic organic pesticides* that eventually replaced the overtly toxic heavy-metal pesticides. However, it's now also known that they, too, have potentially serious negative consequences.

Modern Organic Pesticide Types

Many modern pesticides are known as organic pesticides. This term doesn't mean pure, natural, and untainted as it does with organic food. As applied to pesticides, the word organic means that these compounds contain carbon atoms (generally occurring in chains), and it's these carbon atoms that happen to be the basis of the molecules making up all living organisms. (Actually, organic pesticides also contain hydrogen and may include other elements including oxygen, sulfur, phosphorus, chlorine, bromine, fluorine, and/or nitrogen). Most organic pesticides are man-made compounds derived from petroleum, which itself ultimately originated from microscopic aquatic organisms that lived millions of years ago.

Surprising to many people, organic pesticides first began to be used in 1920s. However, it was not until 1939 when the organic compound *DDT* (*dichlorodiphenyltrichloroethane*), (which had first been synthesized back in 1874) was observed to kill most pests while seemingly not harming humans or the environment, that organic pesticides became popular. Soon, DDT was sprayed on almost everything and everyone with a pest problem, or a potential one. It became known as an inexpensive "chemical wonder." Its success directly inspired the creation of other *organochlorine pesticides* (organic pesticide compounds containing chlorine), primarily between 1940 and 1970.

Other organic pesticides, classified as *organophosphate* types (organic pesticide compounds containing phosphate), were introduced after World War II. Interestingly, these formulations were based on Nazi research.

Modern Organic Pesticides' Toxic Consequences

The effects on humans and other non-pest populations of being exposed to some of the older, natural, toxic, pesticide compounds such as arsenic and heavy metal-based compounds were soon apparent and became fairly well known. However, this was not true with many of the synthetic organochlorine pesticides. Unfortunately, since their introduction, they've been found to have toxic side effects that had for years been unsuspected by most people. Actually, it was Rachel Carson's book *Silent Spring*, originally published in 1962, that helped arouse public concern over the possible environmental consequences (to birds, etc.) of these supposedly "safe" pesticides.

Unfortunately, using synthetic, organic-chemical means to eliminate pests has not only harmed nature, but has had a human toll, which has also become evident. Symptoms vary as to dose, chemical composition, type, length of exposure, and the individual. However, certain organochlorine pesticides have been associated with the onset of *chloracne* (a severe and often chronic type of acne due to chlorine compound exposure), lowered sperm counts, *peripheral neuropathy* (nerve damage not associated with the brain and spinal chord such as in the limbs, feet, and hands), and some forms of cancer. New research now indicates some organic-chemical pesticides may actually mimic natural estrogen compounds. It's speculated that such estrogen-like action may lead to hormonal disturbances, which in turn could lead to a variety of abnormal conditions. (This could account for the lowered sperm counts, by the way.) Despite more product warnings and OSHA (the federal government's Occupational Safety and Health Administration) regulations, occupational physicians continue to see patients who have become ill on the job due to the toxicity of these modern pesticides.

Although most pesticide-poisoning cases are, in fact, linked to actually working in pesticide-producing chemical plants or directly using agricultural pesticides on crops, that's not the full extent of the problem. It seems some pesticide-toxicity cases have turned up with homeowners and their families after their houses were treated for termites or other common pests. Probably most of these subsequent illnesses occurred because the pesticide applications were incompetently done. However, in at least some cases, it appears that illness occurred despite "correct" usage. Interestingly, a number of individuals with Multiple Chemical Sensitivity (MCS) firmly believe that they first acquired their condition as a result of a specific organic pesticide application that either occurred at their home or at their workplace.

Despite having some knowledge that synthetic organic pesticides can be harmful, it seems most Americans still routinely turn to them to solve their household-pest predicaments. It's easy to understand why. Consumer-oriented "bug hotels," rodent pellets, and anti-flying insect aerosol cans are conveniently sold in colorful, handy-sized packages in nearly all hardware, grocery, and discount stores. These products take little physical effort or money to quickly kill many problem creatures. And for widespread or serious pest problems, most people still contract pest-management companies to spray, inject, or fumigate their homes with synthetic organic pesticides.

ALTERNATIVE PEST-CONTROL MEASURES

Fortunately, if you want to use safer, less-toxic pest-control alternatives, there are quite a few available. In the following sections, you'll be introduced to a number of them.

ALTERNATIVE PESTICIDES AND CAPTURE METHODS IN GENERAL

Although most people still prefer the quick, sure effectiveness of synthetic organic pesticides, growing numbers of people prefer to use less-toxic means. As a result, pesticides derived from natural plant extracts are again becoming more available. These include chrysanthemum-derived *pyrethrum* (powdered chrysanthemum flower heads) and *pyrethrin* (a liquid chrysanthemum flower-head extract), as well as a variety of tobacco-based products whose active ingredients are *nicotine compounds*.

In addition, relatively safe powders such as *boric acid, diatomaceous earth* (a fine silica powder made up of the cell walls of microscopic algae), and even *talc* are regaining some popularity as pesticides. Then too, in certain circumstances, high heat or electric shock are being utilized as pest eliminators. Also, a wider range of trapping products are now being marketed and more homemade trapping methods are being devised and used. These include snap traps, live-capture traps, special sticky-substance traps, *pheromone* traps (sticky traps that use sex-attractant chemicals to capture mature adults, usually males), and even lights over water. All these approaches generally target specific pests. They can be placed and removed at any time, and they generally create little or no human or environmental side effects.

ALTERNATIVE PEST DETERRENTS IN GENERAL

Using *pest deterrents*—which are meant to discourage the presence of pests but not designed to kill or capture them—is another less-toxic approach to dealing with household pests. Like the other alternative methods mentioned above, these are nearly always less toxic than using synthetic organic pesticides. Therefore, *oil of pennyroyal* (extract from a mint family plant) and *eucalyptus oil* (oil from eucalyptus trees) are regaining favor. With these particular oils (and similar ones), it's their rather intense natural odor that tends to act as an effective pest repellent in certain situations. (Of course, they aren't uniformly effective against all pests.) Unfortunately, some humans, especially many sensitive individuals, also find their odor repelling.

Another method of deterring pests is using *physical barriers*. Of course, screening and netting are obvious examples of how simple nontoxic mesh fabrics can easily bar mosquito, spider, and other insect entry. However, there are also less-well known barrier approaches. For example, it's been shown that having a pit of 12-grit sand surrounding your home's foundation can act as a fairly effective obstacle to subterranean termites.

Other types of pest deterrents include *ultrasonic units,* which have been promoted to ward off a wide variety of household pest species. Ultrasonic units are said to work because the ultrahigh-pitched whine they emit is almost unbearable to most pest species but isn't heard by humans (or cats and dogs). Ultrasonic units vary in size from small battery-operated pendants to fairly large, freestanding, plug-in models. The very small pet pendants are marketed primarily as flea deterrents, and the similar-sized models for people as mosquito deterrents. However, research has established that ultrasonic pest controls are not effective against fleas, rodents, bats, etc. In fact, the Federal Trade Commission has even stated that they are ineffective.

IMPLEMENTING ALTERNATIVE PEST-CONTROL MEASURES

If you have decided you want to use less-toxic pest-control measures in your household, it's important to have alternative home pest-management information on hand. That way, you'll know what to do immediately if a particular pest shows up. While this book can act as a good basic source, it's probably best that you also have more thorough literature on hand (or know where you can get it quickly) to consult when necessary.

Some examples of good alternative pest-control publications are the low-cost, well-researched household-pest fact sheets available from the **Washington Toxic Coalition**. An excellent, small, inexpensive paperback is *Least Toxic Home Pest Control* by Dan Stein. Probably the most complete low-toxicity pest manual is the voluminous 715-page hardback, *Common-Sense Pest Control* by William Olkowski, Sheila Daar, and Helga Olkowski (This is a book you might ask your library to add to their reference collection, if you don't want to purchase it yourself.). In addition, you might want to contact your county extension agent, which sometimes has free informational materials on less-toxic pest control. Finally, check your local library and bookstore to see what appropriate books they may have.

If you find you need more explicit help, contact the authors of *Common-Sense Pest Control* at the **Bio-Integral Resource Center**. This organization offers less-toxic pest-control consultations to its members. You'll also want to check your classified phone directory to see if there is a less-toxic pest-control company nearby you didn't know about.

Unfortunately, at this point, it must be noted that sometimes you may not be able to use the safer pest-control alternatives you'd like to, especially against termites. Sometimes, banks, mortgage institutions, and insurance companies will *only* authorize the use of the familiar, but toxic, chemical termiticides. Also, in certain cases you may not be able to use safe, effective control measures simply because they haven't yet been legally classified as registered pesticides in your state. Finally, it may turn out that it's just plain necessary to spot-treat with toxic synthetic organic pesticides to successfully eliminate a particular infestation. All this is not meant to discourage you from trying to use less-toxic alternative pest control measures, but rather to let you know of the possible problems you may encounter. The good new is, if you're determined to use less-toxic means to control your household pests, in most cases you'll be able to do so with very satisfactory results.

CONTROLLING SPECIFIC PESTS USING ALTERNATIVE MEASURES

The following sections will cover less-toxic treatment suggestions for some of the most common household pests. The pest-control options mentioned are, for the most part, ones that sensitive individuals have often found both effective and tolerable. However, keep in mind that these are only suggestions—not absolute recommendations that you must rigidly follow. Every pest situation is unique. Therefore, it is you yourself who must ultimately determine the extent of your particular pest problem, what solutions you feel would be acceptable, and, in some cases, finding out what regulations and restrictions will apply to your situation. Remember, killing anything is serious business. Therefore, you'll always want to proceed carefully and with forethought regarding your own personal program for household pest management.

CARPENTER ANTS

Carpenter ants can sometimes cause extensive damage to the wood in homes. To combat this pesky insect, this section will explain some ways of eliminating their infestations.

Carpenter Ant Traits

The term carpenter ant is actually a generic name for several large ($1/4$–$1/2$" long) ant species, which are found in many areas of the U.S. Although their color varies with the species, solid black is probably the most common. As it turns out, most of these ants like living in or near wood.

Interestingly, if a carpenter-ant colony decides that the wood they want to live in is your home, you might hear them moving around within your walls. More likely though, you'll find some fine wood dust on your floors, which they pushed out of their tunnels and nests. It seems that most people assume that the carpenter ants are eating their house. Actually, unlike termites, they can't digest wood. They only use wood to meet their housing needs. Their preferred diet is sweet substances such as nectar.

As a rule, carpenter ants are especially attracted to damp wood. This may be because it's simply easier to bore through than dry wood. However, they will go ahead and cut into dry wood if they find they need to. Carpenter-ant infestations often spread through the creation of new _daughter_ or _satellite_ nests. Therefore, the original source of the _daughter nests_ in your home probably came from a _mother nest_ outside. It's likely the ants were able to enter your house through a crack in an outside wall.

Suggested Carpenter Ant-Control Measures

To rid your home of carpenter ants, you'll first need to locate their nest within your home's walls. You may be able to do this by hearing them scurry around or by seeing wood-dust piles. At any rate, once you've found the nests, you'll need to drill small holes through the walls at those particular sites. After that, you can use a pyrethrin (a chrysanthemum flower head extract) spray such as Tri-Die (**Whitmire Research Labs**) on each nest, utilizing a special injection tube that comes with the product. To buy Tri-Die, you'll want to contact the manufacturer for the nearest dealer.

Another option is to actually have the nest-infested wood cut from your walls and replaced with new, unaffected wood. At the same time, finding and destroying the outdoor mother nest is also a good idea. You might be able to accomplish this by following the ants, from where they enter and leave your home, back to their place of origin, usually in dead wood that isn't too far away. Because they tend to be active at night, locating an outdoor nest can be rather challenging. If you are able to find the mother nest, spray it with the same pyrethrin product you used in the house walls.

After any carpenter-ant invasion, it's important to find and repair all the cracks and separations in your home's foundation. This will help prevent any future carpenter ant problems because there will no longer be any easy entry points through which they can pass in and out.

CLOTHING MOTHS

As most people already know, damage to natural-fiber items can be extensive if proper prevention steps are not taken against clothing moths. Fortunately, there are simple, safe approaches that will usually deter them.

Clothing Moth Traits

Clothing moth is a term applied to several small moth pest species. Of these, perhaps the most common is the *webbing clothing moth*. The adults of this particular variety are pale golden with red head hairs. It's not commonly known, but actually it's the clothing moth's larvae—not the winged adults—that are able to damage your clothing. And the $1/2$" long cream-colored larvae have the ability to eat *all* natural fibers, not just wool. However, despite their capacity to bite off and digest these various fibers, the moth larvae would rather eat the oils and food particles found on them.

Wool and Clothing Moths

Why then is moth damage generally associated with wool? Actually, for a several reasons. One is that wool contains the natural oil lanolin (sometimes called sheep grease). Lanolin is an appealing larval food—one the other natural fibers lack. As it turns out, when the larvae attempt to eat the tasty lanolin, the wool fibers get devoured, too. In addition, wool items are usually cleaned less often than their machine-washable counterparts such as those made of cotton or ramie. As a result, human body oils and food crumbs tend to accumulate more so on wool clothing. These are very appealing to the larvae, so as they attempt to feast on these, the wool fibers get eaten, too. Finally, wool and moth damage are linked together because wool clothing and blankets are often stored in closed drawers or chests for months at a time. This creates the ideal conditions for adult female moths to lay their eggs: dark, undisturbed places on or near potential food sources. Once the clothing-moth larvae hatch, their nest (your wool items with its oils and crumbs) becomes both a serving platter as well as dinner.

Safely Preventing Clothing Moth Damage

To counter any potential clothing-moth damage, be sure to clean your natural-fiber items before you store them. Then immediately after they've been cleaned, place them into tightly sealed bags, containers, or storage units. This is, of course, especially important with your wool items.

However, if for some reason, you're unable to clean and quickly store your natural-fiber items in sealed containers of some sort, as an alternative you can tumble your susceptible things in your clothes dryer for about 15 minutes approximately once a month. You could also simply vigorously shake them out. Either of these methods are usually effective deterrents because clothing moth eggs are not firmly attached to the fabric fibers they're on; thus, they usually fall off rather easily. In addition, high heat in a clothes dryer will apparently kill moth eggs, live larvae, and any adults as well. However, high heat might shrink or tighten some natural fibers even if they're dry, so a low-heat setting may be required for certain items.

Concerns Using Certain Clothing Moth Deterrents

Many people believe they can avoid clothing-moth damage by simply storing a special deterrent substance with their stored items. This would be an easy solution. Unfortunately, neither cedar wood, cedar oil, nor potpourri will kill or effectively repel clothing moths. Worse, using *mothballs* (which are commonly made from *pardichlorobenzene (PDCB)*, *naphthalene*, or *camphor*) can be potentially dangerous to both humans and the environment.

Of course, all these popular anti-clothing-moth measures give off strong odors. After all, their intent is to be extremely unpleasant for moths to be around. However, what's often not seriously considered is how tenaciously the fibers of your clothing and other stored items will absorb and hold onto these very same smells, especially from chemical mothballs. This could make your belongings quite bothersome and perhaps even intolerable to you, particularly if you're a sensitive person. Unfortunately, even repeated cleanings and airings can't always remove all these odors.

(For information on clothing-moth treatments on wool items, see *Wool* and also *Is Dry-Cleaning a Problem?* in *Chapter 3: Clothing*, as well as *Wool Blankets* in *Chapter 4: Linens*.)

COCKROACHES

Most everyone abhors cockroaches. To combat them, here are some less-toxic methods you can use.

Cockroach Traits

Cockroaches are flat, long-legged insects that vary in size. However, many are about $1/2$" long. Although there are many species, only a few varieties usually become household pests. These make nests in your home, scavenge for food, and leave their feces behind.

The most common variety of indoor cockroach in the U.S. is probably the brown German cockroach. Fortunately, cockroaches aren't a continuous problem in most houses. (Exceptions may be some houses in warm or hot climates, poorly kept homes, and certain multiple-dwelling buildings.) However, a large percentage of American homes will likely become infested at one time or another for various lengths of time.

If possible, cockroaches are pests you should try to completely eradicate from your home. Besides being unsightly and destructive to food supplies, there is growing suspicion in the medical community that cockroaches are probably linked to the onset of some human illnesses. Very recent research has also suggested that allergies to cockroaches and their feces may be far more common than previously thought.

Using Boric Acid Against Cockroaches

Once they've gotten in your home, cockroaches often find your kitchen particularly appealing. The food, the convenient dark places to nest and hide, and moisture from perhaps under-sink pipes or water lying in automatic defrost refrigerator drip pans (among other damp places) make for ideal cockroach conditions.

To rid your kitchen of cockroaches using less-toxic means, try putting boric acid powder in a small insecticide bulb dispenser. You may be able to buy one of these in a local hardware store or at a pest control company. Once you've filled the bulb, you simply squeeze it to blow the powder into floor or baseboard crevices. It's especially important to do this behind the stove and refrigerator. If you carefully apply the boric acid powder in this way, there's little chance it will ever become airborne and contaminate your food.

Boric acid is a white crystalline substance also known as *orthoboric acid*. It's commonly derived from borax. You can use the pharmacy-grade boric acid powder (which is primarily sold to be mixed with water to make a mild antiseptic) available at some drugstores, or a lesser-grade dyed boric-acid powder packaged as a pesticide. One popular brand of boric-acid pesticide you might already be familiar with is Roach-Prufe (**Copper Brite, Inc.**). This product is often available in hardware stores. However, you can call the manufacturer to find the nearest dealer to you. Important note: Whenever you apply boric acid powder, wear a protective dust mask to prevent inhaling it.

If you plan to use boric acid against cockroaches, be aware that it will not instantly solve your cockroach problems; it will take a certain amount of time to become effective. This is because the boric acid powder must first be tracked back to the cockroach nest on the legs and bodies of some of the insects. From these carrier roaches, it will eventually end up getting on nearly all the other roaches in the nest. Then, as they begin to preen, they'll ingest the powder. Because it's toxic to their systems, they'll finally die.

As it turns out, boric acid powder lasts almost indefinitely, so reapplications are generally unnecessary. When you are confident that the infestation is over, you can leave the powder in the crevices where it will act as a preventive. However, if you would prefer to clean it up, you can vacuum the crevices using an appropriate attachment while wearing a protective dust mask. You could then thoroughly wash baseboard areas with clear water and a sponge while wearing rubber gloves.

Important note: Although boric acid powder is much safer than typical petrochemical insecticides, it is certainly not a totally harmless substance. Therefore, don't let children and pets get access to it.

Using Sticky Roach Traps Against Cockroaches

An alternative to using boric acid powder against cockroaches is to use *sticky roach traps*. These are usually just small cardboard boxes or sometimes metal containers with an entrance hole and a gluey substance inside, along with a roach-appealing bait. (Note, some sticky roach traps may have a pesticide within them as well.) Once the roaches go inside, they usually become permanently stuck. If you'd like to use this approach, you can try placing three or four traps in each problem area in your home. As they fill up, they should be replaced.

You should be aware that sticky roach traps will not have any effect on the insect nests themselves. Therefore, these traps are more of a reduction measure than an elimination method. The Victor Holdfast (**Woodstream Corp.**) sticky roach trap is one brand that's apparently both safe and effective. It's available at some local hardware and department stores or you can call the company for a nearby dealer. If you'd like to buy sticky roach traps by mail, **N.E.E.D.S.** sells them.

FLEAS

Fleas can be extremely irritating and their infestations can sometimes be difficult to eliminate. Although it may take persistence, fleas can often be controlled without resorting to powerful synthetic organic chemicals.

Flea Traits

If you own a pet, especially a cat or dog that is allowed to be both indoors and out, fleas can become a problem in your home. In hot seasons or year-round warm climates, this can be especially true.

Fleas are actually tiny ($4/100$–$16/100$" long), wingless, bloodsucking insects. The adults are equipped with powerful back legs for leaping. Fleas are common parasites on warmblooded animals. Dog fleas are similar but slightly larger than cat fleas. No matter what kind of fleas they are, they can infest your pet's bedding, as well as your carpets, rugs, and furniture.

Unfortunately, adult fleas actually bite their host, seeking blood. After an adult female has consumed blood, she'll often lay eggs (usually less than ten) on or near the puncture site. The dried blood provides meals for the soon-to-hatch larvae. Most people who are bitten by fleas find it irritating and soon develop small red bumps. However, some individuals experience an allergic reaction in which swelling and other symptoms result. In addition, some human diseases can be transmitted by certain types of fleas. For example, the bacterial toxin causing bubonic plague was transmitted by rodent fleas. Luckily, dog and cat fleas aren't usually associated with human diseases.

Flea Control through Special Pet Care

To minimize flea problems in your home, there are several measures you may want to try. The first is to regularly comb your cats and dogs with a specialized *flea comb*. These combs are designed with very small teeth so close together that when you pull one through your pet's fur, the fleas will be filtered out and caught. (With very long fur, using a flea comb can be somewhat difficult.) Then using your fingernail, you can push the fleas off the combinto a dish of soapy water to quickly kill them. To buy a flea comb, check with your local pet store or your veterinarian. If you'd prefer, you can mail-order one from **Save Our ecoSystem (SOS)** or **Pedigree**.

Another method to help reduce flea infestations is to regularly vacuum your pets using a special dog and cat grooming attachment. These may be available locally in your pet store and they're sold by **Pedigree**. It's also a good idea to vacuum your floors and furnishings frequently, especially during peak flea seasons. Vacuuming is extremely important around your pets' sleeping areas. In addition, wash your pets' bed regularly. When fleas are at their worst, you might even have your pets sleep on old towels, which you could clean daily, if necessary.

Some people have also tried using a variety of herbal and aromatic woods (such as cedar) as flea repellents. Sometimes these are in the form of shampoos, skin applications, or dried material used in bedding. Although some of these may be of questionable value against fleas, the essential oils of *eucalyptus* (a tree in the myrtle family originally from Australia) and *pennyroyal* (a perennial herb of the mint family) apparently can be fairly effective. Unfortunately, some sensitive individuals may find that their pronounced odor too bothersome. If you're interested in herbal anti-flea preparations, check with your veterinarian or pet-supply store to find out what they have available. Several such products can also be mail-ordered from **Pedigree**.

Using Diatomaceous Earth Against Fleas

Still another option is to use naturally mined *diatomaceous earth (DE)* that has not been heat-treated. This powdery material consists of the silica-containing cell walls of millions of ancient *diatoms* (microscopic water algae). Some people suggest that you should simply sprinkle a small amount of DE directly on your pets so that any fleas and eggs present on them will dry up and die. However, others feel that if you do this, it'll also cause an unhealthy drying of your pets' skin. Therefore, a better approach might be to sprinkle DE around your yard or even on your indoor carpeting. If you decide to go ahead and apply it to your carpets, allow it to remain undisturbed for 12–36 hours. Then, vacuum your carpets thoroughly.

It should be noted there are certain human-health concerns that have been associated with using diatomaceous earth. For example, it is often advised never to use heat-treated DE; it apparently has a much greater potential to produce lung diseases such as *silicosis*. (This is a serious lung condition brought on by breathing silica particulates.) Even when using DE that hasn't been heat-treated, it's best to wear a protective dust mask. DE that hasn't been heat-treated may be available from your local veterinarian or pet supply center and can be mail-ordered from **Natural Animal**.

Other Simple Flea-Control Methods

Sometimes cutting your lawn short and keeping it that way will lessen flea problems for your pets, and ultimately inside your home. Interestingly, a very simple flea-killing method is to carefully suspend a lit low-wattage light bulb 6–12" directly above a pan of water indoors at night. (You could also use a sheet of sticky insect paper instead of the bowl of water.) Ideally, this should be near a flea-infestation site in your home. When you do this, it's best to have your pets elsewhere. The fleas will be attracted to the warmth of the light, especially because the warmth of your pet's body is not around. As the fleas jump toward the light, they'll land in the water and drown (or get stuck on the gluey paper).

Another simple anti-flea approach that's widely advertised is using high-pitched sound to ward off fleas. The electronically induced ultrasound is above the hearing range of humans and most pets, but not that of fleas, etc. The noise is supposedly disturbing to fleas (and other insects), so they stay away. Unfortunately, research has shown that ultrasonic flea repellents simply don't work.

(Note: See also *Cats* and *Dogs* in *Chapter 6: Lifestyle.*)

FLIES

Fly is the common name for a range of flying insect species in the order *Diptera*. Included are houseflies, fruit flies, gnats, horseflies, and deerflies among others. Most of these insects are biters or bloodsuckers and, unfortunately, many of them also can carry diseases. Flies are usually attracted to places with poor sanitation. Therefore, having clean surroundings and tight-fitting screens are two of the best deterrents against them.

As everyone knows, it's not uncommon to find a fly (or flies) indoors. Two very safe and effective fly-extermination methods are old-fashioned ones. These are a fly swatter and sticky flypaper. Flypaper has an advantage over a swatter because the dead insects don't have to be handled. If you decide to purchase sticky flypaper, it's a good idea to buy the type made without chemical coatings. With pesticide-free flypaper, the glue itself is the active ingredient. The stuck flies eventually die naturally without the need for poison. Sticky flypaper without pesticides is sometimes available at local hardware stores. One mail-order source is **N.E.E.D.S.**

Unfortunately, swatters and flypaper are capable of eliminating only a few flies at a time. Therefore, if you find a swarm of flies in your home, you'll likely have to try some other tactic. One approach is to simply wait until the swarm rests for the night. Often when they do this, they'll land on the ceiling. When this occurs, you can quickly suction them up with a soft-brush attachment on your vacuum cleaner.

Another anti-fly strategy is to use a Pestlite Insect Trap (Symmetry Technologies Corp.). This unit utilizes an ultraviolet light that attracts flying insects and a small fan that blows the insects down into a tray filled with soapy water where they drown. (This unit doesn't make a zapping noise.) Some local **True Value Hardware Stores** stock it. By mail order, you can purchase one from **Perfectly Safe**.

GRAIN MOTHS

Grain moths can sometimes become a household problem. One common type is the Indian meal moth, which is small (less than $1/2$" long) with gray and copper wings. Unfortunately, grain moth eggs are commonly found in organic grains. Many people have found they can successfully prevent the unnoticeable eggs from turning into unappetizing larvae or live moths by placing their whole grains in tightly sealed, recloseable containers and store them in their freezer.

If grain moths happen to hatch and escape into your kitchen, try using a soft-brush vacuum-cleaner attachment to suck them up. Then thoroughly vacuum around your entire kitchen. By doing this, you'll get rid of any moth cocoons that can be located around ceiling edges, under cabinets, among other places in your kitchen.

You may also want to use a Pestlite Insect Trap (Symmetry Technologies Corp.). Its ultraviolet light will attract the moths and its small fan will blow them into a tray filled with soapy water where they'll drown. Some local **True Value Hardware Stores** handle it. It can also be mail-ordered from **Perfectly Safe**. Another option is to use *pheromone traps*. These are sticky traps that have a species-specific sex attractant on them. In this case, the male grain moths fly to the traps thinking that the odor is coming from female moths. They then get stuck and die. This will prevent females from laying fertile eggs. If you want to try this approach, check with local pest control companies to see if they have these traps available.

MICE

Unfortunately, mice are a common problem. The following sections will offer some less-toxic solutions to deal with these unwelcome house guests.

Mouse Traits

The house mouse (*Mus musculus*) has the widest distribution in the world of any mammal, except for human beings themselves. It's little wonder then that this particular species or other species such as deer mice, harvest mice, and others may from time to time find their way into your home.

Although some people consider mice "cute" and may even keep them as pets, mice should be considered serious pests for a number of reasons. First, certain mice could be carrying viral, bacterial, and/or parasitic diseases that could affect you or your family. (These can be transmitted by direct contact with them, their biting, fleas, or breathing dust from their droppings.) Mice also have the potential to be very destructive. They can gnaw through walls, cabinets, and furniture and get into food supplies and bedding, etc. In addition, their feces can be dropped over a large area of your home's interior, making an unpleasant mess to clean up.

Particularly frustrating is how quickly mice reproduce. Within a few months, two mating mice can easily produce several dozen more mice. This is because many mice species breed four to six times a year and each litter may have four to twelve young. At about eight weeks of age a new mouse generation becomes sexually mature and ready to mate, and so on.

Live Traps for Capturing Mice

Although most people want to eliminate all the mice from their homes, for some individuals this can pose a real moral or philosophical dilemma. While they may feel that killing insects is acceptable, killing mice, it seems, is "cruel." For these people (and others, of course), there are now live traps available which can capture problem rodents. Some models are designed to capture a single mouse, while others can hold several. Live capture traps are usually available in most local hardware stores. In addition, **N.E.E.D.S.** offers them by mail order. When you've captured live mice, they must be released a considerable distance from your home or they'll simply return; that is, unless you're absolutely certain you have sealed up every possible reentry point.

Mouse Extermination Methods

Some persons may simply decide that rodent extermination, rather than live capture is necessary. One possible method is using special poison mouse bait, which is commonly sold in hardware stores and garden-supply centers. Often it's available in small packets that you place in suspected mice areas. These packets appear to be a convenient, effective method for killing mice— a relatively safe way of using a very limited amount of *rodenticide* (rodent-killing chemical).

However, there can be serious problems with using poison bait. Sometimes the mice will scatter the pellets over a fairly wide area around the gnawed-open packets. Unfortunately, this bait can be toxic to small children or pets if ingested. Also, you should be aware that even if mice are the only creatures to consume the pellets, you have no control over where they'll eventually die. Dead mice could end up anywhere inside or outside your home. This could pose real sanitation concerns. Then too, dogs or cats could find and eat the poisoned carcasses.

As medieval as it may seem, the best long-term solution in some situations is often to use old-fashioned snap traps. One very popular brand of these is Victor (**Woodstream Corp.**), which are sold, along with others like it, in virtually every hardware and garden-supply store. Of course, at the same time, make sure all your home's mouse-entry points are sealed so you only have to kill a limited number of mice.

Snap traps are actually designed to kill almost instantaneously by breaking a rodent's spinal chord. Therefore, there's no poison and the dead animal remains with the trap. However, you must be extremely careful where you place snap traps because they can seriously harm fingers and toes. So, make certain that children and pets absolutely do not have access to them.

To make the use of snap traps less unpleasant, you might want to follow this procedure. At the site where you have recently spotted a mouse (or mice), put down a piece of aluminum foil or several layers of paper and situate the trap on top of it. Then, bait the trap using a small dab of peanut butter and carefully set the spring hinge. Once the mouse is caught, you can simply wrap the dead animal in the foil or paper and dispose of it. Incidentally, the foil or paper layers will also stop any splattered blood or bait from getting onto your floors.

MOSQUITOES

Mosquitoes are small, two-winged flies and there are many species of them. Mosquitoes are considered serious pests because the adult females feed on blood. Beside being annoying and often causing swelling, by accessing your blood supply, mosquito bites can be an effective method of disease transmission. *Arboviral encephalitis* (virus-induced acute brain inflammation) and *dog heartworm* are just two of the more common diseases transmitted by female mosquitoes in the U.S.

Fortunately, mosquitoes are usually not found in large numbers in most American homes; that is, if the houses are on properly drained sites, are well-sealed, and have tight-fitting screens in good repair. However, it's certainly true that some locations will naturally just have much greater mosquito populations than others.

To kill a few mosquitoes safely, using a fly swatter works fairly well. To cope with large swarms, you can sometimes suck them up quickly using a soft-brush attachment on your vacuum cleaner. Another method would be to use a Pestlite Insect Trap (Symmetry Technologies Corp.). This unit's ultraviolet light attracts mosquitoes and its small fan blows them into a tray filled with soapy water to drown. If you're interested in buying a Pestlite Insect Trap, some local **True Value Hardware Stores** carry it. You can also mail-order one from **Perfectly Safe**.

Of course, a number of people use herbal oils, such as *citronella oil* (derived from citronella grass), to deter mosquitoes. These are sometimes sold at some health-food stores. Generally, herbal oils have strong natural scents that are meant to repel the mosquitoes, and some of them actually can be quite effective. However, their odors can be bothersome to some sensitive individuals.

A non-odorous deterrent you might try is Love Bug and Love Bug Nite Lite (**Prince Lionheart**). These are devices that electronically mimic beating dragonfly wings. (Dragonflies are natural predators of mosquitoes.) Supposedly, when the mosquitoes hear the noise of their age-old enemy, they quickly retreat. On the other hand, humans may just barely perceive the sound. Both Love Bugs are made of plastic and resemble several-inch-long ladybugs. The Love Bug battery model is self-contained and can be clipped to the fabric of a canopy bed or onto a playpen. The Love Bug Nite Lite is made to plug into a wall outlet. Both the portable and the night light models are said to be effective for up to a 20–30' radius. The Love Bug can be mail-ordered from **Perfectly Safe**, or it can be ordered directly from the manufacturer.

Still another mosquito deterrent you might try is mosquito netting. This can be draped over your bed if you find it necessary. Remember to purchase only types that haven't been treated with chemical repellents or pesticides. There's no need to breathe these compounds while you sleep. To find mosquito netting, check local army/navy surplus stores, camping departments, and perhaps baby departments as well.

SILVERFISH

Silverfish are ugly but they're generally not much of a threat to you or your belongings. However, the following sections offer some ways to safely eliminate them from your home.

Silverfish Traits

Silverfish are actually varieties of *bristletails*. These insects are usually about $1/2$" long with rather flat, soft, silvery bodies. They have two large antennae on their head and three bristles emerging from their rear. Silverfish especially like to be around moisture.

Apparently, silverfish have the capacity to eat natural fibers, paper, and starches. Especially enjoyable to them are starchy glues, such as those used for wallpaper and bookbinding. If only one or two silverfish are in your home, it (or they) should probably not be of much concern. It's generally agreed they don't pose much of a problem to households or the health of you or your family.

Eliminating Silverfish

Occasional silverfish, can be vacuumed using a soft-brush vacuum-cleaner attachment. If you have many of these insects, you'll probably have to do something more than simply vacuuming. As an eradication method, try using boric acid powder. White pharmacy-grade boric acid powder is available at most drugstores, and synthetically dyed boric acid pesticides, such as Roach-Prufe (**Copper Brite, Inc.**), are sold at most hardware stores. To use boric acid powder, carefully sprinkle a narrow line of the powder around the water and drain pipes under your sinks and in the basement. In the kitchen area, it's best to only apply boric acid powder into the crevices between the floor and the baseboard molding using a small squeeze-bulb insecticide applicator. By applying it this way, it's not likely the powder will ever become airborne and contaminate your food. Bulb-type insecticide devices can be found in some local hardware stores or at a nearby pest-control company. To be on the safe side, whenever you apply boric acid powder, it's wise to wear a dust mask.

When the infestation is over, in certain locations you may want to leave the boric acid powder as a permanent anti-silverfish measure. However, if you decide to remove it, you can vacuum up the powder using a crevice attachment while wearing a dust mask. Then thoroughly wash the affected areas with water, wearing rubber gloves. Note: It's important to make sure that pets and children don't get into boric acid powder. Although boric-acid pesticide is relatively safe, it can be harmful to humans and pets if ingested or inhaled.

SPIDERS

Although flies have caused far more human death by acting as transmitters of disease, spiders still create more fear when they're spotted in homes than common houseflies. The following sections discuss truly dangerous spiders and what you can do to rid your home of them if desired.

Spider Traits

Spiders are not insects but eight-legged, carnivorous arachnids. All make silk and most have fangs capable of injecting venom. Generally, in America, you may want to overlook the presence of most spiders in your home. It seems the vast majority are not dangerous to humans, they lead rather secluded lives, and devour pest insects such as flies. However, there are some that are too big, too ugly, or too poisonous to ignore.

Poisonous U.S. Spiders

Fortunately, there are not many really dangerous spiders in America. However, there are at least two with which you should become familiar: the black widow and the brown recluse.

Black Widow Spiders

Probably the best known (at least by name recognition) of the poisonous spiders is the black widow. The females of this species are small ($1/2$" long) and glossy black with a red hourglass marking on the underside of their abdomen. The males are even smaller and have four pairs of red marks along the sides of their abdomen. Interestingly, the males are rarely seen.

Black widow spiders are actually found throughout the continental U.S. They can live in a wide range of indoor and outdoor habitats. Fortunately, however, they're usually not aggressive; that is, except when a female is protecting her egg sac. If bitten, black widow venom can cause spasms and breathing difficulties. Bites may, therefore, become fatal.

Brown Recluse Spiders

Another dangerous spider is the brown recluse. These spiders are small, just under 1/2" long. Despite their name, brown recluse spiders are generally orange-yellow with a dark violin-shaped marking on the backs.

Brown recluse spiders can be found within an area extending from Kansas and Missouri, south to Texas, and west to California. Often, brown recluse spiders make their homes in sheltered spots outdoors as well as in houses. Generally, they're active at night.

Fortunately, bites from these spiders are rarely fatal to humans. However, the skin surrounding a bite site may blacken and die. Sometimes, the complete healing of a bite can take up to several months.

Spider Extermination

A good approach to minimizing spiders is to vacuum regularly and thoroughly around your home's interior. This means under the beds, in the closets, behind the curtains and shutters, in the corners, etc. Vacuuming will not only suck away any live spiders, but it will also rid your house of their webs, nests, and eggs.

If you come across a poisonous spider, be extremely cautious and wear protective clothing and rubber gloves while eradicating it. If you're ever bitten by a suspected poisonous spider, it's important to call for medical help and take the spider, even if squashed, to the emergency room for proper identification. If you suspect you've been bitten by a poisonous spider but didn't actually see it happen, you should seek medical help at once if you begin experiencing symptoms such as abdominal pain or dizziness.

SUGAR ANTS

Seeing an ant or two wouldn't seem like much to worry about. However, a few sugar ants in your kitchen could be a harbinger of a full-scale ant invasion. To help you deal with them safely and effectively, the following sections discuss sugar-ant traits and less-toxic measures to eliminate the ants from your house.

Sugar Ant Traits

Sugar ant is actually a generic term; it includes several small ant species that like nectar and other sugary foods. Generally, sugar ants are only about 1/8" long and dark in color. Sugar ants are social creatures living in colonies that may contain hundreds of individuals.

Unfortunately, sugar ants can become a persistent in-home pest problem. Although their nest may remain outdoors, their daily activity may consist of repeatedly entering your home for food and then leaving to return to the nest. Therefore, be alert whenever you first see a few sugar ants in your house. They are often large female workers searching for food. These scout ants will lay down scent trails that the other ants in the colony will follow.

Talcum Powder for Controlling Sugar Ants

Surprisingly, simply sprinkling *talcum powder* around the areas of sugar-ant activity in your home will often control their invasions. It seems that this powdery material clings to their bodies, preventing normal respiration. (Ants take in air through tiny holes known as *spiracles* along the sides of their bodies.) When their breathing holes become clogged, they suffocate.

Talcum powder (also known as *talc*) is a finely ground magnesium-silicate mineral product. (You may be familiar with it because it's the base material for many bath powders.) You'll generally find you can purchase talcum powder at most pharmacies. Note that, powder of any sort should not be breathed by humans or pets because it could lead to respiratory irritation and/or damage. This is especially true of talc that is a silicate mineral. (Silica can cause *silicosis*, a serious lung disease.) Therefore, it's important to wear a good-quality dust mask whenever you apply talc. In addition, it is wise not to let children or pets get access to the powdered talc.

Pyrethrin For Controlling Sugar Ants

If talcum powder fails to stop sugar ants, the next step is to block their entry into your home. To do this, trace their trail back to where it penetrated your home's exterior. Generally, this is somewhere near the foundation. At that point, caulk or otherwise repair the gap. After that, you can spray a pyrethrin solution around the repaired site and along the exterior foundation wall for several feet on both sides of it. Pyrethrin is a natural insecticide, a liquid extract derived from chrysanthemum flower heads. One brand you might use is X-clude (**Whitmire Research Labs**). If you decide to use it, make certain that you closely follow the written directions on the package. To buy X-clude, you can call the company for the nearest dealer.

If the sugar ants still return, they've obviously found another entry point. Therefore, it might be a good idea to now spray a pyrethrin solution around the entire outside perimeter of your home's foundation. You might also want to seek out and destroy the outdoor sugar ant nest. To do this, trace the ants' path from the exterior-wall entry point all the way back to their nest site. This will likely be frustrating and time-consuming; however, there's a chance you might find it. If you do come across their nest, you can spray it with a pyrethrin solution or drench it with boiling water. By destroying the nest, you will have permanently ended the ant attack; that is, until another scouting party manages to enter your house from another nest.

TERMITES

One word that virtually all homeowners dread hearing is *termites*. This is not only because they fear the tremendous damage termites can do, but also out of concern over having their homes treated with potentially dangerous and potent *termiticides* (termite killers). Therefore, to help you cope more effectively with termites, the following sections introduce you to termite traits, typical treatments, and safer alternative approaches you can use to effectively stop them.

Termite Traits in General

Termites are extremely successful creatures. Throughout the world, there are nearly 1,800 termite species. Many people falsely believe that termites are white ants. Actually they're quite different. Physically, termites lack the very thin wasplike waist that ants have. However, the biggest difference is that termites can eat wood; ants can't. Although some types of ants live in wood (see *Carpenter Ants* above), they're unable to use wood as a food source.

Actually, termites can eat virtually all plant materials, including wood. Although the tough cellulose making up a plant's cell walls is often hard to digest (it's completely indigestible for many creatures), termites have certain bacteria living in their digestive tracts that allow them to easily break the cellulose down. In addition, termites that primarily bore into wood also have a type of *protozoa* (microscopic single-celled organism) living in their digestive tracts that apparently enhances their ability to break down tree cellulose.

In the U.S., three termite species are the most common sources of concern to homeowners. These are the subterranean termite, the drywood termite, and the dampwood termite. As a rule, these are small creatures ($1/2$" or less, in most cases) with white bodies and darker heads. These insects are social creatures living in colonies. The colonies are made up of three types of members: workers, reproductive adults, and soldiers. However, each of the three problem species has its own climate in which it lives and other particular preferences and habits.

Subterranean Termite Traits

Subterranean termites have worker members that are about $1/4$" long with white bodies and darker heads. The soldier termites look fairly similar to these workers, but they're a little larger. On the other hand, the winged reproducing males and females are about $1/2$" long and black.

Subterranean termites are present over much of the U.S. As their name suggests, this species lives in soil. In order to reach wood that is not directly on the ground, these termites often build mud tubes to travel through. These tubes keep their bodies moist by protecting them from the air. This is absolutely essential for their survival, because if they dry out they die.

Dampwood Termite Traits

Dampwood termites workers are about $1/2$" long and are ivory-colored with darker abdomens. The soldiers are about $3/4$" long with larger and darker heads. The reproductive adults are light brown with wings about 1" long.

Dampwood termites are common in the Northwest. As you might have guessed, they live only in or around damp wood, and eat damp wood as well. Therefore, these termites are almost completely dependent on moisture-laden wood in order to survive.

Drywood Termite Traits

Drywood termite workers are white with yellow-brown heads. The reproducing winged adults are dark brown and the soldier termites have light-colored bodies with very large reddish-brown heads. All these forms of drywood termites tend to be $1/2$" long or less.

Drywood termites are found both in the southern U.S. and in California. Interestingly, this species doesn't have the moisture requirements of subterranean or dampwood termites. As a result, they can have nests wherever there is wood, wet or dry.

Typical Termite Controls

In this country, powerful toxic synthetic organic chemicals (See *Modern Organic Pesticides* above) are commonly used to combat termites.

Typical Termiticides

Termites are capable of burrowing into wood and feeding on it. Unfortunately, most U.S. residences are constructed primarily of wood or at least are wood-framed. As a result, termites enter and damage thousands of American homes annually. If a termite infestation should occur in your house, the actual structural destruction of wood joists, studs, etc. tends to occur rather slowly. However, an infestation can go on unnoticed for several years. This could lead to serious damage, which would be very costly to repair. It's not surprising then that most people have used (and continue to use) potent termiticides (termite killers) to protect their homes.

At one time, one of the most popular chemical termiticides was the synthetic organic chemical, chlordane, a chlorinated hydrocarbon. (By the way, the commercially available product was actually 60% chlordane with 40% other ingredients such as the insecticide *heptchor*.) However in the 1970s, chlordane was shown to be *carcinogenic* (cancer-causing) and it has since been removed from the market. Today, synthetic chlorpyrifos-containing pesticides (such as Dursban) are now widely used against termites. These particular termiticides are supposed to be less dangerous, and therefore, safer for humans than chlordane; however, there are negative health effects reported with their use as well.

Despite the increase in public awareness of the potential dangers posed by exposure to many of the synthetic chemical pesticides, most homes are still subjected to these solutions to prevent or exterminate house-damaging termites. Some residences are actually on a regular, routine, reapplication schedule as an ongoing deterrent measure (This is especially true in warm climates such as Florida.). Unfortunately, as a rule, once a synthetic pesticide has been applied to your house, it can't easily be removed. It, therefore, has a long-term presence in your home.

Typical Termiticide Application Methods

There are actually three chemical treatment methods that are popularly used to apply typical termiticides. The type that's utilized depends on the termite species, the extent of the infestation, and the specific termiticidal chemical chosen. Each approach has its particular advantages as well as its potential drawbacks.

In *ground-injection liquid fumigation*, a pesticide applicator inserts a device into the ground around a home's foundation and injects a liquid termiticide. This saturates the soil and kills any termites (usually subterranean termites) that come in contact with the solution. At the same time, it forms a protective barrier against future termite infestations. Apparently, ground-injection liquid fumigation using typical termiticide chemicals can remain active in the soil for ten years or more, depending on the specific compound used. Therefore, if this application method is used, repeated treatments or monitoring are usually unnecessary for at least a few years after it's been done.

Theoretically, if the home's foundations are completely sealed, no termiticide compounds should enter the actual living space to be inhaled or otherwise make contact with the people inside the house. Unfortunately, misdirected injections have entered the walls. However, even if the ground-injection liquid fumigation was properly done, sometimes the chemicals are able to seep into the living space through unsuspected tiny gaps and cracks in a home's foundation.

In *whole-structure gas fumigation,* a house is completely tented with plastic sheeting. During the actual fumigation process, the occupants and pets leave and a powerful gaseous termiticide chemical is allowed to fill the entire structure. This particular method is sometimes used against dry wood termites that can attack any wood in a home, even the attic floors and roof trusses which are far above the ground.

Whole-house gas fumigation must be done very carefully because the harmful chemicals used can easily become inhaled and cause toxic symptoms. Therefore, the pest-control personnel doing the fumigation always wear special protective chemical respirator masks. Also, chemical-detection equipment is generally used to measure potentially harmful gas levels as well as any remaining harmful residues. Unfortunately, if you use this method, anything left inside a house during the fumigation process will be subjected to the fumigating chemicals and, to a certain extent, will be contaminated.

In *spray dispersal,* a professional pesticide applicator uses a portable tank with a wand attachment to spray around a home's foundation and/or specific infested areas. Theoretically, this method could be used against any type of termite. In a spray-dispersal application, there's direct control over the placement of the termiticide. However, how precisely the spray is actually applied depends on the skill of the applicator. It's conceivable that these chemicals might land on heating ducts and seep in between the seams. Typical termiticides that have been sprayed could remain active for up to several years, depending on the type used.

Alternative Termite Controls in General

Although they're not often well-known or commonly utilized yet, a number of safer termite control methods are available other than the typical highly toxic organic-chemical termiticides. Unfortunately, for a variety of reasons, you might be unable to actually use some of these even if you wanted to (see *Implementing Alternative Pest-Control Measures* above). Despite this, many people have been able to use alternative termite controls and, for the most part, they've been very satisfied with their effectiveness. Therefore, the following sections explore some of these methods.

Homeowner Responsibilities Using Alternative Termite Controls

Before you opt for an alternative method to control termites, you should first be aware that most alternative anti-termite controls will require you to take an active role. This means you must consistently and conscientiously monitor your home by routinely inspecting it for evidence of termites. During an actual infestation, your patience will be tried as well. Alternative termiticides may have to be applied several times or a combination of alternative methods might have to be used together until the infestation is eliminated. This may be necessary because most alternative termite-control methods are not as deadly or as long-lasting as their toxic chemical counterparts.

While admittedly time-consuming and sometimes frustrating, you simply can't be lazy or just plain hopeful that termites won't be a problem for your house or that they'll simply disappear after a single less-toxic treatment. The sad truth is, termites will always be nearby and ready to devour your home if they have the opportunity to do so. Unless you're going to inject toxic synthetic poisons around your home's foundation, use toxic gas to fumigate it, routinely spray with toxic chemicals, build your house in a cold climate where termites can't survive, or construct a house without wood, anti-termite measures should be an ongoing and necessary responsibility of home ownership.

Alternative Termite-Control Basics

To determine the best alternative anti-termite method to use, you should learn which species is active in your area. If you already have found termites in your home, capture a few specimens and have a local pest-control company analyze them if you're unsure what type they actually are. The pest company might charge you a small fee, or they may not charge you anything. After all, they're hoping for your business. Once you know what species you're up against, you can go ahead and use the alternative extermination measures you've decided upon.

It should be noted that you need not always treat your entire house. Instead, you often can simply spot-treat the infested areas and still have a successful and effective treatment. Treating only the affected areas will also cost you much less. By the way, even if you find you must eventually use a powerful synthetic pesticide chemical for a particularly tenacious infestation, it is often best to spot-treat rather than subject your whole house to the chemical treatment. By doing this, you'll definitely minimize any potentially toxic pesticide exposure that you and your family might experience.

Specific Termite Species Alternative-Control Suggestions

Because termite damage can be serious, because some chemical applications are potentially harmful, and because alternative-control measures are often unfamiliar, it's very much suggested that you read the sections on termites in *Common-Sense Pest Control* by William Olkowski, Sheila Daar, and Helga Olkowski. In addition, you should seriously consider joining and consulting with the **Bio-Integral Resource Center** (**BIRC**). A personal consultation with the **BIRC**'s alternative pest-control experts (or others like them) is especially important if you're currently experiencing a termite infestation in your house. Although the following sections in this book present a number of available alternative control measures you might use, the truth is, every termite problem is more or less a unique situation that will require very explicit answers: ones that are impossible to always give here.

Subterranean Termite Alternative-Control Methods

Subterranean termites must either travel in protected, hidden cracks and crevices or build mud-tubes to reach wood that's not situated directly on the ground. Because of this behavior, one monitoring method is particularly effective: *termite shields*, which help you spot termite activity around your home. Termite shields are nothing more than continuous sections of thin, bent aluminum or galvanized steel (steel having a zinc coating to prevent rusting) placed on top of the foundation wall around the entire perimeter of your home. It's important that they be correctly installed when a house is being built; they can't be installed in an existing house. When installed correctly, the metal strips block the termites' paths and cause them to build their mud-tubes around the metal—out in the open—in order to reach the wood sillplate, wood joists, and wood studs, etc. Therefore, termite shields allow you to more easily and more effectively inspect for termites because the mud-tubes are going to be more visible than they otherwise would be.

However, it's important to stress that metal termite shields can't stop a termite invasion; they're simply an inspection aid, and actually of little value if you don't regularly check them. However, because they permit you to quickly spot termite mud-tubes, any infestations that do occur will likely be caught and stopped before there's real structural damage.

One apparently effective and certainly a very simple subterranean termite-control method is to use a sand barrier around your home's foundation walls. Interestingly, termites can't tunnel through sand, as long as it is a specific size. To make a termite sand barrier, you need a 4" layer of sand (8–12 mesh) around the entire perimeter of the foundation. It should extend from the footing to the surface of the ground. Although this method is said to provide fairly good ongoing protection against subterranean termites, at this time it's still considered an experimental procedure.

A very effective and relatively safe termiticide substance that can be used on new construction is Tim-Bor (**U.S. Borax and Chemical Corp.**). This powdered borate product (a boric-acid compound somewhat like borax) is diluted with water and sprayed on all the wood framing. Tim-Bor actually penetrates wood all the way through to the heart. Unfortunately, Tim-Bor is water-soluble, so rain and other precipitation can wash it off before the exterior sheathing or siding is in place. If that occurs, the solution will have to be reapplied. (A good way to apply Tim-Bor to a new house is to spray it on all the wood framing after the roofing, siding, doors and windows are in place, all of which will, of course, protect the structure from the weather.) Another concern with Tim-Bor is that any solution that reaches the ground could damage grass or surrounding trees. Therefore, if Tim-Bor is used on your site, make certain that the package directions are followed carefully. Treatment with Tim-Bor is said to provide permanent termite control. To have Tim-Bor used on your new house or room addition, call the manufacturer for the nearest pest-control company that uses it.

In an existing house, it is generally only possible to spray Tim-Bor on wood that is exposed in a basement or crawl space. This may be sufficient to eradicate some termite infestations. However, in some houses, it may not be possible to get to the termite-eaten wood to be able spray it.

For less-toxic spot-treating of subterranean-termite infestations, try using an injectable pyrethrin (an extract made from chrysanthemum flower heads) at the sites of the termite activity. One brand of this is Tri-Die (**Whitmire Research Labs.**). To buy it, call the company for the nearest dealer.

Another spot-treatment method is to use injections of predatory *nematodes* (minute types of roundworms). These creatures are quite effective in attacking and killing termites. The nematodes are mixed in water and the solution is injected into the soil around a house. The tiny nematodes then seek out termites and kill them. If you're interested in this approach, contact a supplier such as **N-Viro Products Ltd.** for an applicator in your area. Note that, applications of both pyrethrin and nematode injections may have to be repeated to be effective and that they don't remain active against termites for extended periods of times.

Dampwood Termite Alternative-Control Methods

Dampwood termites can only live in or around damp wood. Because of their absolute dependence on moisture, drying up all your home's moisture problems will quickly end most dampwood-termite infestations.

Therefore, check to be sure all your gutters and any footing drains are working correctly. If your shrubbery has become overgrown or is too near your home's foundation, you may need to cut it back or remove it. You'll also want to make certain that the ground slopes sufficiently away from your home's foundation on all sides. If you're in an area with a high water table, seriously consider installing a sump pump, if necessary.

In some situations, a dehumidifier can effectively remove excess indoor humidity. Exhaust fans can also be helpful. (See *High Humidity* in *Chapter 9: Indoor Air*.) In addition, check to see that there are no roof problems such as loose or missing shingles. Finally, repair any leaking pipes and drains.

Drywood Termite Alternative-Control Methods

Drywood termites are a species that doesn't have the moisture requirements of subterranean or dampwood termites. As a result, their nests can be anywhere where there's wood. For homeowners, this means that even roof trusses can be at risk. With new construction, you can permanently protect your home against drywood termites by having a preventive borate treatment sprayed on all the wood (for more information on this procedure, see *Subterranean Termite Alternative-Control Methods* above).

A relatively safe approach to dealing with drywood termites in existing homes is to spot-treat any areas that are infested with drywood termites using an injectable pyrethrin (a liquid extract derived from chrysanthemum flower heads) (One brand of this is Tri-Die (**Whitmire Research Labs**)). To buy it, contact the company for the nearest supplier. The solution can either be injected into the affected wood yourself, or you can hire a pest-control company to do it for you. Of course, it should be a company that's willing to use alternative pest-control methods. By the way, the pyrethrin may have to be injected more than once to be effective, and you also should know that it's not a long-term acting termiticide.

Another alternative approach to spot-treating drywood termites in existing houses is *electrocution* (killing by electricity). One electrocuting device designed to specifically do this is Electro-Gun. It will create an electric current capable of killing termites without damaging your home. In the U.S., this machine can be leased by local pesticide companies from **ETEX, Ltd.** For more information on the Electro-Gun, contact the company. (Note that, this method can't be used against subterranean termites or dampwood termites.) It should be mentioned that killing termites by electrocution is immediately effective but it won't provide long-term protection because a new infestation, unfortunately, could begin immediately.

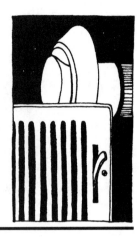

CHAPTER 9
INDOOR AIR

People like to think the air they breathe in their homes is safe and healthy. Unfortunately, this isn't always the case in many American homes. Instead, most of us commonly inhale a tremendous number and variety of pollutants when we are indoors.

But what exactly is indoor air pollution? Defined, indoor pollution is simply the presence within a home's atmosphere of substances that could negatively affect human health (or the health of your pets). These might be from a natural source (pollen, for example) or of man-made origin (the outgassing of synthetic materials). Air pollutants can arise briefly but intensely, as when you use model-airplane glue, or be a long-term low-level chronic situation, as with the release of unvented combustion products from your gas range's burning pilot light.

Ideally, the best defense against indoor pollution is not owning or using any potentially contaminating materials or products in your home. This should be combined with thorough and regular housecleaning using less-toxic, low-odor products (see *Chapter 7: Cleaning*), controlling any serious moisture problems in your home, including high relative-humidity levels, and providing your house with adequate clean-air ventilation. If your home still has somewhat minor air-quality problems after doing all this, in some situations using an appropriate air-cleaning device (air filter, negative ionizer, etc.) can be used to remove any remaining airborne contaminants.

Admittedly, creating a home with unpolluted air can be difficult—at least, all at once. However, if you solve your home's individual air-pollution problems one by one, it's likely you'll eventually have indoor air that will positively, rather than negatively, affect the health of you and your family. And, that's what this book, and especially this chapter, is all about: defining indoor air problems and how you can best cope with them.

COMMON INDOOR AIR POLLUTANTS

The following sections discuss some of the more common indoor pollutants. You'll find that they're classified in several major categories.

INDOOR-AIR-POLLUTION TESTING IN GENERAL

As you read the sections on specific indoor pollutants below, the common testing (and/or monitoring) procedures for several of them are given. It should be said at this point that there are environmental testing companies that do on-site measuring for virtually all the contaminants listed. There are also many home test kits you can buy for yourself.

Because tests and testing companies have now become available, it's not surprising that many people ask, Should I have my house tested for mold (or formaldehyde or whatever)? In the end, that's a decision you must decide for yourself. The truth is, there are certain tests you can perform on your indoor air that are simple, low-cost, and can tell you truly valuable information; for example, radon tests. However, there are others that may be less worthwhile to you.

Actually, how accurate and useful an indoor pollution test will be depends on it's proper setup, the sensitivity of the measuring devices, the correct analysis of the recorded data, and your (or an expert's) knowledge on how to use the results to effectively solve any problems. After all, tests generally can't tell you the actual source(s) of the contaminants they've measured. By the way, it's not unusual for very sensitive persons to find they react negatively to air-pollutant levels considered "safe" or even undetectable by conventionally performed tests. This is often because these individuals are far more susceptible to lower concentrations of particular pollutants than average populations, that their systems are more sensitive than the mechanical devices doing the testing, or that they are reacting to contaminants not even being tested for. Therefore, it seems that a sensitive person's nose can often better determine for him- or herself if a problem is present than air-quality testing.

You should be aware that the cost of having your indoor air tested will vary, depending on who does the testing, the extent of the testing, the degree of test sensitivity, and exactly what's being tested for, among other factors. Therefore, before you decide to hire an environmental testing company, find out how long they've been in business, whether they have any certification or licenses of any type, some professional references, how soon you can expect to have written findings, and what the costs will be.

GASES

As you might have expected, potentially harmful gases usually make up a certain proportion of a home's indoor air pollution. The following sections discuss some of the more common of these.

COMBUSTION GASES

Combustion gases are the invisible gases resulting from combustion (the burning of a substance). Smoke is also released by combustion; it consists of tiny particles and vapors, the visible components of combustion. In homes, combustion gases are created from combustion appliances and equipment such

294

as gas and oil furnaces, gas dryers (see *Clothes Dryers* in *Chapter 8: House-keeping*), gas ranges (see *Gas Stoves* in *Chapter 8: Housekeeping*), gas and oil water heaters, and gas and oil boilers. Others sources of combustion gases include fireplaces, wood stoves, tobacco, kerosene lamps, and even candles (see *Flames* in *Chapter 5: Interior Decorating*).

Combustion of fuels can produce water vapor, *carbon monoxide, carbon dioxide, sulfur dioxide, formaldehyde*, and other gaseous hydrocarbons. Unfortunately, breathing combustion gases can promote respiratory problems. While it isn't healthy to breathe any combustion gases, carbon monoxide (CO) is the most life-threatening.

In your home, keeping your combustion appliances properly maintained and adjusted, ensuring that the chimney functions correctly, and having adequate fresh-air ventilation can all help reduce the level of combustion gases indoors. However, when you burn a fuel indoors, it's often difficult to completely eliminate combustion gases from the living space. (Generally, combustion gases are expelled through a chimney, but not all chimneys function correctly. As a result, in many houses some, or all, of the combustion by-products remain inside the living space.) Therefore, it's important to have a CO detector in your house that will help alert you when deadly CO has reached dangerous levels.

To completely eliminate any concern over combustion gases existing in your home's air, it may be necessary to stop burning all substances within your home. While many people would find this difficult, for some very tightly constructed, underventilated homes and/or for certain very sensitive or acutely asthmatic individuals, this approach might be necessary. Another solution involves using a high-efficiency gas or oil furnace having a *sealed combustion chamber*. These devices do not require a conventional chimney; instead, they use a fan to blow the combustion gases outdoors through a sealed exhaust pipe.

CARBON MONOXIDE

One of the most serious combustion gases in houses is *carbon monoxide* (*CO*), a flammable, odorless, tasteless, colorless gas. It's usually formed as the result of the incomplete combustion of carbon. In homes, high levels of CO can be released from fireplaces (either using wood or natural gas for fuel), coal- or wood-burning stoves; or kerosene, oil, propane, and natural gas heaters, furnaces, hot water tanks, or other combustion equipment. Whenever you burn something, combustion by-products, such as smoke, CO_2, water vapor, and CO, are released. Unfortunately, when CO is breathed into the lungs, it immediately reacts with *hemoglobin* in the blood. CO-saturated hemoglobin is unable to perform its necessary job of transporting life-sustaining oxygen throughout the body.

Commonly, one of the first signs you experience of becoming poisoned by CO is a headache. As you breathe more CO, flu-like symptoms follow, such as muscle weakness, loss of coordination, confusion, and unconsciousness. Death can occur if levels of CO in the body become high enough. Eerily, victims of severe CO poisoning take on a characteristic cherry-red coloring. Each year in this country, hundreds of people die from unplanned, undetected, high carbon monoxide concentrations in their homes, and many more suffer symptoms that they attribute to the flu when in fact they are being poisoned by CO.

Not surprisingly then, some experts believe that ideal healthy houses shouldn't have any forms of combustion taking place inside the living space. However, if your home does have some type of combustion appliance or equipment, it is absolutely essential that it be working efficiently. (When a gas-burning appliance is properly adjusted, CO production is minimized.) Make sure you have regular and professional routine checkups and maintenance performed on both the combustion equipment and the chimney system.

It's also a very good idea to install a *carbon monoxide detector*. (Some local jurisdictions now actually require them in all homes.) These devices continually monitor CO levels in your house. When higher-than-normal CO concentrations are detected, these units will emit a high-pitched alarm sound. Like smoke detectors, some CO detectors are battery-operated, while others are designed to be wired into your home's electrical circuitry. If you're interested in purchasing a CO detector, they're usually handled by most local hardware stores. One popular brand is First Alert (**BRK Electronics Corp.**).

CARBON DIOXIDE

Carbon dioxide (CO$_2$) is a tasteless, colorless gas. It's created through the action of human and animal respiration, decay, and the burning of organic materials. Although it's always present in air (it typically makes up 0.03% of outdoor air), high CO$_2$ levels in homes usually indicate that there isn't enough fresh air indoors. Although CO$_2$ isn't particularly toxic itself, too much can lead to an uncomfortable feeling of stuffiness or closeness, which can add stress to those already having respiratory problems. If fresh air is brought into such a home, the carbon dioxide levels will rapidly diminish, and the stuffy sensation would soon go away.

Unfortunately, high carbon dioxide levels in houses is a growing problem. These days, some new homes are being so tightly built that air can't *infiltrate* (find its way indoors). At the same time, many existing homes are undergoing air tightening measures, such as having new storm windows made for them, having caulk and sealants applied to any cracks or gaps, having weatherstripping put up around their exterior doors, and having added insulation installed. All this is being done for energy efficiency. Although this is usually a good idea, it can create an environment in which outdoor air is no longer able to be easily exchanged for stale indoor air—simply because no planned ventilation system was ever installed. For a more in-depth discussion of ventilation and ways to accomplish it, read *Understanding Ventilation* by John Bower, which is available from **The Healthy House Institute**.

VOLATILE ORGANIC COMPOUNDS

Volatile organic compounds have become a serious health threat in many homes. This section explains what these chemicals are, why some are harmful, and how to prevent them from becoming a problem in your home.

The Nature, Uses, and Potential Health Consequences of VOCs

Volatile organic compounds (VOCs) are actually a class of carbon-based chemicals that have the capacity to rapidly evaporate. Once airborne, many

VOCs have the ability to combine with each other (or with certain other molecules in the air) to create new chemical compounds.

In reality, a great many compounds are classified as VOCs. Some are of natural origin and happen to be relatively benign. For example, a freshly cut orange or onion both give off certain types of VOCs. However, there are also naturally occurring VOCs that can be extremely dangerous such as the toxic VOCs given off by certain molds. Other VOCs, such as *alcohol*, lie somewhere in between.

Usually, however, when the term VOC is used in conjunction with indoor air quality, it doesn't refer to naturally occurring VOCs. Instead, it generally refers to VOCs derived from man-made manufactured products, such as the common solvents toluene, xylene, and lacquer thinner. Other synthetically derived VOCs include formaldehyde and benzene.

Although the negative effects on humans from synthetically created VOCs varies with the particular compound, as a rule they're often harmful to breathe. Many are considered inflammatory to mucous membranes and the respiratory system. The worst of them have been linked to central nervous system damage, chromosomal abnormalities, and even cancer. Interestingly, many sensitive individuals feel that exposure to certain dangerous VOCs is the reason for the onset of their Multiple Chemical Sensitivity (MCS) condition.

Unfortunately today, potentially harmful VOCs are found in the indoor air of many U.S. homes; in some homes they exist at fairly high levels. This is because many typical finishes and coatings (including wall paints), adhesives, cleaning products, and other synthetic materials contain and release at least some of these compounds. It seems that for the most part, the quantity of VOCs in common consumer products and materials is poorly regulated. However, in 1987, California began regulating the VOC content in paint, and a few other local jurisdictions have since passed similar restrictions.

Testing and Eliminating VOCs in Homes

If you want to determine the level of volatile organic compounds (VOCs) in your home, an environmental testing company can be hired to come in and make measurements. But comprehensive testing can cost hundreds of dollars and could easily result in the discovery of a hundred or more different VOCs in the air. While relatively inexpensive test kits are available (one mail-order source is **The Living Source**), it's unlikely that such simple, inexpensive tests will be able to provide you much help. Even a sophisticated test, listing scores of specific VOCs and their concentrations, probably wouldn't offer much use. After all, you still wouldn't know the particular sources from which the specific chemicals had been released.

The truth is, when it comes to VOC levels in indoor air, it's impossible to precisely predict at what concentrations you or your family will become negatively affected. Some people are just more susceptible than others. Therefore, the best defense against the dangers of breathing VOCs is to use in your home only items that don't contain synthetically derived VOCs, or only those items with extremely low amounts of them.

However, it should be noted that newly applied paints and finishes will quickly give off their own VOCs. Also, older items that emitted high levels of VOCs when they were new will eventually release lower and lower amounts of these gases. This is because by their very nature VOCs evaporate quickly. In addition, it's important to stress that good indoor ventilation helps reduce VOC concentrations. Furthermore, *activated charcoal* can be effective in adsorbing higher molecular weight VOCs. (Molecular weight is defined as the total atomic weights of all the component atoms making up a molecule. Larger, more complicated molecules are made up of many atoms, so they tend to have high molecular weights.) For low-molecular weight VOCs such as formaldehyde, specially treated activated-carbon or activated-alumina filters (see below) are effective. However, for certain sensitive individuals, ventilation and/or filters may not be enough to stop reactions if VOC-releasing materials remain within their homes.

(For information on VOCs in your home water supply, see *Industrial Pollution* in *Chapter 10: Home Water.*)

FORMALDEHYDE

These days, one of the most common indoor air pollutants is the VOC formaldehyde. Though it isn't as potentially deadly as CO, its presence can definitely provoke a variety of health complaints. The following sections discuss this well-known contaminant and what you can do to reduce it's level in your home.

The Nature, Uses, and Health Consequences of Formaldehyde

Formaldehyde (HCHO) is the simplest compound in a class of organic compounds known as *aldehydes* (Aldehydes are created through **al**cohol **dehy**drogenation or, in other words, removal of two hydrogen atoms from a primary alcohol.). Formaldehyde is considered a volatile organic compound or VOC. At very high concentrations, formaldehyde is an extremely reactive, colorless gas with a distinctively pungent and unpleasant odor, however, at concentrations typically found in houses, it is virtually odorless.

If formaldehyde is inhaled, it can cause nasal and sinus irritation, respiratory inflammation, asthma, depression, and even menstrual irregularities. Formaldehyde exposure can also cause burning eyes, and has been shown to be *mutagenic* (capable of increasing the rate of cellular mutations) and *carcinogenic* (cancer-causing.) After becoming sensitized to formaldehyde, a certain percentage of the population (probably less than 10%) has been shown to react to smaller and smaller amounts of it. Interestingly, exposure to formaldehyde has been reported by many individuals with Multiple Chemical Sensitivities (MCS) as the suspected reason why they acquired the illness (see *MCS, A New Medical Condition* in *Chapter 1: Getting Started*). Virtually all people with MCS find that they react negatively to extremely low concentrations of it.

Formaldehyde is one chemical that's easy and inexpensive to produce and can be used in a variety of ways. Therefore, in the last few decades it's been routinely used in a wide range of consumer products. A use that once received a lot of public attention was in the formerly popular, then banned, now unbanned *urea-formaldehyde foam insulation.* The urea formaldehyde (UF) resin in this particular product can emit relatively high levels of formaldehyde over several years. But formaldehyde is also found in glues used in man-made wood products, either as urea formaldehyde or phenol formalde-hyde (PF). PF glues emit considerably less formaldehyde than UF glues. PF and UF glues are typically used in plywood, particleboard, medium-density fiberboard, and hardboard (see *Man-made Wood Products* in *Chapter 12: Home Workshop and Garage*).

Formaldehyde is also used in some clear finishes. UF finishes are typically used on kitchen cabinets (see *Typical Modern Cabinets* in *Chapter 5: Interior Decorating*). It's also commonly used as a resin treatment on certain fabrics to give them wrinkle resistance; for example, to create no-iron sheets (see *Typical Cotton-Mill Processing* in *Chapter 2: Clothing*). In addition, formal-dehyde is used in the manufacturing of some paper goods; for instance, in some paper towels to increase their absorbency (see *Paper Goods* in *Chapter 8: Housekeeping*). Besides these particular applications, it's sometimes used in personal-care products, such as certain cosmetics, shampoos, and even toothpaste (see *Typical Modern Ingredients* in *Chapter 2: Personal Care*).

Unfortunately, most of the items containing formaldehyde will release it into the air. In the case of cabinets made with formaldehyde-containing glues and finishes, the formaldehyde will be continually released for years. In fact, the formaldehyde in some man-made wood products has a *half-life* of 3 to 5 years. This means that after the first 3 to 5 years, half of the formaldehyde present will have been released. During the next 3 to 5 years, half of what remains is outgassed, and so on. Interestingly, the amount of water vapor present in your home, as well as the temperature, will affect the rate of the formaldehyde release. Both a higher relative humidity and higher tempera-tures will cause the formaldehyde to be released into the air faster.

Testing and Eliminating Formaldehyde in Homes

What is considered an acceptable, safe, level of formaldehyde in the indoor air is still being debated. However, increasing numbers of concerned experts believe that formaldehyde concentrations should be as low as possible in the air you breathe. So, how much formaldehyde is too much? Clean outdoor air in the country might contain 0.01 parts per million (ppm). Sensitive people often react to levels as low as 0.03 ppm, and levels of 0.05-0.15 aren't un-usual in houses. The World Health Organization recommends that levels be below 0.05 in houses. This is especially important if a house contains young children, asthmatics, or persons weakened by a major illness. On the other hand, levels as high as 0.75 ppm are often allowed in the workplace.

Because of the controversy over the safety of formaldehyde, some people feel it is a good idea to test their home's formaldehyde level. If you'd like to have this done, contact an environmental-testing company or buy a home formaldehyde-level test kit. Mail-order sources for these kits include **The Liv-ing Source** and **The Home Shopper**, among others. Unfortunately, testing may not detect the extremely minute levels that still promote reactions in certain sensitive individuals. And these tests can't pinpoint the outgassing source(s) of the formaldehyde for you.

If you have too much formaldehyde, what should be done? Airing items sus-pected of containing high levels (such as some new furniture) outdoors for a period of time often helps. Special sealant coatings can be applied to wood items such as kitchen cabinets (see *Sealants and Other Acrylic Water-Based*

Wood Finishes in *Chapter 12: Home Workshop and Garage*). However, for many sensitive persons, these remedies just won't help enough. After airing and sealing, your furniture may still remain too bothersome. By the way, it should be mentioned that sealants also can pollute the air with their own chemical odors.

As you might suspect, some air filters can remove formaldehyde from the air. Activated charcoal is often used, but in reality it is not particularly effective. This is because activated charcoal can't adsorb low-molecular weight VOCs like formaldehyde (Commonly, molecular weight is defined as the total atomic weights of all the atoms making up a molecule.). However, specially treated activated charcoal is available that can remove formaldehyde from the air. Activated alumina can also remove a great deal of airborne formaldehyde. Yet, filtering is often not sufficient.

The truth is, permanently removing the source of the formaldehyde, or storing the offending items elsewhere until the amount of formaldehyde they release is undetectable, are the two best solutions. Of course, this can be disruptive, time-consuming, and costly. However, these are the only measures that best ensure your family's health against any possible negative effects from exposure to formaldehyde.

RADON

Within the last decade, researchers have become aware that *radon* gas is present in quite a few American homes at unacceptable levels. Unfortunately, they've also concluded that the presence of radon at high-enough concentrations can lead to serious health consequences. The following sections discuss exactly what radon is, how to detect it, and then introduce ways to reduce it, if it proves necessary.

The Nature and Potential Health Consequences of Radon

Radon (Rn) is an odorless, colorless, radioactive gas. Actually, there are twenty radon *isotopes* (unique atomic forms each having a different number of neutrons). Of these, *radon-222*, which is produced by naturally occurring *radium* in the ground, is the isotope of most concern. It is radon-222 that can cause serious health problems if it becomes concentrated in your home.

Radon-222 can enter homes through foundation cracks and/or through well water. If it's unable to leave freely (for example, through a ventilation system), it's concentration soon rises. Unfortunately, the trapped gaseous radon-222 decays, producing solid *radon decay products*. It's actually this material—and not the radon gas itself—that can become lodged in your lung tissue and eventually lead to cancer. Because of this, radon is believed to be the number 2 cause of lung cancer in the U.S. (smoking remains Number 1.

At this point it should be pointed out that radon gas is a natural part of our environment. Actually, it's been estimated that it makes up more than half of the background radioactivity we are surrounded with every day because it's continually rising up from bedrock, soil, and from some ground water (see also *Radon* in *Chapter 10: Home Water*). However, because of certain geologic conditions, some locales have much higher concentrations of radon than others. In the U.S., for example, known radon "hot spots" include western Pennsylvania and Maryland, among many others. If done correctly, tightening a house can prevent radon from entering. But in some tight houses, radon can enter easily, but has difficulty escaping.

Testing and Eliminating Radon in Homes

It's important for every home to be tested for radon. Because of individual differences in construction and in building sites, there's absolutely no way to predetermine whether or not a specific house will have a high radon level. Even if all your neighbors' homes have low levels of radon, yours might have a high concentration. But what exactly is a high radon level? Currently, the Environmental Protection Agency (EPA) says any reading above 4 pC/l (4 picoCuries of radon per liter of air) is too high, requiring remedial action.

To determine if your home falls above this level, you can buy a simple radon test kit. These are relatively inexpensive and available at most local hardware stores. In addition, **Environmental Health Shopper** is a catalog that offers them by mail order. Radon test kits are really very easy to use. You only need to read the instructions, open the canister in a location suggested, and leave it there undisturbed for the recommended time. Then, seal the canister and fill out a simple form with the time of day the canister was opened and closed and your name and address. Then mail the canister to the address given in the directions and wait for the test results to be mailed back to you.

If an inexpensive radon test indicates a level above 4 pC/l, you'll probably want to buy a costlier, more accurate test kit, or have an environmental testing company perform a more accurate test for you (see *Indoor Air Pollution Testing in General* above). If the result of this test is also high, then radon-control measures (known as *radon mitigation*) will need to be undertaken.

Ridding your house of high radon levels entails either some form of ventilation system to safely direct the radon outdoors or sealing any cracks in the foundation and basement floor to prevent the radon from entering. To help you know precisely what to do, your local board of health may be able to provide information on radon tests, radon-reduction strategies, and perhaps even the names of local companies that specialize in radon-mitigation services. In addition, a number of books have been published about radon. One you might read is *Radon: A Homeowner's Guide to Detection and Control* by Bernard Cohen and the editors of *Consumer Reports*. Although this particular book is no longer in print, it should still be available from your local library. For other books on radon, check your local bookstores and library. Also, it would be a good idea to contact the **Environmental Protection Agency (EPA)** at 401 "M" Street S.W., Washington, DC 20460; (800) 438-4318. The EPA offers several free booklets regarding radon in homes.

It is possible to buy continuously operating radon gas monitors. For example, the Radon Alert Meter takes readings every two hours and flashes a red light if over 4 pC/l of radiation is detected. This unit is portable and can be moved from room to room. If you're interested in purchasing the Radon Alert Meter, it's available from **Ozark Water Service and Environmental Services**.

VAPORS

A *vapor* is a substance in the form of a gas that is usually a liquid at room temperature. The most common vapor in houses is water vapor, which results in *high relative humidity*.

HIGH RELATIVE HUMIDITY

High relative humidity exists in many houses. Unfortunately, this can lead to a host of possible problems. The sections below explain relative humidity and ways you might lower it, if necessary, in your home.

High Relative Humidity Defined and Potential Consequences

Humidity refers to the water-vapor content of air. Therefore, it can be difficult to think of humidity as a pollutant. Yet, if your indoor air contains high levels of water vapor, it can damage your walls, floors, and interior furnishings. Also, high water-vapor levels can cause mold, mildew, and other microbial growth. In addition, it can often increase the rate of formaldehyde release from man-made wood products, etc.

The word *relative* is used with humidity because there's a direct relationship between the temperature of the air and the potential amount of water vapor the air can hold. Simply put, cold air can't hold as much water vapor as warm air. Therefore, if a room at 50°F held 10 gallons water vapor and an identical room at 80°F also held 10 gallons of water vapor, the rooms would have the different relative humidities. The hot room would have a lower relative humidity than the cold room because it had the potential to hold much more water vapor than the cold room. Incidentally, when air at any temperature is saturated and is no longer capable of holding any more water vapor, it's said to have a relative humidity of 100%. At the usual indoor temperatures of American homes, the best relative humidity would be less than 40% in the winter. At 40% relative humidity, mucous membranes usually won't become irritated, the skin won't become dried out, wood won't tend to crack, and mold and mildew aren't encouraged to grow.

With the use of an instrument called a *hygrometer*, you actually can measure the relative humidity in different locations in your home. Inexpensive analog (non-electronic) models are usually sold at hardware stores, and at **Sears Roebuck, and Co.** Electronic versions are available at local Radio Shack stores. A mail-order source is **The Environmental Health Shopper**, which also sells a handy temperature/humidity guide as well.

Eliminating High Humidity in Homes

If your home's air consistently has high relative-humidity readings, check for unsuspected water leakage sources around your house. These could include leaking air conditioners and plumbing lines or damaged roofs. Also look for clogged gutters and foundation drains. In addition, too much shady foliage planted near the house can contribute to problems.

Of course, poor ventilation can easily result in high humidity levels. Therefore, it's a good idea for rooms in your home that commonly generate large amounts of water vapor to be properly vented to the outdoors so that the water vapor can't build up indoors. Ideally, a range hood over your kitchen stovetop, an exhaust fan in your laundry room, and exhaust fans in your bathrooms should be installed and used regularly. All such fans must be vented to the outdoors to be effective.

Bathroom fans can have a simple, manually operated on/off wall-mounted switch, a manually set crank timer, or they can be controlled by a *dehumidistat*. A dehumidistat is simply a device that monitors relative-humidity levels

302

and automatically triggers an electrical switch when a certain preset reading has been reached. In this case, the dehumidistat would turn on a bathroom exhaust fan when the relative humidity gets too high. You might want to install an exhaust fan in your laundry area, and you'll also want to make sure that your clothes dryer is vented to the outdoors. By the way, **Broan Manufacturing Co.** and **Nutone Inc.** are two manufacturers of fans and control switches. Local electrical-supply companies should carry them or similar brands, as well as dehumidistats.

You can also lower a high relative-humidity by using air conditioners and dehumidifiers. Both of these are able to pull water vapor out of the air and condense it into liquid water. Of course, air conditioners and dehumidifiers are available from many local department and appliance stores including **Sears and Roebuck and Co.** Dehumidifiers can be also mail-ordered from **The Environmental Health Shopper**. It should be noted that dehumidifiers can be emptied either automatically into a house drain, or manually. If you decide upon a dehumidifier, it's important to clean it regularly to prevent any mold growth. This is especially necessary with models that must be emptied manually inasmuch as they can contain standing water (see *Mold* below).

BIOLOGICAL CONTAMINANTS

Anything airborne that is presently living, was once living, or was produced by something alive, and has the capacity to create negative health effects is considered to be a *biological contaminant*. Therefore, bacteria, viruses, dust-mite fragments and feces, mold, mildew, and pollen are all biological contaminants. These particular biological contaminants are in *particulate form* (tiny bits of solid matter.) However, most metabolic processes also release a variety of gases including volatile organic compounds (VOCs). Some of the major biological contaminants commonly found in homes are discussed under the following headings.

(For information on biological contaminants in your water supply, see *Biological Contaminants* in *Chapter 10: Home Water*.)

BACTERIA AND VIRUSES

In America, bacteria and viruses are popularly known as *germs*—a word with very negative connotations. Surprisingly though, many bacteria and viruses are actually not harmful to human beings. In fact, some bacteria are actually necessary for life. But, of course, there are also harmful, disease-causing bacteria and viruses in a home's air whose numbers should be minimized or eliminated if at all possible. In the following two sections, information on both viruses and bacteria will be given and suggestions made regarding methods you might try to control their populations within your own home.

Bacteria

Bacteria is a classification of some of the simplest one-celled microscopic organisms on earth. Unlike viruses (see *Viruses* below), individual bacteria are complete entities in themselves and are capable of their own reproduction. In size, bacteria usually range from 0.2–50 microns in length (One micron is one millionth of a meter.). So far, about two thousand species of bacteria have been identified and they have been found to exist virtually everywhere. Interestingly, certain bacterial species have a resting state known as the en-

dospore stage. Bacteria in this form can be among the most indestructible of all living things. Apparently, only long periods of high-pressure steam will cause some endospores to die.

For humans, certain bacteria can pose very real health dangers. For example, staphylococci can cause strep throat, and bacteria known as pleuropneumonia-like organisms (PPLO) can lead to contagious pneumonia. Other *pathogenic* (disease causing) bacteria are responsible for salmonella, Legionnaire's Disease, and botulism. Unfortunately, under ideal circumstances, most bacteria can divide and multiply about every twenty minutes. As a matter of fact, theoretically, one bacterium could produce one-half million descendants within six hours. Therefore, diseases caused by bacteria often have the potential to spread rapidly.

To counter the proliferation of dangerous bacteria in your home, it's extremely important not to create hospitable living conditions for them. Therefore, be sure to store all your food properly, clean your house thoroughly and regularly, and avoid having standing water or persistently high relative-humidity levels in your home. Also make sure that any humidifiers you're using are frequently cleaned, perhaps daily in some cases. It's also a good idea to disinfect your humidifiers from time to time with *hydrogen peroxide* (use the 3% solution sold in most pharmacies) or with some other tolerable disinfectant (see *Controlling Mold and Mildew* in *Chapter 7: Cleaning*).

You may also want to use special air-cleaning equipment. Certain air purifiers and filters, such as *HEPA* filters (which strain out bacteria) and *electrostatic filters* (which cause bacteria to become trapped through electrical-charge adhesion) will help remove airborne bacteria. *Ozone generators* can also counter bacterial levels by actually destroying them with reactive and caustic *ozone* (O_3). In addition, *negative-ion generators* can cause airborne bacteria to leave the air and adhere themselves to walls, etc.

Viruses

Viruses are extremely minute parasites that, by definition, border somewhere between life and nonlife. Viruses are found in several forms, the most distinctive being the *virion*, which basically consists of nucleic acid (reproduction information within a chemical structure) protected with a protein sheath (coating). Virions are the infectious form of a virus as it exists outside host cells. Because of this, the term *virus* often simply implies the virion form.

In reality, viruses differ greatly from one another in size and shape. Most are extremely minute—many being only 3,000 angstroms long (One angstrom is one ten-billionth of a meter.). Viruses are unable to function or reproduce completely on their own and must invade a host species' cells. Once in a compatible cell, the virus injects its nucleic acid into that of the host cell's. This eventually causes the host cell to reproduce the virus. However, although there are hundreds of virus strains, only a limited number are actually a threat to humans. Viral infections that can occur in people include polio, mumps, German measles, chicken pox, influenza, hepatitis, and herpes. Even some cancers are thought to be caused by certain viruses.

In the indoor air of your home, relatively high levels of airborne infectious viruses are present most commonly when a family member or pet currently has a viral disease. Therefore, vaccinations of those family members still unaffected is the best preventive, if vaccinations for their illness is available. By the way, ozone generators may be able to kill certain viruses through the action of the reactive ozone (O_3) gas.

DUST MITE FRAGMENTS AND FECES

Although it's admittedly disgusting to think about, *dust mite* body parts and feces often make up a fairly large portion of house dust. Interestingly, it's the lightweight dead body parts and fecal pellets, and not living mites themselves, that tend to become airborne. For susceptible individuals, this dust-mite debris can trigger asthmatic or allergic symptoms.

Unfortunately, common dust mites are found in virtually every home. But exactly what are these creatures? Dust mites are actually tiny (usually less than 0.04" in length), eight-legged creatures related to ticks and spiders. If you want to test your home for its dust-mite population, a test kit is available from **The Environmental Health Shopper**.

To minimize dust-mite populations and their debris, you should dust and vacuum your home frequently and thoroughly. For dusting, it's a good idea to use a dampened all-cotton flannel cloth that will be able hold onto the dust rather than just spread it around (see *Dusting* in *Chapter 7: Cleaning*). For vacuuming, you might want to use a central vacuum system with an outdoor exhaust or a very efficient, specially filtered, portable vacuum (see *Vacuuming* in *Chapter 7: Cleaning*). Because dust mites thrive at higher relative humidities, they can often be minimized by keeping your house drier.

By the way, many types of air filters are able to trap dust-mite debris. Also, *negative-ion generators* will cause this material to leave the air and adhere to your walls and ceilings, etc.

MOLD

Mold tends to be both ugly and destructive in homes. This section discusses what mold is, possible outcomes, if present in your home, and methods of dealing with it.

The Nature and Potential Consequences of Mold

Mold is a popular term for those fungi having *hyphae* (threadlike filaments). Living mold, dead mold, and mold spores are common airborne *allergens* (substances that trigger allergic symptoms). Molds generally thrive best where moisture levels are relatively high. Under the right conditions, it can actually grow on almost anything. Therefore, tile, grout, wood, paint, plaster, and fabric are all susceptible to mold.

Unfortunately, mold growth is unsightly and can cause permanent staining and damage to walls and furnishings. Sometimes, unpleasant odors also accompany mold growth. These odors are the gases given off from the mold's metabolic processes, which sometimes include potentially harmful volatile organic compounds (VOCs). Sadly, once your belongings become moldy, it's often difficult to completely eliminate the stains or the musty odors.

Testing and Eliminating Mold in Homes

If desired, you can hire an environmental-testing company to test your indoor air for mold content. You can also buy home test kits for mold. Two mail-order mold-testing sources are **The Living Source** and **The Environmental Home Shopper**. However, in certain situations, it's probably questionable what real benefits emanate from testing your home for mold. After all, in most cases, homeowners will already know they have a mold problem from actually seeing or smelling it.

Generally, the best way to guard against mold is to create an indoor habitat that's unappealing for its colonization. This is done by properly storing your food and cleaning your home and clothing frequently (see *Chapter 7: Cleaning*). You should also eliminate any moisture problems in your home. That means fixing leaking water pipes, drains, gutters, and roofs and foundations. Another important step is reducing your home's relative-humidity levels if they're too high. In the winter, when the indoor relative humidity is below 40%, mold growth drops off dramatically.

By the way, very common airborne mold sources in homes are contaminated air conditioners, humidifiers, and dehumidifiers. To help prevent mold growth from starting in your air conditioner, try running just the fan for thirty minutes immediately after you turn the cooling function off. This will help dry out your air conditioner's inner components. For humidifiers and dehumidifiers, your best defense is to keep them as clean as possible. For all these devices, remember to wash their filters often.

If, despite your best efforts, your air conditioner, humidifier, and/or dehumidifier becomes contaminated with mold, you can sometimes get rid of it by doing the following procedure. First, unplug the machine or shut off the electricity running to it and place protective plastic sheeting on the floor. Then, carefully—but thoroughly—spray the waterproof parts (never spray anything on or near the wiring, electronics, and/or controls) with *hydrogen peroxide* in a spray bottle (This is the 3% hydrogen peroxide dilution commonly sold in pharmacies.). After that, clean by hand what you're able to dismantle or easily reach using a sponge soaked in hydrogen peroxide. Afterwards, let the unit dry thoroughly before using. When doing this, remember to wear a chemical respirator mask to protect yourself from inhaling mold particles, as well as rubber gloves to protect your hands from cuts. Of course, if you are allergic to mold, this generally isn't a project to do yourself.

By the way, if the walls of your home or some of your items become moldy, wash off the mold promptly using an appropriate mold-killing solution; that is, one that's tolerable to you and that won't damage what you're trying to clean (see *Mold and Mildew* in *Chapter 7: Cleaning*). Another approach that can work if moisture problems have caused the mold growth is to fix the leaks and high humidity, etc. Then, once the mold has become dormant, vacuum it up while wearing a chemical respirator mask as protection against breathing the mold particles.

Several air-filtering strategies including HEPAs can usually trap airborne mold. Also, ozone generators reduce mold levels by the use of the unstable, highly reactive ozone (O_3) gas they release. In addition, negative-ion generators can cause airborne mold spores to adhere to walls, ceilings, etc. so that they won't be inhaled. However, these particular approaches are certainly not the best to control mold; controlling excess moisture or high relative humidity is always the most effective solution (For information on mold in your water supply, see *Biological Contaminants* in *Chapter 10: Home Water.*).

POLLEN

Pollen grains are actually *gametophytes* of male plants, which is equivalent to sperm in male animals. The amount of pollen produced by different plant species varies enormously. However, most plants produce huge quantities of it. For example, the number of pollen grains from just one pine cone often runs in the millions.

Each plant species' pollen grains are uniquely shaped, but virtually all types of pollen grains are very small. In fact, most pollen grains are between 24 and 50 microns (One micron is one-millionth of a meter.). Interestingly, pollen grains contain proteins and sugars, some of which act as insect and animal attractants. This is because intermediary creatures are necessary to help transfer the pollen to the female flowers.

Of course, pollen grains are natural and necessary substances. Unfortunately, high airborne levels of pollen can be irritating to many people's eyes and sinuses. In some individuals, certain types of pollen grains can provoke allergic symptoms or asthma attacks. If pollen is a health concern for your family, you may want to take measures to minimize its levels inside your house. Obviously, you won't want to bring any flowering plants indoors. Also, it's a good idea not to plant trees or shrubs too near your house because the huge quantities of pollen grains produced from your nearby landscaping could easily enter through doors, windows, and the home's ventilation system.

However, for very allergic individuals, these approaches may still not be enough. Because tiny pollen grains are hardy and somewhat indestructible, they can be blown in the wind for great distances. If conditions are right, tree and plant pollen grains from many miles away could end up in the air outside—and, therefore, eventually inside—your house. Fortunately, there are a number of air-cleaning strategies that help reduce indoor pollen-grain levels. Although pollen grains are small, most are still large enough to be trapped by many types of air-filtering equipment. And, it should also be mentioned that *negative-ion generators* cause indoor airborne pollen grains to adhere to ceilings and walls, etc. so that they won't be breathed in.

MINERALS AND METALS

Harmful minerals and metals are particulate pollutants that are sometimes found in indoor air. Two in this category of which you should be aware are *asbestos* and *lead*.

ASBESTOS

Just saying *asbestos* triggers fear among many people. Although it definitely can cause severe illness, in certain situations in your home it'll pose little risk to you or your family—if you don't disturb it.

The Nature, Uses, and Potential Health Consequences of Asbestos

Asbestos is actually a generic term that's applied to several minerals that occur in a fiber-like form. However, *chrysotile* (the fibrous form of *serpentine*) is usually the particular type meant when the word *asbestos* is used. Unfortunately, if small asbestos fibers become inhaled, minute fragments can become trapped in your lung tissue. This can lead to very serious consequences. In fact, since the mid-1960s, exposure to asbestos in the workplace (asbestos mines, asbestos insulation factories, etc.) has been known to cause *asbestosis* (a severe, debilitating lung disease) as well as lung cancer.

Concern over asbestos exposure since these findings first become known has steadily increased. As a result, in 1971 asbestos became the first regulated material in the workplace by the Occupational Safety and Health Administration (OSHA). Then in 1986, OSHA decided to severely limit the acceptable exposure levels for workers. However, it was not until 1989 that the Environmental Protection Agency (EPA) regulated asbestos beyond the workplace. That year, the EPA ordered that asbestos use, manufacture, and export be reduced 94% by 1996. Asbestos was also completely banned in building materials as well as brake linings.

Yet a tremendous amount of asbestos already is present in our environment. Because asbestos fibers are fire-, heat-, and corrosion-resistant and able to be spun, woven, compressed, or added to other substances, asbestos has been widely used in industry and in commercial and consumer products. For example, it has been an ingredient in brake linings, hard flooring materials (such as certain types of hard-vinyl tiles), some cement and cement products (including cement/asbestos siding and roofing tiles), and even in some drywall compounds. It's also been used as insulation around a lot of ductwork and furnaces, as well as around particular types of electrical circuitry. As a result, many U.S. homes contain at least some quantity of asbestos. The exceptions would be only those houses that have been most recently built.

Testing and Eliminating Asbestos in Homes

It should be pointed out that asbestos in your house may not necessarily be a problem. For instance, asbestos imbedded in older hard-vinyl floor tiles is unlikely to create asbestos dust that can be inhaled. However, one of the worst situations is having deteriorating asbestos insulation surrounding your ducts and furnaces. In this case, the asbestos should be removed completely and as soon as possible. Note, this isn't a job for homeowners or amateurs but one that must be performed by licensed asbestos-removal contractors. During the removal process, there must be a complete sealing off of the contaminated areas, workers must wear hazardous-material protective gear, and special hazardous-material disposal methods are used.

If you suspect any sources of airborne asbestos in your home, call your local board of health, which can advise you on what steps to follow, including testing. If an asbestos problem is confirmed, health officials may be able to suggest approved asbestos-removal companies. In order to get a reliable asbestos-removal firm, it would be wise to obtain several homeowner references from jobs they've previously performed, a written estimate of the total cost and the projected time the removal procedure will take place. You should be aware that asbestos removal can often be quite expensive.

Although other filtering methods might be able to trap asbestos fibers depending on their size, very efficient HEPA filters would be the logical choice to use with such a potentially dangerous material. However, in reality, the best protection is to eliminate any deteriorating asbestos. For more information on asbestos, contact the **Environmental Protection Agency (EPA)** at 401 ""M" Street S.W., Washington, DC 20460; (800) 438-4318. The agency offers booklets addressing issues regarding asbestos in homes.

(For information on asbestos in your water lines, see *Asbestos/Concrete Water Main Concerns* in *Chapter 10: Home Water.*)

LEAD

Lead particles pose a real health threat in far too many U.S. homes. The following sections explain why this is the case.

The Nature, Uses, and Potential Health Consequences of Lead

Lead (*Pb*) is a very heavy, silvery-gray metal that turns a dull blue-gray when exposed to the air. It's also soft, malleable, and has a low melting point. Interestingly, once lead has *oxidized* (tarnished), it becomes corrosion-resistant. It also can be alloyed with many metals (Pewter was originally a combination of lead and tin.).

Lead has been widely utilized over the years. It's been used as a *whitening pigment* (known as *white lead*) in paints—and even in face powders at one time. It's also been widely used as an inexpensive and useful solder. In addition, it's been used to make water pipes, fishing sinkers, molded toys, printing type, and gun shot. Today, lead continues to be an essential component of lead-acid automobile batteries and is sometimes used to create waterproof barriers in certain roofing applications. Furthermore, lead is used in some ceramic glazes, among many other uses. However, deteriorating lead paint is the use that usually poses the most serious health concerns in homes.

Despite its useful qualities, lead has a serious problem: It's poisonous. For a number of years, it was suspected that lead might be responsible for certain workplace-related negative health effects (in lead mines, lead foundries, etc.), yet in amounts once considered safe. Finally, research proved that many of these fears were true. Because of this, the U.S. Centers for Disease Control (the CDC) since the mid-1980s has been steadily lowering what officials there consider the acceptable "environmental lead level."

Actually, what's currently known is that lead and many lead-containing compounds can be toxic when swallowed or inhaled. While lead is absorbed by the human body at a very slow rate, it apparently can gradually accumulate in fairly large amounts because it can't be easily eliminated. Unfortunately, high lead levels can injure the central nervous system and damage the *blood-brain barrier cells* that provide a natural shielding of your brain tissue against potentially harmful chemicals.

Signs of lead poisoning can include loss of appetite, weakness, anemia, vomiting, and convulsive episodes. In some cases, permanent brain damage can result and even death. In children, impaired learning or kidney problems can sometimes be an indication of lead poisoning. In adults, *hypertension* (high blood pressure) can sometimes be a symptom of high lead levels in the body.

Because a variety of studies have documented that children have been made ill by eating and breathing deteriorating lead paint, the federal government banned lead as a paint ingredient in 1977. More recently, lead has been banned in solder. In addition, lead additives in gasoline, such as *tetraethyl lead* and *tetramethyl lead*, have been phased out. In the past, some of these additives probably routinely entered the living spaces of homes with attached garages (see *Controlling Odors within Garages* in *Chapter 12: Home Workshop and Garage*).

Testing and Eliminating Lead in Homes

These days, it's now agreed by virtually all experts that everyone should completely avoid lead dust and lead fumes, if at all possible. Therefore, if you're concerned whether your wall paint contains lead, you might want to perform a lead test on it. Two such simple test kits are Lead Check Swabs (**HybriVet Systems, Inc.**) and Lead Alert (**Frandon Enterprises**). These can be bought directly from the companies (see *Testing for Lead* in *Chapter 5: Interior Decorating*). If you find evidence of lead in your wall paint, contact your local board of health for information on what steps to take. Lead tests can also be used on pottery, dishes, etc. that may be suspected of having lead glazes (see *Glass, Glass-Ceramic, and Pottery Cookware* in *Chapter 8: Housekeeping*).

For more on lead, you can call the **National Lead Information Center** at (800) 532-3394, which is a hotline maintained by the Environmental Protection Agency (EPA). After contacting the hotline, you'll be sent printed materials about lead poisoning and measures you can perform to prevent it, as well as a list of state and local agencies and additional information.

Although air-filtering methods for removing airborne lead might prove somewhat effective, very efficient HEPA-filtered vacuums are one of the most effective methods of eliminating it, for example, if you have deteriorating lead wall paint. However, with such a toxic metal, the best protection is to sufficiently seal the source of the lead or have it professionally removed.

(For information on lead in your water, see *Industrial Pollutants* and *Contaminants from Supply Lines, Pipes, and Solder* in *Chapter 10: Home Water.*)

MIXED CONTAMINANTS

House dust and *smoke* are actually made up of several types of pollutants. The following sections give you information on these two complicated contaminants so you'll be better able to deal with them more effectively.

DUST

Every home contains a certain amount of house dust. But exactly what is it and how do you best deal with it?

The Nature and Potential Health Consequences of Dust

House dust is a generic term that can be defined as fine, dry particles of earth and/or other debris. In homes, dust is usually made up of many components. In fact, it's possible that it can contain some soil, lead, perhaps asbestos, natural or synthetic fibers, *dander* (skin flakes), hair, fur, pollen grains, mold spores, insect parts, and insect feces, both live and dead bacteria, as well as many other things. Actually, the exact make-up of the dust found in each home is quite unique.

Not surprisingly, many people find that breathing dust can be irritating to the nose and sinuses. In addition, certain individuals have asthmatic or allergic responses when they inhale dust—sometimes suffering severely from it. In reality, it's often only one component, or perhaps only a few, in the dust that actually triggers these autoimmune symptoms.

Of course, the best defense against indoor dust is to thoroughly and regularly clean the interior of your home. If you frequently dust using a damp all-cotton flannel cloth, for example, it can help eliminate a great deal of the particulate matter that lands on your tables, lamps, accent pieces, and dressers, etc. If you vacuum often your floors, walls, and upholstered furniture with a central vacuum system with an outdoor exhaust or a specially filtered portable unit, it can also help cut down on the quantity of accumulated house dust. (See *Dusting* and *Vacuuming* in *Chapter 7: Cleaning.*)

To remove airborne dust in your home, you can use one of many air-cleaning and air-filtering approaches designed to remove particulates. Also, negative-ion generators can cause airborne dust particles to leave the indoor air and adhere to your walls, etc.

Duct Cleaning

Furnace and air conditioning ducts commonly acquire a layer of house dust in them over time. Therefore, it's a good idea to clean your home's entire ductwork system from time to time. However, it must be said that cleaning ducts can be a very difficult, if not impossible, job for many homeowners to personally undertake. Fortunately, professional companies now specialize in this field, many of which use a powerful vacuuming procedure.

You may find that some duct-cleaning contractors want to use a *disinfectant* (sometimes scented) in your ducts. The disinfectant treatment is meant to inhibit the growth of biological contaminants such as microbes, dust mites, fungi, and bacteria. And if scented, it's also meant to act as a deodorizing "air freshener." However, it is generally wise to avoid having these chemicals used in your ducts because they can leave odors in them for some time. Naturally, this is an important consideration for sensitive persons.

To find a professional duct-cleaning service, check in your local classified telephone directory. If you don't see any listed, you might ask for suggestions at you local board of health or heating/cooling contractor. If you do find a prospective company, ask specifically about their procedure for cleaning ducts, what cleaning products and chemicals, if any, they normally use, and some homeowner references, as well as time and cost estimates.

SMOKE

Smoke is a surprisingly complex substance whose effects can linger long after the combustion that created it has been extinguished. The sections below explain what's in smoke, and how it can affect you if inhaled, and give you information on smoke detectors.

The Nature and Potential Health Consequences of Smoke

Smoke is a by-product of combustion. It is actually considered a *mixed aerosol* of gases, suspended liquid vapor droplets, and very tiny solid particulates. Unfortunately, if you breathe in smoke, these minute solids can be particularly damaging to your respiratory system, especially your lungs. Interestingly, if the combustion gas sulfur dioxide is also present, the particulates can become even more deeply imbedded in your lung tissue than they otherwise would. In any case, bronchitis, asthma, emphysema, and even lung cancer can result from breathing in smoke. And too much smoke inhaled at one time can easily result in death. The particular effects you'll experience from inhaling smoke depends on the origin of the smoke (wood, tobacco, or synthetic vinyl, for example), its concentration in the air, the length of exposure, and your own personal susceptibilities.

In homes, sources of smoke can include tobacco, kerosene lamps, candles, incense, fireplaces, and wood stoves. Of course, unplanned combustion in the form of accidental fires can be devastating sources of smoke in houses. This is because the amount of smoke produced from even a very small, localized fire can be both massive and pervasive. It's no wonder then that smoke inhalation causes more injuries and deaths in home fires than burns.

Besides the direct health effects, smoke can easily permeate and saturate your clothing, furnishings, walls, and flooring. Unfortunately, smoky odors can often be difficult to get rid of completely. Sometimes, even repeated cleaning and extended airing outdoors may not remove all the smell. However, in certain cases, some individuals have found that ozone generators have been somewhat helpful. Apparently, the very reactive ozone (O_3) is able to break down the compounds that make up the smoky odors.

Many people ask, What's the best air filter to eliminate smoke in the air? (These same persons are often concerned about smoke in their homes from lit tobacco products, wood stoves, etc.) Smoke is a mixture containing both solid particulates and vapors, but it is also acompanied by combustion gases, so it requires an air-cleaning system capable of removing several types of contaminants. Therefore, some sort of device capable of trapping minute particulate material is needed. Actually, because the particles in smoke are often so extremely tiny, HEPA filters are probably be the best type to use. In addition, activated charcoal would also be necessary to adsorb the gases. Note, an air-cleaning system can easily become overwhelmed and rendered more or less useless if the concentration of smoke in the air is very high. Ideally, in a healthy home, there are no sources of smoke whatsoever.

Smoke Detectors

Even in homes where there are no combustion appliances or equipment, no tobacco smoking, and no burning candles or fireplaces, the threat of smoke from unplanned and unsuspected fires still exists. Fires started by lighting, electrical shorts, or when objects are too near electric stovetops, hot water tanks, and heating units can—and do—occur. Because smoke is so dangerous, it's best to continually monitor your home for its presence with smoke detectors. (In a great many locales, their installation is required by law.) These will sound off loudly if smoke is present.

Many experts now believe that smoke detectors should be installed on each floor, including the basement, of every home. When you're ready to mount them, place at least one of them in the hallway leading to the bedrooms. By the way, a good location is the ceiling, away from any air ducts or vents. There should also be a multipurpose fire extinguisher on each floor (see *Portable Fire Extinguishers* in *Chapter 8: Housekeeping*).

Be aware that there are two basic types of smoke detectors. Perhaps the most common variety is the *ionization unit*. These smoke detectors continually release *ions* (an ion is an atom or group of atoms with an electric charge) from their internal *radioactive components*. If smoke is present, the smoke particles will attach themselves to these ions. When this occurs, it reduces the electric flow inside the detector, which in turn sets off the alarm. The other type of smoke detector is the *photoelectric* or *optical unit*. These generate a tiny light beam. If smoke is present, the beam is either blocked or scattered, causing a change in the electric flow that triggers the alarm.

Although the amount of radioactivity released by ionization-type smoke detectors is tiny, it's probably a good idea to avoid having any radioactive sources in your home whenever possible. Unfortunately, most smoke detectors available at local hardware stores are generally the radioactive type. **Baubiology Hardware** and **Ozark Water Service and Environmental Services** offer non-ionizing, photoelectric smoke detectors. It's important that you gently and carefully vacuum the exterior of a photoelectric smoke detector occasionally to remove any dust. You also should test all smoke detectors monthly to see if the alarm is working properly (Most units have a "test" button to press.). In units that use batteries, the batteries should be replaced annually.

It should be mentioned that some smoke detectors run by batteries, while others are designed to be wired into your home's electrical circuitry. (Some units that are electrically powered will also hold batteries.) If smoke detectors are required by law in your locale, the regulations often require that they be connected to electric wiring.

AIR PURIFICATION AND CLEANING

A wide range of products and devices sold today attempt to purify or clean the air—with an equally wide range of effectiveness. In the following sections, many of these types are discussed.

SIMPLE INDOOR ODOR CONTROL

Of course, good ventilation and routine home interior cleaning should help prevent or eliminate many household odors and pollutants. However, extra measures may be necessary from time to time. In certain of these cases, simple, inexpensive, non-mechanical solutions may be all that's necessary.

POTPOURRI

One very popular odor-control method is to use *potpourri*. While some potpourri consists of natural dried herbs, spices, and flower petals, others also have added perfumes, either natural or synthetic. However, no matter what they're composed of, potpourri can only mask unpleasant odors—not eliminate them. Then, too, potpourri's own fragrant emanations can actually be more bothersome to certain sensitive individuals than the original unpleasant odors they were meant to disguise.

If you want to use potpourri, consider the all-natural types to avoid breathing synthetically derived chemicals. Because the odors will permeate and linger, use potpourri only in areas where its odor won't be bothersome for an extended period of time (see *The Problems with Scents* in *Chapter 2: Personal Care*). To purchase potpourri, check in department and health-food stores. In addition, your local library and bookstore may have books that tell how to make your own.

AEROSOL DEODORIZERS AND DISINFECTANTS

Some typical deodorizing sprays are actually little more than diluted, aerated, synthetic fragrances. However, those labeled as *disinfectants* usually have, in addition, chemicals capable of inhibiting or killing certain biological contaminants, especially bacteria and mold.

Of course, the ingredients of these spray products are usually absorbed by your walls, floors, and furnishings—and you yourself, if you breathe them in. Therefore, it may be best to avoid deodorizing and disinfecting sprays, especially if you're a sensitive person. It should be remembered that sometimes the odors created by these sprays can be very long-lasting (see *The Problems with Scents* in *Chapter 2: Personal Care*).

However, one alternative spray you may want to try is Smells Begone. This is a nontoxic, nonstaining, unscented product specifically designed to eliminate many kinds of household odors. Local health-food stores sometimes carry it. If not, you can mail-order it from **The Seventh Generation**.

BAKING SODA AND BORAX

Often, a safe solution to odors in small, confined spaces is simply to use an open box of baking soda. Of course, this has been done for years in refrigerators, but it can also reduce odors in your freezer and in closets. Baking soda is effective at eliminating odors because it actually absorbs them. However, be sure it doesn't get spilled, and remember to replace it from time to time.

Another similar odor solution is to use a small amount of unscented borax in a bowl. As with baking soda, be careful not to tip it over, and to replace it occasionally. Note that, it's important that borax not be ingested, so make certain that small children and pets can't get access to it.

ACTIVATED CHARCOAL

Sometimes, a pie pan filled with activated charcoal helps eliminate odors within a small, confined space. Activated charcoal works because it actually adsorbs odors. In adsorption, odor molecules (tobacco smoke, metabolic products of bacteria, as well as many compounds given off from plastics and other synthetic materials) adhere to the activated charcoal's surface.

If you choose to use a pan of activated charcoal, place it so it can't be easily tipped. You'll also need to replace the activated charcoal occasionally when it can't adsorb any more. Activated charcoal is available from **E.L. Foust Co., Inc.** and many other manufacturers of air filters. It's also often sold in pet stores because of it's use in aquarium filters.

ZEOLITE

Zeolite is the name of a family of naturally occurring minerals. As with activated charcoal, zeolite works by way of adsorption. A real advantage to using zeolite is that it can often be renewed and reused many times. Once the contaminated surface is no longer capable of adsorbing pollutants, zeolite can be placed in the sun and, after only a day or two, most of the adsorbed odors and gases will have freed itself and dissipated into the outdoor air, thus reactivating the adsorbing zeolite surface.

It must be noted that zeolite doesn't work on every airborne pollutant, and different individuals have reported varying success with it. In some cases, people have reported that it's worked "like a miracle," while others have said it seemed to do very little. Obviously, zeolite's effectiveness depends on the type of contaminants in the air, the quantity of contaminants, how big the room is, how contaminated the zeolite is, your personal expectations, and your olfactory sensitivity.

If you want to buy zeolite, Non-Scents (**CWY Products**) is one popular brand. This particular product is sold packaged as a powder, in granules, or in chunks. Call the company for the dealer nearest you. You may also want to try the Molecular Adsorber, a simple canister device that holds zeolite pellets. These units come in several different sizes and refills are available. Two mail-order sources for the Molecular Adsorber are **enviro-clean** and **The Environmental Health Shopper**.

AIR FILTERS

Air filters work by letting air pass through a material (often called *media*) designed to trap certain substances considered pollutants. Many people assume that if they purchase an air filter, it'll solve any indoor air problem they have. This is faulty reasoning. Air filters often aren't powerful enough to decontaminate a home if it has stagnant air, mildew, outgassing carpets and furnishings, or intolerable wall paint. Adequate fresh-air ventilation, proper home repair and maintenance, and the use of less-toxic construction, cleaning, and furnishing materials are always the best techniques to ensure good indoor air quality. What air filters can do is *polish* the air. In other words, they work best if they only have to handle minor air pollution problems or polluting situations of short duration.

It is important not to assume that your furnace filter will do much in cleaning the air. Common replaceable, thin, fiberglass furnace filters do little to actually improve your home's indoor air quality. As such, these are *furnace* filters, not *human* filters, and are meant only to capture very large particles capable of damaging your furnace fan's motor and other parts—not to protect you and your family. However, you might consider some better-than-average alternative furnace air filters that are specially designed to protect occupants from airborne contaminants.

It should be pointed out that sensitive people are often bothered by air filters themselves. Even though the purpose of an air filter is to clean the air, many also add complicating substances to the air. For example, many filters are held together with a resin or glue of some type that has slight outgassing characteristics; some filters give off ozone; and sensitive people sometimes can't tolerate some kinds of activated charcoal.

AIR FILTER TYPES

There are several basic air-filtering strategies with which you should become familiar. Knowing them will help you make more informed choices when you prepare to purchase a filter unit for your own home. An important point to remember is that activated-charcoal and activated-alumina filters can't remove all forms of indoor pollution. Actually, they're primarily capable of adsorbing gases—not solid particles. Other filters with other types of media, for example extended-surface filters with their synthetic filtering media, are designed to trap particles—not gases. Therefore, if you want to capture both gaseous and particulate contaminants, the filter you select should combine both strategies.

In the following sections, the most common filter media and technologies are discussed. Suggestions for specific filter models and brands are listed later in the chapter.

Activated-Charcoal and Activated-Alumina Filters

One of the most common air filters currently being marketed to sensitive people is the activated-charcoal (also known as activated-carbon) filter. These units are designed to remove polluting gases such as volatile organic compounds (VOCs), but they aren't capable of removing all of them. Certain low-molecular weight VOCs, such as formaldehyde, aren't adsorbed by typical activated-charcoal media (Molecular weight is the total atomic weight of all atoms making up a molecule; large, complicated molecules are composed of many atoms and, thus, tend to have high molecular weights. Formaldehyde, is actually a fairly simple molecule, so it has a low molecular weight.).

Interestingly—and something you may not be aware of—research has shown that activated charcoal can adsorb large quantities of certain polluting gases when the air is polluted, then release them slowly back into clean air. While this certainly isn't ideal, being exposed to very low levels of contaminants is probably preferable to experiencing a few large-exposure events. Therefore, despite this characteristic, activated charcoal should still be considered an advantageous filtering material—even for sensitive individuals.

On the plus side, activated-charcoal filters can be relatively affordable. However, their prices can vary depending on the particular model and their specific features. And, of course, the activated charcoal used in filters should be replaced every few months—or whenever it no longer seems to be working effectively (Some devices must have their entire activated-charcoal cartridge units replaced.).

But exactly what is activated charcoal? Defined, it is charcoal (coconut shell is one of the more popular types, but it can also be made from coal, wood, etc.) that's been subjected to a special steam process that causes its surface to become extremely pitted and porous. This creates a tremendously large surface area, resulting in greater adsorption capacity. Adsorption is a chemical-physical process whereby gases adhere to a surface. With great deal of surface area, activated charcoal has a great deal of adsorption capacity. It should also be noted that some particulate matter can become inadvertently trapped in activated-charcoal media.

If formaldehyde needs to be removed from your indoor air, your filter should be equipped with a specially treated activated charcoal or an adsorption material that's capable of actually adsorbing formaldehyde. One substance that's often combined with activated charcoal for this purpose is activated alumina. To make activated alumina, regular granular alumina (aluminum oxide, the compound from which commercial aluminum is derived) is heated. This causes the alumina granules to acquire a very porous, pitted structure. At this point, the granules are capable of adsorbing certain gases. Then the alumina is impregnated with *potassium permanganate* (a dark-purplish, crystalline, water-soluble solid material). The impregnated alumina is able to adsorb an even wider range of gaseous contaminants, including formaldehyde. Of course, like activated charcoal, activated alumina must be replaced periodically as it becomes contaminated.

Activated charcoal, activated alumina, and mixture of the two are available as replaceable filters for use in forced-air furnace or air-conditioning systems as well as in a "loose-fill" form for many types of portable filtering devices. If you're a sensitive person, it would be wise to experiment will several types of adsorption media to find an activated-charcoal or activated-charcoal/activated-alumina mix that you personally find tolerable (see *Testing* in *Chapter 1: Getting Started*). (As it turns out, some people find that they react negatively to certain kinds of charcoal.) To help you determine which charcoal you can tolerate best Carbon Media Samples are available from **E.L. Foust Co., Inc.** This company sells several different types of activated charcoal, as well as impregnated activated alumina.

It should be mentioned that activated-charcoal and activated-charcoal mixes can initially be very dusty. Therefore, if you have a new furnace-type filter containing this material, it is a good idea to vacuum both sides of it before installing it. If you are refilling a portable canister-type filter, vacuum the canister thoroughly after you fill it and before you operate the unit.

Extended-Surface Filters

Extended-surface filters are made of multi-pleated material, usually polyester or fiberglass, held together with a synthetic resin. These filters are often 4–5" thick. The deep-pleated design actually creates a very large filtering surface without greatly increasing the resistance to the air flowing through it—a problem that can occur with many types of filters. Most of the extended-surface filters available require the installation of special housings in which to mount them. These housings are permanently placed in the duct systems of forced-air furnaces and air conditioners. (It should be mentioned that 1"-thick extended-surface filters are also available. These are meant to replace your standard furnace/air-conditioner filter.)

Extended-surface filters are fairly effective as particulate filters (They're actually classified as *medium-efficiency filters.*). They're designed to trap many types of airborne solids, including most pollens. However, they aren't capable of adsorbing contaminating gases. Extended-surface filters are usually moderately priced but often require the services of a professional heating and cooling contractor to install them. As with most filters, the media (the pleated material) must be replaced annually or when it becomes dirty.

One consideration to keep in mind, especially if you're a sensitive person, is that the synthetic materials making up these filters can give off odors. However, some people have found that by putting a new filter in their oven at a low oven temperature (200°F or under) for about two hours, it often helps eliminate most bothersome smells. If you're considering this, first contact the filter manufacturer to see if its product will withstand such a procedure.

If you find it acceptable to go ahead and "bake" your filter, make certain that you have adequate ventilation when you do it. You should close off your kitchen from the rest of the house, open the kitchen windows, and operate the range-hood fan (vented outdoors) on high. Once the filter has finished baking, use hot pads or oven mitts to place it outdoors to cool. However, continue to keep your kitchen windows open and the range-hood fan on for at least 30 minutes and heat the oven up to a temperature high enough to burn off any odors that may have accumulated within the oven itself.

HEPA Filters

HEPA filters are a very special type of *extended-surface filter*. The acronym HEPA actually stands for **h**igh **e**fficiency **p**articulate **a**rresting (or sometimes **a**ir or **a**ccumulator). Interestingly, these filters were originally developed by the U.S. Atomic Energy Commission (AEC) during World War II to trap radioactive plutonium particles in nuclear laboratories.

HEPA filters are generally made of fiberglass or polyester fibers held together by a synthetic resin. These filters have extremely tiny pores, so the airflow through them is very restricted. Therefore, powerful fans are necessary to forcibly push air through them. HEPAs are sometimes termed *absolute filters*, and it's easy to understand why. Most HEPA filters are capable of trapping 97% or more of particles as small as 0.3 microns (a micron is one millionth of a meter); some are designed to be even more efficient. Not surprisingly, vacuums fitted with HEPA filters are used to remove all traces of contaminants during asbestos cleanup operations. In addition, HEPA air filters are commonly used in research laboratories and in the manufacture of electronics. However, although these filters are very effective at removing particulates, they're unable to remove any contaminating gases.

HEPA filters have other drawbacks as well. For example, they're usually fairly expensive. Therefore, to help extend the life of the HEPA filter itself, most filtering units using HEPA technology have one or more prefilters to first capture most of the large particles. With a prefilter, the HEPA media itself will only need to be replaced annually. (The prefilters will need to be replaced more frequently.)

It's important to note that some sensitive individuals find that the synthetic material used in HEPA filters gives off odors they find quite bothersome. In a few cases, despite the advantages of particulate-free air, these odors have proven to be intolerable. However, if an activated charcoal postfilter is added to the HEPA filtering unit, this will usually minimize these objectionable odors. Yet, you also should also understand that most people, even very sensitive ones, often don't require the tremendous efficiency of a HEPA filter anyway. Unless someone smokes in your home, other filtering approaches will generally suffice (see *Smoke* above).

Electrostatic Filters

Electrostatic filters, like electrostatic precipitators (see below), rely on *electrostatic force* to work (Electrostatic force causes like-charged molecules to repel and those with unlike charges to attract.). However, unlike electrostatic precipitators, electrostatic filters rely on simple static electricity rather than live electric current. Electrostatic filters are made of special plastic media, such as vinyl, polyester, or polystyrene, and are about 1" thick. These filters are meant to replace typical standard forced-air furnace/air-conditioning filters (Some companies offer models that fit in windows.).

Electrostatic filters work as a result of air passing through them causing both positive and negative static-electric charges to build up in their synthetic media (Some units are actually precharged, using *electrets*, a special plastic material that has a permanent charge.). In the filtering process, those particulates in the air that happen to be charged are then attracted to—and adhere to—the portions of the plastic media that carry a charge opposite of their own. It should be noted that many pollutant molecules are positively charged although others are negatively charged or uncharged.

Electrostatic filters are relatively inexpensive and constructed so that the air flowing through them is only slightly restricted. While these filters aren't extremely efficient, they're able to capture many mold spores and pollen grains (Electrostatic filters are not capable of trapping gases of any kind.).

Sometimes dirty electrostatic filters can be washed off so that their surfaces are again able to capture particulates. (Of course, this should be done only if the manufacturer allows it.) Most electrostatic filters should be replaced when they're no longer capable of retaining an electrical charge. This will vary with the brand and how dirty the air in question is. It should be noted that the plastic media can sometimes be bothersome for certain sensitive individuals.

Electrostatic Precipitators

Electrostatic precipitators, also known as *electronic air cleaners*, operate differently from the above filters in that they don't require the air to pass through media (such as activated charcoal or a screening material). Therefore, technically they aren't filters, however, they do capture and retain pollutants, so are contained in this section. (Note that, these units will not trap contaminating gases.) Today, most electrostatic precipitators are designed to be permanently installed in the ductwork of forced-air furnace/air-conditioner systems.

Electrostatic precipitators, like electrostatic filters rely on electrostatic force to remove pollutants from the air (Electrostatic force causes like-charged molecules to repel and those with unlike charges to attract.). However, electrostatic filters use static electricity, while electrostatic precipitators require live current to do their job. There are other major differences as well.

Electrostatic precipitators contain metal wires that have a strong electrical charge. As the air passes by these wires, any particulate matter in the air takes on the same charge as the wires. The air (with its now-charged particulates) then passes into a *collection chamber* containing a series of metal plates. These plates have also been charged, but with a charge opposite that of the wires. As a result, the charged particles become greatly attracted to the collection plates and tightly cling to them.

As it turns out, dust and debris clinging to these plates can quickly build up. This causes electrostatic precipitators to steadily, sometimes rapidly, become less and less efficient. Therefore, the metal plates in electrostatic precipitators must be removed and cleaned periodically, sometimes as often as once a week. Fortunately, these plates can be washed satisfactorily by simply placing them in an automatic dishwasher. Hand washing in a tub is also possible.

One notable feature of electrostatic precipitators is that, unlike other filters, they have virtually no restriction to the flow of air. This is because there's no media of any type to hinder the air's passage. There's also no filter media to replace, which is another advantage. However, electrostatic precipitators are relatively expensive, are certainly not as efficient as HEPA filters and can quickly lose much of their effectiveness unless they're regularly cleaned.

Electrostatic precipitators also produce a certain amount of toxic, reactive ozone (O_3) gas when operating. However, a postfilter of activated charcoal can usually adsorb any ozone that has formed. You should also know that electric sparks can be created inside electrostatic precipitators. These can actually free some of the particulate matter from the collection plates so that they end up back in the air you breathe. You should also be aware that some electrostatic precipitators have a tendency to make erratic zapping noises, which can be irritating.

CHOOSING THE RIGHT AIR FILTER

Before purchasing any air-filtration device, it's best to improve your home's air by other means first as much as possible. This is because air filters work best when they only must cope with minor air-pollution problems. Therefore, its wise to eliminate as many known sources of contamination (mold, perfume, tobacco products, noxious cleaners, etc.) as you can. After doing that, you should determine what problems remain in the air. The next step is to buy a filtering device designed to eliminate those sorts of pollutants.

Unfortunately, as has already been mentioned, filtering strategies that are capable of removing particulates such as pollen grains or house dust can't remove gaseous pollutants such as volatile organic compounds (VOCs), and vice versa. Fortunately, quite a few models are now available that combine two or more filtering strategies. This is especially true in portable units.

Besides offering differing strategies, various filtering units come in a variety of sizes. These range from tiny desktop units to permanently mounted, built-in, whole-house models. Obviously, in many situations the very small units are just too small to accomplish very much. On the other hand, whole-house models may be more than you really need; they are probably impractical if you're renting. Therefore, it's important to pinpoint the types of contaminants that need to be removed, as well as areas where they're found in your home. If these areas include most of your house, the whole-house models could make good sense. However, if only your kitchen, or a single bedroom needs improvement, room-size units might be more practical.

In addition, you should consider what special features you desire in a filtering device. For example, how should it be constructed? Many sensitive people will prefer a model with a metal casing, and may also require that the fan be upwind of adsorption filtering media to capture any potentially bothersome odors from the motor. It might also be important to select a unit that's designed to be especially quiet, or has two or more fan speeds.

Of course, you also should consider how much you'll be willing to spend on a filtering unit. And you should honestly evaluate how willing you are to give up convenience in order to insure a unit's reliability. Are you the type of person who would be willing to wash an electrostatic precipitator's collection plates each week? How often are you willing to order and replace your filter's media? Are you the type who doesn't mind going down into the basement occasionally, opening up your furnace, and checking to see if the electrostatic filter is dirty? Finally, you should take into consideration any manufacturers (and perhaps dealers) guarantees or warranties.

Of course, if you're a sensitive person, it would be a good idea to ask for air-filter recommendations from your physician or other health-care professional. Also, talking with friends who currently own air-filtering units should provide some useful information. In addition, to help you choose the right filter, independent consultants are available (for example, **The Healthy House In-**

stitute and **Environmental Education and Health Services**), dealer-consult-
ants (including **Nigra Enterprises**), testing service/dealers (such as **Ozark Water
Service and Environmental Services**), as well as catalogs (**The Living Source,
The Allergy Store, The Environmental Health Shopper, N.E.E.D.S., Nontoxic
Environments, Sinan Co.**, and **The American Environmental Health Foundation, Inc.**, among others). However, bear in mind that most of the above
sources do not have certified staff engineers who can specifically design whole-
house systems for your home. Incidentally, those dealer/consultants and catalogs that handle several brands with different filtering strategies will likely be
more objective and unbiased than those handling a single brand.

It should be stressed that only brief descriptions of certain air-filtering devices are given in the following sections. If you're interested in a particular
model, it's best to contact the manufacturer and/or dealer for more complete
information. Of course, other fine-quality air filters are available in addition
to the ones listed here.

Whole-House Air Filters

Whole-house filters offer the major advantage of cleaning all the air that's
circulated in your home. Some units are actually very simple and are used in
place of a typical standard furnace filter. However, others require a special
housing, and professional installation—and are very expensive.

Before investing in complex and expensive filtering/cleaning units, you probably would find it advisable to speak with an engineer or architect who is
familiar with airflow complexities, solving particular pollution problems, and
the construction of various units. Installation of such equipment should be
undertaken only by knowledgeable individuals. For more information on
whole-house filter options, read, *Understanding Ventilation* by John Bower,
which is available from **The Healthy House Institute**.

Whole-House Activated-Charcoal and Activated-Alumina Filters

If your major air-quality concern is removing gaseous contaminants such as
volatile organic compounds (VOCs), **E.L. Foust Co., Inc.** offers several brands
of 1"-thick activated-charcoal furnace/air-conditioner replacement filters.
These are available in several sizes and some also come in a special mix of
media to remove formaldehyde.

Another approach is the 600 OdorAdsorber (**Pure Air Systems, Inc.**). This
unit can be mounted into a forced-air furnace/air-conditioning system or can
be used alone with its own ductwork. It consists of a metal housing containing a prefilter and a 16"-thick activated-charcoal or activated-alumina filter.
It also comes with a one- or two-speed fan. You should realize that this unit
will likely require professional installation. To purchase one, call the company for the nearest dealer.

Whole-House HEPA Filters

HEPA filters are extremely efficient in removing particulates—probably far
more efficient than you really need. And yet, they're unable to remove any
gaseous contaminants. The big drawback to HEPA filters is that they have a
great deal of resistance to airflow. Therefore, they can't easily be used with
residential furnaces and air conditioners. Individual HEPA filters are made by
the **Farr Co.** and other manufacturers, but they generally require engineering

expertise for an effective installation. If a HEPA filter is installed improperly, it can damage your heating/cooling system.

Combination filters are available that contain a HEPA and a built-in fan to overcome the resistance to airflow.

Whole-House Extended-Surface Filters

A very simple extended-surface filter that does a reasonable job at capturing mold spores, pollen grains, and other larger-sized particulates is the 20/20 filter manufactured by the **Farr Co.** These are 1" thick and designed to replace typical standard furnace filters. To purchase them, contact the company for the nearest dealer.

Even more efficient, larger (about 2' square and 4–5" thick) extended-surface filters are also available. However, these require the installation of a special metal housing to mount them in your forced-air furnace/air-conditioning system. It should be mentioned that these large filters are much more efficient than 1" thick filters, but they're also more costly. Space-Gard (**Research Products Corp.**) is one popular brand of these extended surface filters. Others are manufactured by **Carrier Corp.** and **Honeywell, Inc.** To purchase a filter from one of these companies, call them to find their nearest dealer.

Whole-House Electrostatic Filters

While electrostatic filters are not overly efficient, they can trap some of the more bothersome larger particulates—and they're relatively inexpensive and easy to install. One popular brand is Filtrete (**3-M Do-It-Yourself Div.**). To buy these, contact the manufacturer for local suppliers. Another brand you might consider is Permastatic II (**Allermed Corp.**). These particular filters are washable and come in standard or custom-made sizes. They can be ordered directly from the company.

Also, Enviro-Duct electrostatic filters come in a variety of standard sizes. Custom sizes can be ordered at an extra cost. These filters are available in the standard 1" thick model, and more efficient $1^1/_2$" or 2" versions. In addition, a $3/_8$" prefilter can be purchased for use with them. These electrostatic duct filters are washable and can be returned to undergo "filter reconditioning" in order to regenerate their static charge. The Enviro-Duct is sold by dealers including **Ozark Water Service and Environmental Services.**

Whole-House Electrostatic Precipitators

If you're interested in a whole-house electrostatic precipitator to remove airborne particulates, many brands are available to choose from. Of course, all of them will require special installation. Two brands you might consider are **Carrier Corp.** and **Honeywell, Inc.** Incidentally, **Honeywell** also offers an electronic sensor that lights up when the collection plates need to be cleaned. To purchase these items, contact the companies for their nearest dealers.

Whole-House Combination Filters

Allermed Corp. manufactures a CS-2000 whole-house unit that can be fitted with its own ductwork system or be made to work in conjunction with a forced-air furnace/air conditioner. These units contain a prefilter, 40 pounds of activated charcoal or other adsorption mix, a HEPA filter (two models are available), and a postfilter, plus they have their own fan. Of course, these will have require professional installation. The CS-2000 can be purchased directly from the manufacturer.

In addition, **Pure Air Systems, Inc.** offers the 600 HEPA Shield whole-house filter, which can stand alone or be fitted into a forced-air furnace/air-conditioner system. The metal cabinet houses a prefilter, a 2" activated carbon filter, and a 99+% rated HEPA filter, plus a one- or two-speed fan. If interested, call the company for the nearest dealer. Like the Allermed unit, this filter, too, will likely need professional installation.

Portable Room Air Filters

A large number of portable air-filtration devices are now available. In fact, there are so many that it may sometimes seem overwhelming in deciding on exactly which unit to pick. However, no matter which model you choose, if you're a sensitive person it's best if it has a metal cabinet with any fan motors upwind of the adsorbing filtering media. Filters such as these are usually the least bothersome.

The truth of the matter is, it is sometimes necessary to try several brands or models of filters before finding the one that personally meets all your needs and is tolerable to you. Therefore, it's a good idea to ask the dealer if it's possible to rent, rent-to-buy, or have some type of trial period to determine if a particular filter is right for you before totally committing yourself to one particular model.

Portable Activated-Charcoal/Activated-Alumina Filters

Despite all the choices on the market, many sensitive individuals have found that a simple, single-room, activated-charcoal air filter satisfactorily meets most of their needs. These are units capable of removing many contaminating gases including volatile organic compounds (VOCs), and if their activated charcoal has been mixed with activated alumina, they can remove formaldehyde as well.

One popular activated-charcoal filter is the #160R2 (**E.L. Foust Co., Inc.**). This particular model uses about 7 pounds of regular activated charcoal, or a special formaldehyde-adsorbing mix, held in a cylindrical metal canister. These units, as well as the replacement cartridges, can be bought directly from the manufacturer.

Portable Combination Air Filters

Today, most portable air-filtering units actually combine several types of filtering strategies, so that both contaminating gases and particulates can be removed with one machine. One device of this type is the Aireox air filter (**Aireox Research Corp.**) This filter comes with an all-metal case, activated charcoal, and filtering media capable of removing particles as small as 1 micron. In addition, other filtering options are available including a special activated-charcoal mix that is capable of removing formaldehyde and media capable of capturing 0.5 micron particles. Aireox filters can be ordered directly from the company or from dealers including **N.E.E.D.S.** and **earthsake**.

Air Quality Systems (AQS) makes filters with metal cabinets having "thermal-bonded wood grain finishes" in three model sizes. Each device contains five filters. These include coconut-shell activated charcoal, activated alumina, a polyester prefilter, and two other types of media that act as high-efficiency particulate filters. Combined, these filters are said to provide removal of particulates as small as 0.3 microns, formaldehyde, and other bothersome odors. AQS offers additional filtering options as well. AQS filters are available from dealers including **Ozark Water Services and Environmental Services**.

Another combination portable room air filter you might consider is the enviracaire (**enviracaire**), which has an all-metal case. It has a washable-foam prefilter, a fiberglass HEPA filter to eliminate 95% of 0.3 micron and larger particles, and 10 panels holding activated charcoal to adsorb many types of contaminating gases. These filters can be ordered directly from the company or from dealers such as **N.E.E.D.S.**

Another HEPA filtering unit worth considering is the Healthmate (and the Healthmate Plus) (**Austin Air Systems Limited**). This metal unit contains a cotton retaining filter, a foam retaining filter, a prefilter, and a HEPA filter capable of trapping 99.97% of 0.3 micron and larger particles. There's also about 14 pounds of an activated-charcoal/zeolite mixture. These filters can be ordered directly from the manufacturer.

Still other popular combination filters you might investigate are the Air Sentry and the Series 400 (**E.L. Foust Co., Inc.**), which are available directly from the company. Also, the VH-300 and VH-400 (**Allermed Corp.**) are two more very good combination portable filters. They can be bought from the manufacturer or through dealers including **N.E.E.D.S.** and **Nontoxic Environments**.

Personal Facial Air Filters

Some sensitive and allergic individuals have found it helpful to wear *personal facial filters* when doing tasks that usually provoke negative symptoms in them, such as reading a magazine (to protect against ink and paper odors) or cleaning the house (to filter out dust). Surprisingly, there are actually several types available.

Washable, 100%-cotton masks with replaceable activated charcoal (made from coconut) inserts are sold by **The Living Source**. Similar ones are available from **The American Environmental Health Foundation** and **Nontoxic Environments** both of which offer them in 100%-silk fabric. In addition, **E.L. Foust Co., Inc.** handles one kind of disposable mask capable of trapping pollens, molds, and most dust particles down to 0.1 micron. They also sell 3M Dust/Mist Respirators. These are constructed with a thin, activated-charcoal layer in them and are designed to protect you from both particulates and some minor chemical exposures. Finally, a variety of personal facial filter masks are handled by **The Environmental Health Shopper**.

(Note that, most, but certainly not all, disposable masks are made of synthetic fabrics and materials. Therefore, if you're interested in using a throwaway mask, it's probably a good idea to test several brands to see how well you tolerate them.)

OZONE GENERATORS

Ozone generators produce ozone (O_3) by continually creating electrical discharges. Often the units are designed so that this rate of production can be increased or decreased. But why do some people buy ozone generators as air cleaning devices? After all, ozone is a pungent-smelling, irritating gas. Because it's a very unstable form of oxygen, it's extremely reactive. In sufficient concentrations, it can severely irritate your skin, eyes, and mucous membranes. Ozone can also cause you to have breathing problems.

However, ozone is also a powerful *oxidizing antiseptic* that is capable of killing many forms of bacteria and mold (Unfortunately mold, either alive or dead, can provoke allergies.). It can also reduce smoky odors in a home after a fire. However, to do this effectively, the ozone must be at fairly high concentrations. Therefore, this work is usually left to professional contractors who specialize in fire damage. Such work must usually be done with the family out of the house. Interestingly, a number of sensitive persons have bought ozone generators to purposely break down airborne *volatile organic compounds* (*VOCs*) to which they would normally react. As it turns out, while ozone can break down some existing VOCs in the air, it can also react with existing pollutants and create bothersome new ones. Obviously, ozone's benefits are a mixed bag.

Despite their drawbacks, a few individuals have found that ozone generators have been helpful in certain situations. For example, sometimes an ozone generator has been effective in removing bothersome perfume or other odors when no other solution was readily available. However, if you plan to use an ozone generator, it's extremely important to follow the manufacturer's directions precisely. Also, whenever you operate it, doublecheck the controls to make sure they're adjusted correctly. This is absolutely essential so that excessive amounts of ozone aren't created that could damage your furnishings—and injure you. In addition, regularly ventilate ozoned areas of your home frequently.

One model of ozone generator you might want to consider is the FreshAire 500 offered by **N.E.E.D.S.** Others brands are available from a variety of sources including **The Living Source. The American Environmental Health Foundation, Inc.** also offers ozone generators for either rent or purchase. One ozone generator that's meant to be permanently installed in your forced-air furnace/air-conditioning system is manufactured by **Kleen-Air Company, Inc.** These units are designed to only produce ozone when air is actually flowing through the ductwork. Therefore, the ozone is diluted and distributed evenly throughout the whole house. To purchase this device, contact the company for the nearest dealer.

NEGATIVE-ION GENERATORS

In recent years, *negative-ion generators* have become popular as air-cleaning devices. But exactly what are they? Negative-ion generators are actually specialized electronic devices that are capable of using electric current to create *negatively charged ions*—in this case, *free electrons*. These electrons are immediately spewed out into the air where they quickly attach themselves to airborne particulates, in the process giving them a negative charge. The newly negatively charged particles usually leave the air and cling to surfaces such as walls and ceilings that tend to be positively charged. This adhesion occurs because of the action of natural *electrostatic force* in which like-charged molecules repel but unlike-charged molecules attract.

Although most users of negative-ion generators won't notice it at first, their walls and ceilings will usually become steadily dirtier as the adhering pollutant particles accumulate on them—although the air itself will be less contaminated. Therefore, it's necessary that these collecting surfaces be cleaned from time to time. However, you should realize that this is not only for aesthetic reasons. As it turns out, many pollutant particles will eventually reenter the air as they lose their negative charge. To counter this problem, some negative-ion generators have built-in air filters so that the particles are trapped in the units themselves.

Unfortunately, it's doubtful that negative-ion generators can make very polluted indoor air safe. But in situations where allergic or sensitive individuals are unable to eliminate certain indoor contaminants (perhaps requiring giving up the family pet for example), and/or they can't afford a more efficient air filtering device, negative-ion generators can sometimes be beneficial. To purchase a negative ion generator, check in **Befit Enterprises Ltd.'s** *Cutting Edge Catalog* which offers Zestron ionizers. Negative-ion generators are also handled by **The Living Source**, among others.

HOUSE PLANTS AS AIR CLEANERS

It's become a popular belief that house plants, especially spider plants (*Chlorophytum elatum* variety *viitum*), have the capacity to clean a home's air of most of its airborne pollutants. Therefore spider plants, also known as ribbon plants, have become almost floral celebrities (These common plants have long slender leaves, white flower clusters, and long shoots with tiny new plants attached to the ends of them.). Unfortunately, although they're attractive, the air cleaning capacity of spider plants is a misconception.

Early research suggested that these plants (and also golden pothos *Scindapsusu aureus*) were capable of fairly efficient removal of certain gaseous pollutants (but not particulates). But these initial studies, which were performed by the National Aeronautics and Space Administration (NASA) in the mid-1980s, were conducted under very limiting artificial laboratory conditions. The results from this preliminary work were widely reported in the press.

Then, a few years later, comprehensive research at Ball State University simulating real-life situations contradicted the NASA assumptions. In fact, their studies showed that house plants were far less effective as air cleaners than originally believed, even under laboratory conditions. Therefore, although plants bring a sense of nature indoors and produce oxygen, they won't reduce your indoor air-pollution levels by very much. (See also *Plants* in *Chapter 5: Interior Decorating*.) In fact, they can sometimes actually increase the likelihood of moisture and mold problems (see *High Relative Humidity* above).

VENTILATION SYSTEMS

A ventilation system is an excellent way to bring fresh air into your house. However, their sometimes-extensive technical nature is beyond the scope of this book, especially planned, whole-house ventilation systems. For complete information on all types of residential ventilation systems including *heat-recovery ventilators* (HRVs) (units able to transfer a portion of the heat from the outgoing air to the incoming air, or vice versa), read *Understanding Ventilation* by John Bower, available from **The Healthy House Institute**.

In this book (*The Healthy Household*), local, single-room ventilation is discussed concerning your stove (see *Making your Gas-Range Operation More Tolerable* in *Chapter 8: Housekeeping*), and your bathroom and laundry room (see *High Relative Humidity* and *Mold* above).

AIR HUMIDIFICATION

In dry climates, or during the heating season, it might seem that *humidifying* (adding moisture to) your indoor air would always be the logical, healthful thing to do. After all, if the relative humidity of your home air is very low, your eyes, skin, and mucous membranes could become irritated, your lips might crack—and your wood furniture could become dry enough to shrink and become unglued. However, there are other considerations to keep in mind. Therefore, in the sections below, the actual pros and cons of humidifying your home are discussed, as well as specific methods of humidification you might choose to use.

SIMPLE HUMIDIFYING STRATEGIES

If you feel you want to raise the relative humidity level in your home, there are actually some very simple things you can do to accomplish this. One of these is to merely lower the room's air temperature. The cooler a room is, the higher its relative humidity—as long as it's holding the same amount of water vapor. Other approaches you might try are opening your bathroom door immediately after you shower or bathe to let the moisture-laden air spill out into the rest of your house, boiling distilled water in a pot on your stove, putting distilled water in clean pans on your steam radiators, and misting the air with *distilled water* in a spray bottle. By the way, it is always better to use distilled water than tap water because tap water can add particulates such as minerals or bacteria to the air (see *Distilled Water* in *Chapter 10: Home Water*).

In addition, by merely drinking more water during the winter months, you'll help keep your mucous membranes more moist. Of course, if you use a tolerable body moisturizer and lip balm each time after you bathe, you'll help retain more water in your skin (see *Moisturizers* and *Make-Up* in *Chapter 2: Personal Care*). You might want to use tolerable eye drops to help soothe your eyes as well.

If, despite these measures, your home still feels too dry, you might try adapting to the more arid conditions—in other words, *acclimating* yourself. This may take several weeks. However, if you still find that the low-humidity levels are unsatisfactory, only then will you want to consider using a *humidifier*. This is because several problems are associated with using humidifiers.

HUMIDIFIERS

To increase the relative-humidity level in homes, humidifiers are commonly used. Humidifiers are simply devices purposely designed to increase the air's moisture content. Today, there are actually several approaches to doing this: producing steam, as well as several methods of creating a cool mist. It should be pointed out that different humidifiers are capable of humidifying different coverage areas: a single room, a portion of the house, or the entire house. In addition, humidifiers are equipped with different features—for example, automatic shut off, adjustable vents, etc.—and different price tags.

Unfortunately, many humidifiers have innate problems associated with them. These can include spewing out bothersome odors (from plastic, rubber and vinyl parts or oily odors from fan motors) as well as mold and other biological growth (which can quickly contaminate certain humidifiers). Of course, these are of special concern for sensitive and allergic persons, but they're not healthy for anyone to breathe.

If you opt to go ahead and purchase a humidifier anyway, it would be a good idea to monitor the humidity level of the room(s) often so that excess moisture isn't accidentally added to the air (for information on potential problems resulting from having high humidity, as well as relative humidity measuring devices see *High Relative Humidity* above). You'll also want to use only distilled water, which will be free of mineral particulates and biological contaminants. In addition, you'll want to thoroughly and frequently clean your humidifying unit. Finally, you'll want to avoid using scented additives (and probably the chemical disinfectant additives as well) that some manufactures of humidifiers include with their new units, especially if you're a sensitive person. The odors from these will not only get into the air, but will become absorbed by the humidifier's plastic parts.

HUMIDIFIER TYPES

Several different humidifying strategies are used in humidifiers. The following sections discuss these. (For suggestions on what specific humidifier is best for you, see *Choosing the Right Humidifier* below.)

Steam Humidifiers

For many years electrically operated *steam* (or *vaporizer*) *humidifiers* have been popular to increase indoor humidity. These units contain electric heating elements that boil water to produce steam. Typically, these are room-size models with plastic water reservoirs. However, some steam humidifier devices are now designed for whole-house installations in forced-air furnace ducts; at least some of these are constructed primarily of metal.

Steam's major advantage as a source for humidity in your home is that its high heat destroys virtually all the microorganisms that might be present in the water. However, if you get too close to a portable unit, you could burn your nasal passages, skin, or eyes. At the same time though, it must be said this is unlikely to happen because the steam cools quickly just a very short distance from where it is emitted.

Some people fear that electric steam units might be dangerous because they could tip over and spill out boiling water. However, many, if not most, models are now designed to seal completely, so that spilling is unlikely. Yet, there is always the inherent potential danger posed by any electrical element of overheating and causing a fire. Fortunately, the units generally available today have safety features to help prevent such accidents from occurring, such as an automatic shutoff when the water level in the reservoir is too low and/ or the unit is tipped over.

Remember not to use *hard water* (water with high mineral content) in a steam humidifier or vaporizer, so that the dissolved minerals won't create a mineral scale buildup on the heating element and around the vent opening. If this happens, it will lead to higher energy use as well as inefficient dispersal of the steam. Extremely fine particulate minerals, which aren't good to breathe, can also be spewed out into the air along with the steam. Some manufacturers now recommend that you only use *distilled water* in their units for these very reasons.

As with any humidifier, it should be cleaned regularly. If minerals should build up on the elements, read your owner's manual for suggestions on cleaning. In addition, when your portable steam unit isn't actually in use, unplug it and empty the reservoir.

Cool-Spray Humidifiers

Cool-spray humidifiers spew out unheated water in a very fine mist. They're available in small portable units as well as models designed to humidify your whole house; they tend to be constructed with plastic water reservoirs and other parts. Cool-spray humidifiers eliminate all the potential problems associated with boiling water, steam, and the hot elements of steam humidifiers. However, they don't offer the sanitizing effect of high heat, so microbial growth often contaminates these units. As a matter of fact, as they dispense misted water, they also spray out microbes, dissolved minerals, and anything else that happens to be in that water (see *Common Water Contaminants* in *Chapter 10: Home Water*). Once these contaminants are airborne, you and your family wind up breathing them.

Therefore, if you opt for this type of humidifier, again use only *distilled water* in it. It's also extremely important to clean the unit frequently to prevent any mold problems. Remember to unplug small portable models when not in use and empty the reservoir.

Ultrasonic-Dispersal Humidifiers

Ultrasonic-dispersal humidifiers are actually specialized types of *cool-spray humidifiers.* These are most often seen as portable models, usually made of plastic. Ultrasonic-dispersal humidifiers work by using high-frequency sound waves to shatter water droplets, creating an ultra-fine mist. However, they also break up any minerals and microorganisms that may be present in the water. Unfortunately, the very fine particles of such debris can be potentially injurious if inhaled over an extended period.

Therefore, it's again extremely important to only use distilled water in ultrasonic-dispersal humidifiers. Also, frequent cleaning is necessary to prevent any mold problems. It's also not a good idea to leave water in the reservoir of a portable unit or leave it plugged in when not in use.

Evaporative Humidifiers

Evaporative humidifiers humidify by blowing air across or through some type of water-saturated media and then out into the room. Specific methods to accomplish this differ. For example, some models use a rotating drum, others a conveyor apparatus, and still others use a large wick. The absorbent media are often a synthetic foam or other spongy material. Evaporative units come in both room-size and whole-house furnace installations. The portable units generally have plastic water reservoirs and plastic housings.

Over the years, evaporative humidifiers have become notorious for producing some of the worst problems associated with humidifiers. These include mineral build up as well as microbial growth (mold, bacteria, etc.) contaminating the water reservoir and the media. Of course, all this "stuff" will become airborne and be inhaled by you and your family when these units are operating. It should be mentioned that some units come with an air filter through which the air passes just before entering the room air. However, these filters are usually not very efficient, and they themselves can become easily contaminated with mold, etc.

Therefore, if you're interested in a portable evaporative humidifier, it's very important that you only use distilled water in it. It's also vital that you keep the unit as clean as possible and never leave standing water in the reservoir when the humidifier is not actually in use. Also, remember to unplug the unit when it's not in use as a safety precaution.

CHOOSING THE RIGHT HUMIDIFIER

Before purchasing any humidifier, you should determine the size of the area you plan to humidify (one room or the whole house), have a price range in mind, and evaluate your own inclinations: Are you willing to monitor your room's humidity level, to regularly clean the unit, perhaps daily, and to buy and install any replacement filters, etc.? You also should decide on a basic humidifying strategy. Next, give some though to the actual unit's construction (how easy will it be to fill and clean, as well as what materials will it be made of), its special features (auto shutoff when the reservoir is empty and/or adjustable humidistat capable of turning the unit off if the room air reaches a preset relative humidity level), and the manufacturer's—and possibly the dealer's—guarantees and/or warranties.

Unfortunately, it should be pointed out that there really are not many truly healthy humidifiers to chose from—and this is particularly true from the perspective of sensitive individuals. After all, most humidifiers are constructed with plastic reservoirs and housings, often with internal parts made of various synthetic and rubber compounds. Generally, these materials have the capacity to impart their own odors to the humidified air, especially when the humidifiers are new. Also, frequent cleaning of humidifiers is required to prevent any mold problems.

Then, too, whole-house humidifiers that work in conjunction with furnaces may encourage mold and mildew growth in your ductwork simply by raising the relative humidity levels in them. In addition, if your humidifier doesn't have an adjustable *humidistat* (a device able to detect relative-humidity levels and turn off the humidifier when a preset level has been reached) and you don't regularly monitor your room's moisture level yourself, your humidifier can easily introduce too much moisture into your home. This situation can lead to a number of problems, including damage to your walls and increased populations of microorganisms.

However, if you decide you really need a humidifier, a simple portable *steam/vaporizing unit* is often one of the better choices. Although it'll likely have the usual plastic reservoir, these units tend to have a minimum of other synthetic or rubber components. Also in their favor, the high heat they generate is disinfecting. Note that, when it's new, it's often a good idea to run your steam humidifier (or any other type of new portable humidifier) for sometime outdoors in dry, uncontaminated surroundings until the plastic odors are no longer noticeable in the vapor that is put out. Of course, this is very important to do if you're a sensitive person.

Portable electric steam/vaporizer humidifiers are still relatively popular. Therefore, they can be purchased at many local drugstores, as well as department, discount, and hardware stores. Several DeVilbiss models are also available by mail-order from **The Environmental Health Shopper**. If you decide you'd like a whole-house humidifier that would be permanently installed to work with your forced-air furnace, a steam type would probably be best. Several brands of these are currently available, so check your local furnace installer or plumbing dealer to see what they handle. Naturally, these will generally require professional installation. By the way, one steam whole-house model made of stainless steel is sold by **E.L. Foust Co., Inc.**

DEHUMIDIFIERS

(See *High Relative Humidity* above.)

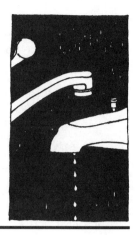

CHAPTER 10
HOME WATER

As everyone knows, good quality water is essential to good health. This chapter discusses some of the more common home water problems and equipment that is available to help reduce or eliminate them.

COMMON WATER QUALITY PROBLEMS

Many people believe that their tap water is simply H_2O. Actually however, it's a very complex solution. In fact, every water sample contains a unique set of minerals in varying amounts, as well as biological life, dissolved gases such as radon, a particular *pH level* (its acidity-alkalinity content), and a certain amount of chemical contamination. It also differs in its *turbidity* (degree of clarity), taste, and smell.

Why does home water vary so greatly? One major reason is that water is a *universal solvent.* In other words, it easily dissolves many of the substances with which it comes in contact. It also puts many other substances into suspension. In addition, water can provide the ideal environment in which certain microbes can thrive. As a result, water composition varies simply because it comes from so many different locales and sources, and everything the water comes in contact with alters it. Water sources can include wells (private or municipal) that tap into *aquifers* (underground geologic formations holding or conveying water), springs, rainwater *cisterns* (holding tanks), rivers, reservoirs, and lakes.

Then too, home water can be altered by local utility departments when they filter it and subject it to *chlorine* or *fluoride* treatments. Furthermore, water can vary because of how it eventually reaches your faucet. Did it travel through cement, asbestos/cement, plastic, cast iron, copper, or perhaps lead pipes? Were the soldered joints between the copper pipes and the copper fittings made with lead-based or lead-free solder?

When you consider all the possibilities, you can start to see how complicated the subject of home water really is. While this book will address some of the more common problems and solutions, you may be interested in learning more on the topic. Therefore, you might want to read *The Home Water Supply: How to Find, Filter, Store, and Conserve It* by Stu Campbell. You also should check with your local library, bookstore, board of health, water utility, and county extension agent for other appropriate books and literature that delve into the complexities of water.

COMMON WATER CONTAMINANTS

The following sections should help you become more aware of contaminants that could be in your water and the potential aesthetic and health consequences of these ingredients to you and your family.

BIOLOGICAL CONTAMINANTS

It's not uncommon for water sources to harbor microorganisms. Fortunately, most of these contaminants are relatively safe. However, some microorganisms definitely pose a health threat such as certain bacteria (*salmonella*, for instance), parasitic worms, amoebae, molds, algae, and viruses, among others. Therefore, water utilities constantly monitor the water they process for its microbial content. As a rule, they add a very reactive purifying substance such as chlorine or sometimes ozone, to kill most of the disease-causing microbes in the water.

Of course, individual water systems such as private home wells can also be biologically polluted. This is especially likely if the home's septic field is too near the well—that is, if it is less than 100' away. It's essential for individual homeowners to accept responsibility for their own personal water system by having their water tested regularly for its microbial content.

By the way, when a professional water-testing laboratory examines a water sample provided by a homeowner, it often checks first for the presence of *coliforms* (*fecal* and/or *total*) and also *fecal streptococcus*. While these bacteria are not particularly desirable components in your water, labs look for them because they're considered *marker species*. In other words, if they're present, then it's likely that even more harmful microbes are also living in the same water.

If it turns out you actually have biological contamination in your home water supply, drilling a new well may be necessary. However, if the situation is less severe, there are home-treatment devices that can sometimes help. For example, certain *reverse-osmosis* units are capable of removing much of the bacteria and other biological contaminants that are present—unless the contaminants are extremely minute. Also, *Kinetic-Degradation-Fluxion (KDF)* units can control microorganisms through *bacteriostatic action*.

However, by far the most effective methods of killing biological contaminants in your water include *water distillation* and *ultraviolet-light purification*. Other purifying approaches that can be used by homeowners include *pasteurization* (heating the water above 150°F for a period of time), *ozonization* (subjecting the water to ozone gas), and adding specific amounts of iodine or silver to the water.

INDUSTRIAL AND AGRICULTURAL POLLUTANTS

Sadly, a growing threat to water everywhere is pollution generated by manufacturing and agricultural products and practices. The sections below discuss this potentially toxic situation.

Industrial Pollution

Unfortunately, experts are now telling us that much of America's water supply has already become contaminated, to varying degrees, with potentially dangerous pollutants originating from poorly managed industries, mines, and dump sites, among others. These *adulterants* can include acids, solvents, cleaning solutions, caustic compounds, dissolved gases, radioactive material, and other poisonous substances including heavy metals. As a result, unacceptable levels of copper (Cu), selenium (Se), cobalt (Co), cadmium (Cd), arsenic (As), and other pollutants are no longer rare occurrences in water supplies.

Each of these pollutants has its own individual negative toxicological effects. Therefore, depending on the particular pollutants, the amounts of them you ingest, as well as your own personal susceptibility, a whole range of possible symptoms could result. In a worst-case scenario, central nervous system problems, birth defects, and even cancer could result from drinking water containing a high concentration of industrial pollutants.

Perhaps surprisingly, one of the more common chemical pollutants in U.S. water supplies is gasoline. It seems that gasoline has been getting into our water supplies for decades by way of leaks from petroleum refineries and underground service-station tanks. However, another major source is from individuals simply spilling or dumping gasoline on the ground.

As it turns out, the gasoline that has already entered into water supplies hasn't merely added dangerous petroleum hydrocarbons to the water content, but also lead (Pb) as well. This is because *tetraethyl lead* and *tetramethyl lead* were used as popular gasoline additives for years and only recently have been phased out. Unfortunately, as most people now realize, lead can be toxic when it's ingested. It's slowly absorbed by the human body and becomes concentrated in the liver and kidneys. Lead can eventually lead to mental retardation in children and hypertension in adults, among many other debilitating conditions.

Agricultural Pollution

Farm chemicals such as fertilizers, pesticides, and herbicides are another growing threat to America's water supplies (Home garden and lawn chemicals also should be included here.). A number of these products contain *nitrates* such as *nitrogen nitrate*. Unfortunately, it seems most nitrate compounds have the capacity to interfere with the ability of our red blood cells to transport oxygen throughout the body. The negative health effects of drinking water with a high concentration of nitrates are particularly bad for pregnant women and small children.

Coping with Industrial and Agricultural Pollution in Water

Fortunately, most utility-supplied water is relatively safe from many types of industrial and agricultural pollution, although the situation varies from utility to utility. However, utility water is usually regularly tested for the presence of certain chemical contaminants. If one of these particular chemicals is found in a high concentration, it's often removed or reduced to acceptable levels through filtration or some other method. But if a utility's water is too contaminated, it may be necessary for them to locate a new less-polluted, source.

Generally, individual home water systems are not continually monitored for industrial and agricultural pollution. Therefore, some could easily contain unsuspected levels of heavy metals and chemical pollutants that may not have been present when the well was originally drilled. Unfortunately, testing—and especially removing—certain agricultural and industrial contaminates from your home water supply can be both difficult and expensive.

Fortunately, however, if the contamination is of a type and concentration that simple methods are able to satisfactorily handle, a homeowner can treat his (or her) water and make it drinkable. For example, *activated charcoal in block form* can be used to remove many kinds of *organic chemicals* (carbon-containing chemicals such as gasoline) that it will adsorb, as well as nitrates and heavy metals that it will strain out. Water distillers and reverse-osmosis units can remove nearly all the nitrates and heavy metals. If Kinetic-Degradation-Fluxion (KDF*)* units are used, they can also effectively remove heavy metals.

At the same time, it must be said that in some cases reducing levels of certain agricultural and industrial pollutants to acceptable limits is just not feasible. In those instances, a new well may have to be drilled or outside water brought in to supply a home cistern (holding tank). Sometimes, however, the water may be safe enough for general-purpose use but not safe enough for drinking and cooking.

SUSPENDED PARTICULATES

A high level of *suspended particulates* in your water indicates that it has *turbidity*. As a result, the water will appear cloudy. The particulates themselves may be anything from bits of soil to bacteria, algae, or mold. Sometimes, the suspended material is actually a combination of different types of solid matter.

To test for the specific water-turbidity level, water-testing laboratories often simply direct a beam of light at the water sample. A measurement is then made of the amount of light that is scattered because of its inability to pass through the sample. This figure is compared to the measurement obtained from clear water undergoing the same procedure. Other tests can then be performed to determine exactly what the suspended particulates are composed of.

If suspended particles are simply dirt or sand granules, they can usually be removed easily by using *settling tanks* or special *turbidity filters*. These low-technology solutions are generally quite effective and are commonly used both by utilities and private well owners. Of course, utilities also disinfect the water with extremely reactive *chlorine* or *ozone* gas to kill most forms of biologic life that could also be contributing to the turbidity.

In home situations, if just a small amount of soil and sand is present in the water, it can sometimes be satisfactorily strained out (not adsorbed) with an activated-charcoal filter—especially one in solid-block form (This is actually a type of *mechanical filtration*.). Reverse-osmosis units will also work; however the grit can be very wearing on reverse-osmosis membranes. Therefore, unless there's an effective prefilter, this approach is definitely not the best one to use. However, distillation will remove virtually all suspended particulates including biological ones.

HIGH CONCENTRATIONS OF COMMON MINERALS AND METALS

Several common minerals and metals (for example, calcium, magnesium, iron, manganese, and sodium chloride) can cause problems when they are found in high concentrations in your water. Interestingly, these same particular minerals aren't considered toxic substances if they're ingested in very small quantities. In fact, all these minerals are actually necessary for proper functioning of the human body. This is true even of manganese. (Note that, many water-quality analysts refer to all these substances as *minerals* rather than classifying some as *metals*.)

Generally, if any of these minerals are above standard, established limits in a utility's water, the utility will use various approaches to reduce their levels. Of course, homeowners with private water supplies can also use treatment methods to lower the level of dissolved minerals in their water. These treatment methods will be mentioned under each heading below.

Calcium

Calcium (Ca) is a lightweight, silver-white metal. Interestingly, if the dissolved calcium levels are high in your water, it's common for dissolved magnesium (and perhaps other dissolved minerals) to also exist in large amounts. By the way, if calcium and/or magnesium are present at a concentration over 120 milligrams per liter of water (mg/l), the popular term *hard water* is typically used to describe it. Interestingly, it's been estimated that over 85% of water in the U.S. is considered hard water.

Unfortunately, water with a high dissolved-calcium content is often troublesome for those using it. This is because it causes soaps to create insoluble scum (soap curds). This happens because the minerals react with the fat and oil ingredients of the soap (see *Soaps versus Detergents* in *Chapter 7: Cleaning*). Also, a crusty scale (lime or lime scale) can form on the interiors of pipes and plumbing fixtures when the dissolved mineral compounds *precipitate* (come out of solution). Even at levels as low as 85 mg/l, problems like these can still be experienced.

Fortunately, water hardness is relatively easy and inexpensive to test for and treat. Often *water-softening devices* using *sodium-ion/calcium-ion exchange* technology will solve most hard-water problems. However, there are also a variety of other alternative water-conditioning approaches to counter the effects of hard water. It should be mentioned that Kinetic-Degradation-Fluxion devices belong in this category. Of course, distillation and reverse-osmosis units are usually capable of removing calcium and other dissolved minerals.

Magnesium

Magnesium (Mg), in its purest form, is a silvery-white metal. In fresh water, both dissolved magnesium and magnesium-calcium compounds are both commonly present together. These two minerals are primarily responsible for *water hardness*. (For more on the problems and solutions to high magnesium content in your water, see *Calcium* above.)

Iron

Iron (Fe) is one of the most common metals on earth. In its pure state, it's a silvery-white solid. However, it's very easily *oxidized*, forming rust. Therefore, a high dissolved-iron content in water will have a reddish-orange color, which, in turn, will stain your laundry, sinks, etc. To complicate matters, *iron bacteria* may also be present. These are often the cause of an orange slime inside your toilet tank, etc.

Fortunately, the iron content in water can be easily tested for. If there's a high level present (above 0.3 mg/l), a typical ion-exchange water softener will generally help lower it. However, special iron-removal equipment is also available. Note that, a high manganese level may accompany a high iron level in your water.

Homeowners who also have iron bacteria in their water supply will probably want to use some sort of filtering unit or a more thorough disinfecting treatment such as an ultraviolet purifier to eliminate them. It should be noted that some reverse-osmosis equipment is able to remove not only the dissolved iron but also much of the iron bacteria as well. Naturally, distillation is more effective and will completely remove both the iron and iron bacteria. Another option would be to use a Kinetic-Degradation-Fluxion (KDF) device. The media used in them can actually alter the problematic dissolved iron into insoluble *ferric oxide* (Fe_2O_3), a solid form of iron. Note, too, that KDF also has a *bacteriostatic effect* (the ability to reduce bacteria populations).

Manganese

Sometimes dissolved *manganese* accompanies dissolved *iron* in water. Manganese (Mn) in its purest state is actually a silvery-gray metal. However, high concentrations of dissolved manganese (above .05 mg/liter) will tend to make the water grayish or brownish-black. Unfortunately, any fixtures and laundry that comes in contact with such water will likely become stained by it. To make matters worse, water with high levels of dissolved manganese can also have an unpleasant taste. *Manganese bacteria* may be contained in the mix as well.

Homes with individual water systems can have their manganese content tested for. If it's too high, often a typical water conditioner using a mineral-ion exchange process can greatly reduce the amount of it present in the water. However, if magnesium bacteria are also living in this same water, some additional type of filtering or disinfecting treatment may be necessary to eliminate them.

By the way, certain reverse-osmosis equipment will remove dissolved manganese and often much of the bacteria, too. Furthermore, distillation will probably completely remove both of them. It should also be mentioned that Kinetic-Degradation-Fluxion (KDF) devices are capable of removing dissolved manganese, but only at a very slow rate. Therefore, KDF is generally not the method of choice for its removal.

Sodium Chloride

Sodium chloride (NaCl) is apparently becoming a more common contaminant in home water supplies. As you probably know, sodium chloride is common table salt. In oceans, sodium chloride makes up about 80% of all the dissolved solids present in the water. Not surprisingly, it's usually ocean water seeping into coastal wells that has caused sodium chloride levels to become excessive in certain areas. Whatever the source of the salt, fresh water containing too much of it is termed *brackish*. Of course, high levels of dissolved sodium in drinking water is generally considered a real health concern. After all, many people with hypertension as well as other medical conditions must restrict their salt intake.

Testing for sodium chloride levels in home water systems is not difficult. (Note, if your water has a chloride level—which would include sodium chloride—above 250 mg/l, it will likely be corrosive and have a bad taste.) If sodium chloride is found at an unacceptable concentration, a homeowner can sometimes use a special whole-house reverse-osmosis unit fitted with a membrane rated for salt removal to take it out of the water. Of course, distillation will remove virtually any salt that happens to be present in the water.

It should be mentioned that sodium chloride is actually used in ion-exchange water softeners. The salt is usually in the form of salt pellets that are added to a special tank. There, they dissolve and become brine. Through catalytic action, the salt's sodium ions are exchanged for the hard water's mineral ions. As a result, while the treated water will have very low amounts of dissolved minerals, it will have elevated levels of sodium. However, using a reverse-osmosis unit with a membrane rated for sodium removal (or a water distiller) in the kitchen will take most of it out of drinking and cooking water.

NATURALLY OCCURRING GASES

There are several naturally occurring—but dangerous—gases that may be dissolved in water. Three of these—radon, hydrogen sulfide, and methane—are discussed below. Often, if utility water has high levels of undesirable gases in it, the utility will remove them through a relatively simple aeration process. Homeowners with problem gases in their individual water systems have other options for dealing with them, as discussed under each heading.

Radon

Radon (Rn) is an odorless, colorless, radioactive gas. While radon has twenty *isotopes* (isotopes are unique atomic forms, each having a different number of neutrons), it's *radon-222*, which originates in *radium* in the ground, that can be a concern to homeowners. This is the isotope that could lead to real health problems if dissolved in well water.

If it turns out that radon is, indeed, present in your well water, the radioactive gas will be released into your home air every time your water is running indoors. If it becomes trapped inside the house, it'll have time to decay into radioactive *radon decay products*. Unfortunately, these solid particles can become lodged in your lung tissue, possibly leading to lung cancer (Radon is now suspected of being the second leading cause of lung cancer in the U.S.). (See also *Radon* in *Chapter 9: Indoor Air*.)

It should then not be surprising that most experts now believe that all home well water systems should be tested for radon. (Well water in the state of Maine often has excessive radon.) Experts recommend that water with levels exceeding 20,000 pC/l, be treated. Typical activated-charcoal filters will adsorb radon gas from the water. However, they can't retain the radioactive decay particles, most of which are short-lived. On the other hand, certain reverse-osmosis units will remove these particles, but not the radon gas itself.

Effective (90% or more) radon removal can be accomplished, according to the Land and Water Resource Center at the University of Maine, by using a specially designed whole-house granular activated-charcoal adsorption filter. These units will not only remove radon, but also retain their decay particulate products as well. (Important note: These treatment devices are much larger than the relatively small activated-charcoal filters used for taste and odor problems in home water supplies.) Granular activated-charcoal units for radon removal range in size, but they're usually around 1.0 to 3.0 cubic feet. The actual size that would be needed for a particular situation would depend on the amount of radon present and the volume of daily water used.

You might find that granular activated-charcoal adsorption tanks are sold and installed by some local plumbers and water-treatment companies. To find local help in dealing with a radon problem in your water, contact your local board of health or **The Water Quality Association** at 4151 Naperville Rd., Lisle, IL 60532; (708) 505-0160. This is the national organization for water-treatment equipment dealers. Additional information on radon in well water is available from the **Environmental Protection Agency (EPA)** at 401 "M" Street S.W., Washington, DC 20460; (202) 260-2080.

Hydrogen Sulfide

Sulfur (S) in its pure form is a yellow, insoluble, solid material. Unfortunately, even a very small trace of it (0.05 mg/liter) in water will usually produce an unpleasant rotten-egg smell. A tiny trace of dissolved sulfur will also be able to tarnish silver items and even corrode metal pipes. Actually, one of the most common forms of sulfur in water is as dissolved *hydrogen sulfide* (H_2S), which is also sometimes known as *sulfureted hydrogen*. This is a toxic, flammable gas that is considered a cumulative poison. As a rule, water tests can easily determine the quantity present in a particular water sample.

If you find you only have a very minute amount of hydrogen sulfide in your water, it can often be safely and effectively adsorbed with an activated-charcoal filter. In addition, it should also be mentioned that Kinetic-Degradation-Fluxion (KDF) devices are capable of altering dissolved H_2S gas into an insoluble compound. For more than a very tiny amount of H_2S in your water, you might require more specialized filters or strategies to remove it.

Methane

Methane (CH_4) can sometimes be found in water sources (This is the gas that makes up about 85% of *natural gas*.). Generally, methane's presence results from the action of *anaerobic bacteria* (bacteria that are able to live without oxygen). These bacteria apparently cause dead vegetable matter to ferment and that fermentation produces the gas. In a wetland area escaping methane is sometimes called *swamp gas.*

Methane is actually a colorless, odorless, as well as tasteless gas. It's also apparently nonpoisonous. But methane is quite explosive, and if it builds up to a sufficient concentration in your room air, it can cause suffocation. Therefore, if tests reveal methane in your water, it may be necessary to vent the water supply to the outdoors. However, very tiny amounts can sometimes be satisfactorily adsorbed by simply using an activated-charcoal filter.

WATER-UTILITY CHEMICAL ADDITIVES

As a result of constant testing and ongoing water-utility treatments, public water supplies are usually safer than many untreated private water sources. However, it should be noted that a water utility's treatments can create their own, unique water-quality problems.

Commonly, utilities disinfect their water by adding *chlorine*. In addition, many U.S. utilities also add *fluoride* in order to lessen dental decay. However, both of these additives are corrosive and highly reactive, and each has negative consequences associated with it. Therefore, both chlorine and fluoride are considered contaminants by many individuals.

Chlorine

Chlorine (Cl) is a heavy, greenish-yellow gas with a distinctive pungent odor. It's an element classified as a *halogen* (a family of certain nonmetallic elements). Chlorine is extremely corrosive and reactive. But, these very qualities make it an effective disinfectant because it reacts with and destroys many types of microorganisms with which it comes into contact.

Since the early 1900s, U.S. water utilities have commonly used a form of chlorine (often *chloride of lime,* also known as *calcium oxychloride*) to *oxidize* (react with) and eliminate waterborne bacterial contaminants. In practice, chlorine is often added twice by utilities. First, the chemical is added to the raw water to kill much of the microbial life thriving in it before other water-treatment processes are performed. Then, chlorine is added again as a final disinfecting treatment before the finished, treated water is piped out to the public. In this last chlorination, the utilities add enough of it so that its concentration remains high enough to effectively kill microorganisms even at the very ends of the water system. As a result, homes near water-utility facilities will have much higher chlorine levels in their water than homes further down the line.

Interestingly, because chlorine is so reactive, it tends to actually corrode the water pipes it flows through. To help counter this, utilities often add *lime* (certain calcium compounds), *soda ash, zinc phosphate,* or other substances along with the chlorine. However, even with these additions, the insides of *galvanized pipes* (steel pipes coated with zinc to prevent rust) carrying chlorinated water can become rough and irregular (Galvanized pipes have been used in some home plumbing lines.). Unfortunately, these irregular surfaces can sometimes attract and sustain bacterial growth. Although they might not prove harmful to people, these bacteria can be destructive to certain types of reverse-osmosis membranes.

In addition, there are other problems with chlorination. Chlorine apparently can react with certain trace metals and nonmetals in the water, forming new compounds. Unfortunately, some of these are harmful, such as *chloroform.* Known chemically as *trichloromethane ($CHCl_3$)*, chloroform is created when chloride of lime reacts with carbon-containing organic matter.

But the question arises, What are the real effects on millions of Americans who drink chlorinated water daily? Is the corrosive chlorine itself a problem? Are the compounds formed in chlorinated water really a cause for concern? For some time now, opponents of chlorination have asked these questions. In

1992 research undertaken at both Harvard University and the Medical College of Wisconsin provided evidence that chlorine-treated drinking water seems to increase incidences of bladder and rectal cancers in men.

Unfortunately, simply taking a bath in chlorinated water can also be a problem because the chlorine can be readily absorbed through your skin. In fact, it's been estimated that your skin will absorb as much chlorine during a typical shower as you would normally take in from swallowing six eight-ounce glasses of chlorinated water—and that doesn't include the chlorine you inhale while showering. Just breathing chlorine can lead to nasal and respiratory irritation, and in certain allergic and sensitive individuals it can cause even more adverse reactions.

Therefore, if your water is chlorinated, you might want to remove the chlorine. This can be done easily using an activated-charcoal filter as well as a Kinetic-Degradation-Fluxion (KDF) device. Apparently, a KDF filter can alter chlorine into a less troublesome zinc chloride compound.

Fluoride

Fluoride compounds are also commonly added to utility water. However, most users of that water know very little about these additives. As it turns out, pure fluorine is a light-yellow gaseous member of the halogen family (a certain class of nonmetallic elements). It's poisonous, corrosive, and very reactive. In fact, fluorine is considered the most reactive element on earth, and fluoride compounds retain much of fluorine's characteristics. The most common fluoride compound added to water supplies is *fluosilicic acid* (H_2SiF_6). It is poisonous, corrosive, and highly reactive.

In the environment, fluoride compounds can be present naturally in some water sources. As it turns out, in the 1930s and 1940s reports were published that cited comparisons between individuals whose drinking water naturally contained high levels of fluoride (from 0.9 to 1.4 parts per million or ppm) with those whose drinking water had very little fluoride. These comparisons seemed to indicate a direct correlation between high fluoride levels and low rates of *dental caries* (tooth decay). Long-term studies were then devised to determine what the effect would be on dental caries rates with water having fluoride artificially added to it. However, before these studies were ever completed, the U.S. Public Health Service, starting in 1950, began approving (and encouraging) public water utilities to add fluoride to their water. Today, about one-half of U.S. public water utilities now add fluoride to reach a level of about 1 ppm in their water.

How does fluoride work against dental caries? Apparently, fluoride is able to prevents tooth decay because it causes calcium to redeposit onto your teeth. This action rebuilds and strengthens your tooth enamel. Despite this positive quality, water fluoridation has been hotly debated ever since its inception.

Today, proponents of fluoridation, such as the American Dental Association and the American Medical Association, point to statistics showing a substantial drop in the average child's dental decay rate since fluoridation's introduction. They maintain there's no convincing evidence that fluoridated water poses any health threats in the concentrations that are legally allowed.

On the other hand, opponents (such as the vocal spokesman, Dr. John A. Yiamouyiannis) contend that fluoridated water is "unsolicited medication" at best, and at worst, a potentially health-damaging substance. The opponents believe there's evidence that fluoride is a "persistent bioaccumulator"—meaning that fluoride levels will continue to build up in your body as you ingest more of it. Unfortunately, some limited findings seem to suggest that internalized fluoride may cause immune system and/or nervous system problems in susceptible persons. In addition, there are some indications that fluoride may be associated with the formation of certain fetal abnormalities and bone cancers. Furthermore, fluoride might play a contributing role in some arthritis, gastric ulcers, migraines, and other maladies.

Still another objection to utility fluoridation of water is the potential for fluorides to corrode pipes and solder. In some cases, this corrosion could cause lead in old lead pipes and in lead solder to migrate into the water supply and end up contributing to lead poisoning. Besides pipes, fluorides could also potentially corrode aluminum pots and pans, therefore, causing raised aluminum levels in the foods and drinks heated in them (This point was brought out in a letter in the January 1982 issue of the British journal *Nature* by researchers in Sri Lanka.). With the link between Alzheimer's disease and aluminum deposits in the brain, this may be a very real and serious concern.

Surprisingly, fluoridation's opponents even dispute the contention that fluoride significantly lessens tooth decay. It is interesting that in 1989 the ADA reduced the estimated tooth-decay reduction rates attributed to fluoridated water from 60% to 25%. Both proponents and opponents agree that fluoride levels of 1 ppm can cause mild *fluorosis* in a very small percentage of individuals (This is a corrosive condition in which fluoride reacts with your teeth and/or bones. Early or mild dental fluorosis generally appears as a slightly mottled discoloration, but more severe cases may show dramatic mottling and even pitting. In severe bone fluorosis, crippling may result.). As a precaution against fluorosis, it's now generally agreed that very young children should probably not use fluoride toothpaste. This is because youngsters often tend to swallow a great deal of the toothpaste placed on their toothbrushes. As a result, they could easily ingest unacceptable levels of fluoride.

Because of the heated controversy over adding fluoride to water, very few new fluoride treatment programs have been initiated by U.S. utilities in the last decade. In addition, most Western European nations (including Great Britain) have already abandoned their water fluoridation programs. Ultimately, of course, you must decide whether you believe that drinking fluoride in your water is beneficial to you and your family, or something you and they should avoid. Books and magazine articles in your local library can offer more information on fluoridation.

It should be stated here that realistically it's unlikely you'll be able to convince your utility to abandon its fluoridation program if you personally decide you don't want fluoride in your water. Fortunately, however, most reverse-osmosis units are able to remove it. You can also remove fluoride with a water distiller.

CONTAMINANTS FROM SUPPLY LINES, PIPES, AND SOLDER

Many people are unaware that the pipes and watermains carrying their water can add their own contaminants. Unfortunately, some of these may cause serious health problems.

Asbestos/Concrete Watermain Concerns

The supply lines carrying your water can affect quality. One concern that's recently been raised is the effect on humans of drinking water that's been transported through concrete water mains containing *asbestos* (a fibrous rock) (see also *Asbestos* in *Chapter 9: Indoor Air*). Could the fibers be getting in the water and, if they did, what effect would they have on the human body? These questions were raised because minute asbestos fibers were already known to be capable of causing severe lung disease if inhaled, so it is logical to wonder what damage they might do if they were ingested. (The reason asbestos is added to concrete pipes is to make them stronger. This type of water main has been particularly popular for years in many parts of the U.S.)

Unfortunately, some recent studies have shown that people who drink water from asbestos supply pipes have an increased incidence of gastrointestinal cancer. However, The World Health Organization (WHO) in its *1993 Guidelines for Drinking Water Quality* concluded that asbestos is not a serious health threat. However, if you want to be on the safe side, you might ask your utility if it has asbestos supply lines in its system. If it does, you may want to remove any possible asbestos fibers that could be in your water. Activated-charcoal filters in block form are able to strain out most asbestos. Asbestos fibers can also be removed very effectively by using reverse-osmosis units and water distillers.

Lead-Pipe and Lead-Solder Concerns

Lead water pipes were once common, especially in ancient times. In fact, *plumbum*, the Latin word for waterworks, is the source for lead's Pb elemental designation. However, lead pipes were once used in this country, too, although they haven't been for some time. Therefore, if you live in an older home, you'll want to check to see if it still has any lead piping. If you do come across lead water pipes, you may want to have them replaced. This is because lead can migrate from these pipes into your drinking water, slowly accumulate in your body, and eventually cause lead poisoning. (For more on lead, see *Chapter 9: Indoor Air*.)

It should also be mentioned that the lead solder used on copper pipes could pose a problem. Actually, this situation is very likely, unless you've just purchased a newly built home. This is because lead solder was commonly used by plumbers until it was prohibited by Federal regulations in 1986. By the way, fluoridated water can increase your lead risk if you have either lead pipes or lead solder. This is because there is some concern that fluoride is capable of corroding pipes and solder joints, thereby allowing lead to more easily enter the water.

Fortunately, activated charcoal in block form tends to strain out most of the lead in your water. In addition, lead can be removed very effectively by using most reverse-osmosis units. Lead can also be completely removed through distillation. Yet another good lead removal method is to use a Kinetic-Degradation-Fluxion device.

Galvanized Pipe Concerns

For those with *galvanized* water pipes (steel pipes coated with zinc to prevent rusting), a special concern arises if they transport chlorinated water. Chlorine can apparently react with galvanized pipes and create irregular surfaces on their interiors. While this isn't a problem as such, these rough surfaces can become homes for *non-pathological* (not causing disease) bacteria that can damage certain reverse-osmosis membranes.

Fortunately, reverse-osmosis units that are equipped with ultraviolet-light purifiers are able to kill these bacteria (and other kinds of waterborne microorganisms). If your reverse-osmosis unit doesn't have a built-in ultraviolet-light purifier, or some other type of *bacteriostatic* (bacteria-reducing) device, you can buy and install a separate point-of-use ultraviolet-light purifier. By the way, a Kinetic-Degradation-Fluxion (KDF) device will also control the bacteria capable of membrane destruction.

Plastic Pipe Concerns

In the last few decades, use of plastic pipes to distribute water has increased sharply. They've become common with both utilities and in residential plumbing. In fact, plastic piping is now considered the norm in many areas of the country. Although several different types of plastic are used to make water pipes, one of the more common is polyvinyl chloride (PVC).

It's easy to understand why the use of plastic pipe has become so widespread. Plastic piping is lightweight and easy to assemble using volatile synthetic glues. In addition, it doesn't rust or corrode easily, and is generally less expensive than metal, tile, or concrete alternatives. Unfortunately, plastic pipes can give the water they carry a plastic-like taste and odor, especially if the pipes have been recently glued together. Although many people may find this unpleasant, some sensitive individuals may find the situation intolerable. Fortunately, activated-charcoal water filters will effectively adsorb most new plastic-pipe tastes and odors.

WATER pH

It's often important to know your water's *pH*. What does this term mean? The pH number tells you how acidic or alkaline a substance is—in this case, your water. (To determine the pH, an analysis is performed to determine the number of *hydrogen ions* (H+) and *hydroxide ions* (OH-) found in the water.) As it turns out, the pH scale ranges from 0 (strongly acidic) to 14 (strongly alkaline). A pH of 7 represents neutrality.

Interestingly, most natural water sources in the U.S. have a pH between 5 and 8.5. It's been determined that water with a pH below 6.5 can corrode metal pipes. On the other hand, a high pH (above 8.5) can mean that certain iron-removal treatments will be less successful, that your water will have a caustic taste, and that *mineral scale* will likely build up inside your pipes. Very high alkalinity (above 11) could be an indication that chemical pollution has contaminated your water supply.

It should be stated that a water sample's pH can be easily determined. If the pH is too high or two low, utilities can add corrective substances at their plant to make the water more or less acidic (or alkaline). With an individual private water supply, a low pH (high acidity) can often be countered by simply adding marble chips or crushed limestone to a special tank. However, a high pH (high alkalinity) may require the addition of *sulfuric acid* (also known as *oil of vitriol*) to the water. Unfortunately, sulfuric acid is an oily, corrosive liquid that is potentially dangerous to handle.

Actually, any pH correction that is done to a home water supply should be specifically designed for you by a water treatment professional. Therefore, you may want to consider contacting **The Water Quality Association**, 4151 Naperville Rd., Lisle, IL 60532; (708) 505-01600. This trade organization can provide you with the names, addresses, and telephone numbers of its nearby members.

WATER TESTING

Many people are concerned about their water's quality, especially if they have a private water supply. Therefore, the sections below introduce you to information on water testing, including testing laboratories, how to take a water sample, and the need for specific tests.

Finding an Appropriate Water-Testing Facility

It's very important to have a private water supply tested regularly. For households on public supplies, you may be glad to know that utilities often test their water several times a month. This water-quality test information should be available upon request from them. It's usually provided free or at a minimum copying charge.

However, if contaminants originate within your home's plumbing system (high lead levels from lead solder, for example), you'll need to test your own tap to detect them. If you have a private water system, you alone are responsible for testing your water. This means contacting a qualified water-testing laboratory, deciding on the extent of the testing, and paying all the costs.

Of course your local board of health may have some suggestions, recommendations, or referrals to help with your water-testing decisions (In some locales they might actually do some basic types of testing themselves.). If you're unable to find an appropriate testing facility, you may want to call the **Environmental Drinking Water Hotline** at (800) 426-4791. This hotline can provide you with the name and phone number of your nearest EPA "certification officer." By contacting your state certification officer, you'll be given the names of water-testing firms in your area that are capable of performing water tests that meet EPA standards.

Still another approach to having your water tested is to contract one of the large, nationwide, water-testing companies. These include WaterCheck (**National Testing Labs., Inc.**), **Suburban Water Testing Laboratories**, and **WaterTest Corporation.** In addition, a water-filter dealer offering water tests you might choose to contact is **Ozark Water Service and Environmental Services**. Or perhaps instead, you might want to purchase a home water-test kit. These are available by mail-order from **The Allergy Store** and **Baubiologie Hardware**, among others (Contact the individual companies for information on the specific types of contaminants their test kits are designed to detect.). Incidentally, **Ozark Water Service and Environmental Services** sells a Radon Water Test Kit.

You may be wondering how much testing costs. Actually, the costs can vary enormously. The price depends on who does the testing, the number and types of tests that are performed, and the sophistication (the smallest amount that can be detected and the accuracy). In the end, the more technology, skill, and analysis that's required, the higher the cost will be.

Water Testing in General

The following sections will provide you with some basic information about water testing.

Frequently Performed Water Tests

The most commonly performed water test is for biological contaminants. This test determines if *pathogenic* (disease-causing) bacteria and perhaps other harmful microbes are present in the water supply. Actually, laboratory technicians will generally check a water sample for the presence of *coliforms* (both *fecal* coliforms and *total* coliforms) and *fecal streptococcus*. The ability of these organisms to live in the water often indicates other more harmful microbes may also be thriving in it.

Other frequently run water tests are called *chemical analysis tests*. These generally determine the levels of iron, calcium, and magnesium in water. But the tests can be expanded to include finding out the levels of lead, chromium, selenium, arsenic, etc. in the water supply. In addition, turbidity tests can be performed to determine the degree of the water's cloudiness. Also increasingly popular are water tests for determining whether volatile organic compounds (VOCs), pesticides, and detergents are present.

Water Test Limitations

An important note of consideration is that water tests have their limitations. After all, they can only find what they're specifically designed to look for. Therefore, if your water tests come back acceptable, there still could be contaminants in your water supply that were simply not tested for. Or, the contaminants may be at low levels that the tests simply did not pick up.

You should also realize that water-supply conditions can change fairly frequently and, as a result, so can the composition of the water (Water supplies can be affected by seasonal changes, droughts, the application of farm chemicals, and other events throughout the year.). Changes in water quality can be especially evident in individual private water supplies. Therefore, the result from a water test will only indicate the water's make-up for that particular sampling day. Not surprisingly, some water experts believe that because of all the possible variables involved, water testing on private water systems should be done several times during the first testing year (when you just move into a house or drill a new well) and then periodically every few years after that.

Furthermore, you need to know that there are several factors that determine the accuracy of a water test. These include the length of time between when the water is drawn from the tap and the time it is actually analyzed, how long the tap was running before the sample was obtained, the competency of the laboratory, and your skill in obtaining the water sample in the first place.

Obtaining a Water Sample

If you need to obtain a water sample yourself, it's very important that you make certain that you don't inadvertently contaminate it. So, guard against letting your hands touch the water being sampled, the interior of the canister, or the interior of the canister's lid. Also, follow all the testing lab's instructions completely (This may include writing down a description of the water's appearance and odor.). Finally, make sure the sample canister is securely sealed before you mail it or drop it off at the laboratory.

Water-Quality Concerns and their Appropriate Tests

The following section covers only some of the more common water problems and gives suggestions for the most likely causes and appropriate tests. Certainly, other explanations for certain water symptoms do exist as well as other types of tests.

It should also be noted that most of the information supplied below applies to those people who have individual home water supplies. However, it's likely that persons who use utility water will also find portions of this chart useful.

<u>Water-Quality Concerns</u>—<u>Appropriate Test(s)</u>

Reddish stains on laundry and/or fixtures—Iron.

Brownish-black stains on laundry and/or fixtures, and/or black flakes in the water—Manganese.

Greenish-blue stains on laundry and/or fixtures—Copper.

White scale on fixtures, and/or soap scum—Water hardness, iron.

Dirty-appearing water—Turbidity, sediment, organic matter.

Bitter-tasting water—Nitrates, sulfates.

Salty-tasting water—Total dissolved chlorides, sodium.

Rotten-egg smell to water—Hydrogen sulfide, sulfur bacteria.

Musty, earthy smell and/or taste to the water—Total coliform bacteria, iron.

Gasoline smell and/or taste to the water—Hydrocarbon scan, aromatic organic chemicals.

Illness from drinking water—Total coliform bacteria, nitrates, sulfates.

Infant in household—Nitrates.

Lead pipes or solder—Lead, copper, zinc, pH.

Corroded plumbing—Corrosiveness, pH, lead, iron, zinc, manganese, copper, sulfates, chloride.

Well too near a septic system—Total coliform bacteria, nitrate, total dissolved solids, chloride, sodium, sulfates, detergents.

Well too near a landfill—Total dissolved solids, pH, volatile organic compounds, heavy metals.

WATER TREATMENTS

All utility water as well as many private home water supplies are treated to improve their quality. This section discusses some common methods used to accomplish this.

COMMON UTILITY-WATER TREATMENTS

Today, most American homes use utility-supplied water. As it turns out, about half of this water comes from surface water sources (rivers, lakes, reservoirs, etc.) and the rest is pumped from wells that tap into aquifers (geological formations that contain or conduct ground water). Regardless of the source, most utilities perform treatments on their water to raise its quality before they pipe it out into their service areas.

Today in the U.S., public water utilities must meet the regulations set out in the 1974 Federal Safe Drinking Water Act and its later revisions. Therefore since 1975, all water systems with more than fifteen year-round connections are under the authority of the National Interim Primary Drinking Water Regulations. These standards cover physical qualities (taste and appearance), microbial content, and chemical make-up (amounts of dissolved minerals, etc.). As a result, virtually all water utilities must carry out several types of treatment on their water to achieve these mandated water-quality levels. Although public water utilities aren't required to perform the same particular set of treatment programs, many of them do, in fact, follow similar procedures. Following are typical steps performed by larger water utilities.

For example, the first step a public utility will commonly perform is *pretreatment* in which the *raw water* simply passes through a screen to remove large debris. Then, a *settlement treatment* is often done in which the water is allowed to remain in a reservoir or tank for about twenty hours. During that time, any suspended silt in the water will sink to the bottom, leaving the water free of larger particles. Next, the first chlorination step is usually performed to kill biological contaminants. Then the water is often subjected to *aeration* in which air bubbles up through the water in order to help remove volatile organic compounds (VOCs) and unpleasant tastes and odors.

Usually the next process is *coagulation* in which certain chemicals such as *ferric chloride* or *lime* (a calcium compound) are added to the water. These compounds combine with most of the water's dissolved minerals and metals forming what is known as *floc*. This mixture then passes through *sedimentation*, in which the floc is simply allowed to settle to the bottom of a holding basin. After that, the water is ready for *filtration* and is strained through sand and charcoal filters that trap the remaining particulates.

Fluoridation is often the next step. It is typically added to the water to raise its concentration to about 1 part per million (1ppm). Then most utilities perform a disinfection treatment, the second chlorination. This is done to disinfect the water mains and pipes between the plant and your house. However, because the chlorine is so reactive, other compounds (lime, soda ash, zinc phosphate, etc.) are often added to counter any potential pipe corrosion.

COMMON HOME WATER TREATMENTS

A number of cleaning and purifying devices are now available to improve the quality of your home's water. The following section defines and discusses some of the more common types (Specific product suggestions are given in *Choosing the Right Water Treatment Equipment* below.).

ACTIVATED-CHARCOAL FILTERS

Activated-charcoal (also known as activated-carbon) filters are one of the most common home water purification methods and generally one of the least expensive. The sections below explain how these popular units can affect your water.

How Activated-Charcoal Filters Work

Activated-charcoal water filters have been used since the mid-1950s and continue to grow in popularity. The media they use—activated charcoal—is actually a form of steam-treated charcoal. The charcoal itself can be derived from a variety of plant materials (or coal can be used). However, whatever its origin, the steam processing causes the charcoal to become extremely pitted. This rugged and uneven texture greatly increases the charcoal's surface area, which results in much greater *adsorption* capacity. This is important because it's primarily through adsorption that activated charcoal works, especially the granular types.

What is adsorption? Adsorption is an electromechanical adhesion process. Because of adsorption, most volatile chemicals (benzene, chlordane, etc.) and nearly all dissolved naturally occurring gases including hydrogen sulfide will adhere to activated charcoal. In this process these contaminants cling tightly to the charcoal's surface and are thus removed from the water supply. This procedure also works with radioactive radon. However, it must be pointed out that typical small activated-charcoal water filters can't adsorb or trap the radioactive particles that radon gas emits. However, there are larger granular activated-charcoal radon filtering systems available to remove both the radioactive radon gas and the radioactive particles that are produced.

Activated charcoal works particularly well at adsorbing chlorine from chlorinated utility water. However, it can also remove tastes and odors released by glue in plastic water-supply pipes. In fact, because activated charcoal is so efficient at removing most unpleasant tastes and smells in water, activated-charcoal filters are often called *taste and odor filters*.

You should be aware that activated-charcoal water filters are generally made in two forms: either in granulated or solid block form. In most cases, the solid block type (also known as *microfine carbon*) is somewhat more effective at removing contaminants than granulated charcoal. This is because the loose granules have spaces between them that allow some of the water molecules to pass by without coming in direct contact with the charcoal. Also, sometimes *channeling* can occur in granulated charcoal beds. This occurs when the water passing through the filter tends to follow the same path. This provides less efficient filtration because much of the activated charcoal is bypassed. The granules that are actually in the channel will adsorb contaminants for a while, but they soon become depleted, so, in a relatively brief amount of time, they're unable to adsorb any more contaminants.

On the other hand, solid blocks of charcoal are made of compressed activated charcoal without the spaces that normally surround granular activated charcoal. Therefore, solid-charcoal blocks force all the water molecules to actually travel through their compressed charcoal. As a result, block type activated-charcoal filters (and granules to a lesser extent) will not only adsorb gases but also strain out many types of suspended particulates. This straining action is known as *mechanical filtration*. Apparently, some lead and asbestos can be removed in this manner. It should be noted that certain solid charcoal blocks are manufactured by compressing charcoal with a plastic material that may be bothersome to some sensitive people.

It's very important for you to know that with any type of activated-charcoal filter, the longer the water is in contact with the activated charcoal, the more effective the removal of the contaminants will be. Therefore, manufacturers have devised two basic strategies to help their filters accomplish this. One is simply to use a large amount of charcoal that the water must pass through. The other is to slow the water's rate of flow through the charcoal. Some units actually combine both of these tactics.

Today, you can purchase an activated-charcoal filter as a whole-house unit or as a point-of-use device (for under your sink, above your sink, or to replace your regular shower head). Filters designed for whole-house use, as well as most of the under-sink models, will generally require some special plumbing installation work. Although some activated-charcoal filtering units have stainless-steel housings, a number of them are made from plastic. In addition, many of the granular activated cartridge refills are also made of plastic. It's likely that the activated charcoal will adsorb any plastic contaminants, odors, or tastes that happen to get into the water from plastic housings. However, some extremely sensitive individuals may want to purchase a stainless steel model that doesn't use plastic cartridges.

The cost of activated-charcoal filter models varies. However, as a rule, many of the simpler units are relatively low priced. The actual cost will depend on the filter's size, its casing material (plastic or stainless steel), whether it requires professional installation, and the replacement schedule and cost for replacement media. You'll find that some units use replaceable cartridges while others require that the entire filtering unit be replaced.

Activated-Charcoal Filter Concerns

It must be emphasized that activated-charcoal filters are not the answer to all water-quality problems. Although they can adsorb many volatile chemicals such as chlorine and naturally occurring dissolved gases, they can't remove most of the other types of contaminants that may be present in your water. This is especially true for activated-charcoal filters that use granular activated charcoal as their media. On the other hand, compressed activated-charcoal block filters do have some capacity to strain out (mechanically filter) a certain amount of particulate matter. Because all activated-charcoal filters become inefficient if they become clogged with particles, they're often combined with a sediment prefilter.

Above all, activated-charcoal filters can't *purify* your water. In other words, they can't kill the bacteria (or other microorganisms) in your water, or remove them effectively from your water (Note, solid activated charcoal blocks can strain some of these out.). In fact, research has found that bacteria can actually build up and eventually thrive inside an activated-charcoal filter, especially if the water hasn't been chlorinated. Even activated-charcoal filters with bacteriostatic additives (compounds that inhibit the growth of bacteria) such as silver can apparently become contaminated if given enough time. Furthermore, activated-charcoal filtering units with *backwashing cycles* (designed to periodically rinse off the media) may not be completely effective in preventing bacterial growth either (In addition, they tend to waste water because the water used in backwashing is flushed down the drain.). However, one bright note is that it does seems that a mixture of granulated activated charcoal and Kinetic-Degradation-Fluxion (KDF) media can remain naturally and effectively bacteriostatic. So these types of filtering devices should remain free of bacterial contamination.

Because of activated charcoal's capacity to support bacterial growth and its minimal ability to remove bacteria from water supplies, some water experts believe such filters should only be used with chlorinated water—that is, if no other purification treatment such as an ultraviolet-light purifier has been used on the water. The oxidizing disinfectant action of chlorine will kill many types of bacteria and the activated charcoal will then adsorb the chlorine. (Note, activated-charcoal units using disinfected or purified water should have their media changed regularly as a preventive measure against any bacterial contamination.)

With all activated-charcoal filters, the activated-charcoal media must be replaced from time to time. This is not just because of possible microbial growth, but also because the media will eventually be unable to adsorb contaminants effectively. In fact, if the activated-charcoal becomes saturated with adsorbed contaminants, it could release these contaminants back into your filtered water supply.

Replacement usually means taking out the old activated-charcoal cartridge and putting in a new one, or actually replacing the entire filtering unit—it depends on the model. Of course, the actual life expectancy for a particular cartridge (or filtering unit) will differ with the type of unit, the brand, the quality of your water, and the volume of water used daily. Generally, a filter manufacturer will give a suggested replacement schedule—perhaps once a month, several times a year, or once a year. However, sometimes these recommendations are somewhat exaggerated and a replacement schedule will often vary from a manufacturer's suggestion.

As a final note, because of their unique capacity to remove tastes and odors, activated-charcoal filters are commonly used in conjunction with other types of water-treatment strategies such as reverse osmosis and distillation.

REVERSE-OSMOSIS UNITS

Reverse-osmosis water treatment can often remove a wide range of particulate contaminants. However, the processing of your water is relatively slow, and the cost can be high.

How Reverse-Osmosis Units Work

To understand how a reverse-osmosis filter works, it's best to understand osmosis and reverse osmosis. *Osmosis* is the natural process in which water spontaneously passes through a *semipermeable membrane* (a very fine material that allows only very small molecules to pass through it). Actually, water goes through such a membrane in only one direction: it passes from a solution containing a low concentration of dissolved substances to a solution containing a higher one. Eventually, this results in the same concentration of water on both sides of the membrane. By the way, osmosis is the process by which water passes from the stems and leaves of plants (sites of low concentrations of dissolved substances) through the cell walls (which are semipermeable membranes) into the actual interiors of the cells (sites of high concentrations of dissolved substances).

Reverse osmosis, on the other hand, isn't a naturally occurring process. Instead, it requires the addition of pressure to create the opposite effect from that of osmosis. In other words, in reverse osmosis, water is forcibly pushed through a semipermeable membrane so that the water goes from a solution containing a high concentration of dissolved substances to one with a much lower concentration. The result is unequal water concentrations on both sides of the membrane. The intent of reverse osmosis is to separate water from dissolved substances.

Through this process, reverse-osmosis (*R/O*) units are capable of treating home-water supplies. In practice, *tap pressure* (the of pressure the water in your water pipes), and sometimes additional pressure, drives a stream of water through a special membrane. If your water supply is chlorinated, the membrane might be made of *cellulose acetate* or *cellulose triacetate*. On the other hand, *polymid resin film* might be used with unchlorinated water (other membrane types are also available).

Interestingly, all reverse-osmosis membranes aren't capable of removing the same-size particulates. In fact, the *pores* (tiny openings) in various R/O membranes are rated as to the largest matter that can pass through them. For example, a typical membrane used in residential units might have a rating of 0.01 microns. Although water molecules under pressure are able to pass through these minute openings, the holes are just too small to let solids over 0.01 microns pass through (Actually, a membrane will not have all pores of the same size. The pores in a membrane with a rating of 0.01 microns might actually range from 0.001 up to 0.01 microns.). When water passes through an R/O membrane, a great deal of the dissolved minerals, heavy metals, asbestos, dirt particles, radioactive particles, fluoride, and bacteria will be left behind. R/O units can be so effective that it's been estimated they're usually able to remove between 80% and 95% of all dissolved solids from the water they treat.

By the way, after the water in a reverse-osmosis unit has passed through the membrane, it then drips into a storage tank and is considered finished, treated water. When this tank is full, some units will automatically stop any further processing until you use some of the water and the level in the tank goes down. The treated water is often dispensed from the storage tank through a special faucet mounted next to your sink. To keep the R/O process working efficiently, most R/O units have a *flushing cycle* in which the semipermeable membrane is routinely rinsed clean with a stream of water. Afterwards, this rinsing water is drained away.

Reverse-osmosis units are available in point-of-use units (for mounting above or below a countertop) or as whole-house devices. Certain R/O units now feature automatic monitors that are designed to check the actual quality of the water (this is more common on whole-house units). Some of these monitors check both the original, untreated water as well as the finished, treated water. If any problem is detected, the R/O unit simply shuts off, thus, helping to guarantee consistently good-quality water.

Reverse-Osmosis Unit Concerns

Although most reverse-osmosis (R/O) units produce fairly clean water and are more convenient to use than a distiller, they aren't perfect. As with other treatment strategies, reverse osmosis is not capable of removing everything you might like to remove from your water supply. For example, reverse osmosis can't separate out any dissolved gases such as chlorine or radon (although it can usually remove the particles that are emitted by radon). In addition, reverse-osmosis membranes can't completely remove all biological contaminants (although certain models are much more capable of removing microbes than others).

Interestingly, if you have a chlorinated water supply that runs through *galvanized steel* pipes (steel pipes coated with zinc to prevent them from rusting), there may be an additional unsuspected problem with bacteria. It seems that irregular areas can develop on the interiors of these pipes from the chlorine reacting with the metal. Certain strains of bacteria can thrive in these rough spots. Although they may not be harmful to humans, they can destroy R/O membranes. Even if you don't have chlorinated water and galvanized pipes, bacterial contamination of a reverse-osmosis membrane can occur.

As a result, to remove bacteria and other types of contaminants that reverse osmosis can't eliminate on it own, R/O units are often sold as a part of a *combined water treatment system*. Therefore, you might find a reverse-osmosis model combined with an ultraviolet-light purifier or an activated-charcoal filter. Another type of R/O system you might come across is one using a Kinetic-Degradation-Fluxion (KDF) device for pretreatment. This is because the KDF media has an innate bacteriostatic action capable of controlling bacterial growth.

It should also be mentioned that some individuals are concerned that reverse-osmosis units are actually too effective in removing dissolved minerals from the water. It seems that this *demineralized* water can be somewhat flat-tasting. It is also called *aggressive*. Aggressive water will seek out and dissolve substances with which it comes into contact. As a result, some people believe that if you drink such water it might seek out and dissolve minerals that are in your body—minerals that your system needs.

There is one problem with R/O units on which everyone usually agrees: Reverse-osmosis treatment requires the use of many gallons of untreated water to create just one gallon of treated water. Surprisingly, as many as ten gallons of water may be flushed down the drain for every gallon of water that is filtered (commonly, the ratio is about three or four to one). The major reason for this wasted water is that the very process of reverse osmosis creates water on one side of the membrane, which contains very high concentrations of dissolved minerals. If too much water passes through the membrane, the removed minerals precipitate out of the water and start to crystalize. Therefore, before the solution becomes too concentrated, the water that remains on the untreated side of the membrane is drained away. Furthermore, the periodic flushing of the membrane, which is done to keep it clean, also uses up water. One way to minimize the wasting of water is to purchase a unit with a tank having an automatic shut-off valve. That way, the R/O process stops until additional treated water is really needed.

You should also be aware that R/O units can be somewhat expensive and tend to work slowly to produce a limited amount of treated water. In fact, many point-of-use models can only produce 5 to 15 gallons of treated water a day. In addition, research has found that reverse-osmosis units function less efficiently if they have to treat cold water rather than warm water.

Furthermore, the pressure of your water supply is a key factor in how well your R/O unit will operate. It seems that most utility water lines are between

40–60 psi (pounds per square inch), a range that happens to be ideal for most reverse-osmosis units. However, if you have a water pressure reading much below 40 psi, you'll probably have to increase the pressure. Fortunately, some reverse-osmosis units are sold with an optional pressure-boosting feature. In addition, the *pH level* (the degree of acidity or alkalinity) of your water supply can affect your R/O unit's performance.

Another matter you may want to keep in mind is that if your home requires whole-house R/O equipment, you'll need a separate water storage tank and a *repressurization pump* (to raise the water pressure high enough to allow the treated water to flow from the tank through your home's plumbing lines). And, because reverse-osmosis water treatment is slow, your whole-house model may have to work continually. If you're a very sensitive person, you may be interested to know that there have been reports that some point-of-use R/O units made of plastic have given the water they've treated a "plastic" taste and odor. This is more likely with brand new units. However, use of an activated-charcoal filter after the R/O unit should be able to solve this problem. As an R/O unit ages, steadily lower amounts of the plastic compounds will migrate into the water.

Of course, reverse-osmosis membranes don't last forever. Generally, they'll have to be replaced every 1–3 years (follow the manufacturer's guidelines with each unit). This is because the original pore openings will have enlarged over time through simple abrasive action. Therefore, as any R/O membrane ages, it allows ever-larger contaminants to pass through it. To help lengthen membrane life as much as possible, reverse-osmosis units often come equipped with a sediment prefilter.

WATER DISTILLERS

Distillation is undoubtedly the oldest form of water purification. As a rule, distillers are relatively inexpensive to purchase, but they're slow and limited in their output.

How Water Distillers Work

All water distillers work in basically the same way: They boil water to create steam. This steam is then captured and allowed to *condense* (become a liquid again). Sediments, dissolved minerals, heavy metals such as lead, asbestos fibers, fluoride, and radioactive particles that were in the original, untreated water are left behind in the boiling chamber. In addition, the high heat kills any waterborne biological contaminants. Obviously, distillation is a very effective water purification method. In fact, it's been determined that about 90% of all the contaminants and pollutants originally in untreated water are no longer present after it's been distilled. (By the way, the boiling tank of a water distiller must be drained and cleaned periodically.)

Generally, water distillers are available as kitchen countertop models, which operate off your house's electric current. However, there are models that can be set up outdoors and run on solar energy. When you're ready to purchase a water distiller, you'll find there are two basic types. *Air-cooled distillers* rely on the room's air temperature to condense the steam back into water. On the other hand, *water-cooled distillers* use a continuous flow of cool tap water to do the same job. In addition, you'll find that many water distillers are made either completely or partially of stainless steel. However, water distillers often contain plastic parts, and at least one all-glass water distillation device is available.

Water Distiller Concerns

You should be aware that although water distillation will remove virtually all the particulate matter from your water, it usually can't remove the volatile chemicals (compounds that rapidly evaporate) that might be in the water. This is because these compounds often evaporate at a temperature similar to that of water. Dissolved gases such as chlorine and radon gas can't be removed either, so they will remain in the treated distilled water, if they were present in the original, untreated water.

To address this problem, an activated-charcoal filter is often used after the water-distilling device as a postfilter. In fact, to better adsorb and eliminate certain volatile chemicals and gases, some models offer activated-charcoal filters for both pre- and postfilters. With the addition of activated-charcoal filtration, distilled water will often remove nearly 100% of the original, untreated water's contaminants.

However, there has been some concern about water that is "too pure." This is because water devoid of minerals can have a flat taste. Perhaps worse, distilled *demineralized* water is considered to be *aggressive*. In other words, it's water which aggressively seeks to pull into solution whatever molecules with which it comes in contact. One view holds that if you drink aggressive water, it will pull needed minerals out of your body.

Another potential problem with certain water distillers is the stainless steel of which some of them are constructed. While stainless steel is generally thought to be an inert material, it seems that a few people feel it is not the best material to use in a distiller. Apparently, there's some concern that certain stainless-steel distilling units may produce water containing elevated levels of aluminum. With Alzheimer's disease being associated with aluminum deposits in the brain, those sharing this view may prefer to own a model made of something besides stainless steel. However, if you prefer to purchase a stainless-steel unit, simply request from the manufacturer any information available as to whether the model you're interested in happens to produce water containing aluminum.

Unfortunately, water distillers have other drawbacks. One big concern is that water distillation tends to be an expensive operation. To determine the exact cost per gallon, multiply the number of kilowatts required to distill one gallon of water (this is usually available from the manufacturer) by your local electricity's per-kilowatt cost (available from your electric utility). To be most accurate, you should include the original cost of the untreated water if you buy it from a utility. (Note: Some water distillers can be powered by the sun outdoors, if sufficient sunlight and heat are available, but they can be inconvenient to use on a daily basis.)

Besides the expense, the output from a water distiller is both slow and limited. Plus, there are no known whole-house water distillers capable of supplying enough water for all uses within a household. In fact, most water-distillation units are designed to be placed permanently on your kitchen countertop. Units of this type are generally capable of producing only 3 to 4 gallons of water per day.

Then too, you should remember that water-distillation units tend to require at least some manual operation and certainly must be cleaned from time to time. Depending on the particular model, the cleaning schedule could be as frequent as twice a month or as little as twice a year. Incidentally, to make cleaning easier, the use of softened water in your distiller has been suggested rather than mineral-laden hard water. That way, you won't have to remove any crusty mineral scale buildup.

KINETIC-DEGRADATION-FLUXION DEVICES

Kinetic-Degradation-Fluxion devices are a relatively new and effective method of water treatment.

How KDF Devices Work

Kinetic-Degradation-Fluxion (KDF) is a water treatment technology that was patented in 1987. The name actually denotes three major characteristics of the KDF media. These devices are *kinetic* (creating electrochemical energy), they go through *degradation* (the material very slowly degrades or is used up through chemical reactions), and they allow *fluxion* (fluids pass through without creating excessive back pressure).

What is KDF? KDF is actually an unique high-purity alloy made up of two dissimilar metals, zinc and copper. As it turns out, this alloy has an inherently high potential for electrochemical reduction/oxidation (redox) reactions (*reduction* is simply the addition of electrons to a molecule, and *oxidation* is their loss). Because of this, KDF filters have the capacity to remove a variety of waterborne contaminants in several ways.

During actual KDF treatment, water passes through the KDF media which are in the form of thousands of irregularly shaped granules (the media are available in other forms, but in most home situations, granules are generally used). As the water flows through, certain problematic contaminants (for example, iron, hydrogen sulfide, and chlorine) spontaneously react with the zinc or copper making up the KDF media and are transformed into "acceptable" compounds. For example, when chlorine molecules come in contact with the KDF media, they instantly react with molecules of zinc to create zinc chloride. In fact, KDF media are so efficient at removing chlorine that they are estimated to be ten times more effective than a similar amount of activated charcoal.

However, that's not the limit of KDF treatment's capabilities. Certain heavy metals in water such as lead are removed by actually becoming electroplated onto the KDF media. In addition, the zinc and copper generate a minute electric current like a battery (0.04 volts) that controls the populations of many microorganisms by disrupting their metabolic functions. Therefore, KDF media are naturally bacteriostatic and so are naturally resistant to bacterial contamination. In fact, KDF media are so effective at controlling certain populations of biological contaminants that the Environmental Protection Agency (EPA) has recently designated KDF units as "pesticidal devices."

KDF media can also alter the physical crystalline appearance and character of the waterborne, insoluble, hard-water compounds of calcium and magnesium. Normally, the compounds are crystals with hard, angular structures that can grow in size relatively quickly. If they happen to grow and accumulate on the interiors of a metal pipe, they form lime scale. However, hard water that passes through a KDF filter no longer has typical hard, angular calcium- and magnesium-compound crystals. Instead, these compounds are transformed into very small, evenly shaped, rounded particles that are unable to grow in size or adhere to metallic surfaces. Therefore, KDF treatment tends to counter hard water scale buildup (a 5-micron filtering device can then be used to remove these fine particles from the treated water).

You can now purchase water-treatment equipment for your home that uses KDF media. Point-of-use models for both your kitchen and shower, whole-house units, and even small portable devices are now available. It should be mentioned that KDF media are nontoxic, and in most forms, recyclable. Generally, KDF devices, especially home-use models, use a mixture of KDF media and granular activated charcoal.

KDF Concerns

As with virtually all water-treatment strategies, KDF media alone can't remove every type of possible contaminant that could be present in your water. That's why, for example, they are commonly used in combination with granular activated charcoal, which is able to adsorb certain volatile chemicals and naturally occurring gases that KDF can't. In addition, KDF devices are sometimes used in conjunction with reverse-osmosis units because they are capable of removing waterborne particulates.

You should also keep in mind that although KDF media are bacteriostatic (able to control bacterial growth) and have been EPA-designated as pesticidal devices, they should only be used in homes with water that has been disinfected by a utility, or in those homes with an individual private water source containing only very minimal nonpathogenic (non-disease-causing) biological contamination. This is because home-use models of KDF devices are not considered water purifiers. An ultraviolet-light purifier or a water distiller are specifically designed for water purification purposes.

It should be noted that the KDF media/granulated activated-charcoal mix used in home KDF devices must be replaced from time to time. Often, the replacement schedule for point-of-use units with replaceable cartridges is about once a year or every 25,000 gallons of water (follow the manufacturer's recommendations for your particular unit). As you might expect, KDF media costs more than activated charcoal. For example, a cartridge of combined KDF media/granulated activated-charcoal will probably cost about one-third more than a similar-sized cartridge containing a compressed activated-charcoal block. Fortunately, there is a "buy-back/recycling program" for some used KDF cartridges (check to see if the program is available from the manufacturer of your particular KDF device).

In addition, you may wish to know that whole-house KDF devices come either as *backwashing* or *non-backwashing* models. A unit that can backwash is capable of cleaning its media of excess oxide compounds and calcium and magnesium solids by simply flushing the granules with water and then draining the water out. However, this regeneration process uses a substantial amount of water, then flushes it down the drain. It's been suggested that backwashing be done approximately three times a week, or more often if high levels of certain contaminants are present in the untreated water.

ULTRAVIOLET PURIFIERS

Ultraviolet (UV) light is a very effective *antiseptic* that, if intense enough, can kill most waterborne bacteria and other biological contaminants. UV light is able to do this because it can penetrate the membranes of microbes and inactivate the protein structures inside their cells. This sounds complicated, but is actually a simple, almost instantaneous process. In operation, an ultra-violet-light purifier directs a beam of UV light into flowing water and this immediately brings on the demise of just about all the living biological contaminants in that water.

Ultraviolet-light purifiers can work effectively for both private individual wells and for water stored in cisterns (holding tanks). Whole-house units and point-of-use models are available. By the way, point-of-use UV-light purifiers are commonly used in conjunction with reverse-osmosis units. It should be noted that UV purification only has germicidal (killing) action on waterborne microbes; it has no effect on other possible contaminants that could be in your water. For example, it can't adsorb dissolved gases or strain out sediment.

SEDIMENT FILTERS

Sediment traps and *sediment filters* (also known as *turbidity filters*) are specifically designed to remove gritty particles from water supplies. Therefore, if some type of biological contaminant such as algae or bacteria are part of the turbidity problem, it must be killed and/or removed by some other device because most sediment filters aren't capable of doing this.

Sediment traps are used for whole-house sediment removal to eliminate heavy concentrations of suspended soil in water. Actually, a sediment trap can simply be a special holding tank. In actual practice, the turbid untreated water is pumped into the tank and held there for about 24 hours. During that time, the soil particles settle to the bottom. Then the clean water at the top of the tank is piped away either to another treatment device or to the rest of the house (this may require use of a *repressurization pump*). It should be noted that sometimes a chemical is added to the sediment trap to hasten the settling process. This might be *aluminum sulfate* (a form of *alum*) or perhaps a certain type of *synthetic polymer compound.*

The other common approach for removing sediment is to use a sediment filter. Sediment filters range in size from fairly large to less than 12" tall. Generally, sediment filters work well if water doesn't contain a large amount of suspended soil (this is especially true for smaller-sized filters). Sediment filters are rated according to the smallest size of particulate they're able to remove. For example, a 15-micron unit will trap all the sediment particles that are larger than 15 microns. Sediment filters are available with ratings ranging from 5 to 25 microns.

Large sediment filters may use media such as *diatomaceous earth (DE)* (fine grains of mostly silica compounds originating from the cell walls of diatomic algae), quartz gravel, filtering sand, limestone chips, or even coal. Often, large units must be *backwashed* from time to time so that they don't clog. In this process, a stream of water is run through the media backwards to pick up the accumulated debris and carry it to a drain. Of course, this backwashing process flushes a certain amount of water down the drain. In small units, one or more layers of paper, or another filtering or screening material may be used, often in the form of a replaceable cartridge. Of course, the replacement schedule will vary according to your water's turbidity, the volume of water your household uses, and the size of the filtering cartridge.

It should also be mentioned that *hydrocylonic separators* may be used as a sediment-removing technology. These devices work by rapidly spinning the incoming water. Then, through *centrifugal force*, the soil and sand particles are tossed against the walls of the separator's interior and drained away. Apparently, hydrocylonic separators are usually quite effective.

WATER SOFTENERS

A *water softener* is popularly defined as any substance or device able to eliminate, or in some way inactivate, *hard-water minerals* commonly found in water supplies. It should be noted that hard water is usually defined as having a dissolved calcium and magnesium concentration at or above 120 mg/liter. However, many people find that a concentration of only 85 mg/liter still creates some of the problems associated with hard water.

What are some typical hard-water problems? One is the crusty white buildup that can occur on the interiors of your plumbing fixtures and water pipes. This *lime scale* is actually made by the minerals *precipitating* (coming out of solution). Another problem is that calcium and magnesium minerals in water can react with the fats and oils in the soaps you use creating an insoluble scum known as *soap curd*. In addition, white fabrics washed in hard water can acquire a grayish tinge.

Although most people use the term "water softener" to mean anything that can counter the effects of hard water, you should be aware that there's a legal distinction between the terms *water softener* and *water conditioner*. Water softeners are devices that add a substance to the water to eliminate or inactivate hard-water minerals, while water conditioners are devices that don't add anything to the water. On the other hand, *water-softening agents* are simply substances (not devices) that can deactivate or eliminate hard-water minerals. (Note: Some water-softening devices help remove or inactivate iron and certain other minerals besides just calcium and magnesium.)

Water-Softening Agents

Certain compounds, when added to hard water (water with a high concentration of calcium and magnesium), act as *water-softening agents*. What these particular substances actually do is to combine with the dissolved minerals, causing them to *precipitate* (be pulled out of solution), creating very minute insoluble solids. This process, known as *water softening through precipitation*, causes the hard-water minerals to be chemically bound up so that they're no longer free to react with soap to form scum (*soap curd*) or to attach themselves to the interiors of pipes, etc. and form *lime scale*.

Today, borax and sodium carbonate are two commonly used precipitating, water-softening agents. For many years phosphate compounds were very popular for this, including trisodium phosphate (TSP). However, because it was determined that phosphates can create water-quality problems in waterways, this is no longer the case (see *Trisodium Phosphate* in *Chapter 7: Cleaning*). In homes, water-softening agents are generally point-of-use products. In other words, they're not typically added to the entire water supply of the house, but usually just to the laundry wash water.

Typical Water-Softening Devices

Water-softening devices were created to provide continuous whole-house water softening. They work through a *cation exchange process* (cations are positively charged atoms). Simply put, positive *sodium ions* are used to replace the positive hard-water *mineral ions* in your water supply. The source of the sodium ions is a brine solution made up of common salt (sodium chloride) and water. Because these units add a substance (salt) to change the hardness of the water, they're not considered *water conditioners*.

In practice, a typical water-softening device is able to soften your water relatively quickly because it also contains a *catalyst* (a substance capable of hastening the speed of a chemical reaction while not being changed itself). Once, *zeolite* granules (see also *Zeolite* in *Chapter 9: Indoor Air*) were commonly used as the catalyst in most home water-softening devices. However, these days, beads of a synthetic resin (*polystyrenated bivinylbenzene*) are much more popular. These catalysts provide the surfaces on which the ion-trading takes place. Because a catalyst is never altered or used up, the synthetic resin beads (or zeolite) never need to be replaced. However, their surfaces will eventually become clogged with mineral ions. When that occurs, the ion-exchange process (the softening process) slows dramatically and a *recharging cycle* becomes necessary.

The recharging process actually includes several steps. First, there is a *backflushing* of the water flow, which loosens the mineral buildup on the catalyst surfaces. Then, there's an addition of fresh brine solution. The final step is a complete rinsing of the tank containing the catalyst with fresh water to remove the loosened minerals. Most home water-softening devices recharge themselves automatically. However, salt will have to be added manually from time to time. The actual frequency for this will depend on your particular water softener, the hardness of your water and the volume of water used daily in your household.

It should be noted that most of the typical water softeners that use salt will produce water that feels slick, suds easily, and creates no mineral buildup (lime scale) on your pipes and plumbing fixtures. However, there are negatives to these units. One is that the recharging process wastes a certain amount of water by flushing it down the drain. Water-softening devices can also be fairly expensive, but some companies offer lease and rent-to-own programs.

In addition, you will have to routinely purchase salt for your softener. Fortunately, arrangements with your softener dealer can easily be made to have salt delivered directly to your home. Some dealers will even fill the salt tank for you. Of course, there's a cost to all this (the cost may actually be included in your purchase or rental price). To save money, you might purchase the salt you need at a local chemical-supply company or a wholesale or discount outlet and periodically fill the salt tank yourself. (To find a chemical-supply company in your area, check your local telephone classified directory.

Still another concern with typical softening devices is that, because they use salt, the treated water will have a relatively high sodium content. This can be a real concern for individuals on a salt-restricted diet. However, if you install a *reverse-osmosis unit* in your kitchen with a membrane rated to remove salt, your drinking and cooking water will contain a much lower salt concentration. Of course, *distillation* will remove virtually all the salt.

A few local jurisdictions (for example, the City of Los Angeles) have apparently prohibited the installation of automatic, self-regenerating (backwashing) water softeners that use salt-ion exchange. This is because the water drained from these devices during their cleaning cycle eventually enters the sewer lines and ends up at water-treatment plants. Treating this backwashing water has proven difficult and expensive. Therefore, check local codes and regulations before purchasing a water-softening device.

Alternative Water Conditioning Devices

Besides typical water softeners, alternative devices are available that are also able to prevent or minimize hard-water problems. These units are considered *water conditioners* because they don't add any substances (such as salt) to your water. Therefore, the water they treat is considered *conditioned*, not *softened*.

Catalytic-Converter Water Conditioners

One interesting water-conditioning strategy involves converting the unstable dissolved calcium and magnesium compounds into the stable compounds they were before they went into solution. In the case of calcium, this would mean causing the calcium, which is in the form of a dissolved *bicarbonate,* to revert to *calcium carbonate*—the stable material found in limestone. It is the dissolved bicarbonate contaminant, not calcium carbonate, that is responsible for creating lime scale (the crusty white buildup inside your pipes and plumbing fixtures).

To convert the bicarbonate molecular forms of calcium into molecules of the carbonate form, the bicarbonates have to lose a molecule of carbon dioxide (CO_2). At least one water conditioner does this by moving untreated water through a narrowing tube (a *venturi*). The water then comes in contact with a catalytic metal rod within a chamber (a catalyst is a substance that hastens a chemical reaction without being altered itself).

The effect of this is that CO_2 molecules are stripped away from the bicarbonate calcium molecules. The resulting calcium carbonate (CO_3) molecules immediately become attracted to, and bond to, the metal rod. The CO_3 molecules are attracted to the rod because it is made of a special alloy with properties that mimic a calcium carbonate crystal. Therefore, the newly formed calcium carbonate molecules "think" that they're bonding to other calcium carbonate molecules when they bond to the rod. In reality, the "deceptive" rod becomes a seed bed for calcium carbonate crystallization.

However, the minute, stable calcium carbonate crystals (also known as *calcite*) that attach themselves to the rod are only able to build up very slightly before they're freed back into the water. Once these microscopic calcite crystals are present in your water supply, they themselves act as seeds for calcium carbonate crystallization. Surprisingly, this causes the existing lime scale in your pipes to eventually disappear because the lime attaches itself to the calcite seeds. As a result, in a few weeks or months, your entire home plumbing system could become virtually free of lime scale.

It's important to note that water treated with a catalytic water conditioner will retain it's original mineral content. This is because the conditioner doesn't remove hard-water minerals, it simply *deactivates* them so that hard-water problems are minimized. One concern to keep in mind though is that the surfaces of the rod within the catalytic converter chamber must be kept free from the buildup of contaminants in order for them to work efficiently. Therefore, you must periodically remove the rod and clean it. By the way, these particular devices are generally designed for whole-house applications.

Magnetic-Physical Water Conditioning

Another alternative water-conditioning approach that attempts to free calcium carbonate from its dissolved molecular form is *magnetic-physical water conditioning*. Some devices based on this process accomplish the calcium compound conversion by use of *permanent magnets* (magnets that retain their strong innate magnetic effect over time), while others use *electrically charged magnets* (magnets using live electric current.) Also, some magnetic-physical water conditioners are installed directly in the water flow, while others are designed as clamp-on devices to be mounted around a water pipe (clamp-on models can be attached to all types of water pipes except those containing iron).

One theory (proposed by Dr. Klaus J. Kronenberg) behind physical-magnetic water conditioning is that certain magnetic fields are able to break the *electrochemical bonds* that hold *water/calcium carbonate clusters* together. This is important because these clusters, which are common in water, apparently "lock" calcium carbonate onto water molecules. Therefore, the imprisoned calcium carbonate isn't free to bond to other calcium carbonate and form minute, stable crystals in the water. Instead, the calcium carbonate/water clusters end up creating a crusty white lime scale on the interiors of your pipes and plumbing fixtures.

Yet, if only about 1 in 10 billion water/calcium carbonate clusters in the water break up, the result would be effective water conditioning. This is because the newly freed calcium carbonate molecules act as seed nuclei for calcium carbonate crystallization, and the remaining water/calcium carbonate clusters would readily bond to these seeds. As a result, many very tiny calcium carbonate crystals soon would be present in the water rather than calcium carbonate/water clusters. Therefore, lime scale could no longer form on the interior surfaces of pipes and plumbing fixtures and, eventually, the existing scale would disappear (the tiny calcium carbonate crystals would pass harmlessly through the plumbing lines).

This is the intended purpose of physical-magnetic water conditioning. In actual practice, water flows at a certain speed past several magnets with *alternating polarity* (positive then negative, then positive, etc.). This creates a *resonating field of magnetic effects*. As it turns out, the specific *resonance* (vibration) that's produced coincides with the innate vibration within just a few of the calcium carbonate/water clusters present in the water. However, the increased resonance within these few clusters causes them to vibrate with great intensity. In fact, the vibration is more than some of the clusters can withstand and, so, they break apart, resulting in freed calcium carbonate molecules that then act as crystallizing seeds.

Certain considerations should be kept in mind if you'd like to try using a physical-magnetic water conditioner. The biggest question is whether or not they even work very well. Some people feel that generally magnetic water-conditioning devices are effective only for about ten feet or less of pipe immediately after the magnet. Others feel they're not effective at all. Yet, others believe that with well-planned placements, physical-magnetic water conditioners can work quite satisfactorily.

Like most other alternative water-conditioning methods, water treated with a physical-magnetic water conditioner doesn't have the minerals removed. Although the water retains its mineral content, the hard-water minerals are deactivated and unable to form lime scale. As a rule, magnetic water-conditioning devices are designed for point-of-use applications only.

Electrostatic Water Conditioning

Electrostatic water conditioners are designed so that water passes through a metal *electrostatic chamber.* There is a negatively charged, Teflon-coated, metal electrode inside the positively charged and grounded metal tank (the normal alternating electrical current in a house is changed to direct current to generate the charge on the electrode). The electrode is coated so the direct charge cannot come in contact with the flowing water. As a result of this setup, an *electrostatic field* (an area charged with static electricity) is generated between the electrode's surface and the tank walls. The actual strength of this electrostatic field is said to be between 10,000 and 12,000 volts. Simply put, this means that inside the tank electrons wind up becoming distributed throughout the water.

This is important because the dissolved calcium and magnesium compounds (mostly in *carbonate* and *bicarbonate forms*) passing though this strong electrostatic field apparently become altered by the electrons. This change hinders their ability to bond together or to other surfaces. Therefore, the treated water prevents a further buildup of crusty white lime scale on the interiors of pipes and plumbing fixtures. In fact, the already existing lime scale will eventually break down and harmlessly pass through the plumbing system. By the way, it should be mentioned that the electrostatic field is also able to lower the water's surface tension so that suds are created more easily (see *Soaps* in *Chapter 7: Cleaning*).

One consideration to keep in mind with electrostatic water conditioners is that they continually use electric power. However, they typically use less energy to operate than a 40-watt light bulb. As with most alternative water-conditioning methods, water treated with electrostatic water conditioners retains its mineral content. Commonly, electrostatic conditioning units are designed for whole-house use.

Kinetic-Degradation-Fluxion Water Conditioning

(see *Kinetic-Degradation-Fluxion Devices* above)

WATER-TREATMENT SUMMARY

Following is a brief listing of all the water-treatment strategies covered in this chapter, along with the contaminants they are most effective in removing (or inactivating). Important note: Some treatment devices combine several treatment methods and, therefore, can actually remove more contaminants than are listed here.

Solid-Block Activated-Charcoal Filters—Chlorine, dissolved gases, organic chemicals. Also sediment, asbestos, heavy metals, and some fluoride.

Granular Activated-Charcoal Filters—Chlorine, dissolved gases, organic chemicals. Also, a limited amount of sediment.

Reverse-Osmosis Units—Minerals, nitrates, fluoride, sediment, heavy metals, asbestos. Also effective at lowering salt concentrations (depending on the membrane rating), and greatly lowering the amounts of many types of biological contamination such as bacteria.

Water Distillers—Sediment, minerals, nitrates, heavy metals, biological contaminants, asbestos, fluoride.

Kinetic-Degradation-Fluxion (KDF) Devices—Chlorine, sulfur dioxide, methane, certain heavy metals such as lead. Also controls most bacteria and microorganisms in the media through innate bacteriostatic action. In addition, deactivates hard-water minerals.

Sediment Filters and Traps—Sand and dirt.

Ultraviolet Purifiers—Biological contaminants.

Water Softening Agents—Hard-water minerals (deactivation).

Water Softening Devices—Hard-water minerals (removal). Will add sodium.

Water Conditioners—Hard-water minerals (deactivation).

CHOOSING THE RIGHT WATER-TREATMENT EQUIPMENT

There are perhaps hundreds of various water filters, purifiers, softening, and conditioning devices now available in the marketplace. Not surprisingly, many individuals as a result feel confused and overwhelmed when they try to choose the right equipment for their home. However, some basic steps can help make this process more manageable. These are discussed below.

BASIC WATER-TREATMENT EQUIPMENT CONSIDERATIONS

When you're ready to consider purchasing a specific piece of water-treatment equipment, it's important to have in front of you any written information you can find about your water. This information should include a variety of data, including whether or not your water supply is from a private source or a public utility. If it's from a utility, get a copy of any recent water-quality tests (mineral content, pH, chlorine, fluoride etc.). Of course, if you have a private well, get out any laboratory reports of the quality of the water. Note: Even if you have utility-supplied water, you should consider having your tap water tested for lead content if you have metal water pipes with lead-soldered joints.

With specific water-quality information in front of you, you can decide to what extent you want certain contaminants removed. Naturally, you'll want to have *pathogenic* (disease-causing) and potentially harmful industrial and agricultural pollutants reduced as much as possible. But perhaps a slightly elevated calcium and magnesium content and the minimal lime scale it would create will be acceptable to you. Your next decision is to choose the water-treatment strategy that is capable of actually removing (or deactivating) the contaminants you've targeted to eliminate.

Once you've decided on a basic strategy, your next consideration is figuring out if you need (or want) a whole-house system or one or more point-of-use units. Perhaps you would like a combination of both. Whether you are renting or own your home will, no doubt, have a bearing on whether a whole-house unit is feasible. If you're renting (especially for only a short time), it's likely you won't want to invest in any system that requires permanent installation. Therefore for renters, simple-to-install point-of-use devices often make the most sense. On the other hand, if you own your home and have determined you only want to remove chlorine from your utility-supplied water, a whole-house activated-charcoal filter will probably be the best and easiest solution for you. In still another situation, you might find that a whole-house water-softening device will be able to rid your water supply of any unwanted hard-water minerals and iron so that your water is satisfactory for bathing and general household purposes. But you may choose to use a water distiller in your kitchen to produce extremely pure water for drinking and cooking—water that's free of the sodium the water softener added. And, so on.

The factors to next take into account are an estimate of the volume of water you and your family use daily, as well as the amount of time you're willing to devote to the operation and maintenance of the water-treatment equipment. Are you honestly willing to change the filter each month if it's recommended? Will you remember to regularly clean a water conditioner's catalytic rod? You'll also need to consider whether you have adequate space for certain water-treatment devices. Do you really have room for a full-size water softener in your utility room? Do you really have the free counter space to keep a water distiller set up? In addition, you should take into consideration the materials of which the equipment is constructed (stainless steel or plastic for example), especially if you're a sensitive person.

Of course, when you're choosing water-treatment equipment, you'll have to consider its *initial cost* (price plus installation charge) and its *operating cost* (replacement membranes or filters, electricity, and any professional maintenance fees, etc.; the cost of utility water is especially a concern with reverse-osmosis units). The final step is finding out about any warranties and/or guarantees from manufacturers and dealers.

FURTHER HELP IN CHOOSING WATER-TREATMENT EQUIPMENT

Obviously, water-treatment equipment is an area where further advice, suggestions, and consultations by knowledgeable persons can be helpful. Therefore, it's a good idea to ask your personal physician and/or other health-care professional if he (or she) has any advice on units that would likely fit your specific needs. You might also contact consultant/dealers including **Pure Water Place**, and **Nigra Enterprises** who may be helpful as well. In addition, specialty catalogs for allergic and sensitive individuals that handle several types and brands of water-treatment equipment devices can be good sources of assistance. A few catalogs of this kind are **The Living Source**, **The Allergy Store**, **The Environmental Health Shopper**, and **N.E.E.D.S.**

And, especially if your home has a private water source requiring a complicated treatment program, you'll want to consider contacting **The Water Qual-**

ity Association at 4151 Naperville Rd., Lisle, IL 60532; (708) 505-0160. This trade association provides you with the names of nearby members. These are companies which are local suppliers of *traditional* water-softening/water-treatment equipment. However, it should be remembered that these companies often don't specialize in working with sensitive individuals and generally don't handle or install *alternative* water-conditioning equipment.

WHOLE-HOUSE WATER-TREATMENT EQUIPMENT SUGGESTIONS

The following sections offer suggestions for whole-house water-treatment equipment you might consider purchasing (certainly other fine choices are available other than the ones listed here). Realize that only a brief description is given for each model, so you'll probably want to contact the individual companies or dealers for more complete information. You should be aware that whole-house water-treatment equipment is permanently installed to connect with your water line immediately after it enters your house. Therefore, professional installation is often required.

Whole-House Activated-Charcoal Filters

For many homes on chlorinated water supplies, a simple activated-charcoal filter is often all that's necessary to create acceptable water. Fortunately, many models are available, but some are made of plastic. Naturally, some sensitive individuals may be concerned about a water filter with a plastic housing. However, because activated charcoal will remove tastes and odors from your water, any plastic contamination will likely be removed. Therefore, plastic activated-charcoal filtering units often prove to be quite tolerable (stainless-steel models, however, are available). Generally, manufacturers of activated-charcoal filters tend to recommend that their units only be used on chlorinated lines to reduce problems of microbial contamination.

You may be interested in knowing that local **Sears, Roebuck and Co.** stores sell several low-priced activated-charcoal filtering units you may want to purchase. One of these is the Model 329-321200, which is simply a plastic housing designed to hold a replaceable, activated-charcoal cartridge. Besides their "taste and odor" granulated activated-charcoal cartridges, other types of media-filled cartridges are available (some Sears cartridges are rated to last for only 1,500 gallons of water, but they can last longer, depending on the concentration of chlorine). Very similar models are offered by Aqua Pure (**Cuno**). This particular brand can be ordered directly from the manufacturer or purchased from dealers including **Nontoxic Environments.**

In addition, **Ametek** offers several sizes of granulated activated-charcoal filters made with either stainless-steel or plastic housings. Some models are combined with a sediment prefilter. The company has a large, long-lasting unit with a suggested life of up to 75,000 gallons. The replacement cartridges should last for at least several months, up to a year, depending on your water usage and the level of chlorine in your water. Ametek filters can be directly ordered from the company or purchased from its local dealers.

The Multi-Micronic Water Treatment System (**Multi-Pure Corporation**) is yet another unit with a plastic housing. This model actually combines a "multiple prefilter," a granulated activated-charcoal filter, and an activated-charcoal block. It can be ordered directly from the company or through its dealers.

Although they're more costly, if you'd prefer a stainless-steel water filter, the Spark-L-Pure (**General Ecology, Inc.**) is one whole-house activated-charcoal unit you might consider. This filter uses *structured matrix* activated-charcoal technology, which is a special type of activated-charcoal block. This particular design is said to be effective at filtering not only chlorine and other volatile chemicals but also many microbes as well. The actual filtering cartridges for this unit are in modules designed for about 30,000 gallons of water and can be cleaned and reused. However, new replacement modules are also available. Spark-L-Pure can be ordered directly from the company or from dealers including **The Pure Water Place** and **Nontoxic Environments**.

The Stabilizer Plus (**Fluid Mechanics**) is a unique combination water-treatment device. It utilizes the company's Stabilizer water conditioner plus a three-media water-filtering system: activated charcoal and two other media. Together, they're able to remove volatile chemicals, chlorine, and heavy metals, among many other contaminants. The unit is designed to filter as much as 200,000 gallons of water.

In addition, other brands of fine whole-house activated-charcoal water filters you might consider include models offered by **The Living Source**, **The Allergy Store**, **American Environmental Health Foundation**, **Ozark Water Service and Environmental Services**, and **Nigra Enterprises**, among others.

Whole-House Reverse-Osmosis Units

For whole-house reverse-osmosis (R/O) treatment, you'll probably want to consult and deal with a local distributor. This is because most whole-house R/O units entail installing relatively expensive and complicated equipment (tanks, repressurization pumps, membranes, etc.), that must specifically meet the needs of your particular situation. Therefore, you might consider contacting **The Water Quality Association** at 4151 Naperville Rd., Lisle, IL 60532; (708) 505-0160 for a dealer near you that handles, installs, and is able to maintain such systems.

Whole-House Kinetic-Degradation-Fluxion Devices

Kinetic-Degradation-Fluxion (KDF) material is generally used in a mixture of granular activated-charcoal in home filtering units. This combination is used in the TerraTower (**Global Environmental Technologies**). Actually, several models of the TerraTower are available, all having sediment prefilters. These units are very effective at removing chlorine, heavy metals, and several other contaminants, as well as minimizing lime scale buildup due to hard water.

All TerraTower units either have a 7" x 35" or 8" x 40" cylindrical polyvinyl chloride (PVC) media-filled tank. The larger tanks are capable of automatic backwashing to periodically clean off their media, so the tanks come equipped with solid-state microprocessors to enable them to use water efficiently during these regular regeneration cycles. This manufacturer recommends that the smaller units without backwashing should have their media-filled tanks replaced each year. Models capable of backwashing only need their media-filled tanks replaced every two years. Interestingly, all media-filled tanks are recyclable through the company's buy-back program. TerraTowers can be purchased directly from the company or from its dealers.

You might also check the KDF media units available from **Ozark Water Services and Environmental Services**.

Whole-House Sediment Filters

If only a very small amount of gritty sediment needs to be removed from your water, **Ametek** offers several sizes of sediment filters that work quite well. They can be ordered directly from the company or from local dealers.

In addition, many other companies make sediment-removal equipment. For example, Aqua Pure (**Cuno**) offers several whole-house sediment filters. These can be purchased directly from the company or from local dealers. By the way, **Culligan International Co.** sells and installs a variety of sediment-removal units. To find a local Culligan dealer, call company headquarters or check your local classified telephone directory. **Sears, Roebuck and Co.** also offers sediment filters.

Before buying any sediment filter, it's a good idea to pinpoint exactly what is causing the cloudiness in your water. If it's neither biological contaminants nor sand and soil particles, other treatments may be necessary to make your water acceptable. And even if gritty sediment is the only contaminant, be sure to purchase a unit with enough capacity to effectively solve your particular sediment problem.

Whole-House Ultraviolet-Light Purifiers

To effectively kill microbial contamination in your water, one very good option is to install an ultraviolet-light purifier. One brand of these you might consider is the Ultra-Hyd Germicidal UV Water Purifier (**Ultra-Hyd**). These units are constructed of stainless steel and require very little maintenance. They can be purchased directly from the company.

Whole-House Water-Softening and Water-Conditioning Devices

Quite a few manufacturers offer salt ion-exchange water-softening devices. Of course, one of the best known is **Culligan International Co.**, which offers several models and has dealers nationwide. To find a Culligan dealer near you, call the company headquarters or check your local classified telephone directory, which will likely list suppliers of other brands as well.

For whole-house alternative water conditioning, consider purchasing The Stabilizer (**Fluid Mechanics**), which uses special catalytic technology. The only maintenance required is cleaning the catalyzing rod approximately every two weeks. The same company also offers The Stabilizer Plus, which combines its water conditioner with three types of water filtration. All their units can be ordered directly from the company or they can be purchased from dealers.

If you'd like to try electrostatic water conditioning, ElectroStatic Water-Treatment conditioners (**ElectroStatic Technologies, Inc.**) are available in a variety of sizes. These units are offered with aluminum or optional stainless-steel tanks. ElectroStatic Water-Treatment conditioners can be purchased directly from the company or from dealers such as **Ozark Water Service and Environmental Services**.

POINT-OF-USE WATER-TREATMENT EQUIPMENT

For some households, whole-house water treatment isn't necessary, desired, affordable, or effective enough in removing contaminants. Therefore, many water-treatment devices are available to meet point-of-use needs. These units can be installed in a variety of ways, such as on a kitchen countertop, under a kitchen sink, or to replace the shower head in your bathroom.

In addition, point-of-use water-treatment equipment is also available in portable form. These small filters are often used by individuals who simply want to remove chlorine from a motel's water when they are traveling, for instance. Special models are also designed specifically for camping in primitive locations or for emergency situations. These particular water filters often come with additional purification methods such as iodine drops to help prevent waterborne illnesses.

The following sections offer suggestions for point-of-use water-treatment equipment you might consider purchasing. Of course, other fine products are available other than the ones listed here. Also, bear in mind that only a brief description is given for each model, so you should contact the individual companies or dealers for more information.

Kitchen Activated-Charcoal Filters

Activated-charcoal filtering units that sit on your kitchen countertop or mount under your kitchen sink are among the most popular point-of-use water filters. One countertop unit you might consider is the TerraTop (**Global Environmental Technologies**), which has a polypropylene housing and can hold either granular- or compressed-block activated-charcoal cartridges. In addition, a number of optional cartridges are available including a KDF/granular activated-charcoal mix. By the way, this same company has a similar below-counter model known as the Subterranean, which can combine up to three different filtering cartridges. Terra filters can be purchased directly from the company or through its dealers.

Another filter brand you might consider is the Seagull IV (**General Ecology, Inc.**), which actually comes in several stainless-steel models. These use a four-step filtration system that combines a special activated-charcoal block with other filtering strategies. As a result, it should be effective at removing chlorine as well as disease-causing bacteria and particulates. Specific units are designed for either countertop or below-counter installation. Seagull IV can be purchased directly from the company or from dealers such as **The Pure Water Place** and **Flowright International Products**.

Also, the EPS Drinking Water Filter (**Environmental Purification Systems**) is another all-stainless-steel unit. It's made to be mounted under the kitchen sink and comes with its own faucet for mounting next to your regular faucet. This particular filter holds over $1^1/_2$ lb. of granular activated charcoal and has a 60-micron stainless-steel postfilter. With this filter there are no replaceable cartridges—the canister is simply emptied and new media are added (it's suggested that the media be changed at least twice a year). EPS filters are available from the manufacturer or dealers such as **E.L. Foust Co., Inc.**

In addition, you may be interested to know that Multi-Pure Drinking Water Systems (**Multi-Pure Corporation**) offers several models with stainless-steel housings. These all use a three-stage compressed activated-charcoal block. Multi-Pure filters can be purchased directly from the company or from its dealers and distributors.

If you're seriously interested in buying a stainless-steel activated-charcoal filter, contact **The American Environmental Health Foundation, Inc., The**

Environmental Health Shopper, N.E.E.D.S., The Living Source, and **Nigra Enterprises**, etc. for information on the brands they're currently handling.

If you'd rather lease an activated-charcoal water filter for your kitchen, check out the under-the-sink unit by Puro (**Puro Corporation of America**) (Puro filters can't be purchased—only rented). This water filter is constructed of stainless steel and combines both granulated and solid-block activated-charcoal filters. As a result, it's able to remove most chlorine as well as sediment and many other waterborne contaminants. One special feature of the Puro filter is its yellow indicator light that lets you know when the filter module must be changed. Interestingly, the company not only installs the unit, but also routinely services it. You'll be charged an initial installation charge and a monthly leasing fee, but all the replacement filtering modules are free.

It should be pointed out that certain companies such as **Culligan International Co.** often have rent, rent-to-own, and direct-purchase activated-charcoal filters designed for installation in your kitchen. Contact the company for information on the specific programs currently offered. To find a Culligan dealer, check your classified telephone directory or contact the company's headquarters.

Kitchen Reverse-Osmosis Units

If you're interested in a kitchen-model reverse-osmosis (R/O) unit, one that produces very high-quality water is the Spacesaver SS-90 (**Aquathin**). This particular unit is designed to suspend beneath an overhead kitchen cabinet, thus, saving you room on your countertop or under your sink. However, if you'd prefer a countertop type, the company also makes the Kitchen KT-90, and for under-sink installations, the Platinum 90 model. All these units combine reverse-osmosis with a special deionization process. Aquathin R/O units can be purchased directly from the company or through its dealers.

Also, Nimbus offers a number of R/O models you may want to consider. The Nimbus units use two pretreatment filters and a stainless-steel *desalinator vessel*. These can be ordered from dealers such as **N.E.E.D.S.** In addition, you'll want to become familiar with the Multi-Pure Reverse-Osmosis Plus II Drinking Water System (**Multi-Pure Corporation**). This particular unit combines reverse-osmosis technology with solid-block activated-charcoal filtration. It may be purchased directly from the company or through its dealers.

Another below-counter reverse-osmosis system you may want to check into is the Everpure Reverse-Osmosis Drinking Water System. This unit combines reverse-osmosis treatment with additional filtration cartridges. Interestingly, a range of media choices is available for these extra cartridges to meet different water-quality needs. Everpure R/O units can be purchased from dealers such as **E.L. Foust Co., Inc.** Still another reverse-osmosis unit you might want to consider is the Aqua-Pure Model 5000 (**Cuno**). These can be ordered directly from the manufacturer or purchased from dealers such as **Nontoxic Environments.**

Also, Nature Spring is another countertop reverse-osmosis unit, designed with a very compact, rectangular 6" x 5" x 16" housing. This particular R/O model uses a sediment prefilter as well as a granular activated-charcoal postfilter. It can be purchased from dealers such as **Ozark Water Service and Environmental Services**, among others.

Another reverse-osmosis unit using ultraviolet light is sold by **The Environmental Health Shopper** (this mail-order firm also handles other reverse-osmosis models as well, including a small, compact countertop unit).

Finally, more reverse-osmosis units are available from **Befit Enterprises Ltd.**'s *The Cutting Edge Catalog*, **Nigra Enterprises**, and **Flowright International Products**, among others.

Kitchen Kinetic-Degradation-Fluxion Devices

One Kinetic-Degradation-Fluxion (KDF) device for kitchen use you may want to know about is the TerraTop (**Global Environmental Technologies**). This unit has a polypropylene housing that can hold a KDF/granular activated-charcoal filtering cartridge. In addition, there is a below-counter model known as the Subterranean.

A number of cartridges are available for these models besides those containing a KDF/granular activated-charcoal mix (for example, the Subterranean, uses up to three filtering cartridges sequentially, each can be filled with different media). By the way, the manufacturer recommends that its KDF/activated-charcoal cartridges be replaced annually. Interestingly, it offers a buy-back recycling program for them.

Still another KDF device from the same company is the TerraFlo CTS. This is a simple countertop model that combines a cartridge with its own self-contained dispenser. These units come with a three-year warranty, after which the entire unit should be replaced. Again the company offers a buy-back plan for these. All Terra filtering units can be purchased directly from the company or through its dealers.

Kitchen and Outdoor Water Distillers

Water distillers are generally placed in the kitchen, so they're considered here as point-of-use water-treatment units. One brand you might consider is the Waterwise (**Waterwise**). This company makes and sells two models. Other kitchen distillation units are sold by **Nigra Enterprises**, among others.

One water distiller of special note is the Rain Crystal (**Scientific Glass Co.**). This unique unit is constructed of Pyrex glass rather than stainless steel or plastic. The manufacturer rates the Rain Crystal at producing 5–8 gallons a day (the rate varies depending on your home's elevation above sea level). This particular water distiller can be ordered directly from the company.

An unusual water distiller that is operated outdoors is the Sunwater Solar Still (**McCracken Solar Co.**). This interesting distiller has the advantage of using free solar energy instead of your home's electricity. It's constructed, as you might guess, in the form of a tilted solar panel. Depending on the model, the climate, and the amount of sunlight, the manufacturer rates the Sunwater Solar Still at producing between $1^1/_3$–2 gallons of distilled water daily. You can buy this unit directly from the company.

Kitchen Sediment Filters

For removing a small amount of sediment from your drinking and cooking water, most activated-charcoal block filters and certainly all water distillers will work quite well. So will reverse-osmosis units, although you may have to replace the membrane more often.

Another approach is the Fullerguard (**Fuller Brush**). It's designed for use with chlorinated utility water and attaches to the kitchen sink's cold water line. This is an activated-charcoal unit that also contains four sediment filters. The Fullerguard has a plastic housing and is designed for a countertop installation. Using an optional converter kit, it can be located under your counter. You can purchase this unit from **Fuller Brush** dealers including **enviro-clean**.

It is not uncommon for a number of point-of-use activated-charcoal filters (especially under-the-sink models) as well as reverse-osmosis units to have built-in or optional sediment prefilters. Therefore, check with individual manufacturers (or dealers) to find out which specific units they offer. Also, check with **Sears, Roebuck and Co.** and **Ametek**.

Kitchen Ultraviolet-Light Purifiers

To kill bacteria and other microbial forms at the kitchen tap, you may want to purchase a point-of-use ultraviolet-light purifier. These are especially helpful if you have a reverse-osmosis (R/O) unit that didn't come equipped with one (some bacteria can destroy R/O membranes). Point-of-use ultraviolet purifier models are available from **Nigra Enterprises**, among others.

Showerhead Activated-Charcoal Filters

Because many people want to eliminate chlorine from the water they bathe with, activated-charcoal filters are now available that have been specifically designed for showerhead use. In fact, they are meant to completely replace your present showerhead. As a rule, most of these units have plastic housings with replaceable filter cartridges. With some models, these cartridges must be replaced fairly often because of their small size and, thus, limited adsorbing capacity. Of course, the actual replacement schedule will depend on the specific brand of filter, the concentration of chlorine in the water, and the volume of water used.

One activated-charcoal showerhead filter you might want to consider is the EPS Shower Filter (**Environmental Purification Systems**). This particular unit has two different filter-cartridge options to choose from. The standard type contains an activated-charcoal-impregnated felt pad. The optional High-Powered Granular Activated-Charcoal Filter Cartridge contains a full $5^1/_2$ oz. of activated-charcoal granules. EPS filters can by ordered from the manufacturer or from dealers such as **E.L. Foust Co., Inc.**

Other fine activated-charcoal showerhead filters are handled by **Nigra Enterprises, N.E.E.D.S., earthsake, Flowright International Products, The American Environmental Health Foundation, Inc.**, among others.

Showerhead Kinetic-Degradation-Fluxion Units

A showerhead Kinetic-Degradation-Fluxion (KDF) device you may be interested in owning is the Hydrolife, offered by **Befit Enterprises Ltd.** in its *Cutting Edge Catalog*. This unit uses a spinning action that helps expose as much water as possible to the KDF media. This particular showerhead filter is said to remove chlorine, heavy metals such as lead, and a variety of other water contaminants.

The TerraSpa (**Global Environmental Technologies**) is another showerhead unit that uses KDF media. It can be ordered directly from the company and from its dealers. The ShowerCleenOne combines three filtration methods including granulated activated charcoal and KDF. This unit can be ordered through dealers such as **Ozark Water Service and Environmental Services.**

Interestingly, a portable travel shower filter using KDF with a spinning action is available from Hydropure. This unit is designed to be especially easy to install and remove. It is sold by **The Environmental Health Shopper.**

Point-of-Use Water Softening and Water Conditioning

Commonly, the laundry is where many households need a method to counter the effects of hard water such as crusty white lime scale, insoluble soap scum, and poor sudsing. To minimize these problems, certain water-softening agents such as borax can simply be added to the wash water directly.

However, another approach would be to use a physical-magnetic water conditioning device. Of course, these could be used in other locations besides the utility room. For example, they could be used to treat the water that's used in an automatic ice maker or in a hot tub.

If you'd like to try magnetic conditioning, one option is the SoPhTec Physical Water Conditioner (**SoPhTec International**). These small devices (some models are only 6" x 6" x 4" in size) come in either in-line or clamp-on models (the Model C-250 is one of the clamp-on types). SoPhTec water conditioners are sold through dealers including **AAA Environmental Products**. They have a 90-day guarantee whereby the full purchase price will be refunded.

In addition, Magnetic Water Conditioners are handled by **The Living Source**. A residential model, an ice maker/dishwasher model, and a swimming pool/spa/hot tub model are offered.

Portable Travel Activated-Charcoal Water Filters

A handy solid-block activated-charcoal filtering unit for travelers is the Trav-L-Pure (**General Ecology Technologies**). This device is completely self-contained. All you need to do is fill it with water. Then simply use a manual pumping action to cause the filtered water to flow out the spout. By the way, this unit comes with its own traveling pouch. The Trav-L-Pure is sold directly by the company and from dealers including **The Pure Water Place, Inc.**

Another portable activated-charcoal filtration option is the Mariner travel filter. This model is only six inches high and also comes with its own travel pouch. The Mariner is handled by **The Environmental Health Shopper.**

Portable Travel Kinetic-Degradation-Fluxion Devices

If you're in the market for a portable Kinetic-Degradation-Fluxion (KDF) device, one you may want to check out is the Global Life unit. This filter uses KDF media in wire form. Also included are purification tablets for water of questionable microbial contamination. While the Global Life was designed for primitive camping situations, it can actually be used anywhere. Note that, the KDF media will remove heavy metals, chlorine, among other contaminants. If the purification tablets are used, harmful microbial life will also be killed. The Global Life unit is sold by **Befit Enterprises, Ltd.'s** *Cutting Edge Catalog*, among others.

In addition, you may want to consider the First Need unit (**General Ecology Technologies**). This model not only uses KDF media, but is also equipped with a replaceable purification chamber containing a micro-fine filtering material that is able to strain out many biological contaminants. The First Need was created for use in primitive camping conditions and for emergency situations. With manual pumping action, you can produce a great deal of potable water. The First Need is available directly from the manufacturer and dealers such as **The Pure Water Place, Inc.**

Still another portable unit you might consider is the TerraFlo WaterWand (**Global Environmental Technologies**). This is actually a small (2.5 oz.), personal-sized water-treatment device using KDF media in wire form. Interestingly, the handle has storage space for iodine purification tablets. As you might suspect, the WaterWand was especially created for camping, hiking, etc. You can order it directly from the company or from dealers.

(For portable KDF showerhead units, see *Showerhead Kinetic-Degradation-Fluxion Devices* above.)

BOTTLED WATER

Sometimes people feel that the water in their home just isn't of high-enough quality to drink and use in cooking. In some cases, this is because their private well has become contaminated in some way. In other households, it's because the occupants don't like the thought of ingesting the chlorine or fluoride in their utility-supplied water, but can't afford to purchase or maintain water-treatment equipment. For whatever reason, more and more Americans are choosing to buy bottled water. Therefore, the following sections offer some basic information on bottled water as well as explanations of the various types of bottled water you might want to consider.

BOTTLED WATER BASICS

In the U.S., the Federal Food and Drug Administration (FDA) has declared bottled drinking water to be a *food* item. This puts many types of bottle water—but not all—under FDA jurisdiction. This is because the legal definition of *bottled drinking water* doesn't cover all types of water that are actually bottled in the U.S. For example, *mineral water* and *soda water,*including both *seltzer water* and *club soda water* aren't included in this limited classification. In addition, any bottled water that's produced and sold entirely within the borders of a single state is also exempt from federal regulations (certain states may have their own regulations regarding bottled water). Unfortunately, bottled water that does come under the authority of the FDA only has to meet a minimum water quality standard.

Interestingly, water for processed bottled drinking water can come from a variety of sources including private wells, naturally rising springs, and even utility-supplied water. Therefore, if you're interested in using bottled water in your home, it's best to carefully read the label on the brand you're considering. That way, you should be able to determine the original source of the water, and, at the same time, find out if any additional treatments were performed on the water at the water-bottling plant. If this information is not provided on the label, contact the bottler and ask them to send you any information on their water. As you probably already know, bottled drinking water comes in two forms, *effervescent* or *still*. Effervescent water simply contains bubbles of carbon dioxide gas.

Note that, if you're a sensitive person, you'll especially want to purchase your bottled drinking water in glass bottles rather than in plastic containers. This enables you to avoid drinking water that contains small amounts of plastic compounds that migrated into the water from the container. In any case, you'll probably want to test several types and brands of bottled water to find the one whose taste you prefer and tolerate the best.

Although you can easily purchase your bottled water directly through your local health-food stores, etc., you should also know that there are companies that will deliver large bottles to your home on a regular basis. Often, this delivered water comes in 5-gallon containers that are placed on special dispensers in your kitchen. To find a company that delivers bottled drinking water in your area, check your classified telephone directory.

BOTTLED WATER TYPES

Although, for the most part, no regulations specifically define the different types of bottled water, the following sections list some of the definitions that are popularly used.

DISTILLED WATER

Distilled water is water that has undergone distillation. This process results in water becoming devoid of minerals and most other types of impurities. This type of water is sometimes described as *aggressive*—meaning that it will aggressively seek out substances to put them into solution. As a result, there is some concern that distilled water does not make for very good drinking water. However, it is often recommended for use in steam irons and humidifiers (see also *Ironing* in *Chapter 7: Cleaning* and *Humidifier Types* in *Chapter 9: Indoor Air*).

DRINKING WATER

Drinking water is simply processed (filtered) bottled water. Therefore, it might simply be utility water that's processed before it's put into sealed bottles. Note that, most bottled drinking water contains very low levels of chlorine.

EFFERVESCENT WATER

Effervescent water is water that contains bubbly carbon dioxide (CO_2) gas. Sometime the CO_2 is naturally occurring and sometimes it is added by a bottling company.

MINERAL WATER

Mineral water is water containing a certain quantity of dissolved minerals. Surprisingly, it can even be utility water that has had "desirable" minerals added to it by the bottler. On the other hand, *natural mineral water* is water from underground sources that naturally contains dissolved minerals (such as calcium, iron, potassium, and sodium) that were leached from the surrounding rock. Note, some natural spring water is effervescent, or sparkling.

SPRING WATER

Spring water is water that reaches the surface from underground sources by its own pressure. *Natural spring water* is unprocessed spring water.

SELTZER WATER

Seltzer water is filtered tap water that has been impregnated with carbon dioxide (CO_2) gas. *Club soda* is the same type of water, but has had minerals added to it by the bottler.

SPARKLING WATER

Sparkling water is water impregnated with carbon dioxide (CO_2) gas. *Natural sparkling water* is water that naturally contains CO_2. Note, some bottlers remove the naturally occurring CO_2 and later reinject it before the water leaves the plant.

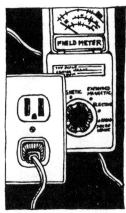

CHAPTER 11
ELECTROMAGNETIC FIELDS

Electromagnetic fields (EMFs) are now considered potential health threats, particularly if your exposure is at high levels for a long period of time. Yet, many Americans are still uncertain how and to what extent these invisible phenomena could be affecting them. In fact, many people don't really know exactly what EMFs are. Thus, this chapter provides some basic information on EMFs and suggests ways you can reduce your exposure to them in your own home.

WHAT ARE EMFS?

To understand electromagnetic fields (EMFs), a good place to start is to understand *electromagnetic radiation* in general.

ELECTROMAGNETIC RADIATION IN GENERAL

Electromagnetic radiation is simply energy that has both an electric and a magnetic aspect. Visible light, infrared radiation, and X-rays are just a few examples of electromagnetic radiation. But beside these, electric current passing through high-voltage power lines, home wiring, and electrical appliances also give off a form of electromagnetic radiation.

Interestingly, all types of electromagnetic radiation travel at the same speed—the speed of light. What actually makes one form of electromagnetic radiation different from another is the length and shape of its wave. Because it has differing *wave lengths*, each type of electromagnetic radiation has its own *wave frequency*.

What is meant by wave frequency? Wave frequency is a term that denotes the number of waves that are able to pass by a given point in a certain period of time. As it turns out, the more waves that are able to pass by, the higher the frequency is said to be. Because of their size, a greater number of shorter waves are able to pass by a point while traveling at the same speed than longer waves. Therefore, the shorter the electromagnetic-radiation wave is, the higher its frequency.

Why is wave frequency an important consideration? Because the higher the frequency, the more potentially dangerous the electromagnetic radiation— the shorter the wave, the more energetic it is. In fact, short, high-frequency waves are so energetic they can actually strip away electrons from some of the stable molecules with which they come in contact. This results in the formation of unstable reactive ions. To gain stability, these newly created ions seize electrons from neighboring molecules in a process known as *free-radical chain reactions* (a free radical is an extremely reactive ion). Therefore, high-frequency radiation is also known as *ionizing radiation.* X-rays and gamma rays (from nuclear reactors, for example) are two types of ionizing radiation.

Unfortunately, if humans are exposed to ionizing radiation (such as X-rays or gamma rays), the resulting free-radical chain reactions take place within their bodies. The snatched electrons come from the molecules actually making up their body tissue. Naturally, this could easily (and quickly) lead to tissue damage, inflammation, and other negative consequences. In some cases, cancer may eventually develop, especially if the length and intensity of exposure is great enough.

Visible light, infrared radiation, radio and television waves (FM, AM, short wave, etc.), and microwave radiation are all different forms of electromagnetic radiation, but they have longer wavelengths and lower frequencies than X-rays and gamma rays. They aren't capable of stripping electrons from molecules, so they aren't ionizing forms of radiation, and, thus aren't considered as dangerous.

ELECTRIC CURRENT AND ELECTROMAGNETIC RADIATION

The principles that pertain to other types of electromagnetic radiation also pertain to flowing electricity. Therefore, the current running in all electric lines travels at the speed of light and it has its own unique frequency—in North America the frequency is 60 cycles per second while Europeans use 50 cycle per second electric current. Fortunately, scientists categorize this frequency as *extremely low frequency (ELF)*. As such, it is classified as *non-ionizing* and as a result, since it can't strip electrons, it has been assumed to be relatively harmless.

However, it turns out that there is more to be concerned about than merely the frequency. Of particular concern are the areas containing *electromagnetic fields (EMFs)* that exist around all wires carrying electricity and all operating electrical devices. These EMFs are actually measurable. Because flowing electricity has both electrical and magnetic aspects, in reality there are two fields: an electrical field and a magnetic field. These fields occur simultaneously and they somewhat overlap each other in space (interestingly, the electrical field surrounds and *oscillates,* or vibrates, 90° to the flow of the electric current, while the magnetic field uniformly surrounds the wire without oscillating). Note that, the more powerful the electric current is, the more powerful the EMFs. Also, EMFs are stronger close to their source than they are further away.

Although the presence of both the electrical and magnetic fields surrounding flowing electricity in home wires and appliances has been well known by electrical engineers, it was felt that these were of no real concern. Unfortunately, relatively recent research seems to suggest that there may actually be real health consequences to being exposed to them, despite the fact that they're produced by nonionizing ELF electricity. This seems to be especially true if your exposure is of long enough duration and the field strengths are strong enough.

Magnetic fields seem to be of special concern. In fact, because it's now felt that magnetic fields pose more potential health risk than electric fields, the term EMF is often popularly used to indicate only magnetic fields. Therefore, in the rest of this chapter, the term EMF will refer to magnetic fields in oder to simplify the discussion.

POTENTIAL HEALTH EFFECTS OF EMFS

Unfortunately, EMF exposure from ELF electricity has been linked to several health conditions. Some of these are minor, while others are much more severe. The following sections will introduce you to some of what's been learned and reported so far on this topic.

POSSIBLE EMF EXPOSURE SYMPTOMS

A variety of symptoms have been linked to EMF exposure. They range from loss of coordination to cancer. Generally, these effects have been associated with long-term exposure to high-voltage electric transmission lines and power stations—sites of very powerful EMF generation. For example, electrical linemen, cable splicers, and others who work around electricity regularly have been shown to have higher rates of diseases such as leukemia, brain cancer, and breast cancer.

However, there are cases where the EMF strength and duration of exposure have been far less and yet certain people still appear to have been harmed. For example, there has been an increased rate of miscarriages reported in women who sleep under electric blankets (especially electric blankets manufactured before 1987) or on electrically heated waterbeds. Unfortunately, some researchers suspect that exposure to EMFs in homes could be causing other problems. For example, in Sweden it's been shown that children who are routinely exposed to EMFs at home have increased rates of leukemia, if the EMFs are strong enough.

Interestingly, a portion of the population appears to be particularly sensitive to the presence of EMFs. Such people are often termed *electromagnetically sensitive*. If these people are in an area where strong EMFs are present, they may respond with any number of symptoms including loss of balance, uneasiness, hearing unusual noises, or mental confusion, among many others. Some of these individuals lose muscle control and actually collapse. Electromagnetic sensitivity appears to be less common than chemical sensitivity, although some individuals have both conditions.

EMF SYMPTOMS, THEORIES, AND RESEARCH

Surprisingly, it's still not known how ELF electricity used in homes could cause ill health. After all, this kind of electricity is *nonionizing*. Therefore, it's supposedly incapable of causing *free-radical chain reactions* that are linked to tissue damage. So, what could explain exactly what happens to certain people when they're exposed to excessive EMFs? Research is underway to find definite answers to these questions. Already, several possible theories have been proposed. However, so far none of these hypotheses seem to adequately explain all the various symptoms that have been associated with EMF exposure.

EMF SYMPTOM THEORIES

One explanation of how EMFs cause negative health symptoms is that they could be disrupting the signals that normally cross cell membranes. It's believed that this "short circuiting" could actually change the normal action of hormones and antibodies—and perhaps even activate certain cancer-inciting molecules.

Another theory is that magnetic fields hinder the deactivation of *free radicals* within the body. Normally, there are mechanisms in the body to squelch free-radical chain reactions to prevent them from continuing long enough to cause severe tissue damage. However, if the body's free-radical defense system is prevented from functioning correctly, free radicals will remain reactive and destructive for longer periods of time. As a result, greater tissue damage would inevitably take place.

A third theory as to how EMFs adversely affect human beings is that they restrict the normal *melatonin* production in the body. This is important because melatonin (a hormone that is secreted by the *pineal gland* in the brain) regulates our body's *biorhythms* (regular cycles of bodily function) and melatonin has anti-malignancy properties. When lesser amounts than normal are present within the body, cancer (among other conditions) can be more likely to develop.

EMF RESEARCH

Because so little hard data is available concerning EMFs (particularly their effects on humans), research is now underway all around the world. In addition, a large American project is currently being undertaken by the **Electric Power Research Institute (EPRI)** (a national association whose membership is made up of electric-power utilities). The EPRI studies are designed to understand the effects, scope, and possible solutions to EMF exposure. If you're interested in learning their findings, contact your power company and ask for copies of recently released EPRI research. For a book that discusses research findings specifically related to EMFs and the human body, read *Cross Currents* by Robert O. Becker.

EMF SOURCES AND REMEDIAL MEASURES

The following sections discuss where high levels of EMFs can be found in homes and what to do to minimize your risk.

WHAT IS CONSIDERED A HIGH EMF IN YOUR HOME?

At this time, most researchers feel that a magnetic-field strength of less than 3 milliGauss (mG) is a reasonably safe level for most people (a Gauss is a unit of magnetic-field measurement; a milliGauss is $1/1000$th of a Gauss). However, there is a very vocal minority who point to research indicating that the safe level is less than 1 mG.

Fortunately, data so far has shown that the average room in an American home has an EMF background intensity about 0.5 mG. However the typical kitchen has an average that's a little higher at 0.7 mG. These averages are below the levels considered unsafe by either faction. However, these are only *average* background intensities. There are areas in virtually all houses where more intense EMFs can be found, such as around certain operating electrical devices and appliances. These are often called *electromagnetic hot spots.*

A major reason for these "hot spots" is because certain wiring configurations actually increase EMF strengths. For example *transformers* and electric motors utilize coiled wires that can have strong EMFs. Both transformers and electric motors are used in a variety of household electrical devices. Also, certain looped wire patterns such as those used in pre-1987 electric blankets and in the floors or ceilings of homes using radiant electric heat will record high EMF levels as well.

By the way, it should be mentioned that some individuals are worried that metal building materials such as aluminum siding or steel framing can create EMFs in their homes. In reality this doesn't appear to be a significant problem. In general, EMFs in houses originate principally from particular wiring configurations and the operation of electrical appliances—not from metal building materials.

COMMON SOURCES OF HIGH EMF LEVELS IN HOMES

All homes that use electric power have electromagnetic fields (EMFs) in them. Fortunately, a great many of these EMFs tend to be of relatively low strength. However, there are also certain situations, and particular areas, in most homes where more intense EMFs usually exist. These are sometimes temporary, such as the strong EMFs generated by using an electric hair dryer, or they can be ongoing, such as the strong EMFs that constantly surround an electric power panel. The following sections discuss some of the more common sources of strong EMFs.

ELECTRIC APPLIANCES AND HEATING SYSTEMS

As has been noted previously, all electrical appliances produce EMFs when they are operating and some of these fields can be of relatively high strength. In fact, research sponsored by the **Electric Power Research Institute (EPRI)** has revealed that the average refrigerator measured at $10^1/2$" away had an EMF level of 2.6 mG. Interestingly, the worst refrigerator (at least in terms of EMFs) had an amazingly high magnetic field strength of 15.7 mG, while the best refrigerator registered a mere 0.1 mG. Of course, in all the other categories of electric appliances measured, there were also a wide range of readings—some much higher than the average EMF level, others somewhat below it. (Actually, these EPRI "averages" were actually *medians* or statistical middle figures.)

As it turns out, EPRI research found that the average electric range had a magnetic field strength of 9 mG at $10^1/2$". The average fluorescent light fixture had a reading of 5.9 mG at this same distance, and the average *analog* (nonelectronic) clock registered 0.8 mG. An average TV measured 7 mG at $10^1/2$". The average microwave oven at $10^1/2$" came in with a whopping EMF strength of 36.9 mG (Note: this is a measurement of magnetic field strength, not microwave radiation). This same research revealed that dimmer switches, electric blankets (especially blankets manufactured before the late 1980s), and electric appliances containing motors generally recorded relatively high EMF readings as well.

One of EPRI's higher EMF measurements was for operating electric radiant heating systems installed either in ceilings or in floors. At $10^1/2$", the average such system had a field strength of 26.6 mG. Furthermore, electric baseboard heaters usually had high EMF readings.

HOUSE WIRING PRACTICES

Besides electrical appliances and heaters, there can be high-strength EMFs generated in homes from certain electrical wiring practices. Many of these practices are common, even though they are in violation of electrical codes. Wiring practices responsible for high-strength EMFs are discussed in the sections below.

Knob and Tube Wiring

Today, most modern electrical home wiring is done with a *single cable* made up of an insulated black wire (the hot wire), an insulated white wire (the neutral wire), and an uninsulated ground wire. Fortunately, as long as the hot and the neutral wires remain close together, they tend to cancel out each other's magnetic fields. If the hot and neutral wires are twisted around each other, they will cancel each other's magnetic fields even more (the ground wire doesn't normally carry any current, so theoretically, it shouldn't produce any fields).

However, years ago home wiring was done much differently. Instead of having the hot and neutral wires bundled together in a single cable, separate individual wires were run from the main electrical panel to the various circuits. These wires were installed about a foot apart from each other and were either supported on ceramic insulators called *knobs* or run through ceramic insulators called *tubes*. Unfortunately, because of the distance between the wires, this type of wiring produced relatively high EMF levels. By the way, the wider the hot and neutral wires are separated, the less the magnetic fields cancel each other out. This is one of the reasons why high field strengths are routinely measured near outdoor power lines that have their individual wires so widely separated from each other.

Cables Carrying High Levels of Electric Current

Of course, the more electric current a wire carries, the stronger the magnetic field that is created around that wire. As a result, the main power cable running between a home's electric meter and the power panel generates a higher EMF level than the smaller wires running from the power panel to typical room receptacles. The wires that run to the electric range or to any electric baseboard heaters will produce EMF strengths somewhere in between those of the main power cable and the smaller wires. As you might suspect, this is because these wires carry less current than the main cable but more than the smaller wires.

Grounding Problems

Perhaps one of the more unsuspected sources of EMFs in homes is from certain *grounding* practices. In grounding, a connection is made between an electric circuit (or electrical device) and the ground itself (the earth) that is capable of conducting electric current. Grounding is very necessary for safety reasons; in fact, all building codes require that it be done. If done correctly, grounding generally doesn't cause any problems.

In actual practice, at the point where the main electric power cable enters a home, the main ground wire is connected to a metal rod that has been driven 8–10' into the soil. However, as an alternative, it might be connected to a metal water pipe. Cable TV lines and telephone lines are routinely grounded in similar ways. Unfortunately, in some cases of water-pipe grounding, the home's entire plumbing system can end up becoming its own complete electrical circuit, a circuit capable of producing EMFs.

To make matters worse, these unplanned metal water-pipe electrical circuits can sometimes connect several homes together. This can occur if two or more houses are hooked to the same electric utility transformer and are connected by metal water mains. It can also happen with homes connected to the same TV cable. These unintentional multi-home interconnections can actually cause the transfer of EMFs from one house to another.

Note that, good electrical wiring practice (as required by the National Electrical Code), states that the ground wires and the neutral wires should be connected together near the main power-panel disconnect switch, and only there. This shouldn't result in the generation of strong EMFs within the house *unless the ground and neutral wires are connected somewhere besides the main power-panel.*

Unfortunately, the neutral wire is often accidentally connected to a ground wire at a receptacle box or at a *subpanel* (a secondary electrical panel located after the main panel). If this is done, some of the electricity that is supposed to travel in the neutral wire travels through the ground wire (or the metal water pipes) instead (some of the electric current travels through the neutral wire and some of it flows through the water pipes). If electricity is traveling through water pipes, the pipes are acting as wires, and there will be EMFs surrounding them. Because the water pipes and the electric wires generally aren't installed close together, the EMFs are as strong as if there were widely separated hot and neutral wires.

Note: Sometimes neutral wires from different electrical circuits are connected together at inappropriate locations, such as at a subpanel. This can also result in strong EMFs. This occurs because the electricity that was supposed to travel only through a single neutral wire is split between two neutral wires. These wires are generally widely separated for most of their length, so strong EMFs are generated.

Power Panels

The bundled wires in the single cables are usually separated inside the main power panel of a house. What is actually done is that the hot wires are run to the individual circuit breakers (or fuses) and all the neutral wires are connected together at a common terminal connection point called a *busbar*. At the same time, the ground wires are also connected together at another, separate busbar.

Because so many hot and neutral wires are separated and also because there are so many wires in one place, the magnetic-field readings are often high at electrical panels.

POWER LINE PROBLEMS

Sometimes strong EMF levels in houses are not actually generated by electrical circuits (either planned or unplanned) within these homes. As it turns out, houses that are within 500–1,000' of high-voltage power lines or that are close to electric-power substations often have higher-than-average EMF background readings. These high ambient EMF levels occur because power lines carry a great deal of current and their wires are widely separated from each other. On the other hand, electrical substations contain transformers that are made up of many wires wound together.

LOWERING EMF RISKS IN HOMES

In almost all cases, it's virtually impossible to avoid strong electromagnetic fields (EMFs) completely in your home. However, there are a number of simple precautions you can take to reduce your risk of exposure. The following sections will discuss how you can minimize your risk by either reducing the strength of the field (this is sometimes difficult to do), or by spending less time near strong EMF sources (this is often relatively easy to do). Of course, those people who are electromagnetically sensitive will have to take more extreme measures.

TESTING EMF LEVELS IN HOMES

Because of different wiring configurations, appliances, locales, and grounding methods, every home's EMF situation is unique. Therefore, to determine what EMF problems actually exist in your house, if any, you should do some EMF testing. Fortunately, this is fairly easy to do. All you need is a meter that can measure magnetic fields (a Gauss meter).

If you like to use mail order, **Befit Enterprises, Ltd.**'s *Cutting Edge Catalog* sells EMF-testing equipment as does **The Environmental Health Shopper**. In addition, **N.E.E.D.S.** offers TriField meters for purchase or rent. And **Baubiologie Hardware** has testers to buy or rent. However, before going ahead and purchasing, or even renting, a meter, first decide how accurate a reading you want. As it turns out, some testing equipment only has small indicator lights to indicate a safe or unsafe EMF level. Obviously, this information may be too vague for many individuals.

However, several kinds of more accurate Gauss meters are available. The different models of these meters have varying degrees of accuracy. The most precise Gauss meters tend to be quite expensive. For residential use, meters that are within 25% of being accurate are popular and reasonably priced. While most electrical engineers wouldn't consider ±25% very accurate, these meters are usually quite acceptable for homeowners who want to determine the EMF risks in their homes.

If you are concerned about EMFs generated by nearby high-voltage electric power lines, transformers, and substations, contact your local electric utility for assistance. Generally, they will come to your home and measure the EMF level resulting from their equipment.

UNDERSTANDING EMF STRENGTH, DISTANCE, AND DURATION

It's unlikely that most people could or would rid their homes of all the electrical appliances and devices in them that happen to emit high levels of EMFs. However, you should keep in mind that just because high EMF readings exist in your house, doesn't mean they're cause for alarm. Negative health problems resulting from EMF exposure depend on three factors: 1) the strength of the field, 2) the length of exposure, and 3) your particular susceptibility. You should also keep in mind that certain parts of your body are likely to be more sensitive to the potential negative effects of EMFs than others. Having your head or reproductive organs subjected to strong EMFs is probably more serious than exposing your feet.

Importantly, the strength of a problematic EMF can often become acceptable by simply adding distance between you and the EMF source. For example, a magnetic field might be very high only 1–2" away from where it originates. But at 3' away, it could easily be at a level generally considered safe. For example, an electrical baseboard heater installed near your headboard might have an EMF reading of 20 mG directly next to the device. But the EMF reading might be only 1 mG near your pillow, just a few feet away. Therefore, if you routinely slept in this particular bed, you would be exposed to reasonably safe EMF levels. However, if you were to sleep on the floor with your head just a few inches away from the heater, the EMF reading now near your pillow might be 5–10 mG—not a very safe level. As it turns out, most of the high EMF fields from electrical appliances in homes decrease so quickly with distance that much lower and safer fields exist only 2–3' away from nearly all of them.

Of course, the actual duration of EMF exposure is also very significant in determining your risk. This simply means the length of time you're actually exposed to high-strength EMFs. Obviously, a few seconds or a few minutes of strong EMF exposure is not nearly as serious as hours, days, or years of exposure at high levels. Therefore, although a portable electric shaver or hair blow dryer might generate very strong EMFs (perhaps over 100 mG) and your head is very close to them while they are operating, you only use them for a few minutes at a time. Because the duration is quite short, many researchers currently believe that the EMF dangers posed by shavers and blow dryers used in this way is probably not very great. Of course, if you had a hair salon set up in your home and you spent many hours every day using a blow dryer as a professional hair stylist, your EMF risks from the blow dryer would be considerably greater.

SPECIFIC EMF REDUCTION STRATEGIES

There are several specific strategies you can do to minimize your risk from certain electromagnetic fields (EMFs) in your home. These are detailed in the sections below.

Coping with EMFs from Appliances and Heating Systems

As has been noted, increasing the distance from their generating source lowers your exposure to EMFs. If your television or microwave oven are problems, for example, you could simply increase the distance between you and them while they're operating. Of course, you might choose to replace some of your older electrical appliances with newer, safer models. As it turns out, in the last few years many companies have begun designing their electrical products so that they generate much less intense EMFs than they did previously. This is particularly true with computer monitors, television sets, and electric blankets.

However, as an alternative to buying a new replacement device, in some cases you might consider buying EMF reduction equipment. For instance, **Safe Technologies, Ozark Water Service and Environmental Services**, and **Nontoxic Environments** all offer EMF-blocking screens for use on various home computers (see also *Electronic Equipment EMF Concerns* in *Chapter 6: Lifestyle*). **The Environmental Health Shopper, Befit Enterprises, Ltd.**'s *Cutting Edge Catalog*, and **Baubiologie Hardware** also handle a good variety of EMF-reduction products.

In some cases, instead of replacing certain electrical appliances and devices with new versions, or modifying them in some way to reduce your EMF exposure, you might simply decide to buy nonelectric substitutes. Of course, these would create no EMFs at all. For instance, you could purchase a windup alarm clock to use in place of your bedroom's electronic clock radio. You could also buy a wire whisk to use instead of a portable electric hand mixer. And so on.

Sadly, if your home has loop-style radiant electric heating cables in its ceilings or floors that happen to emit strong EMFs, this may be a situation that doesn't have a simple, inexpensive solution. If you're truly concerned about these fields, you may have no choice but to shut your radiant heat off and install some other type of heating equipment.

If your waterbed's heater gives off high levels of EMFs, you might try turning it off whenever you're in bed. Then you could turn it back on during the day when you're not in bed. This will usually keep the waterbed at a comfortable temperature, yet significantly reduce your EMF exposure risks.

Incidentally, if you feel that you're electromagnetically sensitive, you might want to shut off all the electric power to your bedroom at night. This can often be done by just switching the appropriate circuit breaker off in your electric power panel (be sure your smoke detector, refrigerator, or freezer aren't on the same circuit or they will be off all night as well!). **Baubiologie Hardware** offers a Demand Switch that is especially designed to shut off all the power to a bedroom at night. Of course, if you're electrically sensitive you'll also want to limit the number and use of all types of electric appliances and devices throughout your home.

Wiring and Grounding Precautions

If you are planning to construct a brand new house, there are a number of relatively easy precautions that can be taken to minimize your exposure to EMFs as far as wiring and grounding are concerned. One of these is to request that twisted electric cable be used. However, it should be pointed out that all modern single-cable wiring has the hot and neutral wires so close together that the twisted cable probably won't make a significant difference in EMF levels.

Another thing you can do to make a real difference in reducing your exposure to high field strengths is to specify that you want the electric wires that will carry high amounts of current installed in such a way that they won't be located in parts of your house where you plan to spend a great deal of time. Such wires would include the main electric cable that runs from the electric meter to your power panel and the wires that run from the power panel to your electric range and electric heaters. For example, these particular wires should be routed in such a way that they won't pass near your bed or favorite reading chair.

If your existing home has its electrical system grounded to your metal water pipes, you'll want to discuss the situation with a licensed electrician (to find one, check your classified telephone book). In some cases, he (or she) may be able to install a section of plastic pipe in such a way that it will stop the unwanted electrical circuit in your plumbing lines from being connected to the plumbing lines in your neighbor's house. In other situations, other remedial measures may have to be taken. However, under no circumstances should you unhook a ground wire because of EMF fears—proper grounding is extremely important and is required by building codes. For more information about EMFs and grounding systems, including some good solutions, you might read, "EMFs Run Aground" in the August 21, 1993 issue of *Science News* (Vol. 144, pp. 124–7).

Unfortunately, sometimes in existing homes, obvious causes for mysterious high EMF levels can't be found. In most cases, such EMFs are likely generated from incorrect connections of neutral wires or unusual grounding situations somewhere in these houses. Sadly, many home inspectors and even licensed electricians simply aren't trained to locate EMF problems, especially unusual ones. However, if you find a home inspector or electrician who is willing to help you, the book, *Tracing EMFs in Building Wiring and Grounding* by Karl Riley contains very good, solid information that he (or she) might use (remember, never to tamper with your electrical system yourself without proper training).

Power Panel Precautions

As has already been noted, all main electrical power panels (both fuse boxes and circuit-breaker boxes) generally produce very strong electromagnetic fields (EMFs), and they do so whenever electricity is flowing through the wires. As a result, it's been suggested by certain experts that you should never locate your home's power panel near where you and/or your family spend a great deal of time. For example, a basement utility room would be a preferred site for your power panel rather than in your family room. Of course, safer siting is much easier to achieve in new homes where you can plan the actual placement of your power panel ahead of time, than in existing homes where it's already in place.

It's important to remember that even if the power panel is in an unused room, you'll still need to consider its potential EMF effects. This is because the magnetic fields can easily extend through the wall on which a panel is mounted (magnetic fields are usually not deterred by a typical home's walls). Therefore, if your power panel is located on an interior wall that is shared by an adjacent bedroom, make certain that the beds in that room are as far away from the electrical panel as possible.

Coping with Site Problems

If you suspect that your building site has a high background EMF level, you'll want to test it *before* any construction begins. If you actually find high-strength fields, it may be possible to avoid them by relocating the house on the lot. Remember, you should build at a safe distance (500' to 1,000') from high voltage power lines or substations. You should also be concerned about ground-level or pole-mounted transformers because they can emit high-strength fields. If you can't find a suitable safe building location, you should seriously consider purchasing another building site.

If you have an existing home with EMF problems due to a nearby electrical substation or high-voltage power line, you'll need to try other strategies. One approach is to use your rooms differently than you have been. For example, you might make your den into a dining room and your dining room into the den, or simply rearrange your rooms' furniture. The goal is to create living areas where you'll spend most of your time that will have only very low field strengths. Unfortunately, if it turns out that every room within your house has high background EMFs due to nearby power lines or an electrical substation, there may not be much you can do to reduce your risk—that is, except to move somewhere else.

FURTHER EMF INFORMATION

To learn more about electromagnetic fields (EMFs), you might read *Warning: The Electricity Around You May Be Hazardous To Your Health* by Ellen Sugarman. Also check out *EMFs in Your Environment: Magnetic Field Measurements of Everyday Electrical Devices* (402-R-92-008) and *Q & A About Electric and Magnetic Fields Associated with the Use of Electric Power,* both from the **Environmental Protection Agency (EPA)**. By the way, the **EPA** now has an EMF Infoline you can call for publications and EMF questions. The telephone number is (800) 363-2383.

Of course, other books and periodical articles on EMFs are available at most local libraries and bookstores. You'll also want to check with your local electric utility for the latest **Electric Power Research Institute (EPRI)** EMF research findings.

GEOMAGNETIC FIELDS

Besides the electromagnetic fields (EMFs) associated with the electric current running in wires, a number of people are concerned with the effects of *geomagnetic fields (GMFs)* within their homes. What are GMFs? GMFs are actually the measurable magnetic fields of the earth itself. According to one theory, they're primarily generated within our planet by an ever-moving layer in the molten core (the *Dynamo Theory*). This particular hypothesis contends that this liquid-rock layer flows in a pattern that results in (*induces*) electric current. The electric current in turn creates the magnetic field.

Fortunately, at this time, most researchers feel that GMFs aren't nearly as significant a cause for concern as exposure to high-strength EMFs. However, there are certain people who adamantly believe that localized *GMF hot spots*—such as from geologic faults, large deposits of igneous rock, and underground streams—have the potential to greatly affect human health. Such

390

individuals note that deformed or stunted trees can often be found on GMF hot spots as proof of their negative effects. Interestingly, some *dowsers* (individuals who claim to find underground water using divining rods or other unconventional devices) are reportedly able to locate not only water, but also problematic GMF sources.

While the health effects of GMFs are probably much smaller than those from EMFs, this is still a very controversial subject. Unfortunately, as of yet, there is almost no in-depth reliable research available concerning GMFs and human health.

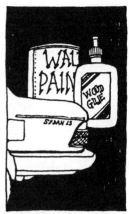

CHAPTER 12
HOME WORKSHOP AND GARAGE

This chapter covers two home environments not often considered problem areas as far as health is concerned: the home workshop and the garage. These two sites often contain dangerous materials and airborne contaminants.

THE HOME WORKSHOP

Many people have designated some area they use as a home workshop. Ideally, a home workshop would be in its own separate structure. Another good choice would be a portion of an insulated, detached garage where the temperature and perhaps the humidity are regulated. However, the reality is that most home workshops are located in basements, utility rooms, and attached garages. In these locations, home workshops can pose potential dangers to the rest of the house and those who occupy it.

As everyone knows, a number of the products and materials commonly found in home workshops have the capacity to cause skin irritation, to be toxic, easily catch on fire, or even explode. Some of them are also quite odorous and hazardous to breathe. Actually, a few really noxious items may have all of these undesirable qualities. Therefore, if your home workshop is located anywhere within your house or its attached garage, the potential for indoor air contamination (and other potentially dangerous problems) can be high.

SAFE HOME-WORKSHOP BASICS

The following sections offer some general guidelines to make your home workshop a safer and healthier environment.

PROPER PRODUCT STORAGE AND DISPOSAL

There are several basic safety measures for any home workshop worth considering. One of these is to always carefully read product labels for the manufacturers' recommendations on the correct storage conditions for their particular products. As it turns out, most paints, clear finishes, adhesives, caulkings, etc. should be stored within a certain temperature range. While keeping within this suggested range guarantees longer product life, in some cases it will also lessen the potential for leaks or even explosions.

Other important aspects of proper storage are good organization and secure shelving. To meet these needs, metal storage cabinets with doors are often ideal. An added bonus is that items stored there are less likely to contaminate the room air with their odors. Of course, cabinets with locking doors (or ones designed to hold a padlock) are best if there are small children around the house. By the way, it's often a good idea to have at least two metal storage cabinets in your home workshop—one to hold odorous paints, caulkings, adhesives, stains, and finishes, and a separate one to hold sandpaper, tools, and protective gear. You'll find that metal cabinets are sold at most office-supply stores, some hardware stores, and some local **Sears Roebuck and Co.** stores, among other places (see also *Household Storage* for other storage ideas in *Chapter 8: Housekeeping*).

Another home workshop storage basic is to store only what you really think you'll actually use again. In other words, rid your shop of old paints and other compounds that were involved in a onetime project or that only have a small quantity left in their container. Although it may seem thrifty to hold on to them, in many cases extended age can cause many products to degrade markedly. They may become contaminated with mold or bacteria or actually change in chemical composition. Then too, long-stored items may simply become dried up or come out of suspension.

However, when you are ready to dispose of unneeded paints, etc., call your local board of heath or sanitation department. They often have established, proper, disposal procedures to follow with certain products—especially ones considered "household hazardous waste." By the way, if you have a considerable amount of a paint in one color that's still in good condition, you might consider donating it to a local charity.

PROPER WORKING CONDITIONS

Proper working conditions are essential for a safe and healthy home workshop. One of the most important of these is to work only with good ventilation. Therefore, when you use paint, glue, mastic, etc., open the room's windows and exterior doors (if possible) and consider using a window fan or a permanently installed fan and blow the odors outdoors (for more on vented fans, see *High Humidity* in *Chapter 9: Indoor Air*).

Of course, proper protective gear is essential for personal safety. Your chemical respirator mask, rubber gloves, neoprene gloves, ear protectors, shop coats, safety glasses, and goggles should be handy, in good condition, and always used when appropriate to do so (see *Protective Gear* below).

In addition, every home workshop should have a multipurpose fire extinguisher in good working order and easily accessible (see *Portable Fire Extinguishers* in *Chapter 8: Housekeeping*). In addition, it's also a good idea to have a small metal canister with a tight-fitting metal lid or a small garbage can with a lid for oily or solvent-containing rags, paper, or other very flammable materials. It's also important to have an operating smoke detector (see

Smoke Detectors in *Chapter 9: Indoor Air.*) Note: Place the smoke detector so it isn't directly over a location where a great deal of dust will be generated because the airborne dust could inadvertently set off the alarm; also, vacuum the alarm regularly.

Keeping your workshop clean is another safety essential. That way, particulate debris will not accumulate and recirculate into the air. Therefore, it's advisable to use a powerful vacuum that's able to clean dirt, grit, and sawdust easily. Another shop basic is to have proper lighting. That means having a good overhead light source as well as a swing-arm lamp(s), flashlights, and electric lanterns for close-up work.

One more safety measure is to keep all your cutting tools sharp. It may seem safer to use dull tools, but in practice, sharp tools slip less and cause fewer accidents. Finally, you'll want to have an easily accessible and well-stocked first-aid kit. Also, an intercom in your shop will permit you to make an easy and immediate call for help to other family members. You may want a telephone as well to be able to make a 911 call quickly.

Important note: It's important to do as much shop-type work as possible in a properly outfitted workshop—or perhaps outdoors. Unless absolutely necessary, it's best to avoid doing any project, especially if it is odorous, potentially dangerous, or just plain messy, within the living space of your home. Of course, certain repairs or remodeling will require that some work be done at a specific site, such as in the kitchen. However, if you must work somewhere besides your shop, continue to follow as many safety precautions as is possible. Above all, be sure to have adequate ventilation and wear appropriate protective gear.

PROTECTIVE GEAR

If you plan to do home projects, it's essential to own, correctly maintain, properly store, and actually use good-quality personal protective gear. But you must use equipment that is truly able to protect you when you're doing a particular job. For example, a thin, inexpensive, disposable paper dust mask could be adequate protection if you plan only to sand one piece of wood for a few minutes, but it simply can't shield you from dangerous solvent odors if you plan to use an oil-based stain. Therefore, before doing any project, analyze what face, eye, ear, hand, respiratory, etc., protection you'll actually need. Then, you should be certain that you have the necessary equipment on hand—and that it's in good working order. Under no circumstances should you ever begin work on a project if you won't be sufficiently protected.

Fortunately, finding protective gear is not difficult. Usually, local hardware stores have fairly good selections on hand. And they're often also willing to order specific items if something is not in stock. In addition, you might want to know about two large national companies that carry an extensive inventory of personal protective equipment. These are **W.W. Grainger, Inc.** and **Orr Safety Corporation**, both of which have local outlets as well as mail-order catalogs.

By the way, **E.L. Foust Co., Inc.** offers several disposable dust masks capable of trapping most large dust particles. The company also handles 3M Dust Mist Respirators, which have a thin, activated-charcoal layer in them. These particular masks are designed to provide protection from not only many types of particulates but also minor airborne chemical exposures as well. In addition, **The Environmental Health Shopper** carries a number of filter masks.

HOME-WORKSHOP MATERIALS AND PRODUCTS

It's important to choose safer materials and products for your workshop projects in order to reduce air-quality problems and other potential risks. Therefore, the following sections discuss typical materials and products, testing procedures, and then suggest specific less toxic brands you might want to use in your next project.

TYPICAL HOME-WORKSHOP MATERIALS AND PRODUCTS

Unfortunately, some typical products and materials used in home workshops are potentially harmful. Many contain petroleum-based solvents and/or other harmful volatile organic compounds (VOCs) that are often dangerous to breathe. In some instances, inhalation of certain VOCs can cause respiratory inflammation or even central nervous system damage (see *Volatile Organic Compounds* in *Chapter 9: Indoor Air*). Then, too, some typical products are very flammable and others have the potential to cause skin irritation. And, unfortunately a number of them are toxic.

You might think that by using only water-based products you'd avoid all such problems. However, this simply isn't the case. It turns out that most latex paint contains some VOCs. In addition, many water-based products contain other very odorous ingredients.

Although health problems with paints, finishes, and other coatings are somewhat familiar to many people, less is known about the risks posed by certain types of wood, wood products, and drywall compounds. But in reality, some wood species release natural compounds that can be irritating to the skin and/or respiratory system. While it's more common to be affected by newly cut wood, certain sensitive individuals find oak, for example, bothersome for several months. In addition, many types of man-made wood products release relatively high levels of formaldehyde (see *Formaldehyde* in *Chapter 9: Indoor Air*). In the case of typical drywall compounds, they generally contain fungicide, antifreeze, adhesive, and other additives that can make walls intolerable for months for some sensitive people.

As hard as it is to believe, the truth is that nearly all typical building products and materials used today have at least some health risk associated with them (for more on this, read *The Healthy House* or *Healthy House Building* by John Bower, both available from **The Healthy House Institute**). These products are often relatively inexpensive, generally easy to work with, and readily available at most local lumberyards and hardware stores. And little, if any, government regulation covers many of them. Therefore, their use has become "standard practice."

But, healthier, alternative products and materials are available. For example, instead of using ubiquitous oak, you could substitute a less irritating solid wood that is not as popular, but nevertheless very attractive, such as maple, birch, or tulip poplar—that is, if you happen to find oak irritating. And you could use these same solid woods in place of formaldehyde-containing man-made wood products. In addition, you can now purchase drywall compounds with fewer chemical additives. Unlike typical brands, these products are usually well-tolerated by many sensitive people, even when wet. There are also less-noxious paints, finishes, adhesives, and lubricants.

ALTERNATIVE HOME-WORKSHOP MATERIALS AND PRODUCTS

Ultimately, it's up to you whether to use alternative materials and products. Because very few government regulations currently cover most building products, the typical unhealthy types will, no doubt, continue to be the norm for many years. As a result, they'll be the products stocked by most local hardware stores, lumberyards, and building-supply centers. They'll also be what most builders and contractors will automatically use. If you want healthier materials to be used in your home projects, it'll be up to you to take the initiative in finding and buying them. The following pages should help you in this regard.

It should be noted that nearly all liquid alternative products are water-based rather than oil- or solvent-based. Formaldehyde, VOCs, and other potentially bothersome or harmful ingredients are usually minimized, or completely omitted. Many liquid alternative products are formulated to have less odor when applied and/or when completely dry. In addition, many such products contain fewer preservatives. Thus, their shelf life may be shorter. Alternative wood products are manufactured without the use of formaldehyde glues.

As you might expect, these alternative products and materials are often more costly than typical brands—but not always. Higher price can be due to smaller production runs and sometimes because the ingredients or materials are of higher quality. You'll find, too, that some alternative items require you to learn new methods of application. For example, alternative ceramic tile grouts can require a special curing procedure.

Because alternative-product manufacturers and distributors tend to be small and the number of dealers carrying these items is somewhat limited, you'll often need to special-order many of these products. However, this isn't difficult. Fortunately, there are a number of fine mail-order sources, including **Nontoxic Environments**, **Simply Better**, and **The Living Source**, among others (for recommendations, see *Specific Suggestions for Alternative Materials and Products* below).

TESTING HOME-WORKSHOP PRODUCTS AND MATERIALS

Although alternative products and materials are safer than their typical counterparts, some items may still be bothersome to you personally. After all, each of us is unique. With products and materials used in home projects (furniture, cabinets, walls, or floors, etc.), testing is particularly important inasmuch as these projects are often large in size and relatively permanent. The expense, time, and stress to redo such projects can be great. Therefore, testing is crucial, especially for sensitive individuals.

You should be aware that different types of products and materials will require slightly different testing procedures. However, these are simply variations of the basic testing procedure described in the beginning of this book (see *Testing* in *Chapter 1: Getting Started*). Of course, it should be stated that testing can reveal more than personal tolerance. It can also help you determine how a clear finish will look, whether a certain glue will adhere well, etc. Remember though, it's important to do your testing sufficiently ahead of the time—before you actually need to use a particular product or material in your project. That way, there will be no panic or work delays if you find you must use something else.

Important note: If you test more than one product at a time, it's a good idea to keep the information you learn in written form, such as in a chart. It's also a good idea to record product prices for a cost comparison. When finished with your tests, you may want to keep the samples and test results for later use. However, you should know that companies tend to change their product formulas periodically. Therefore, the data from a previous test might not be valid in the future. As a result, you must always make new test samples from currently available products.

Testing Paints and Finishes

Before you purchase any large quantity of paint or other finish, it's best to test several first to determine how odorous they can be when wet, their finished sheen, how well they cover, and their true finished color. You'll also want to test for their odor once they're dry to determine how long (if ever) it takes for them to become tolerable. Of course, this is especially important for sensitive individuals. When the samples are completely dry, you might want to test for how washable they are.

After weighing all the information from your testing, you can then confidently choose the best paint or finish for the job you need to do. And you'll also have a good idea how long it will take after it's been applied before it will be tolerable for you. However, you must keep in mind that walls cover large areas, and most samples are very small in comparison. Therefore, an entire room may require a longer time period than a sample, until it's no longer bothersome.

To actually test, all you need do is coat a piece of aluminum foil with a prospective product and label it as to brand name, color and/or sheen, and date of application. Then on a piece of paper, record how the finish smelled when fresh. Then set the sample aside in a dry, uncontaminated place for at least several days. After that, you can very lightly sniff the coated surface once every few days (or weeks) until you can no longer detect any smell. Once odor-free, you'll want to place the test-sample near your pillow. If you're able to sleep normally, the sample is probably tolerable. Of course, you'll need to record the date of tolerability on the sample and on your chart. Finally, you can write down information on how well the finish covered, how the sheen looked, how scrubbable it was, etc.

Testing Adhesives

To test alternative water-based glues and other adhesive compounds, purchase the smallest sizes they come in. Using each product, apply a small amount on a separate piece of aluminum foil each of which has been identified by brand name and application date. On a sheet of paper, record how much each product cost and its peculiar odor when wet. Then, set the samples aside in a dry, uncontaminated area to dry.

The next day, very lightly sniff the samples and repeat this every few days or so until you can no longer detect an odor with one or more of them. At that point, record the date on the foil and on your chart. If you want to be even more sure that a particular product won't be bothersome to you, lay an odorless sample by the head of your bed. If you are able to sleep well through the night, it often means you're able to tolerate that product. As a rule, a small amount of glue often isn't a significant concern. For example, considerably less glue would be used in a furniture project compared to the amount used to adhere floor tile in a large room.

While this procedure will determine personal tolerability, it can't determine how well a certain product will do its job of adhering. To do that, apply the glue or adhesive to a scrap or small section of what you intend to glue, then let it dry. After that, you can examine your test sample for proper, firm attachment. Again, record your results. Although this test can't give you long-term guarantees, it will give you a general idea of whether the product is able to do its job or not.

Testing Lubricants

In most home situations, lubricants are used very sparingly. However, if they happen to be very odorous, they can be bothersome or intolerable to sensitive persons for a very long period of time. Of course, you should realize to begin with that many petroleum-based lubricants have an odor no matter how long they've been exposed to the air. For example, sewing-machine oil can have a long-term odor. However, there are other types of lubricants that you might find worth sampling.

If you want to test a lubricant, you can try the following procedure. First, purchase one or more brands and apply a small amount of each to its own separate sheet of aluminum foil. On the foil, and also on a separate piece of paper, record the date, brand, and cost. Then, very lightly sniff each sample and note the odor. After that, you can lightly sniff the samples over several days. If a sample seems to have no odor, record the date on the foil and on your chart. The odorless sample should then be placed near your bed's headboard. A good night's sleep often indicates that you're tolerating the product reasonably well.

The best way to find out if a product will do a good job of lubricating is to actually use it on something. For example, if you want to find out how well it will work on your kitchen cabinets, apply it to one hinge. After determining how well that seems to work, you can then decide if you want to go ahead and use it on all the other hinges. It might be a good idea to permanently keep the records of your testing for tolerability and effectiveness because lubricant formulas don't tend to change often. Therefore, what you learned could very well be useful in the future.

Testing Woods

To test your personal tolerance for a specific wood species, it's best to get a small section of several different types of wood. Then write the name of the species on each sample and very lightly sniff to determine its odor. Record the results on a separate sheet of paper. Next, sand all four sides of each sample. Vacuum off the dust and lightly sniff again and record your observations. The odor will likely be much stronger.

Next, completely coat the sanded sample with the tolerable paint or finish you plan to eventually use on the wood (see *Testing Paints and Finishes* above).

After waiting for the finish to become tolerable (your previous testing should give you an estimated date), lightly sniff the coated wood and record your findings. Then, put a second coat on each side of the sample so that it ends up getting two coats of finish. Again, wait for the finish to become tolerable, test-sniff, and record your results. This information should give you at least a basic understanding of a particular wood species' initial odor, its odor after being sanded, its odor after one coat of a tolerable finish, and its odor after two coats. Next, take the sample that seems most acceptable and place it near your pillow. If you're able to sleep well, it's likely you'll tolerate that particular wood and finish combination.

While this testing should prove to be of great help, some variables are worth keeping in mind. For example, a small sample is not going to be nearly as potent as one hundred and fifty square feet of newly laid hardwood floor. It isn't unusual for such a large finished project to have more of an odor than you anticipated. Fortunately, however, with age, most wood surfaces lose a great deal of their initial innate odor. Of course, additional coats of finish could be applied to help seal in certain persistently bothersome wood odors if necessary.

Note: For testing alternative particleboard or construction-grade plywood for use in interior applications, you could follow similar testing procedures as described above with solid wood.

SPECIFIC SUGGESTIONS FOR ALTERNATIVE MATERIALS AND PRODUCTS

In the following sections, you'll find suggestions for some specific alternative home-workshop materials and products you might consider using for your next project.

Paints

In most cases, paints have quite complex formulas made up of many compounds. As you already know, there are many types and brands available (see below for a discussion of the differences between oil- and water-based paints). However, only a few of the more popular alternatives will actually be mentioned by brand name, with sources where they can be obtained. These particular paints are generally less bothersome, or have potentially less harmful ingredients, or are designed to be nearly odorless when dry. It should be mentioned that most of these "safer" alternative paints only come in a few off-white or pastel colors.

Whenever you paint, be sure to follow the recommended application directions on the label *exactly*. This is especially important for sensitive people because, for example, if not enough drying time is allowed between coats, it may take longer for the paint to become tolerable. See *Wall Paint* in *Chapter 5: Interior Decorating* for a discussion of paint sheen and suggested application procedures.

Note that, in the following sections, individual paint brands may be mentioned under several headings. For example, Brand X may be listed under both *Alternative Latex Paints* and *Low-Odor Paints*. Thus, Brand X would be an alternative latex paint with low odor. Therefore, it would be a good idea to look under all those headings with qualities important to you and determine which brand(s) best meets your criteria.

Oil-Based Vs. Water-Based Paints

Before choosing any paint, you may want to know more about the two basic types: oil- and water-based. Actually, both types have *pigments* (natural or synthetically derived colorants), *binders* (compounds that hold or bind all the ingredients together), and *vehicles* (liquid base). Of course, a number of other minor ingredients are usually in them as well.

In fact, depending on the particular type and brand of paint, it could also contain antifreeze, *anti-skinning agents* (to prevent a film from forming on the paint's surface in an unopened can), *anti-settling agents* (to keep the ingredients in suspension), biocides, *catalysts* (compounds that hasten chemical reactions without being altered themselves), curing agents, defoamers, *dispersing agents* (compounds that cause the ingredients to disperse uniformly throughout the paint), driers, *emulsifying agents* (compounds that permit minute droplets of one liquid to remain suspended in another), *extenders* (compounds that increase volume or bulk), *fillers* (compounds that simply add solid particles), fire retardants (see *What is Fire?* in *Chapter 8: House-keeping*), fungicides, preservatives, surfactants (see *Soaps Versus Detergents* in *Chapter 7: Cleaning*), thickeners, *thixotropic agents* (compounds that permit a gel to adhere to a vertical surface without running), and many others.

However, it's the vehicle of paint that's primarily responsible for the differences between oil- and water-based paints. (Note: Oil-based paints were once made using natural oils such as linseed oil and soybean oil. However, today they are generally made with synthetic *alkyd resins,* but the term "oil-based" is still popularly used.) Because the oils (or alkyd resins) are very thick, they're combined with solvents to thin them down. Not surprisingly then, it's this oil/solvent vehicle in oil-based paints, or the water vehicle in water-based paints, that greatly determines a paint's odor, it's flammability, cleanup requirements, it's scrubbabilty—and the paint's potential negative health effects. Because significantly more solvents are used in oil-based paints, they release more dangerous volatile organic compounds (VOCs) into the air than water-based paints (see *Volatile Organic Compounds* in *Chapter 9: Indoor Air*).

It's also interesting to know that the oil/solvent (or alkyd resin/solvent) vehicles in oil-based paints don't dry through evaporation. Instead, they cure through a *chemical oxidation reaction process*. Once oil paints have cured, they're very durable. On the other hand, paints using water as their vehicle dry primarily through evaporation. Unfortunately, many kinds of water-based paint are less durable than their oil-based counterparts.

Taking into account all the pluses and minuses, it shouldn't be surprising that water-based products (paints as well clear finishes, stains, etc.) are the type recommended by most health-conscious people over counterparts containing high levels of solvents. That's why you'll find that nearly every alternative paint, clear finish, and stain in the sections below is water-based. (Important note: Even alternative water-based products still require some time after they've been applied to become tolerable for most sensitive individuals.)

Alternative Latex Paints

The most common type of indoor house paint used in America today is probably water-based latex. *Latex* is a natural or synthetic rubber product used as a binder, but today the term latex often refers to any water-based paint—even if it doesn't contain any real latex. As it turns out, most brands of latex paint can provide good coverage, but as a rule, they aren't particularly scrubbable.

Although most typical latex paints contain far smaller quantities of harmful volatile organic compounds (VOCs) than oil-based paints, these substances are still a part of their formulas. Typical latex paints also have ingredients such as preservatives and other additives that tend to be bothersome for many sensitive individuals. Fortunately, a few alternative latex paints have now been developed that you may find preferable. These particular paints have less of the common problem-causing ingredients. (Note that, in most cases, each alternative latex paint manufacturer has reduced or eliminated a different set of ingredients.)

One brand of alternative latex paint you may want to consider is Rubber-Lustre Low Biocide (**Miller Paint Co.**). Unlike most other alternative paints, this brand comes in a range of colors. You can order it directly from the company. Another alternative latex paint option is Murco (**Murco Wall Products**). It's been formulated so that its fungicides and preservatives remain bound up in the dried paint film instead of evaporating into the room air. Murco paint can be purchased from the manufacturer.

A brand you'll definitely want to become familiar with is Best Paint (**Best Paint Co., Inc.**). This is a line of low-VOC (low in volatile organic compounds) alternative latex paint that is tolerated by many sensitive people. You can mail-order it through the company. Another popular brand is Series 2000 (**The Glidden Co.**), which contains no VOCs at all. A real plus with this paint is that it is one of the few alternative paints that is readily available in local stores; it's marketed through Glidden dealers nationwide. Another alternative is the Ecos Paint imported from England and sold by **Simply Better**. Ecos is a zero-VOC alternative latex paint.

Note, latex paints with little or no VOCs generally still contain other ingredients that can be odorous (for paints designed especially for low odor, see *Low Odor Paints* below). As a result, to make latex paints more tolerable, some sensitive people have stirred in a pound of baking soda in each gallon of paint. Although this may somewhat reduce bothersome paint odors, it does have major drawbacks. For example, the added baking soda can affect the paint's durability, texture, and/or color. In fact, this procedure should only be attempted (if ever) with light colors. At any rate, no paint manufacturer recommends adding baking soda to their products. Therefore, if the resulting paint surface ends up unsatisfactory in any way, they take no responsibility.

Alternative Casein Paints

Casein paints are water-based products that use casein (a milk-protein derivative) as the binder. As it turns out, most casein paints are fairly durable. Interestingly, forms of milk and casein paint have actually been used for hundreds of years.

There are a number of persons who consider alternative casein paints to be the best ecological choice as far as paints go. This is because casein paints are made of naturally derived substances. However, there are drawbacks to these paints. First, they are available only in powdered form, so they must be mixed with water before they're applied. Also, because they generally contain no *biocides* to inhibit mold growth, they can't be stored as a liquid for very long or used in damp areas. In addition, casein paints could be intolerable for those with milk allergies. By the way, walls painted with casein paints can retain a faint milky odor for a long time.

If you're interested in using an alternative casein paint, there are at least two brands you should know about. One is Old Fashioned Milk Paint (**The Old Fashioned Milk Paint Co.**), which can be ordered directly from the company. The other is Eco Design (**Eco Design Co.**), which is offered through its catalog as well as **Simply Better.**

Alternative Acrylic Paints

Acrylic paints are water-based paints containing synthetic *thermoplastic acrylic resin* as their binder, but they are sometimes called latex. Acrylic paints are generally very durable and washable. Unfortunately, they are also often quite odorous while being applied.

In fact, alternative acrylic paints commonly remain bothersome to sensitive persons for several weeks after they've been applied (some sensitive individuals find this is the case for up to two months). However, when they've completely dried, they often have very little odor. One brand of low-odor alternative acrylic paint that is often well-tolerated by sensitive people is Enviro-Safe Paint (**Chem-Safe Products**). It has reduced levels of biocides and can be purchased directly from the company.

A few water-based alternative acrylic paints have actually been specially designed as sealants (see also *Sealants and Other Acrylic Wood Finishes* below). One of these is Crystal Shield (**Pace Chem Industries, Inc.**). You can order it from the company or from dealers such as **Nontoxic Environments**.

German Natural Paints

Interestingly, a "natural house" movement in Germany known as *Baubiologie* has spawned several alternative *all-natural* water-based paint lines. Some of these contain turpentine (derived from softwood trees such as pine) and citrus solvents (derived from oranges, lemons, etc.)—substances that sometimes cause a condition known as *painter's rash*. Therefore, in some cases these ingredients have been replaced by less bothersome petroleum-derived solvents. It should be mentioned that these paints often have a strong natural odor when wet. As a result, not all are well-tolerated by sensitive individuals.

There are actually two German natural-paint lines now available in the U.S.: Auro and Livos. Also, paints with a similar formula (Bio-Shield) are manufactured here. If you're interested in these paints, you'll find that Auro is sold by **Osprey Eco-logics** and **Nontoxic Environments**; Livos and Bio-Shield are carried by **Eco Design Co.**, **The Human Habitat**, and **Osprey Eco-logics**. Also check with **Simply Better** for brands it is currently stocking.

Low-Biocide Paints

Biocides are chemicals created specifically to kill life-forms. Normally, small amounts of biocides are added to typical paints (even to some alternative brands) primarily to inhibit mold growth while the paint is still a liquid in the can. This greatly extends the paint's shelf life. Unfortunately, some sensitive individuals react negatively to these additives. Other persons who, for philosophical or other reasons, are uncomfortable with using any product containing biocides inside their homes.

Fortunately, for anyone wishing to avoid paints containing biocide additives, there are now several low- or zero-biocide alternative products available. It should be noted, however, that such paints, especially if they're in liquid form, should not be stored for a very long period of time. In addition, they should probably not be used in damp areas such as bathrooms.

One alternative latex paint with reduced biocide levels you might consider is Miller Paint Low-Biocide (**Miller Paint Co.**), which is available directly from the manufacturer. This particular line contains only 5 to 10% of the amount of biocides found in typical latex paints. Actually, Miller adds no biocides itself. The only biocides present are those that are in the bulk ingredients the company purchases from its suppliers.

Also, Murco latex paint (**Murco Wall Products**) has been specially created so the fungicides and preservatives aren't released into the air. They actually remain bound up in the dried paint. Murco latex paint can be ordered from the manufacturer.

An alternative acrylic paint you might be interested in is Enviro-Safe Paint (**Chem Safe Products**), which contains no fungicides. It can be purchased directly from the manufacturer. Other low- or zero-biocide paints include alternative, powdered, casein brands such as Old Fashioned Milk Paint (**The Old Fashioned Milk Paint Co.**), which you can buy directly from the company, and Eco Design casein paint (**Eco Design Co.**), which is offered through its catalog as well as by **Simply Better**. In addition, some of the German natural paints are low- or zero-biocide as well. You'll want to check with their dealers for specific ingredient information for particular products (see *German Natural Paints* above).

Low-Odor Paints

If you're interested in a low-odor paint, a number of alternative water-based brands are available that might suit your needs. However, you should be aware that each manufacturer tends to have its own definition for "low odor." For example, some alternative paints are purposely formulated to minimize odors during application and drying, such as certain low- or zero-VOC paints. But others are designed to have little or no odor after the paint has thoroughly dried, such as some of the alternative acrylic brands. And a few are intended to do both, such as the alternative casein paints. Therefore, be certain you know exactly what low odor means for the particular brand of paint you're considering buying. Note, virtually all wall paints will have at least some odor when wet, even low-odor brands.

Many sensitive people find that the reduced odors of low-VOC paints are very acceptable paints for them. Two of these you might want to try are Best Paint (**Best Paint Co., Inc.**) and Enviro-Safe Paint (**Chem-Safe Products**), both of which can be ordered directly from the company. Also, a zero-VOC latex paint you might want to use is Ecos Paint. This brand is imported from England and sold by **Simply Better**. Another zero-VOC alternative latex paint you'll want to consider is Series 2000 (**Glidden Co.**) The Series 2000 not only has reduced odor but also the advantage of being sold nationwide through local Glidden dealers.

Another low-odor brand of alternative paint you may be interested in using is SafeCoat (**American Formulating and Manufacturing**). SafeCoat is a water-based paint described by its manufacturer as a "suspended polymer" paint (its binder is made up of plastic particles). You can purchase SafeCoat from AFM dealers including **Simply Better, N.E.E.D.S., The Living Source, Flowright International Products, Nontoxic Environments,** and **The American Environmental Health Foundation,** among others.

It should be mentioned that paints with low- or zero-biocides are sometimes classified as low-odor alternative paints. This is because these types of chemical additives can contribute to a paint's smell. Therefore, one latex paint you might be interested in is Miller Paint Low Biocide (**Miller Paint Co.**). It can be ordered directly from the company or from dealers such as **Nontoxic Environments.** In addition, the fungicides in Murco latex paint (**Murco Wall Products**) are specially formulated so that they remain trapped within the dried paint. Therefore, they can't become airborne. Murco paint is available directly from the company.

It should be noted that, alternative casein paints commonly have much less odor during their application and drying time, compared to other types of paints. However, a slight milky smell can sometimes linger after these paints are dry. Two alternative casein paints are Old Fashioned Milk Paint (**Old Fashioned Milk Paint Co.**), which can be purchased directly from the manufacturer, and Eco Design paint (**Eco-Design Co.**), which is sold through its catalog and by **Simply Better.**

Also, some, but not all, of the German natural paints have reduced odor. A number of people feel that these types of paints have less odor than typical latex paints during their application and initial drying as well as later when they're completely dried. Auro paint is handled by **Osprey Eco-logics** and **Nontoxic Environments** and Livos and Bio-Shield by **The Human Habitat** and **Osprey Eco-logics.**

Clear Finishes

Alternative clear finishes come in a variety of formulas. Most of them are water-based (see *Oil-Based Vs. Water-Based Paints* above). Some are designed to be applied to raw wood and others are for use on other types of surfaces. Naturally, it's important to choose the finish most suitable, durable, and tolerable for the job. As has been stressed throughout this book, test any product first before using it. This is especially a good idea if you plan to use a clear finish on a large area, such as a floor (see also *Testing Paints and Finishes* above and *Hardwood Floors, Unfinished Furniture,* and *Ceramic Tile Floors* in *Chapter 5: Interior Decorating* for suggestions on actually applying clear finishes).

Water-Based Polyurethane

Polyurethane finishes use *polyurethane resin* as their binder. In most cases, polyurethane finishes are clear and work well at protecting wood surfaces. As it turns out, these products create hard-surface finishes that are quite durable, especially the polyurethane products designed for use on wood floors.

However, you should be aware that there are both oil- and water-based polyurethane clear finishes. Of the two, the oil-based types should be avoided.

This is because their solvents are very strong-smelling and potentially harmful when the finish is being applied and while it's drying.

Fortunately, the relatively new water-based polyurethane finishes can easily be used instead of the oil-based versions. These products tend to dry quickly and generally have little or no residual odor after less than a week. As a result, many very sensitive individuals find that water-based polyurethane finishes are quite tolerable. There are other real advantages to using these particular products. One is that they're commonly stocked in local stores. Another is that they're lower in cost than many other types of alternative clear wood finishes.

Two popular brands of clear water-based polyurethane floor finishes you might want to try are Aqua Zar (**United Gilsonite Laboratories**) and Professional Image (**Basic Coatings**). Both of these may be carried by your local building centers or hardware stores. However, there are several other similar brands on the market.

Sealants and Other Acrylic Water-Based Wood Finishes

Clear acrylic finishes can create a hard, durable, low-odor surface. Actually, when they're wet and during their drying period, they're more odorous than water-based polyurethane finishes, despite the fact they're water-based products. Sensitive individuals often report that acrylic finishes take up to two months to become tolerable to them. This is probably due to the synthetic thermoplastic acrylic resin that is used as the binding agent. Generally, clear acrylic finishes are popular for use on wood.

If you'd like to use a clear acrylic product, one you might try is Acrylac (**American Formulating and Manufacturing**). Another is Hard Seal (**American Formulating and Manufacturing**), which, being more durable, is often used on floors. (Hard Seal in particular has been popular with a number of sensitive individuals). Both products are available from AFM distributors, including **N.E.E.D.S.**, **The Living Source**, **Nontoxic Environments**, and **Flowright International Products**.

In addition, you might want to try using either Crystal Aire (**Pace Chem Industries, Inc.**) or the more durable floor finish, Crystal Shield (**Pace Chem Industries, Inc.**). Interestingly, both Crystal Aire and Crystal Shield have been especially created not only as clear finishes but also as *sealants*. In fact, four coats of Crystal Aire can reduce formaldehyde emissions from typical particleboard by up to 92%. Although this is commendable, the remaining 8% is still too bothersome to some people. Once completely dry, Pace Chem products are quite inert. If you want to buy them, they can be ordered directly from the company or from dealers such as **Nontoxic Environments**.

Shellac

Shellac is an ancient finish, first developed in the Far East, which uses purified *lac resin* (a secretion deposited on tree branches by female lac insects) as its binding agent. Lac—and therefore, shellac—varies in color from pale, translucent yellow to dark orange, depending on the variety of tree the lac insects lived on. As it turns out, shellac produces a fairly tough finish that is most commonly used to coat wood. However, white discolorations can manifest themselves rather quickly if water gets on a shellacked surface.

It's important to understand that shellac is neither a water-based, nor an oil-based product. Instead, it uses alcohol as its vehicle. Therefore, *denatured alcohol* is necessary for cleaning up. In fact, because of the alcohol content in shellac, it's quite flammable. It's also very odorous when wet. Fortunately, the alcohol evaporates quickly, and when the finish is completely dry, shellacked items are often tolerable to many sensitive individuals. However, some people have noted that in certain instances a noticeable, a bothersome odor can persist.

Some people consider shellac a completely natural finish. However, most brands likely contain a few synthetic additives. When you're ready to purchase shellac, you'll find that there are usually several brands to choose from in your local hardware and paint stores. One popular brand is Bull's Eye (**William Zinsser & Co.**). An alternative brand you may wish to consider instead is Auro shellac. This particular product is manufactured in Germany, and it's currently sold by **Osprey Eco-Logics** and **Nontoxic Environments**, among others. Note: It's important to test several brands of shellac to see how they look and how well you tolerate them (see *Testing Paints and Finishes* above).

Penetrating Oil Finishes

Some individuals may want to try a natural *penetrating oil finish* on their wood items. Penetrating oil finishes don't leave a thin, hard coating on the surface of the wood, but penetrate and saturate the wood with oil. Therefore, if the wood's surface becomes scratched or abraded, you can simply apply more oil to the damaged area and it will blend in without the need for stripping and refinishing.

However, there is a downside. Many of the oils used as wood finishes are fairly odorous when applied. And they can remain quite odorous for a considerable amount of time afterwards as well. In fact, their smells could continue to be bothersome for up to several months or longer. Of course, this depends on the specific oil, wood, and your personal tolerance but, in general, oil finishes are not often tolerated by sensitive people.

Two of the more popular natural penetrating oils are *tung oil* (derived from the nuts of tung-oil trees) and *linseed oil* (derived from flax seeds). Of these, tung oil is not recommended. This is because it has been implicated in suppressing the functioning of the immune system as well as reactivating chronic Epstein-Barr virus infections.

Linseed oil is available in two varieties: *raw* and *boiled*. While raw linseed oil will not dry properly when applied to wood, boiled linseed oil will. In the past, many manufacturers simply heated raw linseed oil to give it drying properties but, today, most "boiled" linseed oil has not been heat-processed at all. Instead, manufacturers add toxic heavy-metal additives such as lead acetate or cobalt manganese to aid in drying. Fortunately, there are two types of boiled linseed oil still made without these additives. Tried & True Varnish Oil and Tried & True Original Wood Finish are both available by mail order from **Garrett Wade Co.**

If you find you need to use a penetrating oil finish on salads bowls or kitchen knife handles, consider using *virgin olive oil*. Olive oil is not only nontoxic, it's also resistant to becoming rancid.

Wax Finishes

Waxes such as *carnauba wax* (derived from the plant waxes found on certain palm leaves) and *beeswax* (derived from honeycombs) are sometimes used to create clear, natural finishes on wood. Like penetrating oils, waxes provide protection that can be easily repaired if a scratched area should develop. This is because they penetrate and saturate wood rather than form a thin brittle layer that lies on the surface. For some people, natural waxes can be good wood-finishing choices.

However, it's important to know that many natural waxes are somewhat hard in consistency. Therefore, some waxes are heated or mixed with denatured alcohol or another volatile solvent to make them more workable. Of course, solvents could make a wax application intolerable to many sensitive individuals. However, it should be noted that once the solvent has completely evaporated, the finish could be quite acceptable for these very same people. It should be noted that beeswax tends to have a somewhat flowery odor. Although some people may find this attractive, others may find it bothersome. Obviously, testing waxes is important, especially if you're sensitive (see *Testing Paints and Finishes* above).

Often, you'll be able to find carnauba waxes in your local hardware store. One popular brand is Trewax. And you can generally purchase beeswax from local beekeepers. To find one, check your local classified telephone directory. Beeswax can also be mail-ordered from **Dona Designs**.

Water Glass

Water glass is a term applied to certain water-soluble *sodium silicate compounds*. Interestingly, these compounds have a similar chemical composition to ordinary window glass. As it turns out, water-glass solutions used as finishes are transparent and virtually odor-free. This is also true when they're wet. Not surprisingly, these are commonly considered highly tolerable products by sensitive individuals.

Interestingly, water glass was once a popular product. However, since World War II, synthetic sealants have nearly replaced it, but water glass is still sometimes used as an effective gout and concrete sealer. As it turns out, when water glass comes into contact with the calcium (and certain other substances) in these materials, a chemical reaction takes place. The result is the creation of a hard, clear crystalline surface that's very durable. Water glass can also be used to protect your ceramic tile grout joints by applying it carefully to the dry grout joints—not the tile—with a small artist's paint brush.

It should be noted that water glass should not be applied to a concrete floor if you ever plan to apply ceramic tile to it later. This is because the sealed surface would be nonporous. As a result, it would prevent the adhesion of the ceramic-tile mortar. Another consideration to keep in mind is not to use too much water glass when you're applying it. A little goes a long way, and applying too much could result in a film that might peel off.

At least two water glass products are still available today that you might like to try. One is Johnson's SuperSeal (**Johnson's SuperSeal, Inc.**) which might be carried by your local hardware store. If not, call the company for the nearest dealer. The other is Penetrating Water Stop (**American Formulating and Manufacturing**). This particular product is sold by most AFM dealers including

N.E.E.D.S., **The Living Source**, **Flowright International Products**, and **Non-toxic Environments.**

Stains

Many woods look interesting and attractive just as they are. And by leaving them natural, you'll avoid using at least one potentially bothersome product: wood stain. However, if you decide you really want to use a stain anyway, following is some basic information about stains that you may find useful.

Wood stains are generally available in either oil- or water-based formulas. Oil-based types often produce richer, deeper tones than their water-based counterparts. Unfortunately, they're usually somewhat more odorous. They also require paint thinner or turpentine for cleanup (see *Oil-Based Vs. Water-Based Paints* above).

While water-based stains generally don't appear as rich-looking, they do have other distinct advantages. For example, they contain fewer VOCs and don't need solvents for cleanup. As a result, although water-based stains are not odor-free, they're less bothersome than their oil-based counterparts.

If you want to use a water-based stain, it's best to test several brands for appearance and personal tolerance. Of course, tolerance testing is always essential for sensitive persons. By the way, it is best to stain a sample, apply two coats of clear finish, then test for tolerability (see *Testing Paints and Finishes* above). This is important because the clear finish will often seal in any minor odors from the stain. But you won't know for sure until you've actually tested the sample.

Local paint stores often stock typical water-based stains. However, a number of alternative water-based stains can be purchased by mail order. One of these is Duro Stain (**American Formulating and Manufacturing**). This particular brand was originally target-marketed to chemically sensitive people. Duro Stain is available from AFM dealers including **N.E.E.D.S.**, **The Living Source**, **Nontoxic Environments**, and **Flowright Products International**.

In addition, many of the German natural paint companies (see *German Natural Paints* above) also make alternative water-based stains you might want to try (they also usually make oil-based versions, too, so make sure you order carefully). If you're interested in buying these, contact **Osprey Eco-logics** and **Nontoxic Environments** for Auro products, and **The Human Habitat** and **Osprey Eco-logics** for the Livos and Bio-Shield lines. Another source for some German natural products is **Simply Better**, which you should call to find out the brands they currently stock. By the way, alternative natural stains are manufactured in the U.S. under the Eco Design label (**Eco Design Co.**) and are offered through its catalog as well as by **Simply Better.**

Paint Strippers

Virtually all paint strippers in the past were extremely noxious products. This is because they were solvent-based and contained powerful, dangerous chemicals that were harmful if inhaled or came in contact with your skin. Many were also flammable.

Fortunately, a number of water-based paint strippers are now available. Their active stripping agents are *organic esters* (a certain class of carbon compounds).

These compounds are able to dissolve most paints like the solvents can, but tend to require more time to do it.

You should also be aware that wood that's been stripped with a water-based product generally requires an application of a *neutralizing solution*. This is necessary to counter the caustic action of the organic esters. However, this can be easily done by simply sponging on a white-vinegar/water solution. For the correct dilution, follow the label directions for the specific product you are using.

Three brands of water-based strippers you might want to try are Safest Stripper (**3-M Do-It-Yourself Division**), StrypSafer (**Savogran**), and EasyOff (**Klean Strip**). Generally, one of these (or another similar product) should be available at your local paint or hardware store. However, if you're unable to locate a water-based stripper in your area, contact these companies for their nearest dealers.

(For more on how to use paint strippers, see *Antique Furniture* and other appropriate sections in *Chapter 5: Interior Decorating*.)

Adhesives

In the sections below, all types of adhesive products are discussed—everything from tapes to caulkings. Some of these products are quite benign. However, others will require, at the minimum, good ventilation. As always, it's important to carefully read and follow the label directions for the best results. Note: It's always wise to test any prospective adhesive product first for both tolerance and effectiveness before using it on a large project (see *Testing Adhesives* above).

(For information on safe application procedures for certain types of adhesives, see the appropriate sections in *Chapter 5: Interior Decorating*.)

Tapes

Clear plastic tapes are probably the most common household adhesive product. Although tapes are often made of petrochemically derived transparent film coated on one side with glue, they're usually relatively low in odor (see *Plastic* in *Chapter 8: Housekeeping*). However, although clear plastic tapes are extremely popular, if you'd prefer a more natural material, cellophane tapes are still available.

Cellophane tapes are actually made from a transparent film derived from plant cellulose (see *Cellophane* in *Chapter 8: Housekeeping*). Although it's a natural material and virtually odorless, cellophane (and, therefore, cellophane tape) has the drawback of yellowing and degrading with age. As you probably already know, plastic and cellophane tapes are both sold in many drugstores, discount stores, and office-supply stores.

In situations calling for a wider, stronger tape, *aluminum-foil duct tape* can be a good choice. However, you should realize that this type of duct tape isn't the same as fabric-backed duct tape, which is made of a heavy woven fabric with glue on one side and a plastic coating on the other. With time, many low-cost fabric-backed duct tapes tend to lose their ability to adhere and so become unstuck relatively quickly. In addition, fabric-backed duct tape often has an odor that sensitive individuals find bothersome.

On the other hand, aluminum-foil duct tape is generally of higher quality and more costly. It's made of a very thin strip of heavy-duty aluminum foil with glue on one side. Aluminum-foil duct tapes are generally lower in odor because their metal surface seals in most of the adhesive odors from the sticky side. However, although aluminum-foil duct tape usually adheres better than fabric-backed duct tape, the cheaper varieties can also become loose in time.

Aluminum-foil duct tape is actually not difficult to find. Many times it's available in local hardware stores and is generally handled by most heating/cooling-equipment suppliers. One brand that has proven to be especially tolerable for many sensitive individuals is Polyken aluminum-foil tape. It's sold by mail order by **Nontoxic Environments** and **E.L Foust Co., Inc.** Incidentally, an alternative to aluminum-foil tape is stainless-steel tape. One outlet for such tape is **The Living Source**.

Glues

For gluing paper, inexpensive, common *mucilage glue* can work quite well. Interestingly, true mucilage glue is made of gummy plant secretions. However, this term is now also applied to a range of similar, simple liquid glues. Generally, mucilage glues are safe to use and don't have much of an odor. One you might try is Elmer's Mucilage (**Elmer's Adhesives Division of Borden, Inc.**), which is labeled as nontoxic. It and other similar brands are sold in drugstores, office-supply stores, and some discount stores.

White glue, such as Elmer's Glue-All (**Elmer's Adhesives Division of Borden, Inc.**), is another popular, relatively low-odor household product. White glues are chiefly synthetic latex/water solutions or more specifically, *polyvinyl acetate emulsions*. In other words, water is their vehicle and polyvinyl acetate their binding agent. When they dry, the water evaporates, leaving a thin, plastic film.

White glues are designed primarily for gluing paper, cardboard and wood. However, because they're so readily available and convenient to use, many people use them for jobs for which they never were intended. Unfortunately, white glues aren't waterproof. No matter how long they've been dried, they can become liquefied if they ever become wet. Therefore, white glues shouldn't be used on anything that will be exposed to precipitation outdoors or to washing indoors. If you'd like to purchase a white glue, they're available at most local grocery stores, pharmacies, office-supply stores, and discount stores.

Another fairly common household glue is *yellow carpenter's glue*. This type of glue is often very similar to white glue in composition. However, it can contain extra additives that permit better adhesion to woods. Two brands of yellow carpenter glue are Professional Carpenter Glue (**Elmer's Adhesives Division of Borden, Inc.**) and Weld-Wood (**Dap Products, Inc.**). For many years, all carpenter's glues were water-soluble. However recently, some brands now come in waterproof formulations as well. One of these is Weather-Tite (**Elmer's Adhesives Division of Borden, Inc.**). (In some cases, waterproof glues may be more odorous than non-waterproof types.) If you'd like to purchase a carpenter glue, they're generally found in lumberyards, building centers, and hardware stores.

If you need a glue for jewelry or other unusual items, often an *epoxy glue* works well. In fact, epoxy will work on virtually any material: metal, ceramic, wood, and even fabric. Generally, this type of glue comes packaged with two tubes: one containing a catalyst agent, the other containing an epoxy resin. To glue, it's necessary to mix equal amounts from these two tubes together. The combination of these two compounds produces the chemical reaction that results in an extremely strong, durable, and waterproof bond.

Unfortunately, most epoxy glues seem to have a strong odor due to their chemical ingredients. However, Tru-Bond epoxy (**True Value Hardware**) is one of the exceptions to this rule. This particular product has relatively little odor—both when it's wet and after it's had time to cure. But even with this brand of epoxy, make sure to have plenty of ventilation. If you're a sensitive person, you'll also need to set the epoxied item aside a few days until it has no odor at all. To purchase Tru-Bond epoxy, check to see if your local True Value Hardware store stocks it. It may be necessary to call the company headquarters for the nearest authorized dealer or store.

In some situations, you may need to use a *contact cement* in your home. Contact cement is a synthetic adhesive. To use it, both surfaces to be joined are coated with adhesive, the glue is allowed to dry, then the surfaces are brought into contact with each other, creating a permanent bond.

In homes, contact cement is commonly used to attach a hard plastic laminate (Formica is one popular brand) to a man-made wood product (such as particleboard) in order to create a countertop (see *High Pressure Plastic Laminate Countertops* in *Chapter 5: Interior Decorating*). Unfortunately, most typical contact cements have a very strong odor. However, fairly recently, much less odorous and much less hazardous water-based versions have been developed. One you might want to try is Elmer's Saf-T Contact Cement (**Elmer's Adhesives Division of Borden, Inc.**) This particular brand is actually labeled as nontoxic. To purchase it or other similar brands, check your local hardware stores and building centers.

Wallpaper Pastes

When you're wallpapering, you can use one of the wheat or other vegetable-starch wallpaper pastes that are still available at many local wallpaper stores. However, you should be aware that some of these products may contain fungicides that act as mold inhibitors or biocides to deter insects, bacteria, and mold. Unfortunately, some of these chemical fungicides and biocides can be odorous or otherwise bothersome to certain people.

Interestingly, Golden Harvest Wheat Paste (**Golden Harvest**) is one all-natural wallpaper paste that doesn't contain fungicides or biocides. By the way, the company recommends that it not be used with vinyl or foil papers. This is because these types of wallpapers are nonporous and, therefore, the surface can't breathe. As a result, they don't permit the wet wallpaper paste underneath to dry very quickly. Thus, without chemicals to prevent fungal growth, mold problems can quickly develop within the paste. To buy Golden Harvest Wheat Paste, check with your local wallpaper store or call the company for a nearby dealer.

Of course, some people may want to make their own wallpaper paste by simply mixing wheat starch and water. If you do, however, it's a good idea to add one tablespoon of boric acid powder to each quart of paste (this also can be added to any prepackaged all-natural wallpaper paste). Boric acid has innate mold- and insect-inhibiting qualities, yet it doesn't seem to bother most sensitive people.

You'll find you can usually purchase boric acid at your local drugstore. Although it's considered safer than many petrochemical pesticides, you should still realize it's not a totally nontoxic substance. Therefore, children or pets should not have access to boric-acid powder or any of the wallpaper paste containing it.

Drywall Compounds

Many people assume that drywall compounds are simple all-natural, completely harmless substances. Actually, this is not the case. Although drywall compounds are made primarily of gypsum with some mica, talc, limestone, and clay, they also contain vinyl adhesives, fungicide preservatives, and often antifreeze. In addition, up until 1977 some drywall compounds also contained asbestos.

Unfortunately, because of their many ingredients, most typical modern drywall compounds tend to have relatively strong odors, especially when wet. As a result, some sensitive individuals have been bothered for months (or years) by walls coated with typical drywall compounds. (It should be noted that typical drywall compounds are usually marketed as a thick, mud-like paste in plastic tubs.)

Fortunately, alternative drywall compounds are now available. One of these is Murco M100 All Purpose Joint Cement (**Murco Wall Products, Inc.**). It contains no fungicides, preservatives, formaldehyde, or petroleum-derived solvents. Therefore, this particular product is generally well-tolerated by even the most sensitive individuals. In fact, it's almost odor-free even when wet. Murco M100 can also be used to texturize walls and ceilings and for minor spackling jobs.

Unlike many typical drywall compounds, Murco M100 is packaged in bags as a dry powder that must be mixed with water just prior to use. Because it's fungicide-free, once mixed, it should not be stored for more than a day. Important note: This particular product should not be used on walls that will have an alcohol-based paint or sealant coating applied directly over the drywall. Apparently, the ingredients in Murco M100 can chemically react with alcohol. This can eventually lead to cracking and crazing. If you'd like to purchase Murco M100, it can be ordered directly from the company or from **Nontoxic Environments**.

Another alternative drywall compound is AFM Joint Compound (**American Formulating and Manufacturing**), which was originally created for chemically sensitive individuals. AFM Joint Compound can be used for drywall finishing and for spackling as well. It's sold in quart, gallon, and five-gallon sizes. If you'd like to try it, it can be ordered from AFM dealers such as **Nontoxic Environments**, **N.E.E.D.S.**, and **Flowright International Products**.

Thinset Ceramic Tile Mortars

Thinset mortars—also known as dry-set mortars—are cement-like adhesives used to adhere ceramic tile to a base material. Unfortunately, some typical thinset mortars are very odorous because of various additives. The precise ingredients are usually considered trade secrets by manufacturers so it's impossible to say exactly what they are, but they likely include fungicides (to retard mold growth) and a variety of other substances to prevent cracking and crumbling. At any rate, the odors from these ingredients are particularly strong when the thinset mortar is wet. Fortunately, sometimes the ceramic tile and the grout in the joints will successfully seal in any residual odors— but not always.

One brand of thinset ceramic-tile mortar that has often worked well for adhering tile to a variety of surfaces with minimal odor is Multi-Cure (**C-Cure Chemical Co.**). In addition, the company makes other kinds of thinset mortars with fewer additives than Multi-Cure. Although these are more tolerable than Multi-Cure, they can't be used in as many applications. Often, you'll find C-Cure thinsets are sold in local ceranic-tile stores. If you have trouble finding them, call the company for its nearest dealer. Important note: Multi-Cure is made in several factories across the U.S., and some use more noxious additives than others.

If you're interested in specially formulated alternative thin-set mortars, **Nontoxic Environments** handles several you might want to try. One of these is Additive-Free Thinset. If interested in any of these products, call them for more information on what surfaces these can be used, etc.

Important note: If you plan to use Multi-Cure or any thinset mortar, it's extremely important to test it first, especially if you're a sensitive individual. To do this, first purchase a large, odor-free patio block. On its backside, write down the date and the brand of thinset you plan to test (as well as the type of grout and tile). Then, simply apply a layer of thinset mortar to the topside of the patio block. Next, adhere some of the same ceramic tile you plan to use in your upcoming home project. When the thinset mortar is dry, you can then apply the grout to the joints, making sure that none of the thinset mortar is left uncovered around the edges of the patio block. (Of course, if the grout is a type that requires damp-curing, you'll need to mist the tile/grout surface and cover it with plastic sheeting. For more on this, see *Ceramic Tile Installation* in *Chapter 5: Interior Decorating.*)

After the grout has cured, you can then very lightly sniff the surface of the sample block. If there's an odor, wait a week and lightly sniff it again. Repeat this until no odor is detected. At that point, you can put the sample block on your night stand. If you sleep well through the night, it usually means you can easily tolerate the thinset, grout, and tile. Finally, you'll need to note this date on the backside of the patio block.

By the way, a nontoxic grout of water, sand, and Portland cement can be used in many of your ceramic tile projects by following the directions listed in *Healthy House Building* by John Bower. This grout must be damp cured because it has no additives. The book is available from the **Healthy House Institute**. In addition, prepackaged alternative grouts can be ordered from **Nontoxic Interiors**.

Caulkings

Typically, caulkings are usually very odorous, especially while being applied. Unfortunately, the odor can sometimes linger for a long time afterwards. This shouldn't be too surprising upon realizing that most modern caulking products contain a variety of synthetic petroleum-derived ingredients. As a result, a caulking could release acetone, methyl ethyl ketone, methyl porpionate, and a variety of other noxious substances into the air, depending on the exact type and brand.

One hundred percent silicone caulkings are often suggested for sensitive individuals. Silicone is actually a synthetic product consisting of alternating oxygen and silicon atoms. This particular molecular combination results in a material that's both rubbery and very stable. As a result, silicone caulkings are resistant to high temperatures and water. Although most 100%-silicone caulkings are quite strong-smelling when first applied, once they're dry they are often quite inert. However, the main reason they've been recommended to sensitive persons for some time now is that they're quite durable, so they don't have to be replaced for many years. One serious drawback to 100%-silicone caulking is that it can't be painted. Fortunately, some brands are now made in white, brown, and a few other basic colors besides clear. If you're interested in purchasing a 100%-silicone caulking, its usually sold in most local hardware stores and building centers.

An interesting alternative to typical construction-grade 100%-silicone caulkings are aquarium-grade silicone caulkings. These caulkings have been specially formulated so as not to harm fish or plants. Therefore, they are often more tolerable to sensitive individuals. To buy aquarium caulking, check with local pet centers and tropical-fish shops.

In situations where it's desirable to paint the caulking, you might try a latex caulking. However, you should be aware that latex caulkings (which contain natural or synthetic rubber among other ingredients) have a definite odor when they're being applied, which could persist for a few days or a few weeks. As it turns out, a real advantage to latex caulkings is that unlike silicone caulkings, drips and smears can be easily cleaned up with water—that is, if they haven't had a chance to dry yet. But one real disadvantage to latex caulkings is that they're not nearly as durable as their 100%-silicone counterparts. If you're interested in using a latex caulking, virtually all hardware stores and building centers stock them.

A paintable caulking often tolerated by sensitive people is Phenoseal Adhesive Caulking (**Glouster Company, Inc.**). This particular brand is actually a type of polyvinyl-acetate emulsion that is similar to that of common white glues such as Elmer's Glue-All. Like other latex caulks, Phenoseal requires only water cleanup for wet drips or smears, and it too has an odor that can be noticeable for a period of time after it's been applied. However, some people feel that this type of caulk is more acceptable for sensitive individuals than other caulking products.

Around your bathtub and/or sink, you may want to try Kwik Seal caulking (**Dap Products, Inc.**). This particular product has a mildew-resistant formula that is important in persistently wet locales where mold can grow quickly. Of course, some people would prefer to use products in their homes that contained no fungicides. However, around tubs and sinks, the problems arising from inevitable mildew and mold colonization are likely far worse than any that could arise from the antifungal chemicals. Fortunately, you should know that despite containing fungicide additives, Kwik Seal often becomes nearly odor-free within a week. This brand of caulking is sold in many local hardware stores and building centers. However, if you have trouble finding it, contact the manufacturer for its nearest dealer.

Note: Because of the odors and ingredients in most caulkings, it's best to following certain precautions when using them. Above all, have plenty of ventilation when you're applying them. Also, it's a good idea to wear a chemical respirator mask (see *Protective Gear* above). It should be stressed that the actual time that will be required for any caulking product to become odorless will depend on the brand, the amount used, the temperature, the relative humidity (see *High Relative Humidity* in *Chapter 9: Indoor Air*), and your individual tolerability.

Lubricants

Many typical lubricating products are extremely odorous. This is often because they're usually petroleum-based products. Therefore, they're often bothersome or even intolerable to sensitive individuals for months or even years. Fortunately, however, certain lubricants are now available that have very little odor. These can often be used satisfactorily in a number of situations— but certainly not in all.

Some simple low-odor lubricating options to use on your cabinet and door hinges include petroleum jelly, pharmaceutical-grade mineral oil, or natural plant oils such as jojoba. However, although all of these products can lubricate, they can also leave behind greasy stains. In addition, some of them, in time, will become gummy, and some natural oils can eventually become rancid or attract mold or bacteria. However, if you'd like to try one of these options, they're not difficult to find. Petroleum jelly and pharmacy-grade mineral oil are available at drugstores. Jojoba and other plant oils are usually sold in health-food stores, and some cosmetic departments, or they can be mail-ordered from **Common Sense Products.**

As another option, household graphite lubricating products often work well to lubricate hinges and latches. Graphite lubricants are actually composed of fine carbon particles. Generally, pure-graphite lubricants have only nominal odor and never become gummy or rancid. Unfortunately, graphite's big drawback is that it often leaves sooty black dust and smears where it was applied. If you're interested in purchasing a graphite lubricant, check your local hardware store for the brands it carries. Look for a product that contains no oil.

One lubricating product that's very good at stopping metal-to-metal squeaks, and at the same time is often well-tolerated by sensitive individuals, is E-Z-1 Lubricant (**E-Z-1, Inc.**). This nearly odorless, synthetic liquid product comes in small, resealable tubes. E-Z-1 is apparently solvent-free and it can't conduct electricity. It's also able to penetrate a certain amount of corrosion. To top it off, E-Z-1 is biodegradable. You might find this product in local hardware stores. If not, it can be mail-ordered from **E.L. Foust Co., Inc.** or directly from the manufacturer.

For machinery, clocks, or any other mechanical devices that require periodic lubrication, it is often wise to use only the type of lubricant recommended by the manufacturer. Unfortunately, in most cases this means you'll have to use an odorous petroleum-based product. However, if you substitute another kind of lubricant and it doesn't do its job well, it could result in damage as well as voiding of any product warranties or guarantees. Of course, you can place newly lubricated equipment outdoors in dry, uncontaminated surroundings, or indoors in an infrequently used room with good ventilation until they become more tolerable. In cases where the lubricated item remains bothersome (as with a sewing machine), you might consider using a fan situated so that it blows across the machine and away from your face. This should help dispel the oily smells. And a final note: if at all possible, purchase items that never require lubrication.

Foil Barriers

Many times, sensitive people find they need large aluminum-foil sheets to block certain objectionable odors in their homes. This is often for a temporary situation, but it can also be semipermanent. Rather than taping together several strips of heavy-duty household aluminum foil, use *builder's foil*. This is a fairly durable product that is often sold as a *reflective insulation/vapor barrier*. It is actually a "sandwich" consisting of brown Kraft paper with a thin layer of aluminum applied to each side. Builder's foil often comes in 36" wide rolls.

One brand you might want to use is Dennyfoil (**Denny Sales Corp.**), which is offered by mail order from **E.L. Foust Co., Inc.**, **The Living Source**, and **Nontoxic Environments**, among others. In addition, **Nontoxic Environments** also sells KShield Foil. This particular product is approximately twice as heavy as Dennyfoil and comes in two roll lengths and 16", 24", and 48" widths. Of course, you may want to check with local lumberyards and building centers to see what reflective-foil insulation products are carried. These products tend to be more popular in warm, sunny climates. By the way, to adhere builder's foil, simply use aluminum duct tape (see *Tapes* above).

Another foil product that you might want to use is *aluminized sheathing*. This is a much more substantial material than builder's foil. It's constructed of an $1/8$"-thick, gray, cardboard core with an aluminum-foil layer on each side. This foil-faced sheathing generally comes in 4' x 8' sheets. Two brands are Thermo-Ply (**Simplex Products Division**) and Denny Board (**Denny Sales Corp.**). Check your local lumberyard or building center to see if they handle either of these products, or call the companies for nearby dealers.

Wood

Of course, many home projects require wood construction. However, there are some basic guidelines for storing and using wood that are always good to know and follow. First, all wood should be stored flat and in a dry area. This will minimize warping and possible mildew growth. Also, when you sand or saw wood, it's always wise to wear a cartridge-type respirator mask rather than merely a simple, inexpensive paper dust mask (see *Protective Gear* above). This is because newly cut wood can release natural but irritating compounds as well sawdust.

(Note: For more suggestions and precautions for using wood, see the appropriate sections in *Chapter 5: Interior Decorating*.)

Man-made Wood Products

In an ideal healthy home interior, there would probably be no man-made wood products. This means no plywood, no particleboard, and no sheets of wall paneling. Admittedly these materials have real pluses associated with them—they're relatively cheap, often made of wood that would otherwise be wasted (inferior logs, mill scraps, sawdust etc.), they resist warping, and in some cases are stronger than solid wood.

However, typical man-made wood products have health-related drawbacks, especially for sensitive people. For example, they're nearly always made of softwoods (primarily pine or fir) that can release strong-smelling natural terpenes when they're newly cut or sanded. These can be irritating and bothersome to sensitive persons. Even worse, man-made wood products are generally held together with formaldehyde glues. Unfortunately, formaldehyde can cause a wide variety of health problems from nasal irritation and respiratory problems, to menstrual irregularities and cancer (see *Formaldehyde* in *Chapter 9: Indoor Air*).

Sadly, formaldehyde will likely be emitted from man-made wood products for many years. This is because the formaldehyde glues used can have a half-life of 3–5 years. In other words, in three to five years after the cabinets are first made, only half of the formaldehyde that was originally in them will have been released into the air. In the next three to five years, half of the remaining formaldehyde will be emitted. And so on. Therefore, many man-made wood items are ongoing, long-term problems.

However, you should be aware that there are actually two basic types of formaldehyde-based glues. *Phenol-formaldehyde (PF)* glues are generally used in products designed for use outdoors and in construction-grade plywood. As it turns, out PF glues only emit about 10% as much formaldehyde as the other popular formaldehyde-based glue, *urea-formaldehyde (UF)* glue. UF glues are often used for indoor construction and are common in cabinet-grade plywood. Obviously, if you must use a man-made wood product containing a formaldehyde glue, you'll want to choose one that's held together with PF glue rather than UF glue.

You should also know that although typical plywood (construction grade or not) is definitely a source of formaldehyde, typical particleboard is a far worse emitter. That's because much more glue is required to make particleboard than other man-made wood products. Unfortunately, the glue that's usually used is the UF type and the use of particleboard continues to expand. Because it's cheaper than plywood (after all, it's only composed of tiny wood scraps and glue), builders often use it for the sub floor and it is widely used in cabinets. As a result, typical UF particleboard is often a major source of formaldehyde in new homes.

Fortunately, there are alternative particleboard products now available that can be substituted for typical particleboard products, and sometimes typical plywood products as well. Two of these are Medex and Medite II (**Medite Corporation**). These particular particleboard products are actually made with a non-formaldehyde glue. However, the softwood terpenes they release could still make these particleboard products intolerable for certain sensitive individuals. Therefore, if you are thinking of using an alternative particleboard, you'll want to test it for personal tolerance before you purchase a large quantity (see *Testing Woods* above). In the end, you might find that a better choice would be to use a tolerable solid wood whenever you can. If you'd like to try using Medex or Medite II, contact the company for its nearest dealer.

Solid Wood

As a rule, solid wood is often preferable to man-made wood products from an aesthetic as well as a health standpoint. After all, solid wood has an innate beauty that is pleasing to look at and to touch. And being solid, it's not constructed with formaldehyde glues or any other type of glue for that matter. (Of course, individual narrow boards are often glued together to create a wide panel, but this is often done with a less-toxic carpenter's glue.)

However, there are certain drawbacks to solid wood you should keep in mind. First, as compared to man-made wood products, solid wood is relatively expensive. Although you can purchase construction grade wood (which is a more economical grade of solid wood), the boards in this category often have large knots, actual holes, or other deformities in them. Also, you should know that most solid wood is somewhat susceptible to warping and this often creates problems of wasted, unusable lumber.

Of course, another drawback to solid wood is that it's sold as individual boards—not in large 4' x 8' sheets. Therefore, solid-wood boards can't be used to cover large areas quickly. As a result, using solid wood can increase both material and labor costs. Also, solid wood can significantly expand or shrink due to changing temperature and humidity conditions. As a result, people who plan on using solid wood must account for this in their project's design and construction.

If you choose to use solid wood, it's wise to become familiar with the two basic categories: softwoods and hardwoods. Softwoods are *conifers*, or cone-bearing trees, having needles or scalelike leaves. Hardwoods are defined as broad-leafed trees. Confusingly, the terms hardwood and softwood don't always describe the firmness or density of a particular wood. As it turns out, certain hardwoods are actually be softer than many softwoods. For example, balsa is botanically classified as a hardwood. However, as a general rule, most softwoods are softer than most hardwoods.

Common softwood lumber (pine or fir boards) is generally cheaper, comes in more standardized sizes, and is more readily available than hardwood lumber. Therefore, virtually all major construction projects use softwood lumber. Unfortunately, pine and fir can emit strong and sometimes irritating natural hydrocarbon terpenes when they're newly cut or sanded. These odors can be very bothersome to certain sensitive people. Interestingly, some individuals have reported that between pine and fir lumber, fir seemed to be better tolerated. Unfortunately, finding out whether the softwood lumber you're about to purchase is actually pine or fir can be difficult. In most cases, the differences are actually relatively minor.

Generally, if a softwood—whether pine, spruce, hemlock, etc. or fir—is used for framing a house, its odors may not pose a problem because the wood is enclosed inside wall cavities. If *foil-backed drywall* is used to cover the framing and the house is tightly constructed, the odors will be prevented from entering the living space.

If you're bothered by terpene odors, softwood lumber that is used within the living space (such as in cabinets, furniture, and tongue-and-groove paneling, etc.) is of more concern. Fortunately, in time, any emissions from the wood will naturally diminish. But if you want to immediately reduce the terpene odors, you can always apply a sealant finish over any exposed softwood surfaces (see *Sealants and Other Acrylic Water-Based Wood Finishes* above). However, bear in mind that these types of products can't form a 100% seal and they are often very odorous in their own right.

One softwood that's often well-tolerated by some sensitive individuals is redwood. Although redwood is a softwood, it emits fewer irritating odors than other softwood species. This may be because redwood's terpenes are water-soluble, so within a relatively short time after it has been cut or sanded, its odor diminishes greatly. A well-known plus for redwood is that it resists termite damage and rot. If you use it outdoors, for patio furniture for example, it'll weather naturally so no protective finish is actually required, although you might choose to use one anyway if you don't like the weathered, dull-gray color.

In fact, from a health standpoint, redwood is a superior choice for any outdoor project than the more popular *salt-treated* softwood lumber. Few people realize that this benign-sounding descriptive phrase—"salt treated"—doesn't mean table salt (sodium chloride), but a very toxic copper-arsenic salt. During its manufacture, salt-treated lumber has had these salts driven deeply into it through increased pressure. Therefore, this type of wood is also known as *pressure-treated* lumber. Obviously, redwood is a far safer material for you and your family to be around.

Yet, for some projects inside your home, you probably won't want to use redwood. This is because it's fairly soft, making it susceptible to dings, scratches, and nicks. In addition, there are some environmental concerns related to cutting down redwood trees. However, redwood is still commonly used indoors in saunas (see *Choosing Tolerable Sauna Materials and Equipment* in *Chapter 6: Lifestyle*).

If you're bothered by softwood terpene odors, it's often best to use hardwoods for those projects that will be kept inside the living space. Although hardwood lumber costs more than softwood lumber, it's generally far more attractive and durable. Therefore, hardwood lumber is ideal for use in flooring, furniture, wall treatments, cabinets, etc.

However, be aware that certain hardwood species are naturally less odorous than others. Some of these low-odor hardwood species include apple, aspen, basswood, beech, birch, elm, gum, maple, pecan, sycamore, and tulip poplar, among others. Though not always easy to find, these woods are often suggested for some sensitive persons to use instead of the more popular red oak, white oak, and walnut, which have stronger natural odors. Of course, the emissions from all woods will decrease in time, and you can always coat them with a sealant as was described with softwoods earlier.

Tulip poplar is one hardwood with which you might want to especially become familiar. The lumber from this species presents an interesting variegated pattern of tones that's rather similar to pine. Although it's somewhat greenish when newly cut, the wood changes to an attractive tan as it ages. Tulip poplar is also quite affordable, often fairly easy to find (this will vary in different parts of the country, of course), and it's very easy to work with. Therefore, it can be an excellent wood for many projects. However, it is one of the softer hardwood species.

Important note: It's always a good idea to test a wood species for personal tolerance before you use it for a home project, especially if you're a sensitive person (see *Testing Woods* above).

THE GARAGE

Garages are often forgotten places in terms of health. However, they really shouldn't be. As everyone knows, many of today's garages are directly attached to a house. These generally have entry doors that open into a homes' living space. Some houses also have bedrooms that are located directly above an attached garage. Unfortunately, an attached garage can mean health problems if automibile exhaust gases or gasoline odors (among others) migrate from the garage, through tiny openings in the walls, around an unsealed entry door, or even around light fixtures in the garage ceiling and enter the living space (see *Combustion Gases* and *Volatile Organic Compounds* in *Chapter 9: Indoor Air*).

The truth is, the majority of attached garages have not been designed or built to prevent garage-generated pollutants from passing indoors. And this is true no matter the age of the house or how much it cost. In fact, if there is an entry door between the living quarters and the garage, a certain amount of garage air will enter the house whenever the door is opened. Therefore, some safe housing experts believe that healthy houses should have detached rather than attached garages. Of course, with proper sealing techniques, it is possible to isolate the garage from the house, but this is rarely done (for more on sealing, read *Healthy House Building: A Design and Construction Guide* by John Bower, which is available from **The Healthy House Institute**).

If you live in a home with an attached garage, there are several positive steps you can take to minimize any potential air-quality problems. These are covered in the following sections. By the way, some of this information can also be applied to detached garages so that they can become safer and healthier spaces as well. Other sections discuss the environment inside an automobile itself.

GARAGE ORGANIZATION AND SAFETY

One simple way to make your garage safer and healthier is to keep it both clean and well-organized. Doing this will lessen the accumulation of dust and debris, and therefore, potential pest habitats. It'll also lower your risk of tripping accidents. The first step in doing this is to actually discard (or sell, or give away) all the "stuff" you don't really need or will likely not use again. Remember, however, you'll want to properly dispose of any items considered "household hazardous waste" such as pesticides and other petroleum-based products. To learn what procedures to follow, contact your local sanitation department or board of health.

To conveniently store items you intend to keep, consider buying metal cabinets with doors. These cabinets work well at holding tools, hoses, sprinklers, car-cleaning products, etc. You'll find that these are available at most office-supply and discount stores. They're sometimes also sold at **Sears, Roebuck and Co.** stores and some hardware stores. Note: Metal storage cabinets with locking mechanisms or ones that are designed to accept a padlock are excellent choices if children are around your home.

In addition, heavy-duty metal-mesh shelving units designed for mounting on walls can also provide good, solid storage sites. Sometimes these are handled by local hardware or department stores. If not, **Hold Everything** is one mail-order source for them. Then, too, you might consider using sturdy wall-mounted metal brackets to hang your rakes and other long-handled tools. Again, some neighborhood hardware stores may sell them or you can order them through **The Vermont Country Store**, among other catalogs (for more storage ideas, see *Household Storage* in *Chapter 8: Housekeeping*).

Finally, for proper fire safety, you'll want to make sure your garage is equipped with a multipurpose fire extinguisher (see *Portable Fire Extinguisher Types* in *Chapter 8: Housekeeping*). You'll want to keep this in a prominent place. From time to time you'll need to remember to check its gauge to see if it's properly charged.

CONTROLLING ODORS WITHIN GARAGES

Most garages contain a variety of products and devices that can generate polluting odors. However, of all the potential airborne contaminants, gasoline and oil odors, along with combustion gases, are perhaps the most dangerous. These odors are not just unpleasant smelling; they're also toxic (see *Combustion Gases* and *Volatile Organic Compounds* in *Chapter 9: Indoor Air*). In addition, evaporated gasoline can explode if concentrations are high enough. As was mentioned earlier, houses with attached garages will likely have these pollutants entering their living quarters fairly regularly.

Fortunately, you can help lessen these air-pollution problems by following some simple precautions. One is to only fill gasoline-powered machinery outside your garage. Also, start all motorcycles, chain saws, trimmers, and lawn mowers outdoors. In addition, after using any combustion-driven item, shut it off and let it cool outdoors, and only then bring it inside your garage.

Another precaution you might consider is to place vehicular mats under parked cars, trucks, and motorcycles that are stored inside your garage. These can capture oil and other drips of fluid from leaking transmissions, cooling systems, brake lines, etc. before they become absorbed into your concrete garage floor. Such mats are commonly available at auto-supply stores. These mats often need to be replaced or cleaned from time to time.

If oil or other fluids do end up on your garage's concrete floor, you might try sprinkling unscented, clay, cat-box litter on them. The litter material should be left on the floor long enough to have a chance to absorb the liquid, then swept up, and disposed of properly. If you want to purchase unscented, clay cat litter, it can sometimes be purchased at local pet-supply stores. Also, **The Natural Animal** is a mail-order source.

To help minimize auto exhaust odors inside your garage, you might want to follow this procedure. After pulling your car into the garage, turn off the ignition and leave the garage door open for 15–30 minutes. If this isn't possible, you should consider installing in your garage a ventilation fan with its own crank timer. These timers are designed so they can be manually set to shut off the fan after a preset time—say half an hour. Crank timers themselves are generally relatively inexpensive to purchase and install. If you're interested, **Broan** and **Nutone/Scovill** are two ventilation-fan/timer manufacturers. However, there are many others.

If you have a forced-air furnace in the garage, make sure all the ducts are properly sealed. Otherwise, garage odors can be pulled into the leaky ducts and blown into the living space.

Finally, make sure that any entry door that leads directly into your home's living quarters is kept completely shut except when it's actually being used to enter or leave your house or garage. Also, it's important that the door be properly weather-stripped. The doors that often do the best job of sealing have magnetic weather-stripping, like a refrigerator. Check local building-supply outlets for availability.

THE CAR

If you're like many Americans, the interior of your automobile is a place where you spend a lot of time. So, it should be as healthy as possible. The following sections suggest some ways to lessen any problems that could arise.

CAR CARE

Most typical car-care products are odorous and/or potentially harmful. Fortunately, there are healthier alternatives.

Typical Car-Cleaning Products

Many typical products used to clean car interiors and exteriors have formulas containing dangerous petrochemical solvents. These volatile organic compounds (VOCs) can cause a range of negative health effects if inhaled (see *Volatile Organic Compounds* in *Chapter 9: Indoor Air*). Not surprisingly, a great many car-care products are labeled "hazardous" and have a list of warnings on them. If you find you simply must use one of these products, apply it to your car outside the garage while wearing a chemical respirator mask (see *Protective Gear* above).

Unfortunately, one particularly bothersome solution that's hard to avoid is windshield washing fluid. So, if at all possible, never dispense the cleaning fluid if your car's windows or air vents are open even just a little. And once you've squirted it, wait until the fluid has completely evaporated or washed off by rain or snow before allowing the exterior air to come inside again through the vents. Of course, if outdoor temperatures are above freezing, you can simply use water as a windshield washing fluid.

Alternative Car-Cleaning Products

You might be surprised to learn that baking soda and water can harmlessly and effectively perform a number of car-cleaning jobs. For example, a sponge or soft cotton cloth saturated with a solution of 4 tablespoons of baking soda dissolved in 1 quart warm water can clean your car's chrome trim and mirrors. When done, rinse them with clear water. By the way, you can use this same solution (and procedure) to clean your car's vinyl upholstery, wiper blades, and floor mats.

Manufacturers now offer alternative car-cleaning products. Some of these might be handled by auto-supply stores in your area. (Note, remember to read the product labels carefully to see if they really are safer products.) By mail order, **enviro-clean** is one source for a number of "earth-friendly" car-cleaning products. These include car-wash concentrates, upholstery cleaners, and waxes (for other cleaning products and procedures applicable to cars, see appropriate sections in *Chapter 7: Cleaning*).

Rustproofing

As everyone knows, car-rustproofing treatments are done to help prevent corrosion of the steel parts making up an automobile. Although many cars are now automatically rustproofed as part of their manufacturing process, some car owners still feel that additional treatment is necessary. Of course, this is especially true for those people who live in coastal areas and in locations where road salt is commonly used.

No matter who performs the rustproofing, if your car is properly treated, it likely will look good for years, and you're more likely to keep it longer. Being able to keep your car longer is very important for many sensitive individuals. This is because it sometimes can take up to three years for some sensitive persons to become comfortable with the interior of a new car. Unfortunately, after three years, many non-rustproofed cars begin to show rust, so trading them in at this time is common.

While the procedure should make your car last longer, there's also a downside to rustproofing. This is because nearly all rustproofing compounds are thick, greasy or waxy petroleum-based coatings. Not surprisingly, these gummy chemicals release very strong odors. As a result, a newly treated car will end up being surrounded by these odors for several weeks or more. You should also be aware that some rustproofing companies recoat the vehicles annually, rather than merely perform a simple visual inspection on them. Therefore, coping with persistent rustproofing odors could become a yearly event.

Something you might want to consider is having the rustproofing done during the hottest time of the year. This way the very warm air can help dispel the rustproofing odors as quickly as possible. While the odors will end up being more intense than if the treatment was done during colder weather, they'll generally linger for a much shorter period of time. (Note, some sensitive persons would actually prefer that the odors were less intense and lasted longer; this is a definitely a case of personal preference.)

After any rustproofing has been performed keep your car parked outdoors rather than inside your garage for a while, if at all possible. This is for two reasons: 1) so your car can air out faster outside, and 2) you probably don't want to fill you garage with noxious chemical odors if you don't have to. In addition, provide good ventilation within the car while this airing-out process is going on. It should be mentioned that a car air filter may help lessen somewhat any rustproofing odors that seep into the interior (see *Car Interior Air Filters* below).

CAR-INTERIOR ODOR CONCERNS

Car interiors are often unhealthy environments for a variety of reasons. In the sections below, common pollution sources are discussed as well as things that can be done to help improve the air within your car.

New Car Interior Concerns

New car interiors can outgas large quantities of synthetic chemicals, primarily from their stain-proofed synthetic carpets and upholstery. Other sources of airborne pollution are the vinyls and plastics used in dashboards and door and ceiling panels. To help speed up the release of these gases, you might want to consider buying your new car only in a hot-weather month. That way, you may be able to let the car "bake" in the sun with the doors and windows open for extended periods of time.

To help reduce the outgassing from the carpeting, you may want to use a carpet sealant on it. One brand is SafeChoice Carpet Guard (**American Formulating and Manufacturing**), which is handled by most AFM dealers including **Flowright Products International**, **Nontoxic Environments**, **N.E.E.D.S.**, and **The Living Source**. However, you should be aware that carpet sealants can't seal in 100% of the chemicals released by carpeting. Therefore, a sealant simply may not be effective enough for certain sensitive individuals. You also should bear in mind that these products add their own odors to the carpet, which must also air out. This alone could take several weeks or even months, depending on your own personal reaction to them. As an alternative, some sensitive people have simply removed all the carpeting.

Sensitive individuals often deliberate whether to purchase a car with cloth, vinyl, or leather upholstery. Actually, many sensitive persons have found that leather interiors are fairly tolerable to them. Yet for a few, leather interiors are much too odorous (for more on leather, see *Leather* in *Chapter 3: Clothing*). The truth is, there is no simple answer. In the end, each person must ultimately choose the car upholstery material that seems to suit him (or her) best. Of course, sitting in cars with different types of upholstery should help you reach a decision. However, in actuality, most sensitive individuals will find any new car upholstery to be problematic, whether leather, vinyl, or fabric. Unhappily, for them it may take several years before a new car interior is no longer bothersome.

However, there are a few measures you can take to make your car's upholstery more acceptable to you. For example, you could drape cotton barrier cloth over the seats. This is a special type of cotton fabric that's very densely woven so that many odors are unable to pass through it. Mail-order sources for cotton barrier cloth include **The Cotton Place** and **Janice Corp**. Or you might purchase organic 100%-cotton car seat pads from **Dona Designs**. Also, you might be interested in the natural-sheepskin bucket-seat covers and steering wheel covers sold by **The Aussie Connection**. A line of similar sheepskin items is carried by **Heart of Vermont**. Though it can be expensive and time-consuming, some sensitive people have completely reupholstered the interior of their car with less toxic materials.

Car Interior Air Filters and Ionizers

Many sensitive individuals are inclined to use an air filter or ionizer in their car. However, it's important to realize that these devices can only reduce the airborne pollutants found within the car's interior—they cannot totally eliminate them.

Car Interior Air Filters

Several air filters are available for cars that may interest sensitive people. These units generally operate on 12 volts by plugging into the dashboard's cigarette lighter. Some models come with special adapters to allow them to be used on standard 110-volt house current as well. Although it's probably not a good idea to use an adapter on a continuous basis, having one on your car filter could be useful for a stay overnight in a motel room or at a friend's house, for example.

One popular car interior filter is the #160 Auto Air Purifier (**E.L. Foust Co., Inc.**). This unit is essentially a metal, cylindrical canister containing about three pounds of activated charcoal, which is effective in removing many types of chemical odors. If a special charcoal mix is ordered, formaldehyde can be removed as well (see *Activated Charcoal/Activated Alumina Filters* and *Form-aldehyde* in *Chapter 9: Indoor Air*). The #160 unit can be ordered directly from the company.

Another activated-charcoal filtering device is the Aireox Model 22D Car Air Purifier (**Aireox Research Corp.**). This particular filter is constructed with a white-enameled metal housing. It can be ordered directly from the company or from distributors including **N.E.E.D.S.** and **earthsake**.

You might also want to consider an Autoaire II unit (**AllerMed Corp.**). This is a 10" x 10" x 9" metal unit containing two filters (one is an activated-charcoal type) with a two-speed fan. The Autoaire II is designed to remove particulates such as pollen, dust, mold spores, and smoke, as well as chemical odors. You can order it from the manufacturer or from dealers such as **N.E.E.D.S.**, **Ozark Water Service and Environmental Services**, and **Nontoxic Environments**.

Although portable car filters are helpful, they can't eliminate all your car's interior odors, let alone all the smog and combustion gases that enter the car from the outdoors. Therefore, when you're in heavy traffic, it's often a good idea to close your car's exterior air vents and windows. However, you shouldn't keep them closed all the time. After all, you'll need to regularly replenish your supply of oxygen and remove any excess moisture and carbon dioxide generated by breathing.

Car Interior Negative-Ion Generators

A number of people are now purchasing negative-ion generators (also known as ionizers) for their cars. These are designed to reduce the levels of interior airborne pollution. As a rule, negative-ion generators designed for automobiles plug directly into a dashboard cigarette lighter.

All negative-ion generators, including home models, operate by producing large quantities of negatively charged electrons that attach themselves to dust, mold spores, and many minute particles. These ionized particulates then leave the air and cling to the dashboard or ceiling, etc. When these substances become attached to your car's interior surfaces, you won't be able to inhale them. However, this also means it'll be necessary to clean the inside of your car more often to remove the buildup of contaminants. Keep in mind that some of these contaminants will eventually lose their charge and become airborne again. Some ionizers come with filters that are able to trap the particles. (For a more thorough explanation of how ionizers work, see *Negative-Ion Generators* in *Chapter 9: Improving Indoor Air*.)

Sometimes you can find negative-ion generators at local auto-supply stores that are designed to sit on the dashboard or seat. However, these generally have plastic housings. One fairly popular brand of these is Amcor. In addition, there are mail-order sources for car ionizers. For example, the N-2 Car Ionizer is an extremely simple, tiny metal/glass unit. It's actually only a few inches long and somewhat resembles an old-fashioned vacuum tube. It's made to plug directly into the dashboard lighter, so it has no cord. This ionizer is available from **Pacific Spirit**. The Zestron Automobile Model negative-ion generator is a more powerful unit. This particular device is sold through **Befit Enterprises, Ltd.** in its *Cutting Edge Catalog*.

AFTERWORD

Making less-toxic living choices is essential for creating and maintaining a healthy house. Fortunately, there are now hundreds of alternative products on the market to do this. Some are labeled *biodegradable*, some *all-natural*, some *earth-friendly*, some *hypoallergenic*, and still others *scent-free*. There are also a number of alternative products you can actually make at home using simple recipes. In the end though, it's up to you to decide which particular "healthy" values are important to you and your family. Then you can purchase (or make) products accordingly. Especially if you're a sensitive person, you'll want to make sure to test any new product for personal tolerance before you use it.

Obtaining a healthier interior often means trying new procedures for cleaning, storage, and pest control. In addition, it may entail redecorating with natural fibers and materials. It could also include other changes such as installing water and air filtering equipment and taking steps to lower your electromagnetic-radiation risks.

Ultimately, I hope these chapters have shown that creating your own healthy household is not difficult to do. Of course, there are also other books, literature, consulting services, organizations, and catalogs available for further help if you should need it and these are listed in the appendices that follow.

I know that once you've worked towards improving your home's indoor environment, you'll be glad you did. Although this world doesn't hold any guarantees, the odds are that your new healthier household will mean a healthier and perhaps even a happier life for you and your family. What better goals could there possibly be?

Lynn Marie Bower

APPENDIX 1
THE SAFE HAVEN

A number of very sensitive individuals find that they require a *safe haven* within their own home. The following sections discuss what a safe haven actually is and how you can go about making one.

WHY CREATE A SAFE HAVEN?

Some people with severe allergy or Multiple Chemical Sensitivity (MCS) symptoms (see *MCS, A New Medical Condition* in *Chapter 1: Getting Started*) sometimes find it very beneficial to create a single room within their house that is ultra-safe for them. This special place is commonly termed a *safe haven,* a *refuge,* or an *oasis.* A safe haven is an uncontaminated and healthy retreat with better air quality than the rest of the home, in which the sensitive person no longer feels comfortable.

Of course, the actual reason why it's necessary to create a safe haven varies with each individual and the specific circumstances. For example, an individual might just be too ill to convert his or her entire home into a healthy house. In other situations, the other unaffected family members may decide they simply are not willing or able to give up their familiar (but toxic or bothersome) lifestyle in the rest of the home that they all share. In still other cases, a lack of money, energy, or time might prevent more than a only a small portion of a home's living space from undergoing a complete and immediate health-oriented transformation.

Whatever the reason, a safe haven can often result in beneficial effects, not only for the ill person, but also the entire family. Having a personal sanctuary for an ill person generally lessens physical *and* emotional stresses both within the person as well as the rest of the family who must cope with the sick person. Although making a safe haven can be time-consuming, it can be an extremely positive step toward giving the ill person a sense of control over his (or her) own life, and at the same time, recreating harmony within the family as a whole.

MAKING THE SAFE HAVEN

If you're ill with severe allergies or sensitivities, your physician or other personal health-care professional might prescribe or recommend a specific procedure to follow to create a safe haven. Of course, a health-care provider's suggestions will generally take precedence over the suggestions below. However, if you have no idea how to make a safe haven, the procedure given here is one you might find very helpful. (Note, in many cases sensitive people may be too ill to actually create a safe haven themselves, so it may have to be created for them by someone else.)

The first step is to decide *where* to create your safe haven. As a rule, it should be the room where you'll spend the most time. In most situations, that is a bedroom. To create a safe-haven bedroom, choose the one bedroom in the house that's already the least bothersome to you—that is, if that room can actually meet your needs. In other words, your proposed safe haven should ideally be a room that has as few obvious health problems as possible and at the same time is large enough so it that doesn't feel confining. It should be relatively near the bathroom, or better yet, have its own bathroom, as well as its own closet space. Other desirable features are a room with a good source of fresh, outdoor air, one that's fairly quiet, and one that doesn't have any trauma associated with it. This last quality may seem somewhat odd. But if being in a particular room evokes strong memories of an intensely unhappy event, it's doubtful you'll ever feel well in that room—no matter how healthful it is.

Once you've selected the room, remove all the furniture, clothing, wall decorations, curtains, and area rugs that are in it. If there's carpeting, you probably should remove it as well. Naturally, this is especially important if the carpet is new, moldy, musty smelling, or is in some other way known to be bothersome. However, you should know that removing the carpeting could be a major undertaking, especially if it has been glued down. Carpet glue is not only extremely difficult to remove from the floor, but exposing it could also create new intolerance problems that you'll have to deal with. Therefore, it's often a good idea to do some simple investigative work before attempting to remove any carpet. One way to do this is to pull back a corner of the carpeting in an inconspicuous place, such as in the closet to see how it is attached and what is under it.

Even if you find the carpeting is attached to the floor with tacks or tack strips, you'll still have to take into account what is under it. If it turns out that solid, finished hardwood floors are beneath the carpet, you're in luck because the odds are you'll immediately have a fairly attractive and tolerable floor. If concrete is beneath the carpeting, you'll still probably have an acceptable floor. (Because bare concrete is rarely very attractive, you might consider covering it with ceramic tile.) If you remove the carpeting and find a particleboard or plywood subfloor, the subfloor could end up being even more of a problem than the carpeting.

If for some reason you're stuck with an intolerable carpet, subfloor, or some other type of flooring, don't despair. Often, you can still make the room safe by covering the floor with 4' x 8' sheets of aluminum foil-faced cardboard sheathing and taping the seams with either aluminum duct tape or stainless steel tape. Doing this should effectively block most of the odors released by the objectionable floor. (See *Foil Barriers* as well as *Tapes* in *Chapter 10: Home Workshop and Garage.*) Aluminum foil-faced sheating should not be considered a permanate floor covering. While it can last for several weeks, the foil will eventually wear through due to foot traffic.

The next step in creating the safe haven is to consider washing all of the painted wall and ceiling surfaces. If you decide to go ahead and clean them, this will not only help remove any surface grease and dirt, but will also help lessen somewhat the odors of tobacco smoke, fragrances, etc. that they have absorbed. To wash the walls, use an unscented, tolerable product. One that's often acceptable is TSP (tri-sodium phosphate), which is available from most hardware and paint stores. Once the walls are completed, make sure the floor is also clean (see *Cleaning Walls, Vacuuming, Cleaning Hardwood Floors* and other appropriate sections in *Chapter 7: Cleaning*).

If you suspect you have electromagnetic sensitivities, it's best to shut off the electricity to your safe haven at night, if at all possible (see *Lowering EMF Risks in Homes* in *Chapter 11: Electromagnetic Fields*). Also, if the room has forced-air furnace and/or air conditioning registers that may be a source of mold, dust, minute amounts of combustion gases, or other substances to which you could react, temporarily tape them shut with either aluminum-foil duct tape or stainless-steel tape. If you find the room is too hot in the summer, either find a tolerable window air conditioner or use a portable fan. If the room is too cold in the winter, either find a tolerable portable electric space heater or wear heavier clothing and cover yourself with more blankets at night.

Naturally, once you've created your new safe haven, you should keep it as pristine as possible. This means using only unscented personal care products (see *Chapter 2: Personal Care*). Also, it would be wise to use only tolerable natural-fiber clothing, especially for nightclothes (see *Chapter 3: Clothing*). In addition, all your laundry should be washed in tolerable, unscented products (see *Alternative Laundry Products* in *Chapter 7: Cleaning*). Of course, your room should contain only natural, untreated, tolerable bedding (see *Chapter 4: Linens*).

MOVING INTO THE SAFE HAVEN

After emptying out and cleaning the safe haven, it's time to move in. This can be a slow process inasmuch as it involves moving in one item at a time, testing the room's tolerability with that item in it, then moving another item in, and so on. At this point, if you have known food allergies, it's especially important that you only eat tolerable items for a while. Also, if you know you have other allergies or sensitivities, everything should be done to minimize provoking them. That way, if a negative reaction occurs when you move into the room, it can easily be limited to something in the room itself and not to some other exposure. This is the only way to determine if the safe haven will actually be a healthy environment for you.

The first night you actually use the room, you may want to try sleeping with your tolerable bedding directly on the floor. This is especially important if you believe you might have trouble tolerating the bed (perfumey, musty, or otherwise bothersome frames, headboards, mattresses, or box springs, etc.). You might use several untreated 100%-cotton or 100%-wool blankets placed on top of one another to form a thin mattress. You might also consider using a tolerable futon. Another option is using an exposed-metal box spring as a bed foundation. Still another approach is to sleep on a tolerable 100%-cotton canvas cot.

The next morning, you should question yourself about how well you slept and how you generally feel. You may actually feel better. If not, you may want to wait a few days before changing anything. This is because you might still be reacting to some previous exposure that occurred before you moved into the room. After 4–7 days have passed, it is hoped that an improvement in your well-being will have occurred.

If you don't notice any improvement, you might want to bring more fresh outdoor air into the room and/or operate a tolerable portable air-purification device in the room (see *Choosing the Right Air Filter* and also *Negative Ion Generators* in *Chapter 9: Indoor Air*). If you still don't feel better, you might try using different bedding or nightclothes, etc. If that still doesn't bring any improvement, you could tape (with aluminum duct tape or stainless steel tape) reflective insulating builder's foil on all the walls and even the ceiling (see *Foil Barriers* and *Tape* in *Chapter 12: Home Workshop and Garage*). If you haven't already put 4' x 8' sheets of aluminum foil-faced cardboard sheathing on the floors, you might go ahead and cover them with this material, too. If this doesn't help, you may need to wash the aluminum surfaces with a TSP/water solution and then rinse with water (see *Cleaning Walls* in *Chapter 7: Cleaning*). This is because some foil-faced materials have a very slight oil film on them from the manufacturing process, a film that the TSP should be able to remove.

If there's still no improvement, another room in the house could be tried as a safe haven. In some cases, a room or even an entire home may have been unwittingly contaminated with a pesticide or some other substance that causes continual reactions. Therefore, moving out of the room (or perhaps moving out of the house) may be the best solution. It is possible that the overall air quality in the house is simply too bothersome to allow the creation of a safe haven. In that case, you might ask a friend or relative if you can make a safe haven room in his or her home.

Fortunately, most allergic or sensitive individuals end up feeling somewhat better after a few days in a safe haven. If you do, only introduce new items into your sanctuary gradually. Don't move all your old furniture and belongings in at once. Instead, introduce just one item at a time so you can properly test the room for personal tolerance with that item in it (see *Testing* in *Chapter 1: Getting Started*). If an item seems tolerable, wait at least four days before bringing something else into the room. Granted, this can take a considerable amount of time, but it is the best way to determine if everything in your safe haven is tolerable.

By the way, if you introduce an item and it causes a tolerance problem, you can store it somewhere until you feel stronger and then try it again later. Sensitivities change and you may find you will be able to tolerate it in a few months. However, if the item provoked a very strong negative reaction, it might be best to replace it with something less bothersome. This testing procedure will need to be repeated with all your old belongings as well as with any new ones you wish to bring inside your safe haven. In time, at least one room in your house should become a safe, comfortable, and healthy retreat for you. This will give you a place to build up your strength and improve your health.

APPENDIX 2
UTILITY AND GOVERNMENT HELP

This appendix familiarizes you with some of the assistance that's available from public utilities and government agencies that could help you in creating your healthy household.

UTILITY HELP

Often your local utilities can provide you with helpful information, and enroll you in special programs, etc. Take advantage of these if you can.

TELEPHONE COMPANY ASSISTANCE

Some telephone companies will provide a free speaker phone to their disabled customers who are unable to use standard telephones. Also, many telephone companies offer a program for people who are unable to use a phone book. This entails either free directory assistance calls or directory assistance at a minimal flat monthly fee. Often, these special services will apply to sensitive individuals who can't tolerate plastics or printed material. For more information and to see if you qualify, contact your local telephone company. Note, documentation of your medical condition may be required, which usually means merely a letter from your physician.

ELECTRIC UTILITY ASSISTANCE

If you feel your health is in danger due to EMFs from overhead or underground power lines or from a nearby substation or transformer, you can contact your local electric utility and express your concerns. Often, a representative will be sent out to evaluate and test your site for it's EMF level at little or no cost.

Your utility should also have research available on EMFs from the **Electric Power Research Institute (EPRI)**. If not, you may want to contact the EPRI directly at The Electric Power Research Institute, 3412 Hillview Ave., Palo Alto, CA 94304; (415) 855-2000.

GOVERNMENT HELP

Government agencies at all levels often have information, publications, and programs available to help you create your healthier household.

SELECTED FEDERAL GOVERNMENT AGENCIES

The following section is made up of Federal government agencies that will readily provide you information on a number of healthy household issues.

EMF Infoline (800) 363-2383

This is the telephone number of a private company contracted by EPA to provide verbal and published information about electromagnetic fields.

Environmental Drinking Water Hotline (800) 426-4791

This is the telephone number of a private company contracted by EPA. It can provide you with the name of your state certification official (except Texas). Each state certification official has a list of water-testing laboratories that meet the EPA standards and is able perform EPA-required tests.

Environmental Protection Agency (EPA) (800) 424-4000

EPA headquarters' general information number. The full address is EPA, Public Information Center-Mail Code 3404, 401 "M" Street S.W., Washington, DC 20460.

Clearing House on Disability Information (202) 205-8723

This is the U.S. Department of Education's office that provides information on government programs at Federal, state, and local levels for the disabled— including those who are disabled because of MCS. The address is Clearing House on Disability Information, Room 3132, 330 "C" Street S.W., Washington, DC 20202-2425.

National Lead Information Center (800) 532-3394

This is the EPA hotline number at which you can request printed material about lead poisoning and how to prevent it. A list of state and local agencies that have additional information is provided as well.

National Library Service for the Blind and Physically Handicapped (202) 707-5104

This is the division of the Library of Congress that can supply information on becoming a participant in the books-on-tape program. The address is National Library Service for the Blind and Physically Handicapped, The Library of Congress, Washington, DC 20542.

National Pesticide Telecommunications Network (800) 858-7378

This is a EPA-sponsored hotline number that can supply information on various pesticides. Free help is available over the phone or you will be sent printed material at a small fee. The address is NPTN, Texas Technical University-Health Science Center, Thompson Hall Room S-129, Lubbock, TX 79430.

FEDERAL INCOME-TAX DEDUCTION

It may be possible to list, as valid medical-expense deductions, certain home-remodeling expenses and/or items purchased specifically for health reasons. However, these may require a written physician's prescription that such alterations or special purchases are, in fact, medically necessary. All the bills for such items must be carefully documented. This is generally a onetime deduction. (Note that, tax laws are constantly undergoing change.)

For more information, request *IRS Publication #502: Medical and Dental Expenses*. It can be obtained by calling the IRS Forms and Publications ordering number at (800) 829-3676. For answers to your tax questions, call the IRS Information number at (800) 829-1040.

CHEMICAL INTOLERANCE HOUSING DISCRIMINATION

The U.S. Department of Housing and Urban Development has issued a policy statement recognizing Multiple Chemical Sensitivity (MCS) as a disability. For a copy of this statement, contact the National Center for Environmental Health Strategies (NCEHS) (see *Government Advocacy for MCS Individuals* for more on NCEHS below). You may also want to contact the U.S. Department of Housing and Urban Development by calling its general information number at (202) 708-1422.

To understand what housing rights disabled individuals are due, read the excellent guide *What Does Fair Housing Mean to People With Disabilities*. It can be ordered for $3.00 by writing to the Bazelon Center for Mental Health, Attn.: Publications, 1101 15th St. N.W., Suite 1212, Washington, DC 20005. The telephone number is (202) 467-5730.

CENTERS FOR INDEPENDENT LIVING (CILS)

The first Center for Independent Living (CIL) opened its doors in 1972 in Berkeley, California. Its purpose was to focus on helping the disabled function more effectively as independent individuals. The success of this program eventually led to passage of the 1978 Title VII of the Federal Rehabilitation Act, which provided funding to establish CILs across America. Now there are over 350 such centers in the U.S.

Each CIL has disabled persons on its advisory board and staff to better understand the needs of physically and mentally challenged persons. Each center provides a variety of services, which generally includes maintaining files on accessible housing, employment opportunities, appropriate social activities, etc. In addition, training courses are usually offered to help those with disabilities gain independent living skills. Peer (people with the same disability) counseling is also available for many types of disabilities. Furthermore, some centers create individual living plans for each of their disabled clients. These are outlines of specific goals for achieving effective and satisfying life routines and activities.

The extent to which any specific disability is served by a particular local CIL varies greatly. However, if you're disabled by Multiple Chemical Sensitivity (MCS), personnel at some of these centers may be able help you create a less toxic home and lifestyle.

To find a CIL near you, send $10.00 for a complete CIL directory to the Independent Living Research Utilization, 2323 S. Shephard, Suite 1000, Houston, TX 77019. The telephone number is (713) 520-0232. You may also want to contact the Rehabilitation Services Administration's Office of Independent Living at 605 "G" Street N.W., Room 840, Washington, DC 20001; (202) 727-0943. This agency keeps a listing of about 150 CILs that they fund.

ACQUIRING SOCIAL SECURITY INCOME (SSI) BENEFITS

It may be possible for you to acquire Social Security Income (SSI) benefits if you have become disabled by Multiply Chemical Sensitivity (MCS), and as a result, are unable to work. If you qualify, this program will issue you monthly income checks. As it turns out, recipients of SSI are usually then eligible for Medicaid as well as food stamps.

However, acceptance into the SSI program is not automatic. Your household income and the monetary worth of your accumulated assets (usually not including your home or car) must be below a maximum preset total limit. You must also be able to provide compelling medical substantiation for your disability. In other words, you must have convincing evidence that your condition is long term and that you're sufficiently physically and/or mentally compromised to prevent being employed.

Yet, even with a physician's statement, you still might be initially turned down for SSI, especially if you happen to have a controversial condition such as MCS. However, the Social Security Administration does provide a series of appeal procedures to present further evidence and testimony on your behalf if you've been rejected. If you're eventually successful, your benefits will then be granted. For more information on SSI, write the Department of Health And Human Services, Social Security Administration, Baltimore, MD 21235. The telephone number is (800) 772-1213. You may also want to get help on how to apply for SSI at your local Social Security office.

To help you acquire SSI benefits, it's a very good idea to speak with others who have already gone through the process and have qualified. Therefore, if you belong to a local MCS support group, bring this up at one of their meetings or in the group's newsletter. In addition, your personal physician or health-care provider may offer the names of other patients who have received SSI with whom you could speak.

Written information that should help you is available form a national MCS support organization, **HEAL (Human Ecology Action League)** in the form of its *HEAL Resource Data Sheets* (see *Printed Material* in Appendix 3: *Resources for a Healthy Household*). One book that should definitely provide you with useful information is *Social Security Disability Benefits: How to Get Them! How to Keep Them!* by James W. Ross. To receive a copy of this 104-page softbound book, send $12.95 to James Ross, Rt. 3, 118 Forester Rd., Slippery Rock, PA 16057.

OTHER GOVERNMENTAL HELP

There may be still other government agencies that could help you create your healthy household. Therefore, it's a good idea to check in your local classified telephone under "Government-Federal," "Government-State," and "Government-Local." If an agency's name sounds as if it might have something to offer you, call them. They just might be able to supply you with useful information, physical or financial assistance, or refer you to other more appropriate agencies.

GOVERNMENT ADVOCACY FOR MCS INDIVIDUALS

One organization that takes a very active role in governmental advocacy on behalf of those who have become sick from chemical exposures is the National Center for Environmental Health Strategies (NCEHS). It works to urge Federal and state legislatures and agencies to seriously consider the dangers of chemical pollutants. It also documents the experiences of those already made ill. Much of this effort is put forth by NCEHS's founder and president, Mary Lamielle.

NCEHS's thick newsletter, *The Delicate Balance*, is packed with the latest information on governmental acts, programs, benefits, and studies of interest to those with Multiple Chemical Sensitivities (MCS) and other chemical injuries. If you're interested in promoting a safer environment, consider joining this organization. Individual annual dues of $15.00 includes the quarterly newsletter. Contact the National Center for Environmental Health Strategies (NCEHS), 1100 Rural Ave., Voorhees, NJ 08043; (609) 429-5358.

APPENDIX 3
RESOURCES FOR A HEALTHY HOUSEHOLD

This appendix provides the names of books, periodicals, reports, organizations, private consulting firms, catalogs, and product manufacturers that should prove helpful as you create your healthy household. Note, the catalog descriptions given in *The Product Resource* section are partial lists of the merchandise offered.

PRINTED MATERIAL

An Alternative Approach to Allergies by Theron G. Randolph, M.D. and Ralph W. Moss, Ph.D. New York, NY: Bantam Books, Inc., 1980, $4.50, 312-pp. paperback. This book explores causes and treatments of chemical sensitivities and food allergies.

Chemical Exposures: Low Levels and High Stakes by Nicholas A. Ashford and Claudia S. Miller. New York, NY: Van Nostrand Reinhold, 1991, $22.95, 215-pp. hardback. This book is a thorough examination of MCS by an occupational medicine physician and Ph.D. researcher.

The Complete Artist's Health and Safety Guide by Monona Rossol. New York, NY: Allworth Press, 1990, $16.95, 328-pp. trade paperback. This guide delves into the health questions associated with art and craft materials.

Clean and Green by Annie Berthold-Bond. Woodstock, NY: Ceres Press, 1990, $8.95, 163-pp. trade paperback. This book gives methods and recipes for non-toxic cleaning.

Common-Sense Pest Control by William Olkowski, Sheila Daar and Helga Olkowski. Newtown, CT: The Taunton Press, 1991, $39.95, 716-pp. hardback. This mammoth book covers virtually all the available less-toxic pest controls.

The Consumer's Dictionary of Cosmetic Ingredients by Ruth Winter. New York, NY: Crown Publishing Group, third revised edition 1989, $12.00, 284-pp. hardback. This book explains cosmetic ingredients and terms.

Coping with Your Allergies by Natalie Golos and Frances Golos Golbitz. New York, NY: Simon and Schuster, 1979, 1986 trade paperback edition, $12.00, 351 pp. This book provides information on diets and lifestyles for those with allergies or MCS.

Cross Currents by Robert O. Becker. Los Angeles, CA: Jeremy Tarcher, 1990, $19.95, 336-pp. hardcover. This book discusses problems with electromagnetic radiation, and how it can be used beneficially in medicine.

EMF In Your Environment: Magnetic Field Measurements of Everyday Electrical Devises. (402 R–92–008 Dec.1992) from the Office of Radiation and Indoor Air, Radiation Studies Division (6603J). Washington, DC: EPA, 1992, free, 33-pp. booklet. This booklet discusses EMFs in homes.

Environ, Wary Canary Press, P.O. Box 2204, Fort Collins, CO 80522, (303) 224–0083, 4 issues for $18.00. This is a magazine "for ecologic living and health."

Furnishings: Healthy House Report #102. The Healthy House Institute. 430 N. Sewell Rd. Bloomington, IN 47408, (812) 332–5073, $4.50. This is a 12-page report on healthier home furnishings, including a resource listing.

Green Alternatives, Greenkeeping, Inc., 38 Montgomery St, Rhineback, NY 12572, (914) 876–6525, 6 issues for $18.00. This is a magazine for personal "health and the environment." Note, this magazine is no longer published as of Summer 1994. However, back issues may be available from *Informed Consent* (see below), which bought their assets, or through your local library.

Healing Environments by Carol Venolia. Berkeley, CA: Celestial Arts, 1988, $8.95, 225-pp. trade paperback. This book explores healthy interiors from health, aesthetic, and spiritual perspectives.

HEAL Resource Data, Human Ecology Action League (HEAL), P.O. Box 49126, Atlanta, GA 30359–1126, (404) 248–1898. These are low-cost informational sheets, reading lists, and resource listings on a wide variety of subjects. Write for available topics and pricing.

The Healthy Home: An Attic-to-Basement Guide to Toxin-Free Living by Linda Mason Hunter. New York, NY: Pocket Books, 1989, 1990 paperback edition, $10.00, 204 pp. This book provides suggestions and information for healthier homes.

The Healthy House: How to Buy One, How to Build One, How to Cure A "Sick" One by John Bower. New York, NY: Lyle Stuart, 1989, 1991 trade paperback edition, $17.95, 393 pp. This book covers the health consequences of most building materials and provides sources for less-toxic alternatives.

Healthy House Building: A Design and Construction Guide by John Bower. Bloomington, IN: The Healthy House Institute, 1993 trade paperback, $21.95, 382 pp. This book shows the step-by-step construction of a model healthy house, with over 250 photos and illustrations as well as a complete set of house plans.

Home Safe Home Alternatives Fact Sheets. These are three-hole-punched informational reports available on a variety of topics. For a complete listing of subjects and prices, contact the Washington Toxics Coalition, 4516 University Way NE, Seattle, WA 98105, (206) 632–1545.

The Home Water Supply: How to Find, Filter, Store, and Conserve It by Stu Campbell. Pownal, VT: "A Garden Way Publishing Book" of Storey Communications, Inc., 1983 trade paperback, $16.95, 236 pp. This is a thorough guide for home water supplies, with extensive charts and drawings.

The Human Ecologist, Human Ecology Action League, P.O. Box 49126, Atlanta, GA 30359–1126, (404) 248–1898. Membership in HEAL and 4 issues for $20.00. This is the newsletter of HEAL, a national MCS support group.

Human Ecology and Susceptibility to the Chemical Environment by Theron G. Randolph, M.D. Springfield, IL: Charles C. Thomas, Publisher, 1962, $29.25, 148-pp. hardback. This was the first book written by a physician that described the possible causes of Ecological Illness (now known as MCS) and suggested treatments.

Informed Consent, International Institute of Research for Chemical Hypersensitivity, P.O. Box 1984, Williston, ND 58802–1984, (701) 774–7766, 6 issues for $18.00. This is a bimonthly "magazine of health, prevention and environmental news."

Interior Concerns, Interior Concerns Publications, P.O. Box 2386, Mill Valley, CA 94942, (415) 389–8049, 6 issues for $35.00. This is a bimonthly newsletter covering environmentally sound, less-toxic interior design.

Least Toxic Home Pest Control by Dan Stein. Eugene, OR: Hulogosi Communications, Inc., 1991, $8.95., 87-pp. trade paperback. This book covers the essentials of less-toxic pest control.

"Multiple Chemical Sensitivity," by Betty Hileman. *Chemical and Engineering News*, July 22, 1991, 69 (29), pp. 26–42. Reprints available for $10.00 from Distribution, Room 210, American Chemical Society, 1155 16th St. NW, Washington, DC 20036. This is an excellent article on MCS.

The Natural Beauty Book: Cruelty-Free Cosmetics to Make At Home by Anita Guyton. London, England: Thorsons, Harper Collins Publishers, 1981, revised 1991, $14.00, 192-pp. trade paperback. This book contains recipes for cosmetics using readily available natural ingredients.

Natural Healing for Dogs and Cats by Diane Stein. Freedom, CA: The Crossing Press, 1993, $16.95, 186-pp. trade paperback. This book gives remedies for dog and cat complaints using herbs, vitamins, and massage techniques.

The New Reactor, Environmental Health Network, P.O. Box 1155, Larkspur, CA 94977. (916) 432–9448. Membership in the Environmental Health Network and 6 issues for $25.00. This is the bimonthly newsletter of a large California support group for people with MCS.

Non-toxic, Natural and Earthwise by Debra Lynn Dadd. Los Angeles, CA: Jeremy P. Tarcher, Inc., 1990, $12.95, 360-pp. trade paperback. This book provides sources for environmentally friendly, less-toxic products for individuals and their homes.

Our Toxic Times, Chemical Injury Information Network, P.O. Box 301, White Sulphur Springs, MT 59645–0301 (406) 547–2255. There is no charge for membership in Chemical Injury Information Network and 12 issues, but donations appreciated. This newsletter covers issues relevant to human health, with emphasis on those with MCS.

Painting: Healthy House Report # 103. The Healthy House Institute, 430 N. Sewell Rd., Bloomington, IN 47408, (812) 332–5073, $5.50. This is a 16-page report on paints, clear finishes, strippers, and caulks, with sources for safer alternatives.

Q and A About Electric and Magnetic Fields Associated with the Use of Electric Power. Washington, DC: Environmental Protection Agency (order from (800) 363-2383) Free. This booklet is a good attempt to present information without bias.

Radon: A Homeowner's Guide to Detection and Control by Bernard Cohen and the editors of *Consumer Reports*. New York, NY: Avon Trade Paperback, 1989, $3.95, 369-pp. paperback. This book explains radon problems in homes and how to solve them. (Although this is now out-of-print, it should be available at your local library or through the interlibrary loan service.)

Safe Home Digest Healthy Building Resource Guide, Lloyd Publishing Inc. Order from Safe Home Digest, P.O. Box 3420, Saugatuck Station, Westport, CT 06880, (203) 227–1276, $33.00, 120-pp. loose-leaf guidebook. This guide offers sources for a variety of less-toxic building materials.

Social Security Disability Benefits: How to Get Them! How to Keep Them! by James W. Ross. Slippery Rock, PA: Ross Publishing Co., 1984, $12.95, 104-pp. paperback. Order from James Ross, Rt. 3, 188 Forrester Rd., Slippery Rock, PA 16057. This is a step-by-step guide designed to help disabled individuals acquire SSI benefits.

Tracing EMFs in Building Wiring and Grounding by Karl Riley. Tucson, AZ: Magnetic Sciences International, 1995, $30.00, 126-pp. trade paperback. Order from Magnetic Sciences International, HCR-2, Box 850–295, Tucson, AZ 85735, (800) 749–9873, (602) 822–2355. This book explains how to fix EMF problems that are related to house wiring and plumbing.

Understanding Ventilation: How to Design, Select, and Install Residential Ventilation Systems by John Bower. Bloomington, IN: The Healthy House Institute, 1995, $31.95 432-pp. hardback. Using text, photographs, charts, and illustrations, this book thoroughly explains methods of home ventilation and provides resource sections.

The Unhealthy House: Healthy House Report # 101. The Healthy House Institute, 430 N. Sewell Rd., Bloomington, IN 47408, (812) 332–5073, $2.50. This is a four-page report discussing indoor air pollutants and their potential heath consequences.

Warning: The Electricity Around You May Be Hazardous To Your Health by Ellen Sugarman. New York NY: Fireside/Simon and Schuster, 1992, $11.00. 238-pp. trade paperback. This book explains the nature and unexpected dangers of electromagnetic fields and how to minimize them.

The Wary Canary, Wary Canary Press, P.O. Box 2204, Fort Collins, CO 80522, (303) 224–0083, 4 issues for $20.00. This is a newsletter for those with MCS, "allergics, and environmental health advocates."

Your House, Your Health: A Non-Toxic Building Guide by John Bower Unionville, IN: The Healthy House Institute, 1992. 27.5-minutes color VHS video. In this video, the author explains the basic principles of healthy house construction and gives an in-depth tour of a model healthy house.

ORGANIZATIONS AND CONSULTING SERVICES

Note: the acronym is used first if the organization or company generally goes by that term

ACTS (Arts, Crafts and Theater Safety)
181 Thompson St. #23
New York, NY 10012–2586
(212) 777–0062
This organization promotes safer art products and practices. Annual membership is $15.00 and includes a monthly newsletter.

AGES (Advocacy Group for the Environmentally Sensitive)
Heather Miller
543–1515 West Second Ave.
Vancouver, B.C., Canada V6J 5C5
(604) 258–9443
((604)251–4697
This is a Canadian MCS support and advocacy organization. Individual annual dues are $25.00 (Canadian funds) and includes a quarterly magazine.

Asthma and Allergy Foundation of America (AAFA)
1125 Fifteenth St., NW
Ste. 502
Washington, DC 20005
(800) 7–ASTHMA
(202) 466–7643
National support group with local chapters for those with asthma and/or allergies. Individual annual membership is $25.00 and includes bimonthly newsletter.

American Academy of Environmental Medicine (AAEM)
4510 W. 89th
Prairie Village, KS 66207-2282
(913) 642-6062
This is a professional organization of physicians and other health-care workers specializing in the treatment of MCS and food allergies. Listings are available of member doctors by geographic area.

American Academy of Otolaryngologic Allergists
8455 Colesville Rd.
Ste. 745
Silver Springs, MD 20910
(301) 588–1800
This is the professional organization of physician-allergists specializing in the treatment of the ears, eyes, and throat. This society has recognized chemical hypersensitivity and treats it as a valid medical condition.

The American Environmental Health Foundation, Inc. (AEHF)
8345 Walnut Hill Lane
Ste. 225
Dallas, TX 75231
(800) 428–2343
(214) 361–9515
This is a non-profit organization founded by William Rea, M.D. whose main purpose is "to further the practice of environmental medicine." It strives to fund research, disseminates up-to-date information on MCS, and offers health-related products for sale. Annual "friend" membership is $15.00, which includes a newsletter and various other mailings.

Bio-Integral Resource Center (BIRC)
P.O. Box 7414
Berkeley CA 94707
(510) 524–2567
This is an organization focusing on less-toxic pest control. A newsletter subscription and one personal consultation are included with membership. Individual/associate annual dues are $30.00.

DAN (Disabled Artist's Network)
c/o Sanda Aronson
P.O. Box 20781
New York, NY 10025
An organization for information exchange and self-help support between professional artists with disabilities, including MCS. Cost of membership is "letter writing and participation." Newsletter sent out several times a year to active members. Send a SASE for further information.

Eco-Home Network
4344 Russell Ave.
Los Angeles, CA 90027
(213) 662-5207
This is a Los Angeles-based organization promoting healthier solutions to environmental and ecological problems. Individual annual membership is $25.00 which includes a free "eco-home tour," a 10% book discount, and subscription to a quarterly newsletter.

The Electric Power Research Institute (EPRI)
3412 Hillview Ave.
Palo Alto, CA 94304
(415) 855-2000
This is an organization sponsored by local utilities that is currently conducting research on EMFs.

Environmental Education and Health Services
Mary Oetzel
3202 W. Anderson Ln. #208-249
Austin, TX 78757
(512) 288-2369
Private consultant specializing in minimizing indoor pollution.

HEAL (Human Ecology Action League)
P.O. Box 49126
Atlanta GA 30359-1126
(404) 248-1898
National support group for MCS. Quarterly newsletter and fact sheets on a variety of topics. Individual annual dues are $20.00. HEAL maintains a listing of healthier housing consultants. Local chapters are located throughout the U.S. and have their own dues and newsletters. Contact the national HEAL office for the group nearest you.

The Healthy House Institute
430 North Sewell Rd.
Bloomington, IN 47408
(812) 332-5073
This is a private resource company offering books, videos, and consultation services concerning healthy home construction and lifestyles.

Jewish Guild for the Blind
15 W. 65 St.
New York, NY 10023
(212) 769-6200
This is a non-profit organization that provides books on cassettes and CDs to those unable to read. The service is free but it does require a doctor's or social service worker's statement for eligibility.

Kitchens and Baths by Don Johnson
Ste. #1375
Merchandise Mart
Chicago, IL 60654
(312) 548-2436
(708) 548-2436
This is a kitchen and bath certified designer/dealer who sells metal cabinets including units especially manufactured for chemically sensitive individuals.

National Center for Environmental Health Strategies (NCEHS)
1100 Rural Ave.
Voorhees, NJ 08043
(609) 429–5358
This is an organization that actively promotes education, awareness, and advocacy of MCS. Membership includes a subscription to a quarterly newsletter. Individual annual dues are $15.00.

National Foundation for the Chemically Hypersensitive (NFCH)
P.O. Box 222
Olphelia, VA 22530
(517) 697–3989
(804) 454–7538
This is an organization promoting awareness of MCS. Membership includes exchanging experiences coping with chemical sensitivities and occasional mailings. Membership is $20.00.

The National Institute for Rehabilitation Engineering (NIRE)
P.O. Box T
Hewitt, NJ 07421
(800) 736–2216
(201) 853–6585
(914) 986–6557
This is a non-profit organization that provides special technical aids to severely disabled persons (including MCS) at cost. Equipment, labor to adapt them to specific needs, and shipping must be paid by the individual. Annual membership is $35.00 and includes a newsletter subscription.

Nigra Enterprises
5699 Kanan Rd.
Agoura Hills, CA 91301
(818) 889–6877
This is a professional consultant/dealer of air and water filters. Also offered are a variety of less-toxic products.

Recordings for the Blind
20 Roszel Rd.
Princeton, NJ 08540
(609) 452–0606
This is a non-profit organization providing books on 4-track and on CD for those unable to read. The service requires a doctor's statement and a $37.50 registration fee.

Response Team for the Chemically Injured
7343 El Camino Real
Ste. 177
Atascadero, CA 93422
(805) 461–3662
This is a non-profit medical clinic for MCS medical treatment, patient information, referral services, promotion of MCS research, providing a response team to chemical disasters, and patient advocacy.

Share, Care and Prayer
Janet Dauble
P.O. Box 2080
Frazier Park, CA 93225
This is a national support group for MCS with emphasis on mutual support and group prayer. The organization publishes a newsletter. No dues are required, but donations are much appreciated.

The S.T.A.T.E. Foundation (Sensitive to a Toxic Environment, Inc.)
4 Hazel Ct.
West Seneca, NY 14224
(716) 675–1164
This is an organization advocating a non-toxic home community and a research/development program. The group has a catalog of companies offering services and products for MCS persons. Donations are appreciated.

Toxic Carpet Information Exchange
P.O. Box 39344
Cincinnati, OH 45239
This is an advocacy and information exchange concerning the problems of hazardous carpeting.

Washington Toxics Coalition
4516 University Way NE
Seattle WA 98105
(206) 632–1545
This is a Washington organization promoting less-toxic living. A newsletter and low-cost fact sheets on a variety of topics are available. Individual annual dues are $20.00.

The Water Quality Association
4151 Naperville Rd.
Lisle, IL 60532
(708) 505–0160
This is the trade association of local suppliers of water-treatment equipment. Call them for their members near you.

PRODUCT SOURCES

3M Company
3M Center
St. Paul, MN 55144–1000
(800) 842–4946 (3M Do-It-Yourself Division)
(800) 388–3458 (Fitrete Filters)
(612) 733–1110
Safest Stripper paint stripper and Filtrete electrostatic furnace filters

AAA Environmental Products
1772 Ave. De Los Arboles
Ste.115
Thousand Oaks, CA 91362
(805) 492–1755
Magnetic water conditioners and air filters

Adirondack Designs
P.O. 656
350 Cypress St.
Ft. Bragg, CA 95437
(800) 222–0343
Redwood patio furniture

Aireox Research Corp.
P.O. Box 8523
Riverside CA 92515
(909) 689–2781
Aireox room and car air filters

Allens Naturally
P.O. Box 339
Farmington, MI 48332
(313) 453–5410
Allens Naturally Automatic Dishwasher Detergent and other cleaning products

Allergy Relief Shop
4111 W. Beaver Creek Dr.
Powell, TN 37849
(615) 947–5141
Cleaning products, personal-care products, bedding, and household goods

Allergy Resources
P.O. Box 888
264 Brookridge Ave.
Palmer Lake, CO 80133
(800) USE–FLAX
(719) 488–3630
Personal-care products, cleaning products, and natural-fiber bedding

The Allergy Store
P.O. Box 2555
Sebastopol, CA 95473
(800) 824–7163
(707) 823–6202
Cleaning products, personal-care products, and air and water filters

AllerMed Corp.
31 Steel Rd.
Wiley, TX 75098
(214) 442–4898
Containment reading boxes and portable room and automobile air filters

Almost Heaven Hot Tubs, Ltd.
Rte. 5
Renick, WV 24966
(304) 497–3163
Saunas

Alumax-Magnolia Division
P.O. Box 40
Magnolia, AR 71753
(800) 643–1514
(501) 234–4260
Frameless shower doors with no lower track
(Wholesale only, call to locate a nearby
dealer or mail-order supplier.)

Amerec Products
P.O. Box 40569
Bellevue, WA 98015
(800) 331–0349
(206) 643–7500
Saunas

The American Environmental Health Foundation, Inc.
8345 Walnut Hill Lane
Ste. 225
Dallas, TX 75231
(800) 428–2343
(214) 361–9515
Air and water filters, bedding, personal-care
products, and cleaning products

American Formulating and Manufacturing
1960 Chicago Ave.
Ste. E7
Riverside, CA 92507
(909) 781–6860
SafeChoice Super Clean and other cleaning,
personal-care, and building products
(Wholesale only, call to locate a nearby
dealer or mail-order supplier.)

American Olean Tile Co.
1000 Cannon Ave.
Lansdale, PA 19446–0271
(215) 855–1111
Ceramic tile
(Wholesale only, call to locate a nearby
dealer or mail-order supplier.)

Ametek
Plymouth Products Division
P.O. Box 1047
Sheboygan, WI 53082–1047
(800) 222–7558
(414) 457–9435
Whole-house Ametek water filters including
sediment filters

Ampco
P.O. Box 608
Rosedale, MS 38769
(800) 647–8268
(601) 759–3521
Metal cabinets
(Wholesale only, call to locate a nearby
dealer.)

Aquathin Corp.
950 S. Andrews Ave.
Pompano Beach, FL 33069
(800) 462–7634
(305) 781–7777
Aquathin reverse-osmosis water equipment

Ar–Ex Ltd.
156 N. Jefferson St.
Ste. 205
Chicago, IL 60661
(312) 879–0017
Safe Suds dish soap, Chap Cream, and other
hypoallergenic cosmetics

Aroma Manufacturing Co. of America
9245 Brown Deer Rd.
San Diego, CA 92121
(619) 558–6688
Aroma Aeromatic ovens
(Wholesale only. Call for nearest dealer.)

Arctic Metal Products Corp.
507 Wortman Ave.
Brooklyn, NY 11208
(718) 257–5277
Metal cabinets
(Stores in NY and East Coast. Call for nearest location.)

Asko, Inc.
P.O. Box 851805
Richardson, TX 75085–1805
(214) 644–8595
Asko stainless steel-lined dishwashers
(Wholesale only, call to locate a nearby dealer.)

Aubrey Organics
4419 N. Manhattan Ave.
Tampa, FL 33614
(800) 282–7394
(813) 877–4186
Aubrey Organics all-natural cosmetics

Audio Editions
P.O. Box 6930
Auburn, CA 95604
(800) 231–4261
Books on cassettes

Aussie Connection
825 NE Broadway
Portland, OR 97232
(800) 950–2668
(503) 284–2228
100%-wool mattress pads

Austin Air Systems Limited
701 Seneca St.
Buffalo, NY 14210
(716) 856–3704
Healthmate and Healthmate Plus room-size HEPA air filters

Back To Basics, The Catalog Company
1107 West Main St.
Ste. 201
Durham, NC 27701–2028
(919) 682–8611
Smaller and *Plus* catalogs of women's 100%-cotton undergarments

Ballard Designs
1670 DeFoor Ave. NW
Atlanta, GA 30318–7528
(404) 351–5099
100%-cotton slip covers and curtains, and ceramic and plaster tables

Bally Block Co.
30 South 7th St.
Bally, PA 19503
(215) 845–7511
Hardwood butcher-block countertops
(Wholesale only, call to locate a nearby dealer.)

Baron's Window Coverings
325 S. Washington Ave.
Lansing, MI 48933
(800) 248–5852
(800) 537–1895
(517) 484–1366
Metal mini-blinds

Bartley Collection
29060 Airpark Dr.
Easton, MD 21601
(800) 227–8539
Hardwood reproduction furniture assembled and in kits

Basic Coatings
2124 Valley Dr.
Des Moines, IA 50321
(800) 247–5471
(515) 288–0231
Professional Image water-based polyurethane finish

Baubiologie Hardware
P.O. Box 3217
Prescott, AZ 86302
(602) 445–8225
EMF testers, EMF reduction equipment, and books

Eddie Bauer
Fifth and Union
P.O. Box 3700
Seattle, WA 98124–3700
(800) 426–8020
Some all-cotton clothing for men and women

Beam Industries
P.O. Box 788
Webster City, IA 50595
(800) 369–2326
Central vacuum systems
(Wholesale only, call to locate a nearby dealer or mail-order supplier.)

L.L. Bean, Inc.
Freeport, ME 04033
(800) 221–4221
Some all-cotton clothing for the entire family, and the *Home and Camp* catalog offers some natural-fiber bedding

Bedford Fair
421 Landmark Dr.
Wilmington, DE 28410
(800) 964–1000
Some 100%-cotton sweaters for women

Befit Enterprises Ltd.
The Cutting Edge Catalog
P.O. Box 5030
Southhampton, NY 11969
(800) 497–9516
(516) 287–3813
Air- and water-purification equipment, light bulbs, and EMF testers and shields

Best Paint Co., Inc.
P.O. Box 3922
Seattle, WA 98124
(206) 783–9938
Best alternative paints

Bila
1651 S. Santa Fe
Los Angeles, CA 90021
(800) 824–3541
(213) 629–3555
Ethnic-inspired natural fiber (especially rayon) clothing for women

Billard's Old Telephones
21710 Regnart Rd.
Cupertino, CA 95014
(408) 252–2104
Restored metal, wood, and bakelite phones

Block-Tops, Inc.
4770 E. Wesley Dr.
Anaheim, CA 92807
(714) 779–0475
Oak and maple butcher-block countertops

Body Elements/Terressentials
3320 North 3rd St.
Arlington, VA 22201–1712
(800) 541–2535
Nontoxic cosmetics, cleaners, personal-care products, and pet-care supplies

The Body Shop by Mail
45 Horsehill Rd.
Cedar Knolls, NJ 07927–2714
(800) 541–2545
Natural-formula body and hair-care products

Books on Tape
P.O. Box 7900
Newport Beach, CA 92658
(800) 626–3333
Books on cassette for purchase or rent

John Boos and Co.
P.O. 609
Effingham, IL 62401
(217) 347–7701
Hardwood butcher-block countertops
(Wholesale only, call to locate a nearby dealer.)

Robert Bosch Corp.
2800 S. 25th Ave.
Broadview, IL 60153
(800) 866–2022
(708) 865–5200
Bosch dishwashers
(Wholesale only, call to locate a nearby dealer.)

Brass Bed Shoppe
12421 Cedar Rd.
Cleveland Heights, OH 44106
(216) 371–0400
Metal headboards, beds, and daybeds

Bright Future Futons
3120 Central Ave. SE
Albuquerque, NM 87106
(505) 268–9738
All-cotton futons and organic 100%-cotton futons

BRK Electronics Corp.
Division of Pittway Corp.
780 McClure Rd.
Aurora, IL 60504–2495
(708) 851–7330
First Alert carbon-monoxide detectors and fire extinguishers
(Wholesale only, call to locate a nearby dealer or mail-order supplier.)

Broan Manufacturing Co.
P.O. Box 140
Hartford, WI 53027
(800) 637–1453
(414) 673–4340
Ventilation fans and controls

Dr. Bronner
Box 28
Escondido, CA 92033
(619) 743–2211
Dr. Bronner's soaps
(May order directly if disabled or a retail outlet is unavailable. Otherwise wholesale only. Call to locate a nearby dealer or mail-order supplier.)

John O. Butler Co.
4635 W. Foster Ave.
Chicago, IL 60630
(312) 777–4000
Tuff-Spun dental floss
(Wholesale only, call to locate a nearby dealer.)

Caring for You
1139 Cotswald Ct.
Sunnyvale, CA 94087
(408) 296–7968
Cleaning and personal-care products

Carousel Carpet Mills
1 Carousel Ln.
Ukiah, CA 95482
(707) 485–0333
Natural-fiber carpeting

Carrier Corp.
P.O. Box 70
Indianapolis, IN 46206
(800) 227–7437
Whole-house electrostatic precipitators
(Wholesale only, call to locate a nearby dealer.)

Harriet Carter
North Wales, PA 19455
(215) 361–5151
Household gadgets

Carysbrook Mfg.
P.O. Box 57
Fork Union, VA 23055
(804) 842–1108
The Enterpriser long-life incadescent bulbs

Cedarbrook Sauna
P.O. Box 535
Cashmere, WA 98815
(800) 634–6334
Saunas

C-Cure Chemical Co.
16225 Park Ten Place
Ste. 850
Houston, TX 77084
(713) 697–2024
Multi-Cure thinset mortar
(Wholesale only, call to locate a nearby dealer.)

Chempoint Products, Inc.
P.O. Box 2597
Danbury, CT 06813–2597
(800) 343–6588
Citrus-Solv concentrated cleaner
(Wholesale only, call to locate a nearby dealer or mail-order source.)

Chem-Safe Products
P.O. Box 33023
San Antonio, TX 78265
(210) 657–5321
Enviro-Safe Paint alternative paint

Cohasset Colonials
38 Parker Ave.
Cohasset, MA 02025–2096
(800) 288–2389
Note: $3.00 for catalog
Solid-wood furniture assembled and in kits

Colgate-Pamolive Co.
300 Park Ave.
New York, NY 10022
(800) 221–4607
(212) 310–2000
Colgate Fragrance-Free shaving cream
 (Wholesale only, call to locate a nearby
dealer.)

Colonial Garden Kitchens
P.O. Box 66
Hanover, PA 17333–0066
(800) 245–3399
Cookware, metal coat hangers, and house-
hold goods

Common Sense Products
109 Lincoln Ave.
Rutland, VT 05701
(800) 259–7627
Common Sense personal-care products

Confab
601 Allendale Rd..
King of Prussia, PA 19406
(610) 354–0722
New Day's Choice cotton-covered paper
feminine napkins

Copper-Brite, Inc.
P.O. Box 50610
Santa Barbara, CA 93150
(805) 565–1566
Roach-prufe boric-acid pesticide
(Wholesale only, call to locate a nearby
dealer or mail-order supplier.)

Corning, Inc.
Corning-Revere Consumer Information Ctr.
P.O. Box 1994
Waynesboro, VA 22980
(800) 340–5471
(703) 949–9100
Vision glass, Corningware, and Revere stain-
less-steel cookware

The Cotton Place
P.O. Box 59721
Dallas, TX 75229
(800) 451–8866
(214) 243–4149
Untreated natural-fiber clothing for the family, bedding, sewing goods, and household
goods

Cottontails OrganicWear
3684 Hicks Hill Rd.
Friendship, NY 14739
(716) 973–3000
Organic 100%-cotton clothing for men and
women, and San-O-Zon powder odor neu-
tralizer

Cotton Threads Clothing
Rte. 2, Box 90
Hallettsvillle, TX 77964
(409) 562–2153
100%-cotton clothing (including organic) for
men and women

The Country Store
20211 Vashon Hwy. SW
Vashon Island, WA 98070
(206) 463–3655
100%-cotton clothing for the family and personal-care items

Crate and Barrel
P.O. Box 9059
Wheeling, IL 60090–9059
(800) 323–5461
Solid-wood furniture including children's
furniture

Crown City Mattress
250 S. San Gabriel Blvd.
San Gabriel, CA 91776
(818) 796–9101
(213) 681–6356
Organic-cotton mattresses

Culligan International Co.
One Culligan Pkwy.
Northbrook, IL 60062
(800) 285–5442
Water-treatment equipment
(Call to locate nearby dealer.)

Cuno
Consumer Products
400 Research Pkwy.
Meriden, CT 06450
(800) 243–6894
(203) 237–5541
Aqua-Pure water-treatment equipment

CWY Products
4422 54th Ave.
Maspeth, NY 11378
(718) 937–2900
Non-Scents zeolite odor adsorber
(Wholesale only, call to locate a nearby dealer or mail-order supplier.)

The Daily Planet/Russian Dressing
P.O. Box 6441
St. Paul, MN 55164–0411
(800) 324–5950
Natural-fiber ethnic-style clothing for women and men

Dal-Tile Co.
7834 Hawn Freeway
Dallas, TX 75217
(214) 398–1411
Ceramic tile
(Call to locate a nearby dealer.)

Dap Products, Inc.
855 N. Third St.
Tipp City, OH 45371–3014
(513) 667–4461
Kwik Seal caulk and Weld-Wood glue
(Wholesale only, call to locate a nearby dealer or mail-order supplier.)

Davis Products Co.
418 N. Calumette Ave.
Michigan City, IN 46360
(800) 553–2847
(219) 873–0358
Metal cabinets
(Wholesale only, call to locate a nearby dealer.)

Decent Exposures
2202 NE 115th
Seattle, WA 98125
(206) 364–4540
Custom women's 100%-cotton underwear

Deerskin Trading Post
119 Foster Ave.
Peabody, MA 01961–6008
(508) 532–2810
Leather clothing and footwear for men and women

Denny Sales Corp.
3500 Gateway Dr.
Pompano Beach, FL 33069
(800) 327–6616
(305) 971–3100
Denny Foil and Denny Board aluminum-faced building materials

Deva Lifewear
110 1st Ave. West
P.O. Box 4H
Westhope, ND 58793–0266
(800) 222–8024
(701) 245–6668
100%-cotton clothing for men and women

Dharma Trading Company
P.O. Box 150916
San Rafael, CA 94915
(800) 542–5227
Sewing goods and clothing for the family

Dona Designs
825 Northlake Dr.
Richardson, TX 75080
(214) 235–0485
Organic 100%-cotton mattresses, futons, and bedding, and solid wood lawyer's book-cases and furniture

Walter Drake and Sons
Drake Bldg.
Colorado Springs, CO 80940
(800) 525–9291
(719) 596–3853
Household gadgets

Dupont Co.
Corian Div.
Chestnut Run Plaza
P.O. Box 80702
Wilmington, DE 19880–0702
(800) 426–7426
Corian countertops
(Wholesale only, call to locate a nearby dealer.)

Duro-Lite Lamps, Inc.
Duro-Test Corp.
9 Law Dr.
Fairfield, NJ 07004
(201) 808–1800
Vita-Lite full-spectrum fluorescent lamps

Dwyer Products Corp.
418 N. Calumet Ave.
Michigan City, IN 46360–5019
(800) 348–8508
(219) 874–5236
Metal kitchen cabinets

Earth Care Paper, Inc.
Ukiah, CA 95482
(800) 347–0070
Recycled paper for home and office use

earthsake
1805 Fourth St.
Berkeley, CA 94710
(510) 848–0484
Portable alternative portable vacuums, natural-fiber bedding, and air and water filters

Earth Tools
9754 Johanna Pl.
Shadow Hills, CA 91040
(800) 825–6460
(818) 353–5883
Alternative automatic dishwasher detergent, bleach, other cleaning products, brushes, towels, pillows, and natural fiber clothing

Eco Design Co.
1365 Rufina Cir.
Santa Fe, NM 87502
(800) 621–2591
(505) 438–3448
Clothing for the family, brushes, Livos and other alternative paints, and cleaning and personal-care products

The Ecology Box
2260 S. Main St.
Ann Arbor, MI 48103
(800) 735–1371
(313) 662–9131
Personal-care products, cleaning products, and cellophane bags

Eco Source
P.O. Box 1656
Sebastopol, CA 95473
(800) 274–7040
(707) 829–7562
Cleaning products, personal-care products, and paper goods

Ecos Paint
P.O. Box 375
St. Johnsbury, VT 05819
(802) 748–9144
Ecos alternative paint

Ecosport
28 James St.
South Hackensack, NJ 07606
(800) 486–4326
(201) 489–0389
Organic 100%-cotton sweatpants, shirts, and underwear for the family

Ecover
P.O. Box SS
Carpenter Rd.
Philmont, NY 12565
(518) 672–0190
Ecover natural cleaning products

ElectroStatic Technologies, Inc.
2223 Guinotte Ave.
Kansas City, Missouri 64120
(800) 239–2876
(816) 842–0616
ElectroStatic Water Treater conditioners

Elmer's Adhesives
Division of Borden, Inc.
180 E. Broad St.
Columbus, OH 43215
(800) 848–9400
(614) 225–4511 Consumer Response Line
Elmer's Glue products

Engen Drug Allergy Division
Box 218
Karlstad, MN 56732
(800) 648–0074
(218) 436–2485
Personal-care products, cleaning products, alternative portable vacuums, and air and water filters

Enviracaire
747 Bowman Ave.
Hagerstown, MD 21740
(800) 332–1110
Enviracaire portable air filters

enviro-clean
30 Walnut Ave.
Floral Park, NY 11001–2404
(800) 466–1425
Safer-cleaning products catalog

Environmental Health Shopper
P.O. Box 239
Fate, TX 75132
(800) 447–1100
Personal-care items, air and water filters, bedding

Environmental Purification Systems
P.O. Box 191
Concord, CA 94522
(800) 829–2129
(510) 284–2129
EPS activated-charcoal water filters

Enviro Safe Cabinets Co., Ltd.
4250 Dawson St., Ste. 300
Burnaby, BC, Canada V5C 4B1
(800) 668–9778
(604) 298–1050
Enviro Safe 2000 kitchen cabinets without formaldehyde-based glues

Erlander's Natural Products
P.O. Box 106
Altadena, CA 91003
(818) 797–7004
Jubilee washing compound and soaps

ETEX, Ltd.
3200 Polaris Ave.
Ste. 9
Las Vegas, NV 89102
(702) 364–5911
Electro-Gun drywood termite exterminator

Euroclean
Division of White Consolidated Industries
905 W. Irving Park Rd.
Itasca, IL 60143
(800) 545–4372
(708) 773–2111
Euroclean alternative portable vacuums (Wholesale only, call to locate a nearby dealer or mail-order supplier.)

Exotic Gifts
P.O. Box 842
Hermosa Beach, CA 90254
(800) 992–8288
(213) 374–2570
100%-cotton ethnic clothing for women

E-Z-I, Inc.
3500 North Harrison
Shawnee, OK 74801
(405) 275–8110
E-Z-I Lubricant

Farr Co.
P.O. Box 92187
El Segundo, CA 90009
(800) 333–7320
Extended-surface filters and HEPA filters (Wholesale only, call to locate a nearby dealer.)

Faultless Starch/Bon Ami Co.
1025 W. 8th St.
Kansas City, MO 64101
(816) 842–1230
Bon Ami cleaning powder and cake
(Wholesale only, call to locate a nearby dealer or mail-order supplier.)

Paul Federick Menstyle
223 West Poplar St.
Fleetwood, PA 19522–9989
(800) 247–1417
100%-cotton shirts for men

Finnleo Saunas
575 E. Cokato St.
Cokato, MN 55321
(612) 286–5584
Saunas

Flowright International Products
1495 NW Gilman Blvd., #4
Issaquah, WA 98027
(206) 392–8357
Less-toxic carpeting, vacuums, AFM products, and air and water filters

Fluid Mechanics
2789 Klondike Rd.
W. Lafayette, IN 47906
(317) 497–3403
National Sales Office
(219) 486–2888
The Stabilizer water conditioners

Forbo North America
P.O. Box 667
Hazelton, PA 18201
(800) 233–0475
(717) 459–0771
Natural linoleum flooring

Formica Corp.
10155 Reading Rd.
Cincinnati, OH 45241
(513) 786–3525
Formica plastic laminate
(Wholesale only, call to locate a nearby dealer.)

E.L. Foust Co., Inc.
P.O. Box 105
Elmhurst, IL 60126
(800) 225–9549
(312) 834–4952
Portable air filters, activated-charcoal panels, loose-fill activated charcoal, masks, lubricants, and books

Frandon Enterprises
120 W. Beaver Creek Rd.
Unit 16
Richmond Hill, ON, Canada L4B 1L2
(800) 359–9000
(905) 709–1196
Lead Alert lead-testing kits

French Transit Ltd.
398 Beach Rd.
Burlingame, CA 94010
(415) 548–9600
Le Crystal Naturel deodorant crystal
(Wholesale only, call for nearest dealer or mail-order supplier.)

Fuller Brush
One Fuller Way
Great Bend, KS 67530
(800) 522–0499
Natural-bristle hair brushes, carpet sweepers, and water filters

Futon Designs, Inc.
39 Broadway
Ashville, NC 28801
(704) 253–1138
100%-cotton futons

Garrett Wade Co.
161 Avenue of the Americas
New York, NY 10013
(800) 221-2942
(212) 807-1155
Boiled linseed oil without additives

General Ecology, Inc.
151 Sheree Blvd.
Exton, PA 19341
(215) 363–7900
Spark-L-Pure and Seagull water-treatment equipment

The General Electric Co.
GE Appliance Park 6
Rm. 129
Louisville, KY 40225
(800) 626–2000
GE and Hotpoint appliances
(Wholesale only, call to locate a nearby dealer.)

Glidden Co.
925 Euclid Ave.
Cleveland, OH 44115
(216) 344–8000
Series 2000 low-VOC paint
(Call for nearest store or authorized dealer.)

Global Environmental Technologies
P.O. Box 8839
Allentown, PA 18105–8839
(800) 800–TERRA
(215) 821–4901
Terra water-filtration equipment

Gloucester Company, Inc.
P.O. Box 428
Franklin, MA 02038
(800) 343–4963
(508) 528–2200
Pheno-Seal caulk
(Wholesale only, call to locate a nearby dealer or mail-order supplier.)

Gohn Brothers
105 South Main
P.O. Box 111
Middlebury, IN 46540–0111
(219) 825–2400
Some 100%-cotton clothing for the family

Golden Harvest, Inc.
8500 Shawnee Mission Pkwy.
Ste. L-2
Shawnee Mission, KS 66202
(800) 558–5591
(913) 262–2895
Golden Harvest Wheat Wallpaper Paste
(Wholesale only, call to locate a nearby dealer.)

Golden Temple Natural Products
Box 1095
Taos, NM 87571
(505) 776–2311
Nanak's Lip Smoothee unscented lip gloss
(Wholesale only, call to locate a nearby dealer or mail-order supplier.)

W.W. Grainger, Inc.
Safety and Security Equipment catalog
333 Knightsbridge Pkwy.
Lincolnshire, IL 60069-3639
(708) 913–8333
Safety gear and equipment
(Also, local wholesale stores nationwide.)

Granny's Old Fashioned Products
P.O. 660037
Arcadia, CA 91066
(800) 366–1762
Rich and Radiant shampoo, Moisture Guard lotion, Power Plus laundry concentrate, and other personal-care cleaning products
(Wholesale only, call to locate a nearby dealer or mail-order supplier.)

Graphic Dimensions Ltd.
2103 Brentwood St.
High Point, NC 27263
(800) 221–0262
(910) 887–3700
Metal picture frames

Harbinger Carpet
443 Nathanial Dr.
Dublin, GA 31021
(800) 241–4216
Carpeting with reduced outgassing

Heart of Vermont Inc.
Rte. 132
P.O. Box 183
Sharon, VT 05065
(800) 639–4123
(802) 763–2720
Organic 100%-cotton and wool futons, wool mattresses, bedding, solid-wood furniture

Hello Direct
5884 Eden Park Pl.
San Jose, CA 95138–1859
(800) 444–3556
Speaker phones, other phone types, and phone accessories

Hendricksen Natürlich Flooring & Interiors
7120 Keating Ave.
Sebastopol, CA 95472
(707) 829–3959
Wool, jute, and sisal carpeting, and natural linoleum

Hold Everything
Mail Order Department
P.O. Box 7807
San Francisco, CA 94120–7807
(800) 421–2264
Heavy-duty metal closet organizing units

Holland Corp.
Hudsons Cross Rd.s
Selbyville, DE 19975
(302) 436-4375
100%-organic cotton Roman shades

Home Decorators Collection
2025 Concourse Dr.
St. Louis, MO 63146–4178
(800) 245–2217
Some solid-wood furniture, metal furniture, and accessories

Home Etc.
Palo Verde at 34th St.
P.O. Box 28806
Tucson, AZ 85726–8806
(800) 362–8415
Some 100%-cotton woven bedspreads and rug-gripping tape and mats

Home-Sew
P.O. Box 4099
Bethlehem, PA 18018–3809
(610) 867–3833
Selection of cotton lace, trim, and notions

Homestead Paint and Finishes
P.O. Box 1668
Lunenburg, MA 01462
(508) 582–6426
Casein and other alternative paints

Honeywell, Inc.
1985 Douglas Dr. North
Golden Valley, MN 55422–3992
(800) 328–5111
(612) 951–1000
Whole-house electrostatic precipitators and extended-surface filters
(Wholesale only, call to locate a nearby dealer.)

Human Habitat
P.O. Box 491
New Hope, PA 18938
(215) 862–9266
Livos, BioShield, and other alternative paints

HybriVet Systems, Inc.
P.O. Box 1210
Framingham, MA 01701
(800) 262–5323
(508) 651–7881
LeadCheck Swabs test kits

Indian Earth Cosmetics
2967 Randolph Ave.
Costa Mesa, CA 92626
(714) 556–1407
Indian Earth make-up powder

Infinity Herbal Products
Division of Jedmon Products, Ltd.
333 Rimrock Rd.
Downsview, ON Canada M3J 3J9
(416) 631–4000
Heavenly Horsetail all-purpose cleaner
(Wholesale only, call to locate a nearby dealer or mail-order supplier.)

InterMetro Industries Corp.
651 N. Washington St.
Wilkes-Barre, PA 18705
(800) 433–2232
(717) 825–2741
Metal-wire storage and bookcase systems

Jamie Industries
6600 N. Lincoln Ave.
Ste. 400
Lincolnwood, IL 60645
(708) 675–8400
CLR lime remover

Janice Corp.
198 Rte. 46
Budd Lake, NJ 07828–3001
(800) 526–4237
Bedding, cotton mattresses, sewing goods, household goods, personal-care products, and clothing for men and women

Jantz Design
P.O. Box 3071
Santa Rosa, CA 95402
(800) 365–6563
Organic-fiber bedding, 100%-cotton and wool futons, and solid-wood furniture

Johnson's SuperSeal, Inc.
3640 "C" St. NE
Auburn, WA 98002
(800) 994–7822
(206) 941–3910
Johnson's SuperSeal water-glass sealer

Karen's Nontoxic Products
1839 Dr. Jack Rd.
Conowingo, MD 21918
(800) 527–3674
(410) 378–4621
Personal-care, cleaning products, and household goods

KB Cotton Pillows
P.O. Box 57
De Soto, TX 75123
(214) 223–7193
100%-cotton pillows

Walter Kidde
Division of Kidde, Inc.
1394 S. Third St.
Mebane, NC 27302
(919) 563–5911
Kidde portable fire extinguishers
(Wholesale only, call for nearest dealer or mail-order supplier.)

Kitchens and Baths by Don Johnson
Ste. #1375
Merchandise Mart
Chicago, IL 60654
(312) 548–2436
(708) 548–2436
Metal cabinets

Klean Strip
Box 1879
Memphis, TN 38101
(901) 775–0100
EasyOff paint stripper

Kleen-Air Company, Inc.
269 West Caramel Dr.
Carmel, IN 46032
(317) 848–2757
Whole-house ozone generators
(Wholesale only, call to locate a nearby dealer.)

Kurtain Kraft
P.O. Box 12468
Marina Del Rey, CA 90292
(800) 243–9222
Enameled-metal swag hardware

Lands' End, Inc.
1 Lands' End Lane
Dodgeville, WI 53595
(800) 356–4444
Some 100%-cotton clothing for the family

Lee/Rowan
900 S. Highway Dr.
Fenton, MO 63036
(800) 325–6150
Metal-wire closet organizers
(Wholesale only, call to locate a nearby dealer or mail-order supplier.)

The Living Source
7005 Woodway Dr.
Ste. 214
Waco, TX 76712
(800) 662–8787
(817) 776–4878
Personal-care and cleaning products, household goods, bedding, cellophane bags, and air and water filters

Lerner New York
Customer Relations
P.O. Box 8381
Indianapolis, IN 46283–8381
(800) 288–4009
Some 100%-cotton sweaters and other clothing for women

Logona
544–E Riverside Dr.
Asheville, NC 28801
(800) 648–6654
Cosmetics and personal-care items

Lotus Brands
P.O. Box 1008
Lotus Dr.
Silver Lake, WI 53170
(414) 889–8561
Light Mountain henna hair colorants

LS and S Group
P.O. Box 673
Northbrook, IL 60065
(708) 498–9777
Four-track players and tapes

Lumiram Electric Corporation
335 Fayette Ave.
Mamaroneck, NY 10543
(914) 698–1205
Chromalux full-spectrum incadescent bulbs
and fluorescent tubes
(Wholesale only, call to locate a nearby
dealer or mail-order supplier.)

Marketplace of India
1455 Ashland Ave.
Evanston, IL 60201–4001
(800) 726–8905
(708) 328–4011
100%-cotton ethnic clothing for women

McCoy, Inc.
40100 Grand River
Bldg. A
Novi, MI 48375
(810) 476–0111
Saunas

McCracken Solar Co.
329 West Carlos
Alturas, CA 96101
(916) 233–3175
Sunwater outdoor solar water distillers

Medite Corporation
P.O. Box 4040
Medford, OR 97501
(800) 676–3339
(503) 779–9596
Medite formaldehyde-free particleboard
(Wholesale only, call to locate a nearby
dealer or mail-order supplier.)

Miller Paint Co.
317 SE Grand Ave.
Portland, OR 97214
(503) 233–4491
Miller Paint low-biocide paint

The Mind's Eye
P.O. Box 1060
Petaluma, CA 94953
(800) 227–2020
Books on cassette

Modulars, Inc.
6120 South Gilmore
Ste. 202
Fairfield, OH 45014
(513) 868–7300
Cement board for ceramic tile installations
(Wholesale only, call to locate a nearby
dealer.)

Mother Hart's
3300 S. Congress Ave. #21
P.O. Box 4229
Boynton Beach, FL 33424–4229
(407) 738–5866
Bedding, brushes, and household goods

Motherwear
P.O. Box 114
Northampton, MA 01061–0114
(413) 586–3488
100%-cotton nursing-mother clothing

Multi-Pure
21339 Nordhoff St.
Chatsworth, CA 91311
(800) 622–9206
(818) 341–7577
Multi-Pure water filters

Murco Wall Products, Inc.
300 NE 21st St.
Ft. Worth, TX 76106
(817) 626–1987
Murco low-odor paint and drywall joint compound

Nancy's Notions
333 Beichl Ave.
P.O. Box 683
Beaver Dam, WI 53916–0683
(800) 833–0690
Sewing goods

National Blind Factory
400 Galleria
Ste. 400
Southfield, MI 48034
(800) 477–8000
Custom-made discount metal blinds

National Testing Laboratories, Inc.
6555 Wilson Mills Rd.
Cleveland, OH 44143
(800) 458–3330
(2160 449–2525
WaterCheck water tests

Natural Animal
Div. of EcoSafe Products, Inc.
P.O. Box 1177
St. Augustine, FL 32085
(800) 274–7387
All-natural pet supplies and pesticides

The Natural Bath
P.O. Box 97
Haddonfield, NJ 08033
(800) 331–1163
Cotton towels, bathrobes, and natural soaps

Natural Fiber Fabric Club
P.O. Box 586
South Plainfield, NJ 07080
(908) 755–6171
Sewing goods

Natural Lifestyle Supplies
16 Lookout Dr.
Asheville, NC 28804–3330
(800) 752–2775
Personal-care products including Tom's of Maine and Vita Wave, toothbrushes, hairbrushes, combs, bedding, and cookware

Natural World, Inc.
652 Glenbrook Rd.
Stamford, CT 06906
(203) 356–0000
Personal-care products

Nature de France, Ltd.
100 Rose Ave.
Hempstead, NY 11550
(212) 734–2372
Le Stick natural deodorant
(Wholesale only, call to locate a nearby dealer or mail-order supplier.)

The Nature of Things
3956 Long Pl.
Carlsbad, CA 92008
(619) 434–4480
Personal-care and cleaning products

Nature's Colors Cosmetics
424 La Verne Ave.
Mill Valley, CA 94941
(415) 388–6101
Ida Grae Nature's Colors cosmetics and make-up brushes
(Wholesale only, call to locate a nearby dealer or mail-order supplier.)

N.E.E.D.S.
527 Charles Ave. 12–A
Syracuse, NY 13209
(800) 634–1380
Cleaning products, personal-care products, water filters, air filters, masks, books, alternative pest control, builder's foil, bedding, and electromagnetic field meters

Neo-Life Co. of America
3500 Gateway Blvd.
Fremont, CA 94538
(510) 651–0405
Cleaning products
(Wholesale only, call to locate a nearby
dealer or mail-order supplier.)

Neutrogena Corporation
5760 W. 96th St.
Los Angeles, CA 90045
(310) 642–1150
Neutrogena glycerin soap
(Wholesale only, call to locate a nearby
dealer or mail-order supplier.)

Newport News
Avon Ln.
Hampton, VA 23630
(800) 688–2830
Some 100%-cotton clothes for women

Nigra Enterprises
5699 Kanan Rd.
Agoura Hills, CA 91301–3328
(818) 889–6877
Air filters, water filters, and other goods for
those with MCS and allergies

Nilfisk of America Inc.
300 Technology Dr.
Malvern, PA 19355
(610) 647–6420
HEPA portable vacuum cleaners

Nontoxic Environments
9392 S. Gribble Rd.
Canby, OR 97013
(503) 266–5244
Personal-care products, cleaning products,
household goods, bedding, organic 100%-
cotton or wool futons, and solid wood futon
frames

The Noon Family Sheep Farm
R.F.D. Box 630 Sunset Rd.
Springvale, Maine 04083
(207) 324–3733
Organic-wool yarns and stuffing

Nutricology, Inc.
P.O. Box 489
San Leandro, CA 94577
(510) 639–4572
ParaMicrocidin Liquid citrus seed extract

Nutone/Scovill
Madison and Red Band Rd.s
Cincinnati, OH 45227–1599
(800) 543–8687
(513) 527–5100
Ventilation fans, range hoods, and central
vacuum systems
(Wholesale only, call to locate a nearby
dealer or mail-order supplier.)

N-Viro Products Ltd.
610 Walnut Ave.
Bohemia, NY 11716
(516) 567–2628
Nematodes for termite control
(Wholesale only, call to locate a nearby
dealer.)

Old Fashioned Milk Paint Co.
P.O. Box 222
Groton, MA 01450
(508) 448–6336
Old Fashioned Milk Paint casein paint

Orange-Sol, Inc.
955 N. Fiesta, #1
Gilbert, AZ 85233
(602) 497–8822
De-Solv-It concentrated citrus cleaner
(Wholesale only, call to locate a nearby
dealer or mail order-supplier.)

Organic Interiors
Decorating With Fabric
8 College Avenue
Nanuet, NY 10954
(914) 623–2114
Interior decorators using organic materials

Orr Safety Corporation
P.O. Box 16326
Louisvillle, KY 40256–9965
(800) 726–6789
(502) 774–5791
Industrial-quality safety gear and equipment

Orvis
Historic Rte. 7A
P.O. Box 798
Manchester, VT 05254–0798
(800) 541–3541
Some 100%-cotton clothing for men and women

Osprey Eco-Logics
HCR 80, Box 68
Penobscot, ME 04476
(207) 469–3409
Livos, Bio-Shield, Auro, and other alternative paints

Ott Light Systems
28 Parker Way
Santa Barbara, CA 93101
(800) 234–3724
(805) 564–3467
Ott full-spectrum fluorescent lights

Ozark Water Service and Environmental Services
114 Spring St.
Sulphur Springs, AR 72768
(800) 835–8908
(501) 298–3483
Testing services for air and water quality and water- and air-treatment equipment

Pace Chem Industries, Inc.
P.O. Box 1946
Santa Inez, CA 93460
(800) 350–2912
(805) 686–0745
Crystal Shield paint, clear finish, and Crystal Aire sealant

Pacific Spirit
1334 Pacific Ave.
Forest Grove, OR 97116
(800) 634–9057
Alternative health products

Paper Direct
100 Plaza Dr.
P.O. Box 1518
Secaucus, NJ 07096–1518
(800) A PAPERS
Selection of recycled papers

Peerless Imported Rugs
3033 N. Lincoln Ave.
Chicago, IL 60657
(800) 621–6573
(312) 472–4848
Natural-fiber rugs

Peelu-Floss Lifelong Products
6372 Oakton
Morton Grove, IL 60053
(708) 967–9400
Peelu tooth powder

J.C. Penny Company, Inc.
Catalog Division
P.O. Box 100
Atlanta, GA 30390–0100
(800) 222–6161
100% cotton towels and some all-cotton clothing for the entire family

Perfectly Safe
7245 Whipple Ave. NW
North Canton, OH 44720
(800) 837–KIDS
Safe insect deterrents and traps

The J. Peterman Company
2444 Palumbo Dr.
Lexington, KY 40509
(800) 231–7341
Untreated, natural-fiber clothing for men and women

Phoneco, Inc.
207 East Mill Rd.
P.O. Box 70
Galesville, WI 54630
(608) 582–4124
Restored metal, wood, and bakelite phones

Pierce and Stevens
Div. of Pratt and Lambert
P.O. Box 1092
Buffalo, NY 14240
(716) 856–4910
Water-based clear finish

Polar 7 Enterprisers
1237 Nestor St.
Coquitlam, BC Canada V3E 1H4
(604) 944–8001
Dr. Tomorrow's Eclectic Bookstore CD Rom books
(Original version no longer available. New version coming out.)

Pompanoosuc Mills
Attn: Ed O'Keefe
Rte. 5
East Thetford, VT 05043
(800) 841–6671
(802) 785–4851
Solid-wood furniture

Pottery Barn
P.O. Box 7044
San Francisco, CA 94120–7044
(800) 922–5507
Cotton and wool rugs, natural-fiber window treatments, and solid-wood, rattan, and metal furnishings

The Primary Layer
P.O. Box 6697
Portland, OR 97228
(800) 282–8206
Fine-quality 100%-cotton underwear and sleepwear for men and women

Prince Lionheart
P.O. Box 420
Santa Ynez, CA 93460
(800) 544–1132
Love Bug electronic mosquito repellants

Pueblo to People
2105 Silber Rd.
Ste. 101
Houston, TX 77055
(800) 843–5257
(713) 956–1172
100%-cotton ethnic clothing for the family and natural alpaca yarns

Pure Air Systems, Inc.
P.O. Box 418
Plainfield, IN 46168
(800) 869–8025
(317) 839–9135
Whole-house air filters
(Wholesale only, call for nearest dealer.)

The Pure Water Place, Inc.
P.O. Box 6715
Longmont, CO 80501
(303) 776–0056
Water filters

Puro Corporation of America
56–45 58th St.
P.O. Box 10
Maspeth, NY 11378
(718) 326–7000
Leased activated-charcoal water filters

Real Goods Trading Company
966 Mazzoni St.
Ukiah, CA 95482–3471
(800) 762–7325
(707) 468–9214
Alternative light bulbs and lamps

Red Devil, Inc.
2400 Vauxhall Rd.
Union, NJ 07083–1933
(800) 229–9051
(908) 688–6900
Red Devil TSP/90 heavy duty cleaner
(Wholesale only, call to locate a nearby dealer.)

Red River
Arco Iris
Ponca, AR 72670
(No telephone number available.)
100%-cotton menstrual pads

Reflections
P.O. Box 2299
Rt. 2 Box 24P40
Trinity, TX 75862
(800) 852–9273
(409) 594–9019
Organic 100%-cotton clothing for women

Research Products Corp.
P.O. Box 1467
Madison, WI 53701–1467
(800) 334–6011
(608) 257–8801
Space-Gard extended-surface filters
(Wholesale only, call to locate a nearby dealer.)

Rexair, Inc.
3221 W. Big Beaver Rd.
Ste. 200
Troy, MI 48084
(810) 643–7222
Rainbow portable water-filtered vacuum cleaners
(Wholesale only, call to locate a nearby dealer.)

Richman Cotton Co.
2631 Piner Rd.
Santa Rosa, CA 95401
(800) 992–8924
(707) 575–8924
100%-cotton clothing for the family, fabric, and buttons

St. Charles Manufacturing Co.
1611 E. Main St.
St. Charles, IL 60174
(708) 584–3800
Metal cabinets
(Wholesale only, call to locate a nearby dealer.)

Safehouse
724 Welch St.
Ste. #11
Denton, TX 76201
(817) 382–3103
Air and water filters, water tests, and alternative portable vacuums

Safer Alternatives
19674 Day Ln.
Redding, CA 96002
(916) 243–1352
Personal care products, natural-fiber clothing for women, and cleaning products

The Safe Reading and Computer Box Co.
1158 N. Huron Rd.
Linwood, MI 48634
(517) 697–3989
Reading boxes and computer boxes, portable saunas

Safe Technologies
1950 NE 208 Ter.
Miami, FL 33179
(800) 638–9121
(617) 444–7778
Low-EMF computer monitors

Save Our ecoSystem (SOS)
407 Blair Blvd.
Eugene, OR 97402
(503) 484–2679
Pet flea combs and other pet products

Savogran
P.O. Box 130
Norwood, MA 02062
(800) 225–9872
(617) 762–5400
StrypSafer paint stripper
(Wholesale only, call for the nearest dealer.)

Scientific Glass Co.
P.O. Box 25125
Albuquerque, NM 87125
(505) 345–7321
Rain Crystal glass water distillers

Sears, Roebuck and Co.
Sears Tower
Chicago, IL 60684
(312) 875–2500
(Call for nearest retail store.)
Some natural-fiber clothing for the entire family, cotton towels, metal cabinets (not in all stores), and Kenmore appliances

Servaas Laboratories, Inc.
1200 Waterway Blvd.
Indianapolis, IN 46202
(800) 433–5818
(317) 636–7760
Bar Keeper's Friend cleanser
(Wholesale only, call to locate a nearby dealer or mail order supplier.)

The Seventh Generation
Colchester, VT 05446–1672
(800) 456–1177
Personal care products, cleaning products, bedding, paper goods, and clothing for the family

Shaker Shops West
5 Inverness Way
P.O. Box 487
Inverness, CA 94937
(415) 669–7256
Solid-wood Shaker furniture assembled and in kits

Shaker Workshops
P.O. Box 1028
Concord, MA 01742–1028
(617) 646–8985
Shaker-style furniture assembled or in kits

The Silk Collection
P.O. Box 620825
Middleton, WI 53562
(800) 831–0909
Silk clothing for women

Simmons Pure Soaps
Simmons Handcrafts
42295 Hwy. 36
Bridgeville, CA 95526
(800) 428–0412
(707) 777–1920
Simmons Pure Soaps, unscented oatmeal soap, natural scrubbers, combs, brushes, cleaning products, and water filters

Simplex Products Division
P.O. Box 10
Adrian, MI 49221
(517) 263–8881
Thermo-Ply aluminum-faced sheathing
(Wholesale only, call for nearest dealer.)

Simply Better
90 Church St.
Burlington, VT 05401
(802) 658–7770
(No catalog but offers mail-order service)
Alternative paints, stains, and finishes

Sinan Co.
P.O. Box 857
Davis, CA 95617–0857
(916) 753 3104
(Note: Two catalogs are available.)
Cotton and wool futons, rye straw mattresses, natural-fiber rugs, and Auro and other alternative paints

Smith and Hawken
25 Corte Madera
Mill Valley, CA 94941
(415) 389–8300
Solid teak indoor and outdoor furniture

Socks Galore
P.O. Box 748
Rural Hall, NC 27098
(919) 744–1170
Socks for the family

SoPhTec International
930 W. 16th St.
Building E–2
Costa Mesa, CA 92627
(714) 548–7222
SoPhTec Physical water conditioners
(Wholesale only, call to locate a nearby dealer or mail-order supplier.)

Southworth Company
P.O. Box 5006
West Springfield, MA 01090
(413) 732–5141
Southworth cotton paper and envelopes
(Wholesale only, call to locate a nearby dealer or mail-order supplier.)

Suburban Water Testing Laboratories
4600 Kutztown Rd.
Temple, PA 19560
(800) 433–6595
Home water tests

Summitville Tiles Co.
P.O. Box 73
Summitville, OH 43962
(216) 223–1511
Ceramic tile
(Call to locate a nearby dealer.)

Taylor Gifts
355 E. Conestoga Rd.
P.O. Box 206
Wayne, PA 19087–0206
(800) 647–667
(610) 293–3613
Household gadgets

Taylor Wood-Craft, Inc.
P.O. Box 245
Malta, OH 43758
(614) 962–3741
Hardwood butcher-block countertops.
(Wholesale only, call to locate a nearby
dealer.)

TerrEssentials/Body Elements
3320 North 3rd St.
Arlington, VA 22201–1712
(703) 525–0585
Natural cosmetics, alternative cleaners, pet-
care items, and books

Tilley Endurables
900 Don Mills Rd.
Don Mills, ON Canada M3C 1V8
(800) 338–2797
(418) 441–6141
Some 100%-cotton clothing for men and
women

Tom's of Maine
P.O. Box 710
Kennebunk, ME 04043
(207) 985–2944
Tom's natural toothpaste and Tom's natural
shaving cream
(Wholesale only, call to locate a nearby
dealer or mail-order supplier.)

Tom Tom
1810 San Pueblo
Berkeley, CA 94702
(415) 644–3968
100%-cotton winter gloves and scarves for
the entire family
(Wholesale only, call to locate a nearby
dealer or mail-order supplier.)

Trade Wind
P.O. Box 380
156 Drake Ln.
Summertown, TN 38483
(800) 445–1991
!00%-cotton ethnic clothing for the family

Tropical Soap Co.
P.O. Box 797217
Dallas, TX 75379
(800) 527–2368
(214) 357–1464
Sirena Fresh Coconut soap
(Wholesale only, call to locate a nearby
dealer or mail-order supplier.)

True Value Hardware, Headquarters
2310 Gault Ave. North
Fort Payne, AL 35967
(205) 845–2969
Tru-Bond epoxy
(Call to locate nearest retail store.)

Tucson Cooperative Warehouse
350 South Toole Ave.
Tucson, AZ 85701
(800) 350–2667
Organic 100%-cotton clothing and natural
personal-care products

Tweeds
One Avery Row
Roanoke, VA 24012–8528
(800) 999–7997
Fine-quality affordable natural clothing for
women

Ultra-Hyd
361 Easton Rd.
Horsham, PA 19044–2507
(215) 674–5511
Ultra-Hyd ultraviolet water-purification
equipment

United Gilsonite Laboratories
P.O. Box 70
Scranton, PA 18507
(800) UGL–LABS
Aqua Zar clear finish
(Wholesale only, call to locate a nearby
dealer.)

Universal Rundle Corp.
217 North Mill St.
New Castle, PA 16103
(800) 955–0316
(412) 658–6631
Vitreous-china bathroom sink tops
(Wholesale only, call to locate a nearby dealer.)

U.S. Borax and Chemical Corp.
Division of the RTZ Group
3075 Wilshire Blvd.
Los Angeles, CA 90010
(800) 989–6267
(714) 490–6000
Tim-Bor borate temiticide
(Wholesale only, call to locate a nearby dealer.)

USG Industries, Inc.
101 S. Wacker Dr.
Chicago, IL 60606–4385
(800) 347–1345
Cement board for ceramic tile installations
(Wholesale only, call to locate a nearby dealer.)

The Vermont Country Store
P.O. Box 3000
Manchester Center, VT 05255–3000
(802) 362–2400
Socks, clothing for men and women, bedding, vacuum bags, household goods, and coat hangers

Lillian Vernon
Virginia Beach VA 23479–0002
(800) 285–5555
Household gadgets

Vita-Mix Corporation
8615 Usher Rd.
Cleveland, OH 44138
(800) 848–2649
Vita-Vac alternative portable vacuums

Vita Wave Products Co.
7131 Owensmouth Ave.
Ste. 94–D
Canoga Park, CA 91309
(818) 886–3808
Vita Wave less-toxic permanents and hair colorings

WaterTest Corporation
28 Daniel Plummer Rd.
Goffstown, NH 03045
(800) 458–3330
(603) 623–7400
Home water tests

Waterwise, Inc.
26200 U.S. Hwy. 27 S.
Leesburg, FL 34748
(800) 874–9028
(904) 787–5008
Waterwise water distillers

White Consolidated Industries, Inc.
11770 Berea Rd.
Cleveland, OH 44111–1686
(216) 252–3700
White-Westinghouse appliances
(Wholesale only, call to locate a nearby dealer.)

Whitmire Research Labs
3568 Tree Ct. Industrial Blvd.
St. Louis, MO 63122
(314) 225–5371
Tri-Die and X-clude pyrethrin insecticides
(Wholesale only, call to locate a nearby dealer or mail-order supplier.)

Williams-Sonoma
P.O. Box 7456
San Francisco, CA 94120–7456
(800) 541–2233
Kitchen and cooking supplies

Winter Silks
2700 Laura Ln.
P.O. Box 620130
Middleton, WI 53562
(800) 648–7455
Silk clothing for men and women

Winthrop Pharmaceuticals
Division of Sterling Drug, Inc.
90 Park Ave.
New York, NY 10016
(212) 907–2000
Zephiran antiseptic
(Wholesale only. Have your pharmacist order for you.)

The Wooden Spoon
P.O. Box 931
Clinton, CT 06413
(800) 431–2207
Glass storage containers and stainless steel cookware

Woodstream Corp.
69 N. Locust St.
Lititz, PA 17543
(717) 626–2125
Victor mouse traps and Holdfast roach traps
(Wholesale only, call to locate a nearby dealer or mail-order supplier.)

Workshop Showcase
P.O. Box 500107
Austin, TX 78750
(512) 331–5470
Solid-wood Shaker and Mission furniture

World Fibre
P.O. Box 480805
Denver, CO 80248
(303) 628–2210
GoldSpun jute rugs and carpets, and office paper

Yankee Pride
29 Parkside Cir.
Braintree, MA 02184
(800) 848–7610
Some 100%-cotton rugs and all-wool rugs

Yield House
P.O. Box 2525
Conway, NH 03818–2525
(800) 258–4720
Solid-pine furniture assembled and in kits

William Zinsser and Co.
173 Belmont Dr.
Somerset, NJ 08875
(908) 469–8100
Bull's Eye" shellac
(Wholesale only, call to locate a nearby dealer or mail-order supplier.)

APPENDIX 4
RESOURCES FOR INFANTS AND CHILDREN

While much of the information given in this book is applicable to children, this appendix addresses some of the special needs of youngsters.

PRINTED MATERIAL

Allergy Insights, Practical Allergy Research Foundation, P.O. Box 60, Buffalo, NY 14223–0060, (716) 875–0398. Approximately 12 issues per year for $24.00. This is the newsletter of Doris Rapp, M.D. and her associates. It focuses on allergies and MCS with special emphasis on children.

Discovering and Treating Unrecognized Allergies by Doris Rapp, M.D. New York NY: William Morrow and Co., 1992 trade paperback edition, $12.00, 603 pp. A leading pediatric allergist discusses unsuspecting allergy and MCS sypmptoms such as behavioral changes.

Healthy Home, Healthy Kids: Protecting Your Children from Everyday Environmental Hazards by Joyce M. Schoemaker, Ph.d., and Charity Y. Vitale, Ph.D. Washington DC: Island Press, 1991, $12.95, 222 pp. trade paperback. This book reveals how homes can be unhealthy for children and what to do to improve a problem house.

The Impossible Child: In School, At Home by Doris Rapp, M.D. and Dorothy M. Damberg. Buffalo NY: Practical Allergy Research Foundation. 1986, $7.00, 162 pp. paperback. This book helps explain how behavioral problems can often be symptoms of food and chemical intolerances.

Is This Your Child?: Discovering and Treating Unrecognized Food Allergies by Doris Rapp, M.D. NY: William Morrow and Co., 1992 trade paperback edition, $12.00, 626 pp. How you can detect food intolerances in your child and what to do when you find them.

ORGANIZATIONS AND CONSULTANTS

Practical Allergy Research Foundation
P.O. Box 60
Buffallo, NY 14223–0060
(716) 875–0398
*This is an organization established by pedi-
atric allergist Doris Rapp, M.D. It publishes
and sells pamphlets, books, videos, and au-
dio-cassette tapes on childhood allergies and
MCS. Also available are air filters, charcoal
masks, and other equipment.*

PRODUCT SOURCES

For the most part, the catalogs listed below specialize in children's products. However, you
should keep in mind that a number of the catalogs supplied in *Appendix I: Resources for a
Healthy Household* also carry alternative items for babies and children. These include
**Seventh Generation, The Richman Cotton Company, Nontoxic Environments, L.L. Bean,
Inc., Safer Alternatives,** and others. By the way, *Non-toxic, Natural & Earthwise* by Debra
Lynn Dadd contains about 10 pages of healthy resources for children.

After the Stork
1501 12th St. NW
Alburquerque, NM 87104
(800) 333–KIDS
100%-cotton clothing from baby sizes to
children's size 14.

Hanna Anderson
1010 NW Flanders
Portland, OR 97209
(800) 222–0544
100%-cotton clothing in baby and children
sizes.

Earthlings
205 S. Lorita Ave.
Ojai, CA 93023
(805) 646–7770
Infants' & children's organic-cotton clothing.
(Wholesale only. Call for nearest dealer or
mail-order source. Company may have retail catalog soon.)

Lilly's Kids
Lillian Vernon Corp.
Virginia Beach, VA 23479–0002
(804) 430–5555
Some wooden toys.

Motherswear
P.O. Box 114
Northampton, MA 01061–0114
(413) 586–3488
100%-cotton nursing mother clothes, 100%-
cotton diapers, and sheepskin baby blankets
and car-seat covers.

The Natural Baby Catalog
The Natural Baby Company
114 W. Franklin, Ste. S
Pennington, NJ 08534
(609) 737–2895
100%-cotton baby clothes, diapers, and bedding, as well as wooden toys and alternative baby personal-care products.

One Step Ahead
P.O. Box 517
Lake Bluff, IL 60044
(800) 274–8440
Wooden safety gates and some wooden toys.

Perfectly Safe
7245 Whipple Ave. NW
North Canton, OH 44720
(800) 837–KIDS
Love Bug electronic mosquito repellants and other safety equipment for both babies and youngsters.

The Right Start Catalog
Right Start Plaza
5334 Sterling Center Dr.
Westlake Village, CA 91361–4627
(800) LITTLE–1
Tublar-enameled metal children's beds and wooden safety gates.

Tortellini
P.O. Box 2615
Sag Harbor, NY 11963
(800)527–8725
Natural-fiber children's clothing.

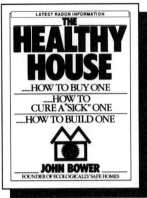
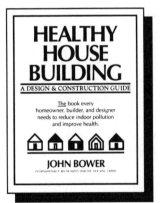

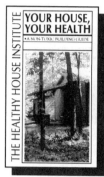
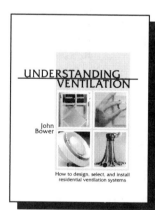

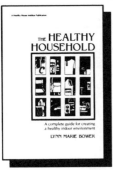

▥ THE
HEALTHY HOUSE
INSTITUTE   430 N. Sewell Road   Bloomington, IN 47408   (812) 332–5073

NAME

ADDRESS

CITY, STATE, ZIP

PHONE ( )   DATE

Qty.	Description	Price Each	Amount

PAYMENT METHOD

☐ Check or   ☐ Master Card   ☐ Visa
Money Order

☐☐☐☐☐☐☐☐☐☐☐☐☐☐☐☐

Expiration date_____

Signature_____

Subtotal	
Indiana residents add 5% sales tax	
Shipping: $3.00 for the first book or video, and $2.00 for each additional book or video.	
TOTAL	

Payment must be in U.S. funds